Transforming
Health Promotion
Practice

Concepts,
Issues, and
Applications

Lynne E. Young, RN, PhD

Assistant Professor
University of Victoria School of Nursing
Victoria, British Columbia

Virginia E. Hayes, RN, PhD

Associate Professor
University of Victoria School of Nursing
Victoria, British Columbia

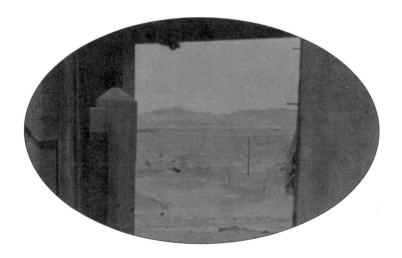

Transforming Health Promotion Practice

Concepts, Issues, and Applications

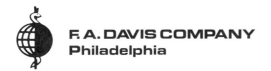

F. A. DAVIS COMPANY
Philadelphia

F. A. Davis Company
1915 Arch Street
Philadelphia, PA 19103

Printed in the United States of America

Last digit indicates print number: 10 9 8 7 6 5 4 3 2 1

Acquisitions Editor: Joanne Patzek DaCunha, RN, MSN
Cover Designer: Louis J. Forgione
Cover Photography: Virginia E. Hayes, RN, PhD

As new scientific information becomes available through basic and clinical research, recommended treatments and drug therapies undergo changes. The authors and publisher have done everything possible to
make this book accurate, up to date, and in accord with accepted standards at the time of publication. The
authors, editors, and publisher are not responsible for errors or omissions or for consequences from application of the book, and make no warranty, expressed or implied, in regard to the contents of the book. Any
practice described in this book should be applied by the reader in accordance with professional standards
of care used in regard to the unique circumstances that may apply in each situation.

Library of Congress Cataloging-in-Publication Data

Young, Lynne E.
    Transforming health promotion practice : concepts, issues, and applications / Lynne E.
    Young, Virginia E. Hayes.
        p. cm.
    Includes bibliographical references and index.
    ISBN 0-8036-0814-4 (alk. paper)
    1. Health promotion. 2. Medical policy. I. Hayes, Virginia E. (Virginia Ellen) II. Title.

RA427.8.Y68 2001
613—dc21

                                                                    2001042156

To the individuals, families, and communities
that consistently guide us to deeper understandings
of health and health promotion
and
to our students who teach us so much about learning.

FOREWORD

If we wish to advance nursing's understanding of health promotion, whether we think of it as a concept, a process, and/or an outcome, we are required to take chances and to maintain a flexible and open mind. The remarkably brief and rapidly evolving history of health promotion compels us to continually reinvent and reinterpret its meaning for, and manifestations within, the profession. Just as routes to safe harbors are lined with sunken ships, knowledge and understanding advances by taking risks and positions and making decisions that may or may not stand the test of time. This book represents such risk taking and its author eloquently state the positions and decisions that a variety of nurses and scholars have taken during points in their evolving understanding of this important topic.

Transforming Health Promotion Practice: Concepts, Issues, and Applications is both a practical guide to help nurses and others understand health promotion and a historical record of our perimillennial understanding of health promotion. As such, this compilation of articles represents a set of particular views that are largely, but not exclusively, based on a post-modern perspective. This perspective has as some of its hallmarks, the use of critical reflection, a desire for emancipation from past ideologies (most notably in this context, the more traditional views of Western science and positivism), the primacy of personal experience, and an emphasis on placing all things within a wider sociopolitical context. Post-modernism will no doubt advance our understanding of health promotion; however, this perspective, like all of the perspectives previously used to understand health promotion, is already becoming part of the intellectual historical record. This observation is not meant to be dismissive; indeed, it is quite the opposite. The authors in this book are making and recording history. They provide us with a unique opportunity to examine current perspectives on health promotion and much of what they profess will no doubt find a safe port.

What is most impressive in this volume is the obvious passion and enthusiasm of the authors as they reveal their personal, and evolving, struggles to develop and apply health promotion primarily within the profession of nursing. A significant proportion of the authors are relatively early on in their academic careers and their scholarly critiques and experience-based observations are imbued with both theoretical and philosophical currency and practice-based wisdom. It should be noted however that, whether seasoned in academe or not, it is clear that all of the contributors are well versed in the challenges nurses face in bringing the promise of health promotion into reality. They convey an undercurrent of impatience with the failure of health care systems, health professionals at all levels, and governments to move beyond paying lip service to all that health promotion has to offer. However, rather than give into frustration, they have directed their energies toward developing new ways of thinking about, and enacting, health promotion. At the heart of it, this is a book written by committed individuals who will undoubtedly inspire students and nurses to take up the challenges they describe so well.

The book itself is organized in a way that will make it a valuable text for nursing students at all levels of preparation. The early chapters lay out the historical and theoretical perspectives that inform much of our current understanding of health promotion. A host of concepts and topics, which include ethics, consumerism, therapeutic relationships and communication, self-care, and advocacy, are all explored in relation to health promotion. Having set the stage in the opening chapters, the remainder of the book illustrates the ways health promotion is enacted in a variety of clinical, educational, and research settings.

I am very impressed with the inclusion of a final chapter that serves to critique all that comes before. This chapter, which is co-authored by one of the most influential writers, thinkers, and researchers in the field of health promotion, Lawrence Green, demonstrates the intellectual integrity of the book in a tangible way. This text is a "bully pulpit" for making a post-modern case for the need to move health promotion to a new level and, as such, it critiques much of what has come before. Thus, it should not be surprising if it leads to spirited debate and even causes a degree of consternation among those that hold different views. I doubt the editors or contributors would want it any other way. I also have no doubt that this text will help illuminate and stimulate new ways of thinking and practicing health promotion.

J. Howard Brunt, RN, PhD

Brief Biography of Dr. Brunt

Dr. Brunt is the Associate Vice President Research and a Professor of Nursing at the University of Victoria, Victoria, British Columbia, Canada. His educational preparation includes a PhD in Epidemiology and Community Health (Calgary, 1990), a MSN in Cardiovascular Nursing (Yale, 1983), an ADN (Vermont, 1978), and a BA in Sociology (Florida). He has conducted a wide range of research related to heart health promotion, most notably in the Hutterite community of Alberta, Canada. In addition, he has investigated risk factors for falls in the elderly, seniors' impact on health policy and, most recently, hospice care. He is the recipient of research awards of excellence from the Canadian Association for Nursing Research and the Registered Nurses Association of British Columbia. Dr. Brunt serves on a number of national research-related peer review committees and is a Trustee of the Canadian Health Services Research Foundation.

Why a book on health promotion in nursing? Writing in the field has escalated in recent decades, with more than 4000 articles addressing this topic cataloged in the *Cumulative Index of Nursing and Allied Health Literature* (CINAHL) by the end of the twentieth century. When compared with a single article appearing in the 1970s, and about 350 on this topic to the end of the 1980s, the currently well over 4000 indicate that health promotion in nursing is a topic whose time has come. Health promotion is a long-established element of nursing care that is at least as old as the writings of Florence Nightingale, and yet how nurses practice health promotion, with whom, and in what settings is far from clear. This book attempts to explore and expand those relevant concepts, issues, and practical applications for a health promotion practice that is transformative for both nurses and their clients or patients.

Health promotion as a professional practice is discussed in terms of varying definitions of health. Health promoters who view health as the absence of disease write on topics such as smoking, injury prevention, and immunization. Those taking a broader view of health may address topics such as nutrition, pain, exercise, and violence. Although there is no doubt overlap among views on health promotion, what the editors of this book responded to was a call from Western Canadian nurse educators and personnel at F. A. Davis Company for a book on health promotion that held to the views that, fundamentally, health is a resource for daily living, and that health promotion is an interdisciplinary activity that increases patients'/clients' control over their health and their lives.

Building on concepts developed in the Ottawa Charter of Health Promotion (WHO, 1986), the authors in this book of collected works introduce patient/client-centered care and the social, political, and ecological influences on health promotion in nursing. We illustrate our views with practice-based examples of nursing *care* and research. We delve into processes that enable people to increase control over, and improve, their own health,

and explore health promotion mechanisms such as advocating, enabling/empowering, and mediating for clients or patients in the diverse settings in which nurses practice. In this book, you will find strategies for promoting health that include but extend beyond the "bedside": building healthy public policy, creating supportive environments, strengthening community action, developing personal skills, and reorienting health services.

The book is designed with undergraduate and graduate students and practitioners in mind. The chapters may be read in almost any order, though we recommend starting with the first two. Theoretical and practice-oriented chapters may be used singly or in combination, in theory or clinical courses. In a specific course, chapters may be paired effectively—that is, a theoretical chapter with a practice-based one. For example, a chapter from the Key Concepts section (Section Two) may be paired with a chapter from the sections addressing Challenges and Controversies (Section Three) or Health Promotion Research (Section Four). Chapter 3 about relational practice can be paired with Chapter 17, students' experiences in learning to practice in hospitals, or Chapter 7 on transformational leadership can be paired with Chapter 21 about seniors' empowerment in preventing falls. A variety of settings for health promoting nursing practice are introduced, but in every case, these present applications to different populations. The 32 Canadian and American authors from nursing and related disciplines have endeavored to challenge thinking, address controversies, and raise issues—a project that we hope will provoke discussion in your classes, seminars, or work settings. Hence, the reflective questions found in each chapter will be an asset. Instructors can use the issues and controversies raised by the authors to frame class or seminar discussions or to design essay questions or suggest topics that evaluate students' learning.

The chapters are grouped into five themes. Section One, Foundations of Health Promotion Practice, lays the groundwork for understanding how the book's authors think about health promotion. Knowledge in this area, as we noted earlier, has advanced significantly since the 1970s. In Chapter 1, *Transforming health promotion practice: Moving toward holistic care,* Lynne Young charts the development of thought in health promotion relative to its location in dominant paradigms of thinking. She argues that health promotion practice that seeks to understand and serve the interests of patients and clients (individuals, families, communities, and populations) is a resource for living and a practice that facilitates patients'/clients' control over their health. In the second chapter, *Health promotion: Historical, philosophical, and theoretical perspectives,* Marjorie MacDonald provides an overview of health promotion: what it is, where it has come from, and where it is going. It is, more than anything, a critique of the notion of health promotion. The author raises critical questions for further thinking about health promotion.

In Section Two, Key Concepts for Transforming Health Promotion Practice, the contributors delineate strategies for health promotion practice applicable to care for individuals, families, communities, and populations. In Chapter 3, *Beyond interpersonal communication: The significance of relationship in health promoting practice,* Gwen Hartrick challenges dominant assumptions underlying relational practice by drawing on complexity theory to demonstrate how practice might be reconstituted to be more in keeping with a philosophy of an emancipatory health promotion practice. In Chapter 4, *Health promoting interactions: Insights from the chronic illness experience,* Sally Thorne critically examines the ways in which nurses help or hinder health promotion, supporting key points with examples from her program of research on the chronic illness experience. These two chapters ground the human interaction component of health promotion practice in the foundational experience of human communication. Extending this, Rosalie Starzomski moves the discussion of health promotion to the community level in Chapter 5, *Listening to multiple voices: Public participation in health care decision making.* She provides a critical review of the role of consumers in health care decision making. She presents the historical background of the concept "consumer partici-

pation" and argues that public participation in health care is not well conceptualized or defined. Madine VanderPlaat, a sociologist, addresses health professionals' roles as advocates in Chapter 6, *Emancipatory politics and health promotion practice: The health professional as social activist.* This chapter provides readers with a comprehensive overview of the theoretical and philosophical principles embraced in emancipatory health promotion, with examples from practice used to highlight key points. The chapter is intended to challenge readers to see themselves as both nursing practitioners and potential social activists who have the capacity to contribute in a very significant way to meaningful social change and social justice. In Chapter 7, *Transformational leadership for health promotion practice,* Gail Cameron develops the notion of transformational leadership by exploring how the philosophical characteristics of health promotion and transformational leadership resonate. By reading this chapter, readers will understand how power relationships can be equalized between leaders and the nurses with whom they work, and come to appreciate that this process can be health promoting. This section concludes with Chapter 8, *Nurses influencing health care policy: International perspectives,* in which Nora Whyte uses a case study approach to highlight practical strategies employed by nurses in three countries (Japan, South Africa, and Brazil) in their health policy initiatives. Although the circumstances are different in each country, nurses experience common challenges worldwide and draw upon similar competencies as they participate in initiatives for change.

In Section Three, Challenges and Controversies: Revisiting and Re-creating Knowledge for Transformative Health Promotion Practice, the discussion shifts to the challenges and controversies inherent in health promotion practice, with authors frequently offering recommendations for moving forward. In Chapter 9, *Self-care: Re-examining the myth,* Deborah Thoun Northrup updates a previously published article of her own, and provides us with a spirited critique of the concept of self-care. The chapter provides a critical examination of a significant health promotion concept. In Chapter 10, *Health promotion, moral harm, and the moral aims of nursing,* Joan Liaschenko continues the critique of health promotion by alerting us to the moral nature of health and health promotion. She suggests that these are troublesome concepts and urges us to explore how we think about health, health promotion, and the moral aims of health promotion practice. In Chapter 11, Margaret Kearney synthesizes evidence from selected qualitative studies and suggests ways that women realize their health risks and take action to reduce those risks. *Defining and managing health risk: Snapshots of women's strategies across the lifespan* not only identifies women's own ways of dealing with threats to their health at different developmental stages, but also explores how cultures and life situations affect a woman's health experience. Kearney demonstrates that the largest obstacle to women's achievement of high-level wellness may be others' unwillingness to assist them to attain their own health-related goals, or evolve culturally consistent goals for achieving optimal well-being.

In Chapter 12, *Mental health promotion,* Catherine Willinsky and Bonnie Pape clarify the idea of mental health promotion by contrasting it to related concepts. This discussion evolves into a model to guide practice. Building on concepts of the model, the authors offer numerous strategies for mental health promotion practice. Chapter 13, Nursing support with family members of the critically ill: A framework to guide practice, also presents a framework for thinking about practice. Its author, Virginia Vandall-Walker, explores the nature of caring for families in critical care settings, where a condition of a family member poses a unique threat to the health of the family unit and its members. This chapter presents a first publication of a framework to guide family nursing in critical care situations, and includes case scenarios from the author's practice to illustrate dimensions of the framework. Following this, Mary Ellen Purkis challenges our complacency and taken-for-granted notions of professional practice in *Governing the health of populations: Conversations in the clinic.* Illustrated by selections of transcripts from an ethnographic study of nursing in a community health clinic, Purkis makes the often invisible elements of practice visible through a perceptive critique of nurses' conversations with mothers. She uses Foucault's notion of governmental rationalities to illustrate how a child's

health is "processed" in the clinic, and regulated by practices socially embedded in established "health promotion" practice strategies. Chapter 15 is a timely re-publication of the *Human genome project: Implications for nursing practice* by Cindy Munro. In it, readers are introduced to the Human Genome Project and its importance to nursing. Directions for health promotion practice within the nursing and genetics field emerge from the discussion. The last chapter in this section, *What is quality care? A hospital health promotion perspective,* is an exploration of what constitutes quality care in hospitals. Alex Berland and Lynne Young propose an innovative way to think about estimations of quality from both patients' and providers' points of views. They systematically explore ways to address the differences in perspectives of quality care between these two groups, and provoke us to consider ways to bring consumers' and professionals' ideas of what is important in quality care closer together.

In Section Four: Health Promotion Research, the authors provide examples of the generation of knowledge for health that is patient/client centered and directly applicable to the improvement of health for various participant groups. Marcia Hills (Chapter 17) begins the discussion by providing exemplars from nursing students' stories to illustrate the article's title, *Perspectives on learning and practicing health promotion in hospitals: Nursing students stories.* Here, analyses of dialogues between instructor and students reveal aspects of learning nursing within an undergraduate curriculum where the concept of health promotion is central. Student nurses were also participants in a study reported by Anne Bruce, Lynne Young, Linda Turner, Rena van der Wal, and Wolfgang Linden in Chapter 18. In *Meditation-based stress reduction: Holistic practice in nursing education,* the authors report their evaluation of a mindfulness-based stress reduction program (MBSR), in which students and faculty collaborated in a community development initiative aimed at reducing the students' stress. Although the chapter highlights the theoretical and philosophical underpinnings of the MBSR, the participatory quantitative and qualitative evaluation is also described.

While conducting an ethnography of midlife women's experiences of their changing bodies, Elizabeth Banister learned more than she expected; her individual participants activated their collective power to galvanize around an issue that was important to them. Banister describes what happened in Chapter 19, *Midlife women's empowerment process within a group*—the participants co-opted the research process and turned it into a venue for political action. In Chapter 20, *Family health promotion within the demands of pediatric home care and nursing respite*, Virginia (Jinny) Hayes and Pamela McElheran present a component of a grounded theory they developed. The mini-theory explains how families deal with the significant demands of caring at home for children that not only have complex or medically fragile conditions, but also require adjustment to the presence of respite nurses within their family circle. Concentrating on family-level health promotion, the authors move to an analysis of the need for health care policy change to promote family health. Shifting to the other end of the developmental spectrum, Elaine Gallagher, Elizabeth Lindsey, and Victoria Scott in Chapter 21 reflect on the progress and processes of promoting health through PAR in their article, *Promoting health through participatory action research: Lessons learned from STEPS* (Study of Environments that Promote Safety) and what seniors and researchers alike learned from the STEPS Project. Aimed to map and reduce slips, trips, and falls in public places, this project also resulted in a group of seniors empowered, through PAR, to create change through coalition building, advocacy, and political action. Empowerment is also an outcome of a project conducted collaboratively with First Nations' communities (Chapter 22). In *More than just questions! Implementation and evaluation of an arthritis self-management program in aboriginal communities*, Patrick McGowan presents a project in which qualitative and quantitative methods were combined in a participatory research process that facilitated a relevant health promotion partnership. The research provided a meaningful opportunity for collaborative program planning, intervention, and evaluation that ad-

dressed a widespread health challenge, arthritis. Marcia Hills and Jennifer Mullett conclude this section with a methodological piece (Chapter 23), a "how to" description of cooperative inquiry, a practical, usable method consonant with the health promotion approach we put forward in this book. In *Enhancing health promotion through cooperative inquiry*, they detail the rigorous iteration of action and reflection, and illustrate it using their own and others' research experiences.

The last section of the book, A Critique of Transformative Health Promotion Practice, contains the final chapter, *Transforming practice, dodging false dichotomies, and avoiding ideological quicksand*, written by Lawrence W. Green and Mark Daniel, that continues the spirit of critique. Here, the authors offer constructive criticism of previous chapters from the perspective of "outsiders." They provoke us to think more deeply and broadly, offering a counterpoint to various contributors' ideas, and serving to extend dialogue on health promotion in nursing.

This book evolved from our (the editors') three decades of practice in nursing and several years of thinking about, teaching, writing about, and investigating health promotion. The collective wisdom and widely varied experiences of all the contributors add up to a powerful statement about the interdisciplinary and unique-to-nursing dimensions of health promotion. Our hope is that this book will provide the impetus for the development of health promoting nursing practice, and stimulate scholarship in the field. We encourage all nurses to continue to tackle, together with their clients, the complex and diverse challenges that health promotion presents— by listening respectfully, implementing, and evaluating well-designed and thoughtfully conceived health promotion strategies, and by working collaboratively to address the cultural, social, and political factors that influence health.

Lynne E. Young
Virginia E. Hayes

ACKNOWLEDGMENTS

The idea for a book about health promotion for use in nursing education originated with Mary MacDonald, Professor of Nursing at the University of Saskatchewan School of Nursing, and then some years later, with Gail Cameron, nursing faculty at Okanagan University College. Both Mary and Gail discussed the idea independently with Sue Pringle, F. A. Davis Educational Sales Representative, who kept the book idea alive in spite of a lapse of several years when it lay fallow.

We wish to acknowledge as well Nora Whyte and Alex Berland for their invaluable input into discussions of the book concept in its earliest stages of development (1991–1993). When the time was right to undertake such a project, Sue Pringle connected us with Joanne DaCunha, F. A. Davis Nursing Acquisitions Editor, who supported us with skill, enthusiasm, and encouragement during the preparation of the prospectus and throughout our work on the manuscript.

Marilyn Kochman, F. A. Davis Developmental Editor, was assigned to the project and worked closely with us toward completion of the book with good humor and competence. We wish to acknowledge our University of Victoria contributing authors who met, encouraged, and designed the book with us, and Janet Storch, Director of the University of Victoria School of Nursing, for her encouragement and ongoing support.

Behind the scenes, Phaedra Bennett, Project Secretary, was a pillar of support. Phaedra attended to the numerous details encountered when tracking the work of more than 30 contributing authors and approximately 55 reviewers. In her absence, Katrina Pandak and America Blasco, secretaries at the University of Victoria, School of Nursing, Lower Mainland Campus, managed the myriad details.

Although the individuals above supported the entire project, others have played roles in developing specific aspects of it. We would like to recognize three University of Victoria School of Nursing colleagues who read and commented on selected chapter manuscripts aside from the formal review process: Elaine Gallagher, Gwen Hartick, and Rosalie Starzomski. Virginia Hayes and Pamela McElheran thank Janet Radford for pushing their thinking and reviewing their manuscript. Joan Liaschenko would like to acknowledge Marjorie MacIntrye, Lisa M. Skauge, and Scott Weber for their contributions to the development of her chapter.

Virginia Vandall-Walker is grateful to Dave Walker and Eleanore Vandall for their input into her work. Madine VanderPlaat acknowledges Yolande Samson, Evaluation Consultant, Health Promotion and Programs Branch (Atlantic Region) and Pauline Raven, Regional Coordinator, Annapolis Valley-Hants, Community Action Program for Children. Collectively, we extend our gratitude to all whose time and effort contributed to this book project.

Institutions also played a role in supporting our efforts, and we would like to acknowledge this. The University of Victoria and its School of Nursing fosters a scholarly environment in which nontraditional views and innovative ideas can be explored and developed. The Heart & Stroke Foundation of Canada (HSFC) and BC & Yukon HSFC funded Lynne Young's doctoral and post-doctoral studies, grants that supported the development of her knowledge about health promotion, and allowed her time to work on the book project. Finally, we have appreciated F. A. Davis's organizational responsiveness.

The editors acknowledge those mentors whose guidance and inspiration is invaluable. Lynne Young recognizes Sally Thorne, Lawrence W. Green, and Susanna Cunningham. In addition, we recognize the University of Victoria staff and faculty, especially Paddy Rodney and Rosalie Starzomski, whose ongoing interest in our work and easy availability to discuss book-related matters, was not only helpful but invigorating as well.

Lynne Young would like to recognize the on-going support and encouragement of her family, especially her daughter Lani Maxwell, son Bruce Maxwell, sisters Barbara Young and Pat Hunt, mother Hilda Young, and brother-in-law Rob Holton. Our families and friends have encouraged and sustained us.

We thank you all for your understanding and believing in the importance of preparing this volume about health promotion in nursing.

Lynne E. Young
Virginia E. Hayes

CONTENTS

SECTION ONE
FOUNDATIONS OF HEALTH PROMOTION PRACTICE

SECTION TWO
KEY CONCEPTS FOR TRANSFORMING HEALTH PROMOTION PRACTICE

SECTION THREE
CHALLENGES AND CONTROVERSIES: REVISITING AND RECREATING KNOWLEDGE FOR TRANSFORMATIVE HEALTH PROMOTION PRACTICE

SECTION FOUR
HEALTH PROMOTION RESEARCH

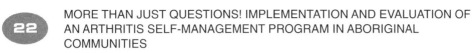
SECTION FIVE
A CRITIQUE OF TRANSFORMATIVE HEALTH PROMOTION PRACTICE

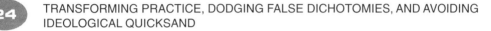

CONTRIBUTORS

Elizabeth Banister, RN, PhD, R Psyche is an Assistant Professor at the School of Nursing, University of Victoria. She has degrees in nursing, counseling psychology, and educational psychology. Her research focuses on health-related issues of women at midlife and adolescent girls. At the undergraduate level, she teaches group process, helping relationships, nursing practice, and research methodology. She also teaches theory and interpretative inquiry in a multidisciplinary master's program. She is currently conducting a participatory action research project that focuses on facilitating adolescent girls' abilities to handle relationships.

Alex Berland, RN, BScN, MSc, CHE is a senior manager and planner who has worked in all sectors of health care, in education and community development, and in government. Currently working for the British National Health Service on acute care policy, he was previously chief executive at teaching and community hospitals in British Columbia, Canada. Alex is also a Clinical Assistant Professor at the University of British Columbia and served as non-executive board member of a primary care group for many years.

Anne Bruce, RN, PhD(c) is a doctoral candidate in the School of Nursing at the University of British Columbia. She is conducting research into the experiences of people living with life-threatening illness who practice mindfulness meditation as a practice of living with dying.

Gail Cameron, RN, MSN teaches health promotion, community development, political action, and group process to BSN students at Okanagan University College. Her nursing practice includes program planning, community development, and advocacy for seniors. She uses a participatory action research methodology to work with community groups—the most recent study considered multiple perspectives to influence change in an organizational culture.

Elaine M. Gallagher, RN, PhD is a Professor in the School of Nursing at the University of Victoria. She is also an Affiliate Researcher in the Center on Aging at the University of Victoria and an Adjunct Professor at Simon Fraser University. Dr. Gallagher's research has examined aging and built environments in a variety of contexts, ranging from prisons to private homes and long-term care settings. Her most recent work has centered on injury prevention in later work where she has examined a variety of factors that contribute to falls and injuries among the elderly.

Lawrence W. Green, PhD and **Mark Daniel, BSc, MSc, PhD** bring to their commentary varied experience in Canadian, American, Australian, and European health promotion, as well as Dr. Green's growing portfolio of responsibility for the Centers for Disease Control global tobacco control efforts in developing countries. They collaborated while at the University of British Columbia's Institute of Health Promotion Research and Department of Health Care and Epidemiology on the development of the Royal Society of Canada Guidelines on Participatory Research and on community studies of diabetes prevention and control in indigenous populations. Dr. Daniel is now Assistant Professor of health behavior and health education and of epidemiology in the school of public health at the University of North Carolina at Chapel Hill.

Gwen Hartrick, RN, PhD, R Psych is an Associate Professor in the School of Nursing at the University of Victoria in British Columbia, Canada. She has an interdisciplinary background (registered nurse/registered psychologist). Her research interests include relational practice, health promotion, family health, women's health, and interdisciplinary practice.

Virginia E. Hayes (Jinny), RN, PhD is an Associate Professor in the School of Nursing at the University of Victoria, Vancouver campus. Her research program centers on the impact of children's chronic conditions on families, and includes basic and applied approaches, qualitative and quantitative methods, and program evaluation. She is involved in policy background research at the national level, particularly in the delivery of services to children with long-term health concerns and their families, such as respite care and family-centered care. She is also interested in participative approaches in education, research, and community development, and has a number of publications in related areas.

Marcia D. Hills, RN, PhD is a Professor in the School of Nursing at the University of Victoria, a Director of the Canadian Consortium of Health Promotion Research, and President of the Canadian Association of Teachers of Community Health. She is the founder and the Director of the Community Health Promotion Coalition, a research unit dedicated to engendering collaborations between government, community groups, and academics in order to expand research methodologies aimed at improving healthy communities. She provided leadership in the development of an innovative curriculum that is currently offered collaboratively in ten post-secondary institutions throughout British Columbia, and is committed to teaching and research that are collaborative and action oriented.

Margaret H. Kearney, RN, PhD is a nurse researcher and faculty member at Boston College in Chestnut Hill, Massachusetts. She holds degrees in nursing from Columbia University (BS), Boston College (MS), and the University of California at San Francisco (PhD). A women's health nurse practitioner, Maggie has used the grounded theory approach in a series of qualitative studies on women drug users' management of sexuality, pregnancy, and mothering, and she has been a pioneer in approaches to synthesizing qualitative findings across studies.

Joan Liaschenko, RN, PhD is an Associate Professor in the School of Nursing and Center for Bioethics at the University of Minnesota Twin Cities. Her primary area of interest and research is the ethical dimensions in the everyday work of nursing. She is concerned with what nurses identify and articulate as ethical concerns and how they respond to them.

Wolfgang Linden, PhD is a Professor in the Department of Psychology at the University of British Columbia. He has an extensive research program studying physiological responses to stress and stress management trials, particularly as this relates to cardiovascular disease.

Elizabeth Lindsey, RN, PhD is Professor Emeritus, School of Nursing, University of Victoria, Victoria, BC. Her areas of interest include health promotion, community health, community development, HIV/AIDS, chronic illness, and quantitative health research. She has collaborated on various health and social service studies using participatory action research methods. In addition, she has undertaken many community development projects in Canada and developing countries. She currently works as a consultant to educational institutions and health organizations, and for the World Health Organization on issues related to HIV/AIDS, home care, nursing, and midwifery care and counseling. She has taught public health, community health and community development to undergraduate and graduate nursing students.

Marjorie A. MacDonald, RN, PhD is an Assistant Professor at the School of Nursing, University of Victoria. She holds a doctorate in interdiscipli-

nary studies in health promotion from the University of British Columbia. Her research and practice focus is in community and public health nursing with specific interests in school and adolescent health, particularly related to alcohol, tobacco, and other drug use. She also has a background in health policy and program evaluation. Marjorie has taught courses in health promotion theory and practice, nurses influencing change, community health nursing, program evaluation, and a senior-level consolidated practice course.

Pamela J. McElheran, RN, MSN is currently a Clinical Nurse Specialist at Sunny Hill Health Center for Children in Vancouver, British Columbia. Sunny Hill is a pediatric rehabilitation facility that is part of the Children's and Women's Health Center of British Columbia. Pamela has a broad range of experience working with children with medically fragile conditions and their families. She has previously been employed as a community health care nurse in Home Care (working with children and families, and in a home IV program) and in the Nursing Support Services Program. She was a co-investigator with Dr. Hayes on the study evaluating the British Columbia Nursing Respite Program.

Patrick McGowan, MSW, PhD has been working with community groups in health promotion projects for over twenty years. The main areas of his work has been on projects addressing health concerns in aboriginal people, coping with chronic health conditions, medication use among seniors, and projects that encourage self-help and self-care activities. Currently, he is the Assistant Director of the Institute of Health Promotion Research at the University of British Columbia.

Jennifer Mullett, BA, MA, PhD is a community psychologist and assistant professor in the Faculty of Human and Social Development at the University of Victoria, a Research Scholar funded by the BC Health Research Foundation and the Director of Research at the Community Health Promotion Coalition. She works with non-profit agencies and health regions on community-based research approaches to enhance health and capacitate social action.

Cindy L. Munro, RN, ANP, PhD is an Associate Professor at Virginia Commonwealth University, where she teaches undergraduate, masters, and doctoral students. Dr. Munro's doctoral work centered around molecular genetics and microbiology. Her current research focuses on oral health and associated systemic illness including ventilator-associated pneumonia (VAP) and endocarditis. She practices as an Adult Nurse Practitioner in a community health center. She has published several articles and book chapters about implications of the human genome project, has taught honors' courses focused on the impact of genetics on health and on society, and teaches in a multidisciplinary graduate scientific integrity course where human genome issues are discussed.

Deborah Thoun Northrup, RN, PhD is a faculty member at the University of Victoria since 1996. Prior to joining UVic, she worked as a nurse scientist and Clinical Nurse Specialist in mental health, and consultant in nursing theory-based practice and research. The focus of Dr. Northrup's practice and research is health and quality of life from the person's perspective. Her research interests include the evaluation of nursing theory-based practice and qualitative explorations of humanly lived experiences from a human science perspective. Current research initiatives investigate the meanings of "time passing" for persons with HIV disease, "facing the unknown" for Canadian military nurses deployed on peacekeeping and humanitarian missions, and "living with traumatic brain injury." Financial support for research endeavors has been received from the Department of National Defense and internal research and development funds within research-affiliated organizations. Dr. Northrup is an elected member of Phi Kappa Phi and serves on the Board of Directors of the Registered Nurses Association of British Columbia.

Bonnie Pape, BA, MEd, MES is Director of Programs and research at the Canadian Mental Health Association, National Office. She has been instrumental in developing and implementing the association's mental health promotion policy model, "A Framework for Support." The model emphasizes the importance of informal supports and inclusion for people with mental illness. Bonnie has led workshops and presentations on this model by invitation throughout Canada as well as internationally in Ireland, Scotland, and Japan. She has written numerous articles and documents on consumer participation, self-help, and mental health policy development.

Mary Ellen Purkis, RN, PhD completed doctoral studies at the University of Edinburgh. She began working at the University of Victoria at the completion of those studies in 1993 and is now the Director. She has taught courses on the development of knowledge in nursing practice. Her research focuses on ethnographic studies of nursing practice in a variety of practice settings. She is presently engaged in writing projects that explicate the contingencies of nursing practice as a social accomplishment.

Victoria J. Scott, RN, PhD is an Assistant Professor at the University of Victoria School of Nursing. She is co-director of the Adult Injury Management Network as well as a member of the Board of Directors of the British Columbia Paraplegic Association. Vicky's research interests include the role of the public environment in falls among older adults and the policy implications of injury prevention. Most recently she has been involved in a community-development project for the promotion of injury prevention initiatives with older adults in their communities and the development of a data collection tool for injuries occurring in long-term care facilities.

Rosalie C. Starzomski, RN, PhD is the Associate Director of the University of Victoria School of Nursing, an ethics consultant at the Vancouver Hospital and Health Sciences Center, and a Faculty Associate at the University of British Columbia Care for Applied Ethics. Rosalie is listed in the *Who's Who of Canadian Women* and her research and scholarly interests focus on health care ethics, health policy, organ transplantation, and nephrology. She is interested in interdisciplinary collaboration and public and health care provider involvement in health care decision making. She has served as a committee member and volunteer for many organizations, including: the Kidney Foundation of Canada, British Columbia Ministry of Health, Health Canada, the World Council for Renal Care, the Canadian Nurses Association, and Canuck Place.

Sally E. Thorne, RN, PhD is a Professor at the School of Nursing, University of British Columbia. She has a program of research in the field of chronic illness and cancer experience, and is particularly concerned with the influence of health care ideology and service delivery on the lives of those who live with ongoing health challenges in our society. She is the author of *Negotiating Health Care: The Social Context of Chronic Illness* (Sage, 1993).

Linda Turner, RN, MSN is a Clinical Nurse Specialist in pain management. She is a Mindfulness-Based Stress Reduction program facilitator committed to evidence-based practice.

Virginia A. Vandall-Walker, RN, PhD(c) has been an Assistant Professor at Athabasca University for the past five years, providing instruction by distance to students across Canada in courses related to trends and issues in nursing, physical assessment, home health nursing, and guided advanced study. She has worked across the spectrum of health service delivery including outpost, emergency, and critical care nursing, and senior nursing management, as well as in nursing education, in numerous Canadian geographical locations. Virginia is currently a doctoral candidate at the University of Alberta with a research focus on nursing support with families of the critically ill.

Madine VanderPlaat, RN, PhD is an Associate Professor of sociology at St. Mary's University in Halifax. She teaches in the areas of research methods and data analysis, social action research, and theories of feminism. Her research interests include health promotion and emancipatory evaluation strategies. She has worked extensively with the Health Promotion and Programs Branch of Health Canada.

Rena van der Wal, RN, MN is a Professional Practice Director and specialist in wound management. She has a record of researching stressful conditions in nursing.

Nora B. Whyte, RN, MSN is President of PHC Consulting Ltd., Vancouver, Canada, and Adjunct Professor, University of British Columbia School of Nursing. In her consulting practice, she assists health organizations in developing community-based health services, based on primary health care principles. As a voluntary consultant for the Canadian Nurses Association's International Bureau, she has worked with nursing associations in Nepal and South Africa; she has also consulted and conducted workshops for the Japanese Nursing Association.

Catherine Willinsky, RN, MS has been interested in the area of mental health promotion for a number of years. Her research for a masters degree in health promotion at the University of Toronto in 1997 formed the basis of her chapter. She continues to research and write about mental health promotion, and recently completed a practical guide, called the Mental Health Promotion Tool Kit, for the national office of the Canadian Mental Health Association.

Lynne E. Young, RN, PhD is an Assistant Professor at the University of Victoria School of Nursing and MRC/HSFC Post-Doctoral Fellow at the University of Washington School of Nursing. Her research and scholarly interests center on health promotion topics, with a primary focus on families and cardiovascular care in community and acute care settings. Dr. Young's research at the University of Washington is concerned with the interface between risk behaviors and risk conditions for athlerosclerotic cardiovascular disease. Dr. Young teaches undergraduate courses at the University of Victoria, Lower Mainland Campus, that address nursing practice in community and acute care settings.

REVIEWERS

GAYLE ALLISON, RN, BSN
Practica Coordinator
University of Victoria School of Nursing
Vancouver, British Columbia

JOANNE BARTRAM, FNP, MS
Department of Pediatrics
Lovelace Health Systems
Albuquerque, New Mexico

FAYE BEBB, RN, BSN, MA
Director, Education Services
Planned Parenthood Association of British Columbia
Vancouver, British Columbia

LYNETTE BEST, RN, MScN, CHE
Professional Practice Leader
Providence Health Centre, St. Paul's Hospital
Vancouver, British Columbia

ANNE BRUCE, RN, BSN, PhD(c)
Sessional Instructor
University of Victoria
Vancouver, British Columbia

BRENDA CANITZ, BScN, RN, MSC, BA
Nursing Consultant & Program Manager
Nursing Support Services and At-Home Program
British Columbia Ministry for Children and Families
Victoria, British Columbia

SUSANNA CUNNINGHAM, RN, BSN, MA, PhD
Professor
University of Washington
School of Nursing
Seattle, Washington

TERRY DAVIS, RN, MEd, PhD
Professor
University of Alberta
Faculty of Nursing
Edmonton, Alberta

DARLENE DAWSON, RN, BN
Patient Care Coordinator, Cardiology
Foothills Medical Center
Calgary, Alberta

JANET DEATRICK, RN, BSN, MSN, PhD, FAAN
Associate Professor and Co-Director, International
    Center of Research for Women, Children & Families
University of Pennsylvania
School of Nursing
Philadelphia, Pennsylvania

ODETTE DOYON, RN, Med, PhD(c)
Professor
Universite de Trois Rivieres
Trois Rivieres, Quebec

CRISTINA FOLLADOR, RN, BSN
Staff Nurse
British Columbia's Children's Hospital
Vancouver, British Columbia

LUCIA GAMROTH, RN, BSN, MPA, MS, PhD
Associate Professor
University of Victoria
School of Nursing
Victoria, British Columbia

SIMONE GARDEZY, RN, BSN
Community Health Nurse
Victoria, British Columbia

DEBORAH R. GARRISON, RN, PhD
Assistant Clinical Professor
Texas Woman's University
College of Nursing
Houston, Texas

KARA GEORGE, RN, BSN
Staff Nurse, Burns and Plastics Unit
Vancouver Hospital and Health Sciences Center
Vancouver, British Columbia

JOYCE HENDERSON, RN, BScN, MPH
Nursing Faculty, BSN Program
Okanagan University College
Kelowna, British Columbia

SUSIE JANOSEK, RN, BSN
Staff Nurse
British Columbia's Children's Hospital
Vancouver, British Columbia

CAROL JILLINGS, RN, BS, MSN, PhD
Associate Professor and Associate Director
University of British Columbia School of Nursing
Vancouver, British Columbia

TERESA S. JOHNSON, RN, PhD, FAAN
Assistant Professor
University of Wisconsin Milwaukee
School of Nursing
Milwaukee, Wisconsin

TONI KARLE, RN, MN, C-FNP, CV-CNS
Assistant Professor
Marshall University
Huntington, West Virginia

RUTH LAMB, RN, MScN, CHTP
Manager Health and Human Services and
    Center for Holistic Health Studies
Langara College
Continuing Studies Department
Vancouver, British Columbia

MARY MacDONALD, RN, BScN, MCEd
Professor, School of Nursing
University of Saskatchewan
Saskatoon, Saskatchewan

JANICE McCORMICK, RN, PhD
Assistant Professor
University of Victoria
School of Nursing
Vancouver, British Columbia

MARJORIE McINTYRE, RN, PhD
Associate Professor
University of Calgary
Faculty of Nursing
Calgary, Alberta

LIAN McKENZIE, RN, BSN
Staff Nurse
St Paul's Hospital
Vancouver, British Columbia

ANNE McMURRAY, RN, BA, MEd
Dean, Faculty of Nursing and Health
Griffith University
Brisbane, Australia

DONNA MEAGHER-STEWART, RN, BScN, MHSc,
  PhD(c)
Associate Professor and
Associate Director Graduate Program
Dalhousie University
School of Nursing
Halifax, Nova Scotia

BARB MOFFAT, BScN, RN, MSN
Project Director
University of British Columbia
School of Nursing
Vancouver, British Columbia

ELLEN OLSHANSKY, RN, DNSc, RNC
Professor and Chair, PhD in Nursing Program
Duquesne University
School of Nursing
Pittsburgh, Pennsylvania

STEPHEN PARKER, RN, BSN
Nurse Clinician
St. Paul's Hospital
Vancouver, British Columbia

JUDITH BARBERIO POLLACHEK, PhD(c), RN, CS,
  A/GNP
Undergraduate and Graduate Faculty
Rutgers, The State University of New Jersey
Newark, New Jersey

PADDY RODNEY, RN, MSN, PhD
Assistant Professor
University of Victoria School of Nursing
Vancouver, British Columbia

KAREN SAMSON, RN, BSN
Community Health Nurse, Early Childhood Program
Vancouver/Richmond Health Board
Vancouver, British Columbia

INGRID SEE, RN, MEd
Clinical Nurse Specialist
Palliative Care
Simon Fraser Health Board
Burnaby, British Columbia

MAUREEN SHAW, RN, MSN, CNS
Clinical Nurse Specialist
Vancouver Hospital & Health Sciences Center
Vancouver, British Columbia

CAROLE SHEA, RN, PhD, FAAN
Professor and Associate Dean for Academic Affairs
Northeastern University
Bouve College of Health Sciences
Boston, Massachusetts

HAL SIDEN, MD, MHSc
Assistant Clinical Professor
University of British Columbia
Faculty of Medicine Department of Pediatrics
Vancouver, British Columbia

VICKI SMYE, RN, PhD(c)
Doctoral Program
University of British Columbia
School of Nursing
and
Consultant Staff
Mental Health Evaluation and Community Consultation
  Unit (Aboriginal Mental Health Working Group)
Department of Psychiatry
University of British Columbia
Vancouver, British Columbia

HASSAN SOUBHI, MD, PhD
Post-Doctoral Fellow
University of British Columbia and BC's Women's and
  Children's Hospital
Department of Health Care and Epidemiology
Vancouver, British Columbia

LYNNETTE LEESEBERG STAMLER, RN, PhD
Associate Professor & Director
Collaborative BScN Program
Nippissing University
North Bay, Ontario

NANCY SYMMES, RN, BSN
Faculty
Northern Collaborative Baccalaureate Nursing Program
College of New Caledonia
Prince George, British Columbia

ROSEMARY THEROUX, PHD, RNC, NP
Faculty
University of Massachusetts Lowell
Lowell, Massachusetts
Women's Health Nurse Practitioner
Framingham, Massachusetts

LAURA THIEM, RN, CS, MSN, FNP
Adrian Rural Health Clinic
Family Nurse Practitioner
Adrian, Missouri

GAYLE M. TIMMERMAN, RN, PhD, CNS
Associate Professor
The University of Texas
Austin, Texas

ELAINE UNSWORTH, BS, MSN
Nurse Clinician
Geriatric Assessment Unit
Vancouver-Richmond Health Board
Vancouver, British Columbia

MAUREEN VAN DEN DOOL, RN, BSN
Staff Nurse
Children and Women's Health Center of British Columbia
Vancouver, British Columbia

RENA VAN DER WAL, BSN, RN, MN
Professional Practice Director
Vancouver Hospital & Health Sciences Center
Vancouver, British Columbia

SUZANNE WARITZ. RN, MSN, FNP
Family Nurse Practitioner
Open Door Clinic
Roseburg, Oregon

K. LYNN WIECK, RN, PhD
Associate Professor
Texas Woman's University
College of Nursing
Houston, Texas

HEATHER MACLEOD WILLIAMS, BPE, MPE
Research Consultant
MTM Research
North Vancouver, British Columbia

APRIL WILLISCROFT, RN, BSN
Staff Nurse
British Columbia Cancer Agency
Vancouver, British Columbia

ANGELA WOLFF, RN, BScN, MSN
Continuing Education Coordinator
Registered Nurses Association of British Columbia
Vancouver, British Columbia

LYNN WOODS, RN, BSN, PhD
Senior Instructor
University of Washington, Bothell Campus School of
  Nursing
Seattle, Washington

JACQUELINE C. ZALUMAS, RNC, PhD, FNP
Principal Investigator and Assistant Professor
Corrections Technical Assistance and Training Project
Emory University
School of Medicine
Atlanta, Georgia

Foundations of Health Promotion Practice

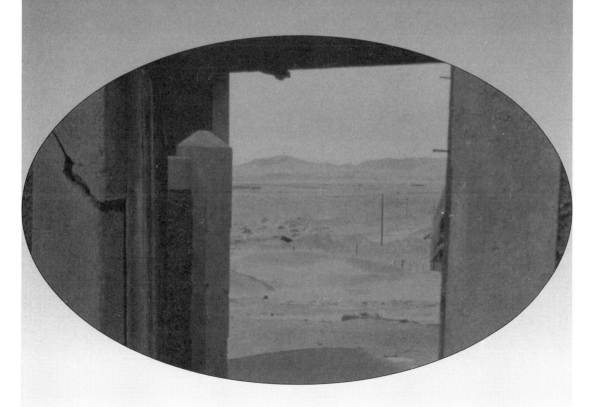

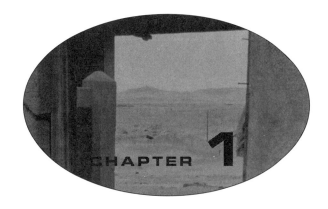

CHAPTER 1

Transforming Health Promotion Practice: Moving Toward Holistic Care

LYNNE E. YOUNG

When Tracy was 45 years old and had her first gallbladder attack, her problems with obesity and hypertension came to my attention. I attempted therapeutic intervention. A couple of years later, her stone-laden gallbladder was removed and we renewed our efforts to control her elevated blood pressure and excessive weight. By this time, her blood sugar and lipid profile were also mildly elevated. Because all these factors were interrelated and potentially amenable to lifestyle and dietary changes, she was urged to increase her exercise and she was referred to a dietitian. Although she herself didn't smoke, she lived in a home with a chain-smoking husband. Both of her parents had myocardial infarcts in their 50s, so it was important to intervene in these areas to reduce her risk for cardiovascular disease.

Last year, at age 55, Tracy had an anterior myocardial infarction (MI) and subsequent triple bypass surgery. I remember her response when she learned of her MI. . . . "I guess I deserve this . . . you have been warning me long enough." I replied, "You are still alive, you survived. It's not too late to make sure that it doesn't happen again."

When Tracy was recuperating from surgery, we could see that she was now determined to "make sure it didn't happen again." So, what has gone wrong? Tracy is educated and was able to understand the advice of the dietitian, yet her weight remains unchanged. Her blood pressure, diabetes, and lipid profiles are near normal but only with the help of medication. It was hoped that lifestyle changes alone would make a significant impact on these laboratory measurements. In regular follow-up visits with me and an internist, her "numbers" have become normal (BP, glucose, cholesterol levels), but we haven't made any solid impact on her **self-care** *practices. Or, maybe we have?*

Tracy insists that she has dramatically changed her eating patterns. The snowy winters in our town preclude year-round, brisk outdoor walking, so Tracy has purchased, and insists that she uses, indoor exercise equipment. We have bombarded her with educational materials and reinforced this information at each follow-up visit. Every indication is that Tracy is compliant with her medications. Her husband has even been convinced to smoke indoors in one specially ventilated room that they have remodeled on Tracy's behalf. It is my hope that dialogue with others about health promotion practice will provide us all with more ideas about how to more effectively help other clients like Tracy in our communities. (Account prepared by a medical colleague.)
McGowan & Young, 1999,
Appendix, p. 7

Health promotion is a professional practice of those concerned with health, such as nurses, physicians, dentists, and nutritionists. The goal of health promotion practice is to improve and maintain health. Although this sounds simple, health promotion is a highly complex professional practice that has evolved in recent years as scholars, researchers, and practitioners address its complexities. Like the health professional in the opening scenario, many of us search for ways to improve our health promotion practice.

Traditional approaches to health promotion practice, as exemplified in the scenario, are rooted in long-held values, beliefs, and assumptions about what is health and what is health promotion.

Health promotion practiced from a traditional behavior change and lifestyle perspective, as apparent in the scenario, is effective in some circumstances and with some people but not with others (Evans & Stoddard, 1990; Glanz, Lewis, & Rimer, 1997; Winkleby, Flora, & Kraemer, et al., 1994). Behind the practice-based decisions of the health professional in the above vignette is the assumption that providing clients with information about how to change health-related behavior, and reinforcing this, will lead to change. The health professional telling of his experience, like many others, is dismayed and somewhat cynical that the "therapeutic interventions" with Tracy were not effective in preventing her eventual heart disease.

Practice experiences, such as the one described here, have inspired health promotion practitioners and scholars to critique the values, beliefs, and assumptions of traditional health promotion as the first step in constructing innovative approaches. They ask, what can we do differently, why, and how? The authors in this book grapple with such questions, and explore health promotion as a transformative process. A *transformative* approach to health promotion is a collaborative process, one in which the health professional works with clients (defined as individuals, patients, families, communities, and populations) to gain insights into social, organizational, political, and personal patterns that strengthen or disrupt health and wholeness, and to take action toward improved **health.**

This chapter focuses on the theoretical basis of transformative health promotion practice. It

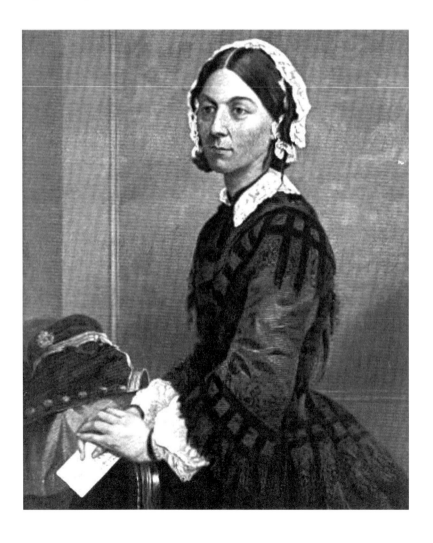

begins with an overview of the roots of health promotion and charts the evolution of theory development in the field since the 1970s with a focus on select theories. The chapter concludes with a discussion of the characteristics of transformative health promotion practice.

The Roots of Health Promotion

To understand health promotion, it is helpful to understand its roots. The earliest records of community health practices were described by the Chinese, Egyptians, and Babylonians (Green & Ottoson, 1999). In China during the Xia and Shang dynasties (21st to 11th centuries BCE), inscriptions on tortoise shells indicate that people dug community drinking wells. In Egypt, excavations near the Nile revealed extensive community rain collection and sewage drainage systems. In 1745–1650 BCE, Hammurabi,[1] a powerful king of Babylon, the world's first metropolis, formulated a set of laws to govern society, the Code of Hammurabi. Some laws governed the distribution of possessions, whereas others were designed to prevent unnecessary deaths and institute care for those with illnesses.

The "modern" era of health began in the mid-1800s in response to the work and writings of influential persons such as Florence Nightingale (Meleis, 1991). In this era, organizing ideas of health progressed through several phases: the miasma phase (1850–1880), in which communities emphasized cleanliness as the key to disease control; the bacteriology phase (1880–1910), during which the prevention of the spread of germs was key; the health resource phase (1910–1960), during which services for illness care expanded; the social engineering phase (1960–1975), during which improving access to health services was a focus; and the health promotion phase (1970s to present), in which policy shifted from disease care to health promotion (Green & Ottoson, 1999). The overwhelming focus on illness care that followed World War II challenges nurses to clarify what health promotion means for nursing.

[1]For a discussion and presentation of the Code of Hammurabi, refer to: http://www.lawresearch.com/v2/codeham.htm.

After World War II

Illness care gained prominence in North America after World War II with the introduction of technological advances in medical care. An infrastructure developed that was "primarily biomedical rather than health in its orientation"(Green & Kreuter, 1991, p. 6). Health promotion was therefore eclipsed for several decades (Green & Kreuter, 1991; Rachlis & Kushner, 1994). This move toward high technology and the hospital-based resources to support it proved costly (Green & Kreuter, 1999; Somers, 1976). As costs escalated, analyses of Canadian and American health care systems indicated that **effectiveness** for improving the public's health was not increasing as expenditures increased (Evans & Stoddard, 1990; Green & Kreuter, 1991; Somers, 1976). Analysts pointed out that the public's health is determined primarily by conditions of living: nutrition, housing, working conditions, neighborhood cohesion, and preventive practices (Illich, 1975; McKeown, 1971). During this time, nursing's voice was a continual reminder that illness care is not necessarily health care.

In the mid-1970s in both the United States and Canada, public health professionals raised the issue that mortality, illness, and disability, key indicators of the health status, did not reflect the expenditure of dollars on health care. In spite of increasing health care expenditure, and greatly increased access to health care for Canadians and Americans, the health status of citizens showed few, if any, signs of improvement (Green & Kreuter, 1991; Somers, 1976). Further, in the United States, the immunization rates for preschool children decreased in the decade between 1963 and 1973 (Somers, 1976). Of concern to public health professionals in the early 1970s was the lack of attention to prevention practices in preference to biomedical cures. They expressed concern that lack of attention to preventive practices had the potential to result in an escalation of premature deaths from heart disease, accidents, cirrhosis of the liver, suicide, and homicide, sequelae held to be related to lifestyle choices that could be influenced by health education (Somers, 1976). During this time, of increasing concern to nurses was the value placed on the biomedical cure and the relative invisibility of nurses' health-related work (Passau-Buck & Jones, 1997).

Society, it was argued, was becoming increasingly dependent on therapeutic medical interventions (Somers, 1976). Public health professionals lobbied for reorientation and refocusing of health care services under the umbrella term "health promotion." In the United States, central to this reorganizing effort was the development of health objectives (Raeburn, 1992; U.S. Department of Health and Human Services, 1980). Health behavior was at the center of health promotion (Glanz et al., 1997). In Canada, the Lalonde Report, *A New Perspective on the Health of Canadians* (1974) (hereafter called the Lalonde Report) shifted the focus from illness care to health care, reconstructing a vision for health care in Canada. This report introduced lifestyle and environment as key determinants of health, thereby reintroducing the idea that health is tied to overall conditions of living, a longstanding stance of the public health tradition (Lalonde, 1974).

The central argument of this report was that health is not achievable solely from health care but rather from the interplay of determinants from four health field elements: human biology, lifestyles, the environment, and health care (Labonte, 1994). Nurses in Canada welcomed this vision for health, one that resonated with nursing's definition. At McGill University, nurse scholars under the leadership of Moya Allen responded by designing a model in which health promotion was the central nursing activity, the McGill Model for Nursing, (Gottlieb & Rowat, 1985). Thus, the health promotion movement was launched in North America and resonated with similar movements instituted throughout the world (Green & Ottoson, 1999).

Since both the Lalonde Report (1974) in Canada and the National Health Consumer Information and 1976 Health Promotion Act in the United States called for a shift away from cure to health care, the appropriate focus for health promotion has been the center of much debate, theory development, and thoughtful critique. During this same period, philosophers and scholars throughout the world destabilized the assumptions of science formulated in the 16th century through their re-envisioning of what counts as knowledge and reality. Kuhn (1970) launched a particularly influential critique, noting that bodies of knowledge such as the sciences are based on shared meanings held by a community of scientists

or scholars. He pointed out that these shared meanings have to do with what a society or community of scientists and scholars consider appropriate, and have more to do with shared understandings than individual actions (Hacking, 1981; Kuhn, 1970).

Kuhn pointed to the scientific review process as an institutionalized strategy that ensures advancement only of science or knowledge considered appropriate by a community of scholars. In the following decades, scholars in health promotion and nursing, schooled in critique of traditional views of knowledge and reality, crafted new theories and philosophies of health promotion. Their work is characterized by a re-envisioning of what counts as knowledge and reality. Current knowledge in health promotion and nursing derives both from the work of scholars holding to traditional (modern) views and those who have critiqued the assumptions of traditional practices to arrive at a new set of assumptions and a different practice (post-modernists). In the next section, these two views of the world and their applications in the health promotion field are discussed.

Modern and Post-Modern Worldviews of Health Promotion

A modern worldview emerged in the 16th century in the writings of Bacon, Descartes, Newton, and Locke, to name the most notable few (Borgmann, 1992; Capra, 1982; Maxwell, 1997a). This intellectual movement, characterized by the development of what we know as the scientific method, was launched to counter metaphysical thinking, the dominant way of knowing at that time. In the 20th century, scholars of what is known as the Vienna Circle extended the attack on metaphysical thinking by declaring all statements meaningless that could not be verified by the scientific method (Morrow, 1994). Popper contested the notion of verification, suggesting that proving theories wrong (falsification) was more appropriate (Morrow, 1994). The influence of the Vienna Circle and Popper infused inquiry in the social sciences (Morrow, 1994). The modern worldview assumes that there is a reality that can be discovered through observation and the scientific method; that scientific knowledge describes and explains reality for the purpose of predicting causal relationships; that there is a single truth; that universal laws govern human matters; that the individual is the appropriate unit of consideration; and, that the mind and body are separate functional entities. Science and practice based on this worldview are characterized by: (1) knowledge as fact; (2) reality as knowable; (3) a focus on the individual; (4) a mechanistic view of the human body; and (5) valuing expert knowledge over other kinds of knowledge (for example, experiential knowledge) (Allen, 1992; Campbell & Bunting, 1991; Harding, 1987; Hartrick, 1994). Because of its roots in the physical sciences, sciences within this worldview are held to be "value free" (Tuana, 1989). Although the science practiced within the modern worldview is the foundation of knowledge development in the social sciences, critics suggest that the doctrine of the modern worldview marginalizes other types of knowledge (Morrow, 1994).

Disenchantment with health promotion practiced within the modern worldview led to critiques of health promotion and the subsequent emergence of what could be characterized as post-modern health promotion. Post-modernism, like health promotion, is not a single entity but a complex way of thinking that is not amenable to succinct descriptions (Miller, 1997; Morrow, 1994). (Readers are referred to other sources for in-depth discussions of post-modernisms.[2]) Although there is no general agreement on the characteristics of post-modernism, there is agreement that it is a period that represents a reaction to, or departure from, modern assumptions about the nature of reality (ontology) and the nature of knowledge (epistemology) (Miller, 1997; Morrow, 1994). Reality here is viewed as a historical, cultural, and gendered social construction. There is, therefore, no single truth but rather multiple socially constructed realities. Post-modern scholars, researchers, and practitioners seek to understand how value and meaning shape constructions of reality (McCormick & Roussy, 1997; Miller, 1997; Sprey, 1990). Rather than assuming an explanatory po-

sition in the manner of mainstream science, post-modern theories are "critical" and "emancipatory" (Sprey, 1990; Thorne, 1997). The central aim of post-modern work is to critique social structures to generate new understandings that will transform the dominant social order (Alexander, 1987; Hacking, 1981; Lupton, 1992; McCormick & Roussy, 1997; Miller, 1997; Sprey, 1990).

Modernism in Practice: Freire's Influence

As one who grew up in poverty, Freire committed his life's work to addressing issues of living in poverty in South America. His work and related publications were seminal. In 1970 he wrote his most cited work, the *Pedagogy of the Oppressed*, in which he described how the "culture of silence" contributes to the oppression of the poor. He noted that political, social, and economic domination kept the deprived "silent," a silence interpreted by the privileged as lethargy and ignorance. Working from the assumption that every human is capable of looking critically at the world in which he or she is immersed, and that this facilitates critical appraisal, Freire convened groups of poor women for the critical discussion of the circumstances of their deprivations for the purpose of consciousness-raising. Through discussion, the women uncovered hidden agendas of the powerful that contributed to their oppression. Then, they articulated a focus and plan for social change that was later implemented.

Freire (1992) commented on his work: "This work deals with a very obvious truth: just as the oppressor, in order to oppress, needs a theory of oppressive action, so the oppressed, in order to become free, also need a theory of action . . . only in their encounter of the people with their revolutionary leaders—in their . . . **praxis**—can this theory be built" (p. 185). Praxis, the process of reflecting on the world toward emancipatory action, is a post-modern strategy. Freire's theory for social change is characterized by its value for lived experience, and its critical and emancipatory intent.

Henderson (1995), a nurse, describes a health-related application of this approach. She was a member of a planning group with a mandate to design a therapeutic drug treat-

[2]See McGowan, J. (1991). *Postmodernism and its critics.* Ithaca, NY: Cornell University Press. Thorne, S. E. & Hayes, V. E. (1997). *Nursing praxis: Knowledge and action.* Thousand Oaks, CA: Sage.

ment program for women. The committee's purpose was to plan the women's program. However, implementation of a participatory methodology moved the group beyond planning. By engaging in dialogue and advocacy, the women raised their consciousness about the social and historical contexts of their lives thereby changing their realities—a process of transformation. The women engaged in self-reflection and theorizing, a process entitled "enlightenment" by Henderson. Individuals in the group made new links between their challenges and struggles and those of others, a process that supported their own theorizing. To create social change, postmodernists hold that it is not enough to theorize, action must be taken. In this project, as members spoke up during group work, made public presentations, articulated their rights and needs, and clarified priorities, they experienced "empowerment." Enlightenment and empowerment are thought to act in concert to create emancipatory experiences (Henderson, 1995). **Emancipation** is a state in which people have come to know who they are and collectively determine the direction of their existence. Planning and implementing the women's program were emancipatory experiences. As a group, the women's growing awareness and connectedness was the force behind their capacity to create a space for social change. (See Chap. 6 by M. VanderPlaat for a critical discussion of the concept of "empowerment.")

Theories and Models for Promotion: An Evolving Field

An overview of theories and models in the field developed since 1970 reveals how health promotion is evolving, with researchers and scholars contributing to its evolution. Theoretical ideas are used in practice, and researched and reported or discussed in the literature, then critiqued, and further developed. The complexities of this body of knowledge cannot be underemphasized because it reflects the contributions of thought developed over the past 150 years. Further, multiple and diverse disciplines have contributed to knowledge development, each leaving its unique mark on the whole, and thereby creating an interdisciplinary project. Critical turning points in the

evolution of thought in health promotion are identifiable, in particular, the Lalonde Report (Lalonde, 1974), the Ottawa Charter for Health Promotion (Ottawa Charter for Health Promotion, 1986), and the U.S. *Healthy People 2000* movement (U.S. DHHS, 1980, 1991).

Current literature suggests that a wide range of theoretical perspectives on health promotion influence practice. The challenge for practitioners is to critically appraise theories in common usage and then to select an appropriate theory for a particular circumstance. Understanding how and why knowledge has evolved in the field is the first step in the critical appraisal process. To this end, I present a brief overview of select theories in common use in health promotion highlighting strengths and limitations, and providing select examples of applications. In this chapter, space allows for only brief commentary on select theories and models.

An overview of the Health Belief Model is presented as an example of a health promotion theory concerned with health behavior change. Then, overviews of ecological models of health promotion, models for family health promotion, and models for health promotion with communities and populations are discussed. For a more comprehensive overview of theories of health promotion, readers are referred to primary and secondary sources for further reading (Andeasen, 1995; Bandura, 1986; Glanz et al., 1997; Green & Kreuter, 1991; Janz & Becker, 1984; Pederson, O'Neill & Rootman, 1994; Prochaska & DiClemente, 1984; Rogers, 1983).

Health Behavior Change: A Traditional Health Promotion Strategy

Health promotion focused on behavior change has roots in the health education movement. Health education proved its effectiveness as a health promotion strategy in the 1960s as public health campaigns increased the number of people seeking immunizations, and through the patient education and self-care initiatives of the early 1970s. The mandate of health education was to influence people to voluntarily change health-directed behavior[3] with a view

[3]The conscious pursuit of actions for the protection or improvement of health (Green & Kreuter, 1999, p. 506).

to reducing their overutilization of medical services (Green & Kreuter, 1999). Health education was practiced in communities, schools, and patient care sites, with a specific focus on individual behavior change. Theories developed to guide health education practice assumed an individual-behaviorist perspective. These theories were subsumed into the health promotion movement, and are used widely to guide health promotion practice, evolving over time in response to critiques of health promotion and new understandings of the determinants of health.

The Health Belief Model (HBM), one of the most widely used theories that addresses individual behavior, exemplifies the individual-behaviorist perspective on health promotion (Glanz et al., 1997; Nutbeam & Harris, 1998). Because of its widespread acceptance, concepts from the HBM are evident in influential nursing models for health promotion (Pender, 1996) and family health promotion models for nurses (Loveland-Cherry, 1996). Thus, the HBM model can be considered fundamental to the development of thought in health promotion in nursing. Further, the HBM exemplifies how theories evolve over time in response to critique and prevailing views.

Health Belief Model

The HBM was developed in the 1950s by social psychologists to explain why people did not participate in tuberculosis screening programs. It is one of the most widely used conceptual frameworks in the health education and health promotion fields (Glanz et al., 1997; Green & Kreuter, 1991; Nutbeam & Harris, 1998). The HBM originally combined operant theory and cognitive theory. In response to growing awareness of its limitations, authors added the concept of **self-efficacy** to the model, a concept borrowed from **social learning theory** (Strecker & Rosenstock, 1997). The development of the HBM exemplifies how theories in health promotion have evolved.

Theory development in health promotion advances as an outcome of the work of a group of scholars who combine existing theories or theoretical perspectives to create a new theory. In the case of the HBM, health promotion scholars combined operant theory with cognitive theories. Operant theory originated from the work of B. F. Skinner (1938), whose

hypothesis that the frequency of behavior is caused by reinforcements generated enormous amounts of research and numerous related theories (Rosenstock, 1974; Strecker & Rosenstock, 1997). Cognitive theory posits that behavior is related to an individual's expectation that a particular behavior will achieve a particular outcome (Strecker & Rosenstock, 1997). Simply put, the HBM comes from a theoretical position that an individual will change behavior to reduce risk for disease when a "cue" to change is reinforced by a positive outcome.

The HBM holds that individuals will take action to ward off, to screen for, or to control an ill-health condition if:

1. They regard themselves as susceptible to the condition.
2. They believe it to have serious consequences.
3. They believe that a course of action available to them would be beneficial in reducing either the susceptibility to or severity of the condition.
4. They believe that the anticipated barriers to (or costs of) taking action are outweighed by its benefits (Glanz et al., 1997).

Health here is defined in terms of disease, and behavioral action is held to be the key to health (see Table 1–1).

A review of research on this model in 1974 was promising, and subsequently, health professionals adopted the HBM as an important theoretical perspective. In the following decade, critiques of individual-behaviorist perspectives appeared in the literature. Meanwhile, there was a growing awareness that those who were educated and financially secure made the most lifestyle improvements (Labonte, 1995). Individual-behaviorist models, like the HBM, were criticized for lack of attention to social, political, and economic influences on health. In 1984, the authors revised the HBM to account for other influences (Janz & Becker, 1984). To increase the explanatory potential of the HBM, they incorporated the concept of self-efficacy into the HBM, a concept introduced by Bandura (1977a, 1977b, 1986).

The introduction of self-efficacy represents an important shift in thinking about what influences health behavior (Green & Kreuter, 1991). Self-efficacy, or the belief in one's competence to take action, implies a state of be-

TABLE 1—1

KEY CONCEPTS AND DEFINITIONS OF THE HEALTH BELIEF MODEL

Concept	Definition	Application
Perceived susceptibility	One's opinion of chances of getting a condition.	Define population(s) at risk, risk levels; personalize risk based on a person's characteristics or behavior; make perceived susceptibility more consistent with individual's actual risk.
Perceived severity	One's opinion of the seriousness of a condition and its aftereffects.	Specify consequences of the risk and the condition.
Perceived benefits	One's opinion of the **efficacy** of the advised action to reduce risk or seriousness of impact.	Define action to take: how, where, when; clarify the positive effects to be expected.
Perceived barriers	One's opinion of the tangible and psychological costs of the advised action.	Identify and reduce perceived barriers through reassurance, correction of misinformation, incentives, assistance.
Self-efficacy	One's confidence in one's ability to take action.	Provide training, guidance in performing action. Use progressive goal-setting. Give verbal reinforcment. Demonstrate desired behaviors; reduce anxiety.

Source: From Strecher, V., & Rosenstock, I. M. (1997). The Health Belief Model. In K. Glanz, F. Lewis, & B. Rimer (Eds.), *Health education and health behavior: Theory, research, and practice* (p. 41). San Francisco: Jossey-Bass, with permission.

lieving that one can take control of one's environment (Green & Kreuter, 1991; Nutbeam, 1985; Strecker & Rosenstock, 1997). It expresses the notion that people can self-regulate their environment, a departure from operant conditioning's theoretical position that behavior is a one-way product of environmental influences (Green & Kreuter, 1991).

Self-efficacy is an often-used orienting concept in planning health-related self-management programs such as a joint protection program for people with rheumatoid arthritis. Because the premises of the self-efficacy concept resonate with the definition of health promotion in the Ottawa Charter for Health Promotion (1986), "the process of enabling people to increase control over, and to improve, their health" (Ottawa Charter for Health Promotion, pp. iii–iv), it is attractive to health promotion practitioners and researchers (Green & Kreuter, 1991). With the addition of self-efficacy to the HBM, the theory provided a

theoretical representation of how beliefs and expectations influence an individual's health behaviors, and opened the door to thinking about what is key to taking health-related action.

Yet, the HBM still fell short. Although people do indeed have some control over what affects their health-related actions, an extensive body of research indicates that health, and an individual's capacity to take action, may be primarily determined by socioeconomic status (Angell, 1993; Pincus, Esther, DeWalt, & Callahan, 1998; Raphael, in press). Including the concept of self-efficacy may have increased the explanatory and predictive potential of the HBM, but it further contributed to its victim-blaming potential.

Since the HBM was first conceptualized in the 1970s, its reach has extended well beyond its original application to encompass preventive actions, illness behaviors, and sick-role behaviors. A considerable body of evidence accumulated over three decades confirms the usefulness of the HBM in particular situations (Green & Kreuter, 1991; Strecker & Rosenstock, 1997). Health behavior change theories, when used to guide practice, are viewed by some as a step away from the "expert" model of care, an approach in which the provider relies on health information and professional status to convince patients to change, and therefore a step toward patient-client centered care (Elder et al., 1994). Health professionals often use the HBM in combination with a health promotion planning model like the PRECEDE-PROCEED model, which is discussed later in this chapter (Strecker & Rosenstock, 1997). The HBM has been used to guide the development of educational interventions as diverse as childhood asthma self-help programs (Bruhn, 1983), interventions to reduce risk for the human immunodeficiency virus in runaway adolescents (Booth, Zhang & Kwiatkowski, 1999), arthritis self-management programs (Hammond, Lincoln & Sutcliffe, 1999), and community heart-health programs (Ebbesen, Ramsden, Reeder & Hamilton, 1997).

The HBM has its critics, however. As a theory located in the individual-behaviorist perspective, the HBM and research validating its worth are criticized for lack of attention to contextual factors; for its victim-blaming potential, for its gender and color blindness; for its ethnocentricity; and, for its limited definition of health.

Let us return to the opening vignette of this chapter. Using the theoretical constructs in the HBM to understand Tracy's health-related situation, Tracy, it seems, believes that her health condition is severe; that she is highly susceptible to heart disease; and that taking action will improve her health. She reports that the primary barriers to change have been dealt with and she thinks she can take action (self-efficacy). Yet, she does not change her behavior. How can this be explained? What are the consequences to Tracy of not demonstrating behaviors that fit the theory? Some health professionals might blame Tracy for failing, others might attack her beliefs, possibly giving up on her by withdrawing their support or care. Although theories such as the HBM may be useful in guiding practice with some patients or clients, for others, such as Tracy, its application may have detrimental or ineffective results (Green & Kreuter, 1991; Guidotti, 1989; Syme, 1986a).

Ecological Models of Health Promotion

Individual-level theories for health promotion, such as the HBM, are primarily focused on individual behavior and are not designed to explicitly address broad contextual factors (Syme, 1986b). Health promotion programs based on such models may be ineffective because people have difficulty changing long-held patterns of behavior, and as previously noted, there are differences in people's access to resources and services to support health. Further, individual-level programs have minimal, if any, impact on population-level health indicators because they do not address community factors that continually produce new people at risk, calling into question the contribution of these programs to society as a whole (Syme, 1986b). In contrast, ecological models in health promotion do much to highlight broad contextual factors influencing health (Green & Ottoson, 1994; Green, Richard, & Potvin, 1996; Green & Kreuter, 1999; McLeroy, Bibeau, Steckler, & Glantz, 1988; Richard, Potvin, Kishchuk, Prlic, & Green, 1996).

Ecology is concerned with the relationships between organisms and their environment (Kleffel, 1991a, 1991b), and social ecology is concerned with the nature of the relationships between humans and their social, institutional, and cultural worlds (Herrin & Wright, 1988; Stokols, 1992). Health promotion from this perspective presents health as the consequence of the interdependence between the individual and the family, community, culture, physical, and social environments (Green et al., 1996; Green & Kreuter, 1999; Moos, 1979; Syme, 1986b). Health promotion practiced from an ecological perspective is directed toward developing interventions that target interpersonal, organizational, community, and public policy factors that influence health (Green et al, 1996; Green & Kreuter, 1999; McLeroy et al., 1988). Models for health promotion that address families, communities, and populations take an ecological perspective on health promotion. PRECEDE-PROCEED is one example of a

PRECEDE

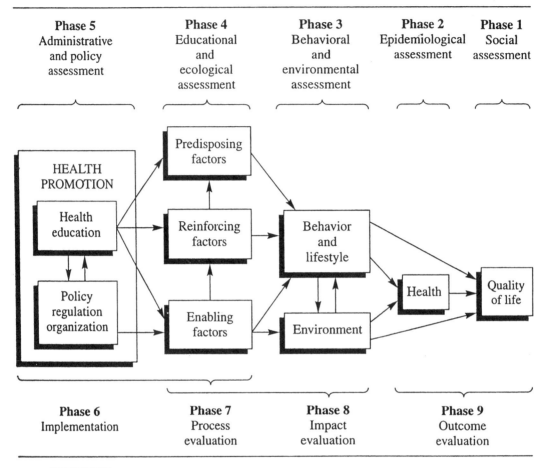

FIG. 1–1. The PRECEDE-PROCEED model of health promotion program planning was originally designed to address utilization of health services. (Green & Kreuter [1999], with permission.)

model that accounts for a myriad of factors influencing health (Strecker & Rosenstock, 1997) (see Fig. 1–1, Green & Kreuter, 1999, p. 35).

PRECEDE-PROCEED

The PRECEDE-PROCEED model of health promotion program planning is built on a quarter century of work by Lawrence W. Green and colleagues at the University of California at Berkeley, Johns Hopkins University, the U.S. Public Health Service, the University of Texas, the Kaiser Family Foundation, and the University of British Columbia (Green & Kreuter, 1999). Like the HBM,

the PRECEDE-PROCEED model was designed to address the utilization of health services. In 1974, it was designed to guide the evaluation of the cost effectiveness of a patient education intervention to reduce the use of emergency room services by adults with asthma (Green, 1974). The model is designed to delineate the essential constructs and relationships in an educational and ecological approach to health promotion for the purpose of guiding the design and evaluation of interventions planned to influence behaviors and the living conditions that influence them and their consequences. Since it first appeared, in response to knowledge development in the field, this model has evolved to its current form (see Fig. 1–1). Applied, tested, studied, extended, and verified in hundreds of published studies and thousands of unpublished projects in community, school, clinical, and workplace settings, this model is theoretically robust (Green & Kreuter, 1991; Green & Kreuter, 1999).

According to the PRECEDE-PROCEED model, health education and policy development are cornerstones of health promotion. Further, the model is designed to guide a relational process that encompasses the health professional, the client, and the social and policy environment in which they are located. It is designed explicitly to serve the interests of the client while addressing the common good. Green and Kreuter (1991) write:

Health education provides the consciousness-raising, concern arousing, action-stimulating impetus for public involvement and commitment to social reform essential to its success in a democracy. Without health education, health promotion would be a manipulative social engineering enterprise. Health education of the public keeps the social change component of health promotion accountable to the public it is supposed to serve. Without the policy supports for social change, on the other hand, health education is often powerless to help people reach their health goals, even with successful individual change efforts. (p. 14)

In this model, health is defined in terms of health-related behavior of individuals, families, groups, communities, and organizations that influence "patterns and conditions of living—housing, eating, playing, working, and just plain loafing" (Green & Kreuter, 1999, p. 11). Health promotion is defined as "the combination of educational and ecological supports for actions and conditions of living conducive to health" (Green & Kreuter, 1999, p. 27). The PRECEDE-PROCEED model draws on theories located in the disciplines of epidemiology; the social, behavioral, and educational sciences; and health administration.

Planning and evaluation for health promotion, according to this model, is an iterative cycle of assessments (Richard, Potvin, Kishchuk, Prlic, & Green, 1996). Phase 1 of the cycle encourages consideration of quality of life, which is accomplished by engaging people in dialogue about their needs and aspirations. Quality-of-life indicators, according to this model, are defined by people themselves, and may include such factors as comfort, hap-

piness, and self-esteem. Phase 2 is the one in which specific health goals or problems that may contribute to those goals are identified. Phase 3 consists of identifying the specific health-related behavioral, lifestyle, and environmental factors. Phase 4 identifies factors that influence health behavior within three broad groupings: predisposing, reinforcing, and enabling factors. *Predisposing* factors are concerned with characteristics of the individual such as knowledge, attitudes, beliefs, values, and perceptions. *Enabling* factors deal with skills and resources or barriers that can influence behavioral and environmental change. *Reinforcing* factors are the rewards and feedback the individual receives from others following the adoption of a behavior. The rewards and feedback may encourage or discourage continuation of the behavior. Phase 5 involves the assessment of organizational and administrative capabilities and resources for the development and implementation of a program. The model guides users to attend to the policy context of health. Phases 6, 7, and 8 are the implementation and evaluation components of the model. The endpoint of this model is also the beginning point—people's own perceptions of their quality of life. The question central to this model is: "How did the intervention or program change the quality of life of participants from their perspective?"

While health promotion is criticized on the basis that it is a movement or ideology that does not lend well to practice, O'Neill and Cardinal (1994) note that the PRECEDE-PROCEED model is unique in its usefulness to guide practice. Health promotion, according to this model, is an integrated process of planning and evaluation designed to serve the health-related interests of the client(s) from their perspectives. These authors note that this model addresses a central need in health promotion and health education: comprehensive planning. With its focus on educational, organizational, and regulatory factors, health promotion programs guided by this model may be conceived as social transformation processes (Richard et al., 1996). This model has been applied to health promotion situations and questions at the individual and community levels in projects as diverse as determining the willingness of patients to pay for an asthma self-management program (Barner, Mason, & Murray, 1999), diabetes prevention programs with aboriginal communities (Daniel et al., 1999), and moral and health education for elementary and pre-school children (Huang, Green & Darling, 1997). As an explanatory model, it can be located within the modern worldview. How-ever, with its focus on democratic social re-form achieved through consciousness-raising and participation, and its central value for the lived experience of health, the PRECEDE-PROCEED model resonates with post-mod-ern perspectives.

Returning again to Tracy, health educa-tion in this case did make a difference. Tracy learned that second-hand smoke increases risk for cardiovascular disease and, seemingly, Tracy or her husband took action to ensure a smoke-free environment for her. However, according to the health professional, the health education approach was far less effective than anticipated. Such cases, and their related frus-tration for health professionals, have stimu-lated much thought about the assumptions of a health education approach. Mystified about why the health education approach is inade-quate for some people, scholars have turned to the post-modern worldview to address this practice issue (Butterfield, 1990; Drevdahl, 1995; Hartrick, 1994; Labonte, 1989; Thorne, 1993).

Before moving on to a discussion of family and community theories for health promotion, I invite you to review the section in this chap-ter on modern and post-modern views and dis-cuss with others how the assumptions of the post-modern worldviews might influence your health promotion practice with someone in Tracy's situation.

Family Health Promotion

Because family is a key social context for health, models of family health promotion fall within an ecological view of health promotion. How-ever, relatively little has been written about family health promotion; hence, theories for family health promotion are in the formative stage (Bomar, 1990; Maxwell, 1997b). Since Nightingale identified family as a central con-cern of nursing, family has been a focus for nursing practice (Doherty & Campbell, 1988; Nightingale, 1859). Wright and Leahey's (1984, 1994) theory of family nursing and the McGill Model for Nursing (Gottlieb & Rowat, 1985), with its focus on family as the appropriate unit

for health promoting nursing practice, have provided nurses with tools for family nursing practice. It is the family unit through which resources for healthy living are or are not ac-cessible to members: food, housing, materials and modeling for active living or leisure-time activities, supportive relationships, caregiving, and an array of other factors. Thus, as the social unit at the interface between individuals and the wider society, the family is foundational to health and an appropriate, if not essential, focus for health promotion (Maxwell, 1997b).

Family health promotion may be concep-tualized as a process that enables people to address cultural, social, and political factors to increase control over and to improve their health. Family health promotion, so defined, is a mediating strategy between people and their environment (Hartrick, Lindsay, & Hills, 1994). In this section, a discussion of a model for fam-ily health promotion congruent with this view is provided, the Hartrick and coauthors' model for Family Nursing Assessment.

In this model, family is conceptualized in terms of descriptive practices that are the everyday communicative processes through which realities are produced and made mean-ingful (Holstein & Gubrium, 1994). For Har-trick and associates (1994), family is viewed as a polyphonic novel in which there is a composition of numerous, independent, and unmerged voices and consciousness. Every-day family communicative processes are a central focus for health promotion (Hartrick et al., 1994; Hartrick, 2000). The health pro-moting nurse, according to this model, has specific areas of responsibilities:

1. Maintaining a neutral yet inquisitive stance
2. Fostering a caring and collaborative rela-tionship with family members
3. Working toward establishing a context for change rather than prescribing change
4. Using conversations to foster critical aware-ness and pattern recognition
5. Respecting and trusting the family and its members to discover and choose direction as they see it

The health promoting nurse whose practice is guided by this theory begins by listening to the family's story. As family members discuss their issues and raise concerns, they are in the process of gaining critical awareness. Active listening assists the nurse and family members to understand the meaning of their health experiences. Through talking and listening processes, the family and its members become experts in understanding their situation and discovering possibilities for improving it. Another strategy used by the health promoting nurse is to engage the family with herself and each other in "participatory dialogue." Here, the nurse poses questions to bring forward diverse perspectives within the family as the first step in assisting the family to identify everyday patterns. Through dialogue, the family and the nurse co-create a picture of the family's health experiences, clarifying values and beliefs, gaining new insights, and identifying new possibilities for action. The nurse-family interaction is a transformative process (evolving consciousness) that moves the family from disruption to wholeness (Newman, 1999). Health is no longer viewed in terms of a mind-body disconnect. Rather, health is a pattern of the whole, and wholeness is health (Newman, 1999; Rogers, 1970). This theory, located squarely within the post-modern worldview, delineates a transformative process that is, in and of itself, healing (see Table 1–2).

TABLE 1–2

HEALTH PROMOTING FAMILY NURSING ASSESSMENT: THE FRAMEWORK

Components	Strategic Elements	Health Promotion Principles
Listening to the family	Elicit diverse family perceptions.	Every person lives within a social/historical context that helps shape social relations.
	Understand the family story.	Family members are experts in their own health experiences.
Participatory dialogue	Pose circular questions to elucidate taken-for-granted family patterns.	Diversity is positively valued; empowerment describes our intentional efforts to create more equitable relationships and interactions such that there is greater equity in resources, status, and authority.
	Family members critically reflect on circular questions and pose questions of their own.	
Pattern recognition	In collaboration, identify the family's behaviors; recognize family's patterns and themes relative to their values and beliefs.	Professional expertise and skills are used in new ways.
	Co-create the family's story.	Expanded view of the family history opens the family to new possibilities for wholeness.
Envisioning action and positive change	Make informed choices; take action; reflect on actions taken; take renewed action.	People involved are the chief actors.

Source: Adapted from Hartrick, G., Lindsay, E., & Hills, M. (1994). Family nursing assessment: Meeting the challenges of health promotion. *Journal of Advanced Nursing, 20*, 89, and Newman, M. A. (1999). The rhythm of reading in a paradigm of wholeness. *Image: The Journal of Nursing Scholarship, 31*, 227–230, with permission.

✳ Reflective Questions

1. How might a nurse use this model to guide practice with a patient in Tracy's situation?
2. How could a nurse use this model to guide practice when she/he has only 20 minutes for family health promotion?
3. What are the implications for using this model to guide practice when only some family members are present?
4. What are the implications for using this model to guide practice when the nurse and family do not share cultural roots?

Models for Health Promotion with Communities and Populations

In contrast to the paucity of models for family health promotion, there are numerous health promotion models and theories to guide practice with communities and populations. Communities can be characterized in several ways: a functional unit that meets basic needs for sustenance (e.g., a town); a unit of patterned social interaction (e.g., an Internet community); and symbolic units of collective identity (e.g., a religious affiliation) (Minkler & Wallerstein, 1997). Populations are categories of people, for example, seniors, prisoners, low-income, single mothers who may or may not identify themselves as a community (Green & Ottoson, 1999).

Strategies that support community and population health promotion include community-based programming, community development, and policy development, to name a few (Freire, 1992; Labonte, 1989; Labonte, 1995; Minkler & Wallerstein, 1997; Wharf & Clague, 1997). Since the 1860s and the writings of Nightingale, nurses have addressed health issues from a community perspective (Cloutier-Lafferty & Craig, 1995). For example, in the early 1900s, Lillian Wald incorporated community participation and development in her practice of community health nursing (Buhler-Wilkerson, 1993). Such approaches resonate with current community development approaches.

Community Development

Community development models of health promotion provide a way of thinking about how community resources can be mobilized to improve quality of life or standards of living in communities or whole populations. Mobilizing resources in communities or populations is about redistributing resources, a process that turns on how access to resources is structured (English, 1995; Green & Ottoson, 1999; Minkler & Wallerstein, 1997; Nutbeam & Harris, 1998). In community development, citizens are engaged in a decision-making process in which they map out community strengths and deficits. Central to this critical appraisal of the community is access to excellent information, and professionals play a key role in ensuring citizens' access to quality information to support their critical appraisal and decision-making processes (Honadle, 1996).

Because community development is essentially about addressing power inequities and issues related to access to resources, community development is a complex, lengthy, and often political process that has ethical implications (Lotz, 1997). In the community development literature, scholars and practitioners grapple with questions such as: Should community development focus on deficits or strengths? How can technology be used to improve access to information to support the community development process? What are the gender and cross-cultural implications of a community development approach? How can sectors collaborate when they have national or state/provincial alliances?

WHO Healthy Cities

A frequently cited health promotion initiative that fits the community development model is the WHO Healthy Cities Project (WHO, 1988). Initiated in 1988, the WHO Healthy Cities movement catalyzed city governments to take a multisectoral approach to health promotion planning (English, 1995; Green & Ottoson, 1999). Citizens representing diverse sectors within the community, for example, recreation and social services, are engaged in a process wherein they explored how policies and social environments contribute to health and quality of life in the community. This pro-

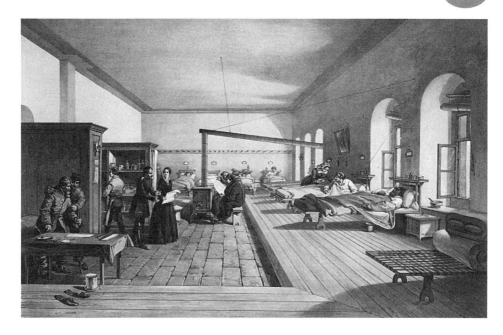

cess is fundamental to identifying disparities. Once disparities are identified, it becomes clear what actions are needed to ensure more equitable access to health-related community supports and services (English, 1995; Green & Ottoson, 1999). The WHO Healthy Cities Movement is now embraced widely in the developed world. With a focus on empowerment and a value for critical awareness, community development fits the perspectives of the postmodern **paradigm.**

WHO HEALTHY CITIES MOVEMENT

Healthy City pioneers define a healthy city as: one that is continually creating and improving those physical and social environments and strengthening those community resources which enable people to mutually support each other in performing all the functions of life and achieving their maximum potential.

They identified 11 parameters of a healthy city:

1. A clean, safe, high-quality physical environment (including housing quality).
2. An ecosystem that is stable now and sustainable in the long term.
3. A strong, mutually supportive, and nonexploitative community.
4. A high degree of public participation in, and control over, the decisions affecting one's life, health and well-being.

5. The meeting of basic needs (food, water, shelter, income, safety, work) for all the city's people.
6. Access to a wide variety of experiences and resources with the possibility of multiple contacts, interaction, and communication.
7. A diverse, vital, and innovative city economy.
8. Encouragement of connectedness with the past, with cultural heritages, and with other groups and individuals.
9. A city that is compatible with and enhances the above parameters and behaviors.
10. An optimum level of appropriate public health and sick care services accessible to all.
11. High health status (both high positive health status and low disease status). (Aicher, 1998)

http://www.amulet.nb.ca/
designinghealthycities/homepage.htm

✳ Reflective Question

In the opening scenario, Tracy's care is delivered at the individual level. However, many people in Tracy's situation receive care at the aggregate level as participants in a cardiac rehabilitation program. How might participants in a cardiac rehabilitation program be engaged as a community to address barriers to change such as a lack of safe walking paths in their community?

Health Promotion Practice for Nursing: A Transformative Process

Nursing has been involved in health promotion since Nightingale charted modern nursing's course. Nurses today, even those who work in the most highly technical and "disease-oriented" settings, consider health promotion an "everyday thing" (Berland, Whyte, & Maxwell, 1996; Hung, 1998). Because of the interdisciplinary nature of health promotion, nursing is challenged to find its unique contribution to health promotion.

A review of the theoretical development of health promotion since the 1970s indicates a paradigm shift characterized by a re-envisioning of what constitutes knowledge and reality. Post-modern health promotion scholars, some of whom are nurses, view knowledge as a historically and culturally grounded and gendered social construction. Further, they challenge the belief in a mind-body dichotomy. For post-modernists, history, culture, and gender shape meaning and therefore perceptions of what counts as knowledge and reality. Health is no longer dichotomous; rather, health is *wholeness*. These foundational shifts in thinking have implications for health promotion practice and research.

Health promotion practice founded on these assumptions is a transformative process in which the nurse as partner engages clients in consciousness-raising characterized by a respect for the dynamic relatedness between people and the environment. This view of health promotion is nursing's unique contribution to knowledge development in the health promotion field. Currently, nurses are exploring the value of transformative health promotion practice in a wide range of settings: from work with seniors or families of chronically ill children to critical care and global nursing. This approach to practice is in its early stages of development with initial findings showing promise (Newman, 1999).

Because of the complexity of health promotion, and its interdisciplinary nature, nurses need to be knowledgeable about and skilled in applying a wide range of health promotion theories that are borrowed from other disciplines, and those that are unique to nursing. The challenge for practitioners is to have the critical capacity to match a particular theory to a specific health promotion situation. In practice, the complexity of health promotion situations may demand that health professionals use a combination of theories.

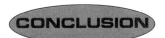

CONCLUSION

In this chapter, I have demonstrated how theories for health promotion practice are ever-evolving in response to dominant views. Theories evolve as critiques are raised and integrated into new theoretical formulations of health promotion. Each theory or model reviewed has strengths and limitations. What is important for health professionals is to be knowledgeable about the wide range of theories, and to select theories to guide practice based on a critical appraisal of the field.

This chapter has presented theories anchored in both modern and post-modern thought, beginning with theories aligned with modernist perspective and progressing to those located within the post-modern views. With critical and emancipatory intents, post-modern theories of health promotion are arguably most relevant for practice with the marginalized or disenfranchised. Further, theories that focus on lived experience and meaning transformation when used to guide practice show promise as professional tools to promote health and healing, a process especially important for nurses. Ongoing and future research and critical scholarship will reveal the strengths and limitations of transformative health promotion practice, thereby shaping this health promotion theory as ongoing critique and research has shaped others. In reading and thinking about the ideas in this volume, you, the reader, are invited to jump into the critical fray.

✳ Reflective Question

Now that you have read this chapter and given some thought to theories of health promotion, from the perspective of the health promoting nurse, how would you care for Tracy?

REFERENCES

Aicher, J. A. (1998). *Designing healthy cities: Prescriptions, principles, and practice.* Florida: Kreiger Publications.

Alexander, J. C. (1987). The centrality of the classics. In A. Giddens & J. H. Turner (Eds.), *Social theory today.* Palo Alto, CA: Stanford University Press.

Allen, D. G. (1992). Feminism, relativism, and the philosophy of science: An overview. In J. L. Thompson, D. G. Allen, & L. Rodrigues-Fisher (Eds.), *Critique, resistance, and action: Working papers in the politics of nursing* (pp. 1–20). New York: NLN Press.

Andeasen, A. R. (1995). *Marketing social change: Changing behavior to promote health, social development, and the environment.* San Francisco: Jossey-Bass.

Angell, M. (1993). Privilege and health—What is the connection? *New England Journal of Medicine, 329,* 126–127.

Bandura, A. (1977a). Self-efficacy: Toward a unifying theory of behavior change. *Psychological Review, 84,* 191–215.

Bandura, A. (1977b). *Social learning theory.* Englewood Cliffs, NJ: Prentice Hall.

Bandura, A. (1986). *Social foundations of thought and action: A social cognitive theory.* Englewood Cliffs, NJ: Prentice Hall.

Barner, J. C. Mason, H. L., & Murray, M. D. (1999). Assessment of asthma patients' willingness to pay for and give time to an asthma self-management program. *Clinical Therapeutics, 21,* 878–894.

Berland, A., Whyte, N., & Maxwell, L. (1995). Hospital nurses and health promotion. *Canadian Journal of Nursing Research, 4,* 13–31.

Bomar, P. (1990). Perspectives on family health promotion. *Family and Community Health, 12*(4), 1–11.

Booth, R., Zhang, Y., & Kwiatkowski, C. (1999). The challenge of changing drug and sex risk behaviors of runaway and homeless adolescents. *Child Abuse and Neglect, 23,* 1295–1306.

Borgmann, A. (1992). *Crossing the postmodern divide.* Chicago: University of Chicago Press.

Bruhn, J. (1983). The application of theory in a childhood asthma self-help program. *Journal of Allergy and Clinical Immunology, 72,* 561–577S.

Buhler-Wilkerson, K. (1993). Bringing care to the people: Lillian Wald's legacy to public health nursing. *American Journal of Public Heath, 83,* 1778–1786.

Butterfield, P. G. (1990). Thinking upstream: Nurturing a conceptual understanding of the societal context of health behavior. *Advances in Nursing Science, 12*(2), 1–8.

Campbell, J. C., & Bunting, S. (1991). Voices and paradigms: Perspectives on critical and feminist theory in nursing. *Advances in Nursing Science, 13*(3), 1–15.

Capra, F. (1982). *The turning point: Science, society, and the rising culture.* Simon & Schuster: New York.

Cloutier-Lafferty, S., & Craig, D. M. (1995). Health promotion for communities and aggregates. In M. Stewart (Ed.), *Community nursing: Promoting Canadian's health* (pp. 125–145). Toronto: Harcourt-Brace.

Daniel, M., Green, L. W., Gamble, D., Herbert, C., Hertzman, C., & Sheps, S. (1999). Effectiveness of community-directed diabetes prevention and control in a rural aboriginal population in British Columbia, Canada. *Social Science & Medicine, 48,* 815–832.

Doherty, W. J., & Campbell, T. L. (1988). *Families and health.* (Vol. 10). Newbury Park, CA: Sage.

Drevdahl, D. (1995). Coming to voice: The power of emancipatory community interventions. *Advances in Nursing Science, 18*(2), 13–24.

Ebbesen, L. S., Ramsden, V., Reeder, B., & Hamilton, T. (1997). Heart health in rural Saskatchewan. *Canadian Nurse, 93*(2), 27–30.

Elder, J. P., McGraw, S. A., Stone, E. J., Reed, D. B., Harsha, D. W., Greene, T., & Wambsgans, K. C. (1994). CATCH: Process evaluation of environmental factors and programs. *Health Education Quarterly* (Suppl. 2), S107–127.

English, J. (1995). Community development. In M. Stewart (Ed.), *Community nursing: Promoting Canadian's health* (pp. 513–531). Toronto: Harcourt-Brace.

Evans, R. G., & Stoddard, G. L. (1990). Producing health, consuming health care. *Social Science & Medicine, 31,* 1347–1363.

Freire, P. (1992). *Pedagogy of the oppressed* (M. B. Ramos, Trans.). New York: Continuum.

Glanz, K., Lewis, F. M., & Rimer, B. (Eds.). (1997). *Health behavior and health education: Theory, research, and practice* (2nd ed.). San Francisco: Jossey-Bass.

Gottlieb, L., & Rowat, K. (1985, October 21). *The McGill Model of Nursing.* Paper presented at the Conference on a Professional Approach to Nursing Practice: The McGill Model, Montreal, Quebec.

Green, L.W. (1974). Toward cost-benefit evaluations of health education: Some concepts, methods, and applications. *Health Education Monographs, 2*(Suppl.1), 34–64.

Green, L. W., & Kreuter, M. W. (1991). *Health promotion planning: An educational and environmental approach* (2nd ed.). Toronto: Mayfield.

Green, L. W., & Kreuter, M. W. (1999). *Health promotion planning: An educational and ecological approach* (3rd ed.). Mountain View, CA: Mayfield.

Green, L. W., & Ottoson, J. (1994). *Community health* (7th ed.). Toronto: Mosby.

Green, L., & Ottoson, J. (1999). *Community health and population health*. Toronto: McGraw-Hill.

Green, L. W., Richard, L., & Potvin, L. (1996). Ecological foundations of health promotion. *American Journal of Health Promotion, 10*, 270–281.

Guidotti, T. L. (1989). Health promotion in perspective. *Canadian Journal of Health Promotion, 80*, 400–405.

Hacking, I. (1981). *Scientific revolutions*. New York: Oxford University Press.

Hammond, A., Lincoln, N., & Sutcliffe, L. (1999). A crossover trial evaluating an educational-behavioral joint protection program for people with rheumatoid arthritis. *Patient Education & Counseling, 37*, 19–32.

Harding, S. (Ed.). (1987). *Feminism and methodology: Social science issues*. Bloomington, IN: Indiana University Press.

Hartrick, G. (1994). *Transforming family nursing theory: From mechanicism to contextualism*. Unpublished manuscript, University of Victoria School of Nursing, Victoria, B.C.

Hartrick, G. (2000). Developing health promoting practice with families: one pedagogical experience. *Journal of Advanced Nursing, 31*, 27–34.

Hartrick, G., Lindsay, E., & Hills, M. (1994). Family nursing assessment: Meeting the challenge of health promotion. *Journal of Advanced Nursing, 20*, 85–91.

Henderson, D. (1995). Consciousness raising in participatory research: Method and methodology for emancipatory nursing inquiry. *Advances in Nursing Science, 17*(3), 58–69.

Herrin, D. A., & Wright, S. D. (1988). Precursors to a family ecology: Interrelated threads of ecological thought. *Family Science Review, 1*, 163–183.

Holstein, J. A., & Gubrium, J. F. (1994). Constructing family: Descriptive practice and domestic order. In T. R. Sarbin & J. I. Kituse (Eds.), *Constructing the social* (pp. 232–250). Thousand Oaks, CA: Sage.

Honadle, B. W. (1996). Participatory research for public issues education: a strategic approach to a municipal consolidation study. *Journal of the Community Development, 27*, 15–22.

Huang, Y. W., Green, L. W., & Darling, L. F. (1997). Moral education and health education for elementary school and preschool children in Canada. *Journal of the National School Health Association, 30*(3), 23–35.

Hung, T. Y. (1998). *Private hospital nurses' knowledge, attitudes, and practices of health promotion*. Hong Kong: University of Hong Kong.

Illich, I. (1975). *Medical nemesis: The expropriation of health*. Toronto: McClelland and Stewart.

Janz, N. K., & Becker, M. H. (1984). The Health Belief Model: A decade later. *Health Education Quarterly, 11*, 1–47.

Kleffel, D. (1991a). An ecofeminist analysis of nursing knowledge. *Nursing Forum, 26*(4), 5–18.

Kleffel, D. (1991b). Rethinking the environment as a domain of nursing knowledge. *Advances in Nursing Science, 14*, 40–51.

Kuhn, T. (1970). *The structure of scientific revolutions*. Chicago: University of Chicago Press.

Labonte, R. (1989). Community and professional empowerment. *Canadian Nurse, 3*(2), 23–30.

Labonte, R. (1994). Death of a program, birth of a metaphor. In A. Pederson, M. O'Neill, & I. Rootman (Eds.), *Health promotion in Canada* (pp. 72–90). Toronto: W. B. Saunders.

Labonte, R. (1995). *Health promotion and empowerment: Practice frameworks* (Issues in Health Series #3). Toronto: Centre for Health Promotion.

Lalonde, M. A. (1974). *A new perspective on the health of Canadians*. Ottawa: National Ministry of Health and Welfare.

Lotz, J. (1997). The beginning of community development in English-speaking Canada. In B. Wharf & M. Clagues (Eds.), *Community organizing: Canadian experiences* (pp. 37–54). Toronto: Oxford University Press.

Loveland-Cherry, C. J. (1996). Family health promotion and protection. In P. J. Bomar (Ed.), *Nurses and family health promotion concepts, assessment and interventions* (2nd ed., pp. 15–23). Baltimore, MD: Williams & Wilkins.

Lupton, D. (1992). Discourse analysis: A new methodology for understanding the ideologies of health and illness. *Australian Journal of Public Health, 16*, 145–150.

Maxwell, L. (1997b). *Family influences on individual health-related decisions in response to heart-health initiatives*. Unpublished doctoral dissertation, University of British Columbia, Vancouver.

Maxwell, L. (1997a). Foundational thought in knowledge for social change. In S. Thorne & V. E. Hayes (Eds.), *Nursing praxis: Knowledge and action* (pp. 203–218). Thousand Oaks, CA: Sage.

McCormick, J., & Roussy, J. (1997). A feminist poststructuralist orientation to nursing praxis. In S. Thorne & V. E. Hayes (Eds.), *Nursing praxis: Knowledge and action*. Thousand Oaks, CA: Sage.

McGowan, J. (1991). *Postmodernism and its critiques*. Ithaca, NY: Cornell University Press.

McGowan, P., & Young, L. (1999). *Supporting self-care: A workshop for nurse and physician educators*. Vancouver: University of British Columbia Institute of Health Promotion Research and University of Victoria.

McKeown, T. (1971). A historical appraisal of the medical task. In T. McKeown & G. McLachlan (Eds.), *Medical history and medical care* (pp. 12–20). Oxford: Oxford University Press.

McLeroy, K. R., Bibeau, D., Steckler, A., & Glanz, K. (1988). An ecological perspective on health programs. *Health Education Quarterly, 15*, 351–377.

Meleis, A. I. (1991). *Theoretical development in nursing: Development and progress*. New York: J. B. Lippincott.

Miller, S. (1997). Multiple paradigms for nursing: Postmodern feminisms. In S. Thorne & V. E. Hayes (Eds.), *Nursing praxis: Knowledge and action* (pp. 140–156). Thousand Oaks, CA: Sage.

Minkler, M., & Wallerstein, N. (1997). Improving health through community organizing and community building. In K. Glanz, F. Lewis, & B. Rimer (Eds.), *Health education and health promotion: Theory, research, and practice* (pp. 241–269). San Francisco: Jossey-Bass.

Moos, R. H. (1979). Social ecological perspectives on health. In G. Stone & F. Cohen (Eds.), *Health psychology—A handbook* (pp. 523–547). San Francisco: Jossey-Bass.

Morrow, R. (1994). *Critical theory and methodology*. Thousand Oaks, CA: Sage

Newman, M. A. (1999). The rhythm of relating in a paradigm of wholeness. *Image*: The Journal of Nursing Scholarship, 31, 227–230.

Nightingale, F. (1859). *Notes on nursing*: What it is and what it is not. London: Edward Stern & Company.

Nutbeam, D. (1985). *Health promotion glossary*. Denmark: WHO.

Nutbeam, D., & Harris, E. (1998). *Theories in a nutshell*: A practitioners guide to commonly used theories and models in health promotion. Sydney, Australia: University of Sydney.

O'Neill, M., & Cardinal, L. (1994). Health promotion in Quebec: Did it ever catch on? In A. Pederson, M. O'Neill, & I. Rootman (Eds.), *Health promotion in Canada* (pp. 262–283). Toronto: W. B. Saunders.

Ottawa Charter for Health Promotion. (1986). Ottawa Charter for Health Promotion. *Canadian Journal of Public Health, 77*, 426–427.

Passau-Buck, S., & Jones, E. M. (1997). Omnipotent omniscient paternalism. *Revolution*: The Journal of Nurse Empowerment, 4, 53–54, 70–71.

Pederson, A., O'Neill, M., & Rootman, I. (1994). *Health promotion in Canada*. Toronto: W. B. Saunders.

Pender, N. (1996). *Health promotion in nursing practice* (3rd ed.). Stamford, CT: Appleton & Lange.

Pincus, T., Esther, R., DeWalt, D. & Callahan, L. (1998). Social conditions and self-management are more powerful determinants of health than access to care. *Annals of Internal Medicine, 129*, 406–411.

Prochaska, J. O., & DiClemente, C. C. (1984). *The transtheoretical approach*: Crossing traditional boundaries of therapy. Homewood, IL: Dow Jones Irwin.

Rachlis, M., & Kushner, C. (1994). *Strong medicine*: How to save Canada's health care system. Toronto: HarperCollins.

Raeburn, J. (1992). Health promotion with heart: Keeping a people perspective. *Canadian Journal of Health Promotion, 3–5. 83 Suppl 1:520–4.

Raphael, D. (2001). From increasing poverty to social disintegration: How economic inequality affects the health of individuals and communities, pp. 17–195. In P. Armstrong, H. Armstrong & D. Coburn. (Eds.), *Unhealthy times: Political economy perspectives on health and health care*. Toronto: Oxford.

Richard, L., Potvin, L., Kishchuk, N., Prlic, H., & Green, L. (1996). Assessment of the integration of the ecological approach in health promotion programs. *American Journal of Health Promotion, 10*, 318–328.

Rogers, E. M. (1983). *Diffusion of innovations*. (3rd ed.). New York: Free Press.

Rogers, M. E. (1970). *An introduction to the theoretical basis of nursing*. Philadelphia: F. A. Davis.

Rosenstock, I. M. (1974). Historical origins of the Health Belief Model. *Health Education Monographs, 2*, 328–335.

Skinner, B. F. (1938). *The behavior of organisms.* Englewood Cliffs, NJ: Appleton-Century-Crofts.

Somers, A. (Ed.). (1976). *Promoting health*: Consumer education and national policy. Germantown, MD: Aspen.

Sprey, J. (Ed.). (1990). *Fashioning family theory*: New approaches. Newbury Park, CA: Sage.

Stokols, D. (1992). Establishing and maintaining healthy environments: Toward a social ecology of health promotion. *American Psychologist, 47*, 6–22.

Strecker, V., & Rosenstock, I. M. (1997). The Health Belief Model. In K. Glanz, F. Lewis, & B. Rimer (Eds.), *Health education and health promotion*: Theory, research and practice. San Francisco: Jossey-Bass.

Syme, S. L. (1986a). Strategies for health promotion. *Preventive Medicine, 15*, 492–507.

Syme, S. L. (1986b). The social environment and disease prevention. *Advances in Health Education and Promotion, 1*, 237–265.

Thorne, S. (1993). *Negotiating health care*: The social context of chronic illness. Newbury Park, CA: Sage.

Thorne, S. (1997). Introduction: Praxis in the context of Nursing's developing inquiry. In S. Thorne & V. E. Hayes (Eds.), *Nursing praxis*: Knowledge and action. Thousand Oaks, CA: Sage.

Tuana, N. (Ed.). (1989). *Feminism and science*. Bloomington, IN: Indiana University Press.

U.S. Department of Health and Human Services. (1980). *Promoting health and preventing disease*: Health objectives for the Nation. Washington, DC: U.S. Government Printing Office.

U.S. Department of Health and Human Services. (1991). *Healthy people 2000*: National health promotion and disease prevention objectives. (DHHS Publication No. PHS 91–50213). Washington, DC: U.S. Government Printing Office.

Wharf, B., & Clague, M. (1997). *Community organizing*: Canadian experiences. Toronto: Oxford University Press.

Winkleby, M., Flora, J., & Kraemer, H. (1994). A community-based heart disease intervention: Predictors of change. *American Journal of Public Health, 84*, 767–772.

World Health Organization (1988). *Promoting health in the urban environment*. (WHO Healthy Cities Paper #1). Copenhagen: FADL.

WHO. (1984). *Health promotion: A discussion document on the concept and principles*. Geneva: WHO.

Wright, L., & Leahey, M. (1984). *Nurses and families*. Philadelphia: F. A. Davis.

Wright, L. M., & Leahey, M. (1994). *Nurses and families: A guide to family assessment and intervention* (2nd ed.). Philadelphia: F. A. Davis.

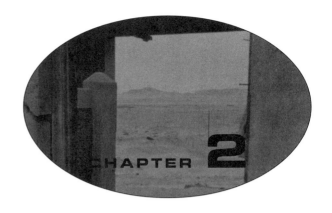

CHAPTER 2

Health Promotion: Historical, Philosophical, and Theoretical Perspectives

MARJORIE A. MacDONALD

What does health promotion mean to you? On the first day of class in a course on community health promotion practice, third-year nursing students in a baccalaureate program offered the following definitions and comments about health promotion in response to the preceding question:

Health promotion means educating people to make healthy lifestyle choices.

Health promotion is a way of being with clients. It's more a philosophy of practice than something specific you do.

Health promotion means taking action on the determinants of health—things like poverty, discrimination, marginalization, and so on. It means getting politically active.

Everything nurses do is about promoting health. There isn't something specific that is health promotion.

Health promotion is too idealistic. It isn't reflected out there in the real world of nursing practice.

The diversity of responses led me to wonder how different students who have come through the same program, based on a specific philosophy of health promotion, come up with such varied understandings of the term. An exploration of the historical development of health promotion in nursing may help to explain this phenomenon.

Nursing has laid claim to a major role in health promotion (Norton, 1998; Williams, 1989). Novak (1988) has argued that health promotion is the social mandate of nursing, with historical roots in

the teachings of Florence Nightingale. Hills and Lindsey (1996) also claim that the origins of nursing were founded on health promotion principles until discovery of the germ theory steered medicine and nursing toward a biomedical orientation. Lowenburg (1995) believes that nursing is in the vanguard of health promotion development, and therefore nurses have a strong leadership role to play. Some schools of nursing have implemented new curricula based on a health promotion philosophy (Caraher, 1994; Duncan, 1996; Hills & Lindsey, 1996; Hills, 1998; Robinson & Hill, 1995).

But what is health promotion, and what are its principles and philosophy? There is no agreement on the answers to these questions. At the same time that nursing has staked out its territory in health promotion, the concept itself is contested within the discipline (Maben & MacLeod Clark, 1995) and the basic principles are open to debate. The nursing literature reflects considerable diversity in the interpretation and underlying ideologies of health promotion, yet many authors appear to assume that there is a widely shared understanding of the term. Nurses, and others, define health promotion in very different ways, but even when two people use the same definition, one person's interpretation may contradict the other's.

Because health promotion is an interdisciplinary enterprise, some nursing theorists might question whether nursing should derive its guidance for practice from the theories of other disciplines, especially given the historical emphasis on health promotion in nursing. Conversely, some authors ask why nursing has contributed so little to the interdisciplinary development of health promotion, given that it is widely accepted as an important focus of nursing practice (Gottleib, 1992; Hagen, O'Neill & Dallaire, 1995; Smith, 1990).

The purpose of this chapter is to explore the historical development of health promotion through two major eras, as both an interdisciplinary enterprise and in nursing. The meaning of health promotion, and its philosophical and theoretical foundations cannot be understood independently of its history because these are intertwined. Critique has played, and will continue to play, an important role in the evolution of health promotion's development. As health promotion has developed over time, there have been significant, if not radical, shifts in its underpinnings, in part the result of thoughtful critiques. A basic premise of this chapter is that it is important for nurses to critique, and understand health promotion in relation to current and historical nursing practice.

There are three reasons why such a critique is important. First, the lack of clarity about the philosophy, nature, and focus of health promotion in nursing creates confusion for practice in a discipline that claims health promotion as its core purpose. As Rush (1997) points out, nursing has not done a critique of the health promotion movement. Yet it is through critique that we more fully understand what we are embracing. Second, because health promotion is a global development that has had a significant impact on national and international health policy, and thus on organizational mandates, nursing must articulate its own understanding of the concept and its role vis à vis these developments. Otherwise, nursing's role and contribution to health promotion will remain invisible. Finally, the day to day practice of nursing provides opportunities to contribute to the development of health promotion theory, both for nursing and for other disciplines, through an exploration of health promotion's enactment. In practice, many of the dilemmas and challenges of health promotion are confronted and managed and thus the knowledge that emerges from nursing practice can make an important contribution.

My purpose is not to write the definitive historical review because there is no singular experience of health promotion's development. Furthermore, many such accounts have been written by others (Badgley, 1978; Green, 1994; Green, 1999; Health Canada, 1998; Kickbush, 1994; Labonte, 1994; Novak, 1988; Rafael, 1999; Robertson, 1998). In exploring the history of health promotion, I am not assuming that health promotion is always beneficial; nonetheless, in this chapter I will not review the literature on the impact of health promotion strategies on health status. Although the question of health promotion's effectiveness is an important one, an exploration of this question is beyond the scope of this paper. My intent is simply to relate the development of health promotion in nursing to influences in the wider arena of political, social, and economic developments at national and international levels. Although I attempt to present an international perspective, my construction is necessarily colored by my own experiences within the Canadian context.

The Era of Health Promotion as Lifestyle Modification

The term *health promotion* entered the official political discourse with the publication, in 1974, of a Canadian government discussion paper entitled, *A New Perspective on the Health of Canadians* (Lalonde, 1974). The Lalonde Report, as it came to be known, was acknowledged by writers in other countries, from a variety of disciplines, as heralding the official birth of health promotion internationally (Bunton, 1992; Kickbush, 1994; Kulbok, Laffrey & Goeppinger, 1995; Parish, 1995; Raeburn, 1994; Seedhouse, 1997).

The term health promotion had been used by practitioners in several disciplines, including nursing, before it was coined officially by Lalonde. Early nursing theorists identified "health" rather than "illness" as the focus of nursing practice. As such, any nursing intervention was intended to promote health. In fact, health promotion has been deemed by some as the primary goal of professional nursing practice (MacLeod Clark, 1993; Smith, 1990). As both Novak (1988) and Rafael (1999) have pointed out, there is a long tradition of health promotion in nursing dating back to Nightingale and the early public health movement in the United States as exemplified by Lillian Wald, and in Canada as reflected in the work of the Victorian Order of Nurses.

This tradition has not been acknowledged in the current discourse on health promotion.

Since publication of the Lalonde Report and the subsequent interdisciplinary development of health promotion as a field of inquiry and practice, the term has taken on new meaning within and outside of nursing. The confusion for nurses appears to arise, in part, because some nursing authors today continue to use the term health promotion in a generic sense, while others use it to refer to a specific approach to practice that derives from a particular philosophical or theoretical perspective. The approach to health promotion that emerged following release of the Lalonde Report, however, focused on lifestyle modification. This approach expanded on the health education and disease prevention work that had been done for years in Canada and other developed countries by practitioners of various disciplines, including nursing (see Badgley, 1978; Kulbok et al., 1995). Until Lalonde, this work had been overshadowed by the growth of biomedicine and the efforts in the late 1950s and early 1960s to deal with issues of access to health care.

The Lalonde Report has been both revered and reviled, but its impact is evident in the subsequent development of public health policy in other countries, including the United States, New Zealand, Australia, the United Kingdom, Sweden and other European countries (Baum, 1990; Hancock, 1985; Parish, 1995; Pinder, 1994;). Tables 2–1 through 2–4 summarize the key milestones in health promotion's history in Canada, the United States, the United Kingdom, and the World Health Organization. The basic thrust of the Lalonde Report was that health status is determined by four general factors: human biology, the environment, lifestyle, and health care. The report sought explicitly to break down the widely held public perception that health was the result of medical intervention and institutional care. Instead, Lalonde argued that future increases in **population health** status

---

TABLE 2–1

CANADIAN MILESTONES IN HEALTH PROMOTION

Year	Milestones
1974	Publication of the Lalonde Report, *A New Perspective on the Health of Canadians.*
1981	First National Conference on Health Promotion. Ottawa, Canada.
1984	Beyond Health Care Conference. Toronto, Ontario. Introduction of the concepts of Healthy Public Policy and Healthy Cities.
1986	First International Conference on Health Promotion. Ottawa, Canada. Release of Ottawa Charter on Health Promotion. Publication of *Achieving Health for All: A Framework for Health Promotion.* J. Epp. Health and Welfare Canada.
1994	Publication of *Strategies for Population Health: Investing in the Health of Canadians.* Report of the Federal, Provincial and Territorial Advisory Committee on Population Health. Health Canada.
1996	Publication of *Population Health Promotion: An Integrated Model of Population Health and Health Promotion.* N. Hamilton & T. Bhatti. Health Promotion Development Division. Health Canada. Publication of *Action Statement on Health Promotion.* Canadian Public Health Association.
1998	Publication of *Taking Action on Population Health.* Ottawa: Population Health Development Division. Health Canada.

TABLE 2–2

UNITED STATES MILESTONES IN HEALTH PROMOTION

Year	Milestones
1976	Task Force on Consumer Health Information and Health Promotion. National Institutes of Health and the American College of Preventive Medicine.
	Publication of *Forward Plan for Health, FY 1978–82, Review.* Washington, DC: U.S. Public Health Service.
	Passage of the *National Consumer Health Information and Health Promotion Act.*
1979	Publication of *Healthy People: The Surgeon General's Report on Health Promotion and Disease Prevention.*
1980	Publication of *Promoting Health/Preventing Disease: Objectives for the Nation.* Washington, DC: U.S. Public Health Service.
1986	Publication of the *1990 Objectives for the Nation: A Midcourse Review.* Washington, DC: U.S. Public Health Service.
1990	Publication of *Healthy People 2000: National Health Promotion and Disease Prevention Objectives.* Washington, DC: U.S. Public Health Service.

lay in improving the environment, modifying self-imposed risks due to personal health behaviors, and increasing knowledge of human biology. Although biology, the environment, and lifestyle were given equal attention in the document, it was the lifestyle element that came to be most closely associated with the Lalonde Report. It was also the element that captured the attention of governments, and was reflected in the practice of professionals.

The appeal of the Lalonde Report to western governments was not surprising, given the economic and political climate of the day. It emerged at a time when governments of developed nations were beginning to realize the impending crisis of cost related to illness care, and had come to acknowledge the limits of medicine in dealing with the increasing burden of chronic illness. This realization occurred in the wake of the mid-century epidemiological transition (Terris, 1976) in which the major causes of morbidity and mortality shifted away from infectious to chronic diseases. At the same time, the women's health movement and other social movements were challenging the medical establishment, and

environmental health risks were on the rise. The Canadian government, having recently passed legislation to support a publically funded scheme of universal health insurance was grappling with the potentially open-ended expenditures related to a fee-for-service reimbursement plan for physicians and "high-tech" advancements in hospital treatments. Lalonde's health education and social marketing strategy, defined as health promotion, emphasized persuading the public to change their personal behavior and to assume more responsibility for their own health. This had enormous appeal for governments as a potential avenue for reducing health care expenditures.

In the years that followed Lalonde, those working in the field struggled to make sense of the meaning of health promotion and to understand whether and how it was different from health education. If health promotion was about influencing individual health-related behaviors, it was indeed difficult to distinguish it from what had always been done in the name of health education (Labonte, 1994).

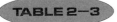

TABLE 2—3

UNITED KINGDOM MILESTONES IN HEALTH PROMOTION

Year	Milestones
1976	Publication of *Prevention and Health: Everybody's Business.* Department of Health and Social Security.
	Publication of *Priorities for Health and Personal Social Services in England.* Department of Health and Social Security.
1981	Publication of *Care in Action: A Handbook of Policies and Priorities for the Health and Personal Social Services in England.* Department of Health and Social Security.
1986	Publication of *Primary Health Care: An Agenda for Discussion.* Department of Health and Social Security.
1992	Publication of *The Health of the Nation.* Department of Health and Social Security.
	Publication of *The Health of the Nation . . . and You.* Department of Health and Social Security.

International Impact of the Lalonde Report

Despite a lukewarm reception in the land of its birth, the ideas reflected in the Lalonde Report were given voice in the United States in a report of the *Task Force on Health Promotion and Consumer Health Education* (1976), sponsored by the National Institutes of Health and the American College of Preventive Medicine. In the same year, the U.S. Congress passed the National Consumer Health Information and Health Promotion Act, which provided funding for programs emphasizing illness or accident prevention that could be controlled through individual knowledge or behavior change (Crawford, 1977).

Also in 1976, the U.S. Department of Health, Education and Welfare (1976) produced the *Forward Plan for Health,* which argued that the greatest health benefits were likely to come from efforts to improve the personal health habits of Americans and the environment in which they lived and worked. In *Healthy People: The Surgeon General's Report on Health Promotion and Disease Prevention* (U.S. Department of Health, Education and Welfare, 1979), the government set national objectives for disease prevention, health protection, and health promotion. Thus, the new three-pronged U.S. public health policy was based on three of

the elements in Lalonde's health field concept (Kulbok et al., 1995).

The development of health promotion in the United Kingdom shared a similar history, although the establishment of national goals and objectives for health promotion did not come until the 1990s. In 1976, the governments of Northern Ireland, Wales, England, and Scotland produced a policy document entitled *Prevention and Health: Everybody's Business* (Department of Health and Social Security, 1976). Much like the Lalonde Report in Canada and the Task Force report in the United States, this British document attempted to reorient health care services away from treatment toward prevention. The report emphasized the provision of preventive services such as screening and immunization, and the importance of personal responsibility for adopting healthy behavior patterns (Parish, 1995).

Health Promotion and Nursing in the Post-Lalonde Era

The lifestyle model of health promotion that emerged following the Lalonde Report was reflected in the health policy of various nations. For the most part, nursing adopted this

TABLE 2—4

WORLD HEALTH ORGANIZATION MILESTONES IN HEALTH PROMOTION

Year	Milestones
1977	13th World Health Assembly. Adoption of Health For All Program.
	Alma Ata Conference on Primary Health Care—Alma Ata, Kazakhstan. Release of *Alma Ata Declaration on Primary Health Care*. Geneva: World Health Organization.
1978	Publication of *Alma Ata Declaration on Primary Health Care*. Geneva: World Health Organization.
1981	Publication of *Regional Strategy for Attaining Health for All by the Year 2000.* Copenhagen: World Health Organization. Official launch of the WHO Health Promotion Program.
1984	Publication of *Health Promotion: A Discussion Document on the Concepts and Principles.* Copenhagen: World Health Organization.
1985	Publication of *Targets for Health for All.* Copenhagen: World Health Organization.
1986	First International Conference on Health Promotion. Ottawa, Canada. Release of Ottawa Charter on Health Promotion.
1988	Second International Conference on Health Promotion. Adelaide, Australia. Release of Adelaide Recommendations for Healthy Public Policy.
1992	Third International Conference on Health Promotion. Sundsvall, Sweden. Release of Sundsvall Statement on Supportive Environments.
1997	Fourth International Conference on Health Promotion. Jakarta, Indonesia. Release of the Jakarta Declaration on Leading Health Promotion into the 21st Century.
1998	51st World Health Assembly. Resolution on Health for All for the 21st Century, and Resolution on Health Promotion, confirming the Jakarta Declaration.
	Publication of *Population Health—Putting the Concept into Action.* H. Zollner & S. Lessor. Copenhagen: World Health Organization.

lifestyle approach, perhaps because its premises and underlying ideology were consistent with the prevailing ethos in nursing. Health education, which had always been a special province of nurses (Novak, 1988), was a key strategy in lifestyle modification. During the 1970s, the wellness movement had also gained ground, and the emphasis of that movement on self-actualization and high-level wellness was reflected in various nursing approaches to health promotion.

In 1982, Nola Pender published the first edition of her influential book *Health Promotion in Nursing Practice* in which she presented a health promotion model for nursing. This model integrated constructs from social psychology, especially **expectancy-value theory** (Feather, 1982) and social learning theory (Bandura, 1986), within a nursing perspective on holistic human functioning. Pender's model clearly was influenced by the structural organization of U.S. public health policy into the three areas of health promotion, health protection, and preventive services. She defined health promotion as "activities directed toward sustaining or increasing the level of well-being, self-actualization, and personal fulfillment of a given individual or group" (Pender, 1982, p. 42).

In 1983, Brubaker reviewed the literature on health promotion to explore current uses of the term. She found that the nursing literature did not deal extensively with health promotion. Where it was discussed, Smith's (1981) four models of health had strongly influenced a nursing perspective on health promotion. Accordingly, *health as self-actualization* was deemed to be the "highest" definition of health, in contrast to *health as adaptation, health as the ability to perform social roles*, and *health as the absence of illness*. Brubaker found that the primary emphasis of health promotion in the nursing literature of the time was on personal responsibility, lifestyle behavior change, and high-level wellness, focusing on individuals whose health had reached a state of stability. This emphasis has carried into the present in much of the nursing literature, particularly in the United States and Britain (e.g., Bright, 1997; Kulbok, Baldwin, Cox, & Duffy, 1997; Pender, 1996), although critiques of this approach have more recently begun to emerge.

Critiques of Health Promotion as Lifestyle Modification

Even as the behavioral approach to health promotion was getting off the ground in the developed world, an emerging critique was challenging the assumptions and foundations of the fledgling enterprise. Criticisms of behavioral health promotion emerged from both ends of the political spectrum. At the conservative end of the spectrum, health promotion critics have argued that the state has no right to interfere in the daily lives of its citizens by promoting lifestyle modification (Wikler, 1978), and that health promotion policies and programs are tools of an authoritarian "nanny state" that restricts personal autonomy. Variations of this argument from the right have been put forth at various times throughout the history of health promotion, and continued into the 1990s (Davies, 1991; Lupton, 1995; Skrabanec, 1992).

From the left emerged the structural critique of health promotion (Allison, 1982; Brown & Margo, 1978; Crawford, 1977; Labonte & Penfold, 1981) which was based on feminist and **neo-Marxist** thinking. This critique incorporated earlier challenges raised by American critics (e.g., Ryan, 1971) that the liberal ideology reflected in the U.S. social policy of the 1960s resulted in an implicit policy of victim-

blaming. The Lalonde Report was taken to task for its potential to contribute to "victim-blaming" because, although Lalonde criticized the medical model, he did not challenge its basic paradigm (Labonte, 1994). As in medicine, the health field concept defined illness and disease as characteristics of individuals. Thus, the "victim" is blamed, at least implicitly, for being sick, and is held responsible for unhealthy lifestyle choices, unhealthy emotional styles, and unhealthy responses to stressful situations (Donahue & McGuire, 1995).

Crawford (1977) argued that health promotion initiatives, such as *Healthy People*, which emphasized personal responsibility and individual behavior change, served a critical ideological function in the political economy. This ideology challenged public expectations for social programs and justified a government retreat from ensuring the public's right and entitlement to medical-care access. At the same time, it diverted attention away from the social production of illness by industrial and commercial interests. Early health promotion thus shifted responsibility to the individual.

To be fair, however, the U.S. social policy of the 1960s, particularly the War on Poverty initiatives of the Johnson administration, did reflect concerns with equity, social justice, and the need for public participation. Despite criticism of the *Objectives for the Nation*, they did encompass strategies for change that included policy, legislation, and institutional change, not just individual change (Minkler, 1989). Approximately one third of the objectives focused on environmental issues such as pollution, occupational health, and safety. The problem, as observed by Green (1994), was that U.S. policy had drawn a clear distinction between health promotion, health protection, and preventive health services. Health promotion focused primarily on individual behavior and lifestyle change, health protection focused on the physical environment (not the social and economic environment), and preventive health services dealt with issues like screening and immunization in clinical practice. This division had the unfortunate effect of narrowing the focus and vision of health promotion in the United States.

Although Green (1994) has convincingly challenged the international stereotype of American health promotion as being dominated by a focus on changing individual behavior, this stereotype is unfortunately reinforced by a body of literature that exemplifies this emphasis. This continues to be true in much of the American literature on health promotion even to this day, especially in nursing. Minkler (1989) and others (e.g., Becker, 1986; Williams, 1989) have observed that this emphasis can be traced to western and uniquely American value systems reflecting a neoliberal ideology, grounded in a radical **individualism.**

A feminist perspective on health promotion also runs counter to the individualist ethic inherent in the focus on personal behavior change. The women's health movement, for example, sought to contextualize women's health within the social, economic, and political conditions affecting their lives, thus making the personal political. The movement also sought to implement strategies that would facilitate a collective rather than an individual response and to challenge governments and institutions to assume their social responsibility for the health of women and the population as a whole. As with the structural critique, feminists have argued that women are assigned responsibility for their own and others' health without recognition that they have a relative lack of power to effect change. The paradox of this "responsibility without power" has been criticized as being at the core of many health promotion programs directed at women (Daykin & Naidoo, 1994).

Despite the debate generated by the structural critique of health promotion in the decade following the release of the Lalonde Report, nursing authors initially were uncritical of this approach and uncritical of the government policy documents that were spawned as a result. This uncritical stance has continued in much of the current nursing literature on health promotion, and has been lamented by Brown and Piper (1997). Major nursing criticisms of the lifestyle approach to health promotion did not emerge until the end of the 1980s and into the 1990s, but did not become more than a marginal position in nursing until the late 1990s. There were, however, some exceptions in the earlier post-Lalonde period. For example, Dreher (1982) criticized the conservative perspective in nursing that adopted an individualistic approach to care. She argued that psychological theories, developed in a white, middle-class, Euro-American context, had been embraced by nursing even though they had limited applicability to the health of disadvantaged and socially diverse populations. The wholesale adoption of psychological theories to explain patterns of health and illness implicitly situated the problem in the beliefs, attitudes, and perceptions of individuals. The role of the nurse was therefore to "penetrate and alter the client's negative perceptions" rather than to challenge or change the system that created inequities in health. Maslow's concept of self-actualization, which is an important concept in many nursing definitions of health and health promotion, was criticized for not considering the issue of unequal access to opportunities to achieve this highest of goals. Similarly, Dreher argued that Erikson's developmental theory did not consider the conditions under which developmental tasks might not be achieved among disadvantaged populations.

Health for All and Primary Health Care

Both inspired by the Lalonde Report and going beyond it, the World Health Organization (WHO) proposed its vision of *Health for All by the Year 2000* (WHO, 1977) at the 30th World Health Assembly. A year later, at the WHO conference in Kazakhstan, of the former Soviet Union, the Alma Ata Declaration on primary health care (WHO, 1978a) was released. Primary health care (PHC) was envisioned as the means for achieving health for all citizens of the world. *Health for All* was thus the first of a series of health promotion initiatives by WHO over the next 15 years; however, there was very little mobilization around PHC implementation in the industrialized world in the decade following Alma Ata. Primary health care does not represent a separate era in the development of health promotion. It is, however, distinct from the proposals of the Lalonde report, yet not fully reflective of the principles of the subsequently developed Ottawa Charter (WHO, 1986). Thus, PHC is discussed here as an intermediate stage in the global development of health promotion even though it emerged during the time frame of the lifestyle-modification era.

Recognizing that there were massive inequalities in health within and between countries, despite technological achievements and the resources devoted to the health care system, WHO proposed that *Health for All* should be the main social goal of governments. Health was declared a fundamental human right. While the Lalonde Report was based implicitly on a definition of health as absence of disease, the Alma Ata Declaration affirmed the expanded WHO definition of health as a positive concept (WHO, 1978a). This move was congruent with nursing's belief that health, not illness, was the primary focus of nursing practice.

The most significant feature of PHC was the recognition that health was determined primarily by social and environmental conditions that lay outside the traditional purview of the health sector and thus required intersectoral cooperation to improve health status. Primary health care is about equity in access to health and health care through the provision of community-based health services that emphasize disease prevention and health promotion. Community participation and socially acceptable, affordable technology are critical features. Thus, the seeds of a social definition of health promotion were sown with *Health for All.* As will be demonstrated later in this chapter, it is clear that the principles of PHC are central features of the "new health promotion." At that time, however, there was a lack of congruence between the vision of PHC with its implied collectivist approach and the individually focused approach reflected in the personal responsibility and behavior change focus in the health policy of many developed countries. As Baum and Sanders (1995) pointed out, western countries, despite being signatories to the Alma Ata Declaration, quickly retreated from the goals of PHC to a more selective and targeted approach that stressed medically and behaviorally defined goals.

Nursing's Response to *Health for All*

The *Health for All* initiative was strongly endorsed by the International Council of Nurses (ICN), which encouraged nursing in all member countries to develop a primary health care system that capitalized on the strengths, capacities, and potential of nurses, and responded to the unique health care needs of each country (WHO, 1978b). Despite the leadership of ICN,

primary health care was off to a slow start in most industrialized countries. Ten years after Alma Ata, Maglacas, then chief nursing scientist for WHO, challenged nursing by stating that "nursing's response to the health for all challenge has been fragmented, sporadic, unplanned and uncoordinated, and has involved few, if any, other disciplines or sectors" (Maglacas, 1988, p. 67).

Maglacas' charge certainly appeared to be true in Canada, Britain, and the United States. A Canadian study by Edwards and Craig (1987) found that only 31 percent of nursing educators were aware of the Alma Ata Declaration, and that only 20 percent had ever read the Canadian Nurses Association (CNA) position statement on PHC. In the United States, driven by political and professional support for the *Objectives for the Nation* (U.S. DHEW, 1980), health promotion as lifestyle modification was becoming entrenched in nursing practice and the development of PHC made little headway. Even today, there are few American nursing texts that discuss the principles of PHC, even in community health nursing, although there are exceptions (e.g., Anderson & McFarlane, 1995; Hitchcock, Schubert & Thomas, 1999). More recent writings by American nurses that critique the current primary care system in the United States have emerged (e.g., Schoultz & Hatcher, 1997).

The Era of Health Promotion as "The New Public Health"

As a result of the structural critique, the perspective on health promotion began to shift in Canada, and internationally. In 1980, at the First National Conference on Health Promotion, in Canada, the structural critique was given voice (Labonte & Penfold, 1981) and, as a result, many practitioners began to question Lalonde-style health promotion. As the new decade of the 80s began, the WHO European office embarked on the development of a new social model of health promotion (Kickbush, 1994), which was to go beyond the individualistic model that had emerged in the post-Lalonde era, while at the same time encompassing it. This "new health promotion" (Robertson & Minkler, 1994), sometimes called "the New Public Health" (Kickbush,

1989; O'Neill, 1997) was an attempt to integrate a "systems" perspective with an "individual" perspective. The term *lifestyle,* introduced to the health promotion discourse by Lalonde, was the source of much debate and opposition in the development of the new health promotion (Coreil & Levin, 1984). Because of this debate, Kickbush (1994) says that WHO reclaimed the concept of lifestyle in the way that Max Weber (1948) had used it a century before, and drew upon a primarily European social philosophy for its grounding.

For Weber, lifestyle was a social and not an individual concept, a "process by which social identities and sense of self are constructed from available political, economic, and cultural resources" (O'Brien, 1995). Weber argued that divisions in society arise, not from social class based on economic relationships, but rather from status. A status group is distinguished by the honor accorded it by others, and by its particular style of life comprising symbols and symbolic acts. Thus, lifestyle is not just about patterns of behavior, but is the very apparatus by which power is wielded (Veal, 1993). To live a particular style of life was to respond to the broad social divisions in society (O'Brien, 1995). It is clear that this view of lifestyle is congruent with the ethos of the social model of health promotion put forth in the Ottawa Charter (Frohlich & Potvin, 1999). It contrasts markedly with the understanding of "lifestyle" that came to be associated with Lalonde's approach to health promotion. In this approach, lifestyles were individual characteristics, as reflected in social psychological approaches that dominated health education and health promotion research in the 1970s, 80s, and into the 90s.

In 1986, the European office of WHO, Health and Welfare Canada, and the Canadian Public Health Association co-sponsored the First International Conference on Health Promotion, which produced the Ottawa Charter on Health Promotion (WHO, 1986). At that conference, the Canadian government released its own similar discussion document: *Health for All: A Framework for Health Promotion* (Epp, 1986). The Ottawa Charter defined health promotion as " . . . the process of enabling people to increase control over and improve their health" (WHO, 1986). It embodied a social model of health, which meant that "an individual or group must be able to identify and realize aspirations, to satisfy needs, and to change or cope with the environment." In this definition, health is not an end, but rather the means, a resource for everyday living that emphasizes social and personal resources and physical capacities.

Expanding on the concept of "social determinants" implicit in the Alma Ata Declaration, the Ottawa Charter explicitly identified the prerequisites for health to include: peace, shelter, education, food, income, a stable ecosystem, sustainable resources, social justice, and equity. The health promotion mechanisms of advocating, enabling, and mediating were defined as the central processes for health promotion practice. Advocacy aims to create the social and environmental conditions that are favorable for health. The process of enabling, later conceptualized as empowerment, is aimed at reducing inequities in health and ensuring equal opportunities for achieving health potential. This is accomplished by providing a supportive environment and assisting people to take control over those things that influence their health and well-being. Because health promotion demands coordinated action from many sectors, health professionals as well as social and professional groups have a responsibility to mediate between different interests in the pursuit of health. Five major strategies for promoting health were identified: building healthy public policy, creating supportive environments, strengthening community action, developing personal skills, and reorienting health services.

The Ottawa Charter succeeded in politicizing health and health promotion in a way that Lalonde and Alma Ata did not, by laying out a broad agenda for social and health reform. In many ways, health promotion as the new public health was a radical agenda (Kickbush, 1994), in that it implied a real shift in power, from bureaucracies and professionals to the people (Green & Raeburn, 1988). It called for very different ways of working, with professionals as facilitators, mediators, advocates, and supporters rather than as experts in control of the situation. The Ottawa Charter takes an explicitly ecological perspective in which health is produced in the continuous interaction of people with their environments. It shifts the emphasis from individuals or systems to communities and places a new focus on collective responsibility for health.

Nursing and the New Health Promotion

The response of nursing to the new health promotion must be considered within the social and political context of each country in which it occurred. The paradigm shift implied by this new way of conceptualizing health promotion progressed (or not) at different rates in different countries. It depended, in part, on the extent to which health promotion, defined as "individual behavior change," had become entrenched in policy. In the United States and Great Britain, the diffusion of a new definition of health promotion occurred very slowly, particularly in nursing. This was a testament to the power of national policy, which made it more difficult to talk about health promotion as being something other than what had been officially defined. In Canada, the Lalonde Report had never reached official policy status. Furthermore, Canada was actively involved with the European office of WHO in the background work for the Ottawa Charter (Kickbush, 1994; Raeburn, 1994) and released its own framework for health promotion at the same time (Epp, 1986) amidst much fanfare and publicity. These events might explain the fairly rapid diffusion of the Ottawa Charter ideas within the Canadian government health bureaucracy, among the professional nursing associations, and by task forces and commissions for health reform across the country. This is not to say that these ideas diffused as rapidly to the front lines of practice, or that there were not gaps between rhetoric and reality.

In Canada, the official nursing response to health promotion occurred within the context of the philosophy of primary health care. Following release of the Ottawa Charter, between 1987 and 1993, there was a major professional mobilization in nursing in relation to PHC (Roger & Gallagher, 1995), and the new health promotion. The Canadian Nurses Association (CNA) developed a position statement on PHC in Canada and recommended strategies for achieving *Health for All* (Canadian Nurses Association, 1988). In 1989, CNA developed a five-year plan to guide the implementation of PHC strategies in nursing. In 1990, the community health nursing section of the Canadian Public Health Association produced a definitional statement on community health nursing in Canada, which established PHC as the conceptual foundation for practice (Canadian Public Health Association, 1990) and identified health promotion, as defined in the Ottawa Charter, as the primary goal of practice. A policy statement on health promotion, in keeping with the Epp framework (Epp, 1986) was released by CNA in 1992. At the provincial level, professional associations across the country produced position statements and discussion documents on PHC (Alberta Association of Registered Nurses, 1989; Registered Nurses Association of British Columbia, 1990) and health promotion. The Registered Nurses Association of British Columbia (RNABC), for example, promoted the Ottawa Charter approach to health promotion within the context of their New Directions for Health Care policies and programs. In 1992, RNABC produced a document entitled *Determinants of Health: Empowering Strategies for Nursing Practice* (Little & Labonte, 1992), which provided a socioenvironmental framework for health promotion practice that included strategies directed at individual, family, small group, community, and societal levels (Little & Labonte, 1992). Since that time, publications have appeared in the nursing literature demonstrating the application of that framework to nursing practice (Clarke & Mass, 1998; Duncan, 1996; Ritchie, Boutell, Buchan, Foster, & St. Aubrey, 1995).

Developments in nursing during the post-Ottawa Charter period signaled the beginning of a paradigm shift to the new health promotion. The structural critique of Lalonde-era health promotion, that had appeared earlier in the interdisciplinary writing, emerged in the nursing literature in the late 1980s (e.g., Butterfield, 1990; Williams, 1989) but was articulated in relation to nursing concerns. Williams (1989), for example, challenged the individualistic health promotion models in nursing and proposed an alternative feminist conceptualization, based on assumptions of human interdependence and reciprocal responsibility. Williams' proposal is entirely consistent with the socioecological perspective on health promotion in the Ottawa Charter. The structural critique by nursing authors continued with more intensity into the 1990s (Brown & Piper, 1997; Rush, 1997) as the new health promotion has gained ground.

At the same time, nursing scholars had initiated a general critique of traditional nursing theory. This critique was consistent with the concepts and ideas central to the new health promotion, but did not fall under that rubric. Rather, the approach to nursing reflected in these critiques was referred to variously as upstream nursing (Butterfield, 1990), critical social nursing (Stevens & Hall, 1992), and emancipatory nursing (Kendall, 1992). There were two stages in this critique. In the first stage, beginning in the mid 1980s and proceeding into the 1990s, several nursing authors challenged the narrow conceptualization of nursing's foundational concepts (i.e., person, environment, health, and nursing) and proposed theoretical expansions to these concepts that were congruent with the new health promotion. For example, several nursing writers (Chalmers & Kristjansen, 1989; McKnight & VanDover, 1994; Sills & Goeppinger, 1985; Shultz, 1987) explored the notion of client or person as "more than one." Although the concept of community-as-client had long been a focus for community health nursing, most nursing theories refer to person in the singular. This expansion of "person" to include collective clients made it possible for nurses in areas other than community and public health nursing to focus beyond the individual. This is consistent with the Ottawa Charter view of health promotion, in which the community is the center of gravity and the location where individual and societal interests come together. It is also consistent with a feminist critique of the individualist bias inherent in the concept of client (Sherwin, 1992).

Similarly, the concept of environment, although central to nursing theory, has tended to focus on the immediate psychosocial environment of individuals rather than on the social, political, and environmental contexts that influence health and health care (Chopoorian, 1986; Kleffel, 1991; Starzomski & Rodney, 1997; Stevens, 1989). These nursing authors have proposed an expansion of the concept of environment in nursing to incorporate the broader sociopolitical environment, arguing that existing nursing theories are inadequate to guide practice in light of "inequitable health care access, impoverishment, and ecological destruction" (Stevens & Hall, 1992, p. 3). Although Stevens and Hall do not cite the Ottawa Charter, their ideas are very consistent with it. With respect to the concept of health, nursing has long defined its focus as being on health rather than illness; however, health is typically represented in nursing theory as a personal construct. This notion has been challenged by Jones and Meleis (1993) and others (Thorne et al., 1998) who argue that health is more than a personal matter and that nursing must develop a contextualized definition of health congruent with societal needs.

Expanded Concept of Nursing

If the foundational concepts of health, environment, and person must be expanded to reflect the social mandate and mission of nursing (Jones & Meleis, 1993), then the concept of nursing must also be expanded to encompass nursing action that is relevant to individual and collective clients whose health is experienced within and is affected by the broad sociopolitical context. This expanded notion of nursing implies an important focus on social action and not just personal care. Several nursing authors have voiced the need for nursing to expand its focus to incorporate social activism, policy development, and political action (Butterfield, 1990; Kendall, 1992; Moccia, 1988; Watson, 1990). Such a focus is very much in keeping with the Ottawa Charter, which proposes that it is important to take action on the broad social and environmental influences on health.

The second stage of theoretical development in nursing related to health promotion began in the early 1990s, and also reflected the concepts inherent in the Ottawa Charter. These include such concepts as empowerment (Brunt, Lindsey, & Hopkinson, 1997; Gibson, 1991; Jones & Meleis, 1993; Rodwell, 1996; Skelton, 1994; Styles, 1994), participation (Hudson-Rodd, 1994; Jewell, 1994), collaboration (Clarke & Mass, 1998), and partnership (Courtney, Ballard, Fauver, Gariota, & Holland, 1996). These concepts were not necessarily discussed within a specific model or framework for health promotion, but more as concepts that were directly relevant to nursing theory and practice in particular settings or with particular client groups. The view that concepts inherent in the Ottawa Charter are integral to nursing theory is consistent with the findings of at least one study in Britain (Maben & MacLeod Clark, 1995), which suggested that nursing students define health promotion primarily as lifestyle modification. Students do, however, understand the concepts of empowerment, participation, collaboration, and equity as theoretical concepts in nursing rather than in health promotion.

It is in relation to these core concepts of health promotion (or nursing), that nursing has potential to contribute to the interdisciplinary development of health promotion. As O'Neill (1997) points out, it is nurses who represent the greatest number of professionals involved in health promotion practice. Because nurses have on-the-ground experience with these concepts, it is possible to expand our theoretical understanding of the concepts of participation, collaboration, empowerment, and partnership. For example, the study by Brunt and associates (1997) raised some important questions about the potential ethnocentricity of empowerment when working with certain populations and they challenged some basic assumptions about this concept. It is this type of challenge that can contribute enormously to the continual refinement and development of health promotion concepts both within and outside of nursing.

Despite the beginnings of a paradigm shift to the "new health promotion" in nursing, traditional conceptualizations remain predominant in practice although there is more diversity in nurses' understandings of health promotion now than there was at the time of Brubaker's (1983) concept analysis. At that time, health promotion was viewed primarily as lifestyle change. More recently, Maben and MacLeod Clark (1995), drawing from diverse sources and studies, have identified six different ways that health promotion is being understood by nurses. These authors consider the first four to be traditional views, and the last two to be "new paradigm" approaches.

Six Views of Health Promotion

First, health promotion is viewed by nurses as an umbrella concept, in which any nursing action is seen to be directed at promoting health. This generic view of health promotion dates back to the pre-Lalonde era. Second, health promotion is frequently viewed as being synonymous and interchangeable with health education. This is found more frequently in those countries that have established educational

programs for and a discipline called "health education." Third, health promotion is sometimes seen as the marketing or selling of health, with some nurses reporting that health promotion "involved the promotional tactics of selling, pushing, or advertising the health message" (Maben & MacLeod Clark, 1995, p. 1160). Fourth, health promotion is defined as lifestyle modification, which appears to be the most common understanding in the recent nursing literature. Fifth, health promotion is sometimes viewed as "health education plus," meaning that in addition to information-giving, life skills teaching, and self-empowerment, health promotion means engaging in social and environmental change. Finally, health promotion is viewed by some nurses as being an approach that encompasses a particular set of values, which include concepts of empowerment, equity, collaboration, participation, and encompasses a "bottom-up" strategy. In this last view, health promotion is less concerned about who the client is or the setting in which it is practiced but rather, is concerned with how it is done. These last two conceptualizations are consistent with the Ottawa Charter definition of health promotion but, according to Maben and MacLeod Clark (1995), are infrequently identified by nurses in their definitions of health promotion.

Emerging Critiques of the New Health Promotion

Despite the warm fuzziness of the Ottawa Charter, it had not been the new kid on the block for long before the critics emerged. If health promotion is the goal of professional nursing practice, then it is important to understand the criticisms of health promotion. Critique helps us to reflect on our practice by surfacing issues that we may not be aware of, thereby contributing to practice improvement. It forces us to challenge our assumptions on an ongoing basis and thus is essential to praxis. Critique not only guides us in changing our practice when necessary, but also provides us with information we need to counter misperceptions about health promotion, so that we may reaffirm and justify our own approach. It helps us to clarify our values, beliefs, and principles in relation to health promotion. At a more abstract level, critique contributes to the theoretical development of health promotion.

The major critiques of health promotion are categorized under four major headings, none of which is entirely distinct: (1) the structural critique, (2) the rhetoric critique, (3) the epistemological critique, and (4) the surveillance critique. I have already reviewed the basic elements of the structural critique, which was targeted mainly at the lifestyle modification approach to health promotion. As you now know, this critique led to the emergence and development of the "new health promotion." The other three critiques are aimed primarily at the health promotion of the post-Ottawa Charter era, although aspects of the surveillance critique are also directed at the behavioral approach.

✳ Reflective Questions

Take a few moments now to reflect on your own concerns about, and criticisms of, health promotion. What are these? Give some thought to the following questions:

1. What criticisms of health promotion have you heard from your peers? Your teachers? Your colleagues in practice?

2. What is your assessment of the criticisms you have heard from others?

3. In looking at the names of the three critiques of health promotion listed above that we have not yet discussed, what do you think these might be about?

The Rhetoric Critique

The rhetoric critique argues that there are major gaps between health promotion practice and its rhetoric. This has been a major criticism of the new health promotion in the post-Ottawa charter era. For some critics, health promotion is thus condemned as inherently flawed (e.g., Kelly & Charleton, 1995), and this is one of the most frequent criticisms I hear from students. In seeing the lack of congruence between the ideals of health promotion and its absence in practice, many students question its relevance. For others, however, this incongruence is less a criticism of health promotion principles and its philosophy, and more a criticism of its enactment. A basic premise of the rhetoric critique is that there are a number of barriers at international, national, organizational, professional, and individual levels that make it difficult to enact health promotion in practice.

At the international and national levels, the global economy, with its emphasis on economic rationalism, places constraints on what any single country can do in the way of health and social policy (Labonte, 1993). Baum and Saunders (1995) argue that these constraints have resulted in an approach to health promotion that strays far from the original radical agenda of *Health for All* and the Ottawa Charter. Instead, powerful global forces have led national and state/provincial governments to adopt a more conservative approach that emphasizes individually focused rather than collective strategies. Governments have set goals and targets that aim to change individual behavior because these goals are more manageable and easier to measure. Thus, despite the rhetoric of a shift to collective responsibility for health, governments default to a focus on individual responsibility.

Within such a "goals-and-targets" approach, governments and organizations can use health promotion rhetoric as a bureaucratic tool to serve their own ends. The language of health promotion is co-opted to serve and sustain the status quo. For example, the concept of empowerment is used to justify cutbacks in community services and resources, in the name of community self-reliance. Bunton (1992) says that the support of governments for health promotion is largely symbolic rather than real. In fact, the broad definitions of health and health promotion, put forth by WHO, "allow national and local governments to effect a crusading zeal with little actual risk or commitment" (p. 5).

Whatever the rhetoric of health promotion as a radical agenda for reform, the reality for health professionals working within the bureaucracy is that the conservative ethos of organizations makes it very difficult to challenge the status quo and work toward radical change from within (Stevenson & Burke, 1992). Health professionals are often disempowered within their own organizations (Labonte, 1993), and to be true to the rhetoric of health promotion may have to "bite the hand that feeds them" (Green et al., 1996), thereby placing themselves at risk for sanction, and even job loss.

Green and Raeburn (1988) observed that the Ottawa Charter implied a radically reconceptualized role for health professionals in which power was to be transferred to the community. They suggested that health professionals might have difficulty giving up their expert roles and transferring power. In the end, they might only pay lip service to this notion. The findings of a study of health promoting practice among nurses support this observation, in which O'Brien (1994) concluded that the radical dimensions of health promotion are subverted in practice. In marked contrast to the ideology of health promotion, with its emphasis on client empowerment and collective action, O'Brien found that nurses actively constrain and curtail collective action, by virtue of their own unacknowledged prior agendas, as well as their explicit and implicit models of practice. It seems that leaders in nursing expected that the official adoption of a health promotion philosophy would result in a shift in the perspectives of individual practitioners. This shift did not happen because, O'Brien argues, nurses are already embedded in a system and guided by models of practice that do not support such a shift in perspective, let alone changes in practice. The introduction of health promotion concepts into traditional health care settings, led to nurses using the language of health promotion to justify and carry on with their prior agendas. This reinforced the conservative **individualism** inherent in contemporary health care provision and supported an expert model of practice. The result was that health promotion, as it was enacted in that setting, did not facilitate a transfer of control to the patient. Instead, it took on a controlling and manipulating character that was masked by health promotion rhetoric.

Perhaps it is unreasonable to expect nurses to shift their practice to reflect a health promotion perspective without the educational and institutional supports that will facilitate them in doing so. The nurses in O'Brien's study were not necessarily educated about health promotion. Given the diverse understandings of health promotion, even among those who have been educated about it, we should not be surprised that there may be challenges in translating rhetoric to practice. Hills (1998) has explored the extent to which nursing students, educated in a curriculum based on the Ottawa Charter philosophy of health promotion, are able to practice from a health promotion perspective in a hospital setting. The findings demonstrate that students are able to integrate the ideals of health promotion into their care and interactions with patients in hospital. Student narratives powerfully reflect their integration of the concepts of empowerment and caring in their practice. The challenge they struggle with is the difficulty practicing from a health promotion perspective in settings where their nursing colleagues do not share or support such a perspective. In the current climate of increasing patient acuity, staff shortages, and health care reform, this challenge may be particularly acute.

The Epistemological Critique

The epistemological critique challenges the integration of the social and individual views of health promotion in the same global model. Hagan, O'Neill, and Dallaire (1995) state that health promotion, as it is currently envisioned, emerged from two distinct streams that then merged in the articulation of the Ottawa Charter. One stream came from health education, which had focused on the voluntary adaptation of individual health-related behaviors and drew primarily from a theoretical base of social psychology and behavioral epidemiology. The other stream emerged from a more sociological and political vision, which argued that the main determinants of health lay in social, political and economic structures that placed constraints on individual behavior. This merger has not been without dissent.

In the wake of the Ottawa Charter, Green and Raeburn (1988) predicted that people would retreat into separate ideological camps, one supporting an individualistic model of health promotion, and the other a social model. Just because the Ottawa Charter tried to merge disparate perspectives did not make it so. Some authors question whether these two approaches, based on different sets of assumptions, different research traditions, and different ideological bases can truly be integrated (Green & Kreuter, 1993; Whitelaw, McKeown & Williams, 1997). Clearly, the assumption of the Ottawa Charter is that it can be done.

For many people, the Ottawa Charter is simply a merging of these two approaches. In reality, it may be impossible to merge them without some reconceptualization of either and a theoretical basis for understanding the relationship between the two. Typically, an individually focused perspective views individual cognition and the freedom to choose as paramount influences on human action. A social perspective, at its most extreme, is deterministic and portrays the individual as buffeted by the forces of the system and social structures, with little ability to influence those or to choose freely. The social model does not adequately conceptualize the individual within the environmental context and thus ignores the potential for the influence of individual action on the production and reproduction of societal structures. The individual model ignores the social structural influences on health status and thus is at risk of making assumptions about the possibilities for disadvantaged and marginalized groups to take action and to choose freely among options. The result may be the implementation of racist, **sexist, ageist,** and other discriminatory strategies.

Whitelaw and colleagues (1997) argue that the radical concepts of health promotion can be readily accepted by governments because the proposed frameworks have been inclusive and comprehensive, thus neutralizing the radical dimension. Their argument is that the creation of global models of health promotion, such as the Ottawa Charter, inhibits constructive debate around alternative perspectives on health. There is no need for governments to reject these radical elements, thereby alienating particular groups of professionals and community members. Rather, the existence of all-encompassing models allows governments to focus on those elements in the model that fit with their political and ideological perspectives while paying lip service to the more radical dimensions. In such attempts to integrate, tensions and oppositions are smoothed out, simplified, and made to appear unified. This accommodation of different perspectives eliminates genuine debate and key issues in health promotion are depoliticized. Global models tend to imply an equal weighting of all elements in the model. The authors argue, however, that a bias toward individualistic approaches emerges in practice when global models are invoked.

The epistemological critique explains, in part, the rhetoric versus reality dilemma raised earlier.

The ecological model of health promotion, which has been more clearly elaborated in the 1990s (e.g., Green et al., 1996; Stokols, 1992) presents its view of health as the interdependence among individuals, groups, and collectives and their social, physical, and political environments. Individual actions in the world are shaped and constrained by the social and environmental context in which the action occurs. At the same time, the actions of individuals change the larger environmental context, which, in turn, influences subsequent action. Thus, proponents of this view do not see an inherent contradiction in the integration of individual and social systems perspectives on health promotion. Nonetheless, there are limitations of the ecological model, not the least of which is that its complexity makes it difficult to articulate a clear set of strategies (Green et al., 1996) or to set priorities (Whitelaw et al., 1997).

Health promotion theorists have begun to engage seriously in working through "the individual versus social systems" issue (see Poland, 1992), but to date, no firm resolution has been articulated clearly. Considerably more theoretical development is required. In nursing, recent studies of health promotion practice by community health nurses may help to sort out this dilemma. In 1988, Green and Raeburn argued that the distinction between individually focused and community-focused practice was largely an academic distinction that was not born out in the real world of practice. Unfortunately, few researchers have examined this assertion empirically. Recent nursing research, however, has demonstrated that nursing practice with individuals and families is essential for providing the grounding for community or population-focused practice (Bent, 1999; Diekemper, SmithBattle, & Drake, 1999; SmithBattle, Drake, & Diekemper, 1997). Nurses draw on their practical skills and situated knowledge of individuals and families to change policies, and develop programs for the benefit of the larger population, and to build responsive communities. The distinction between individual and community level practice may have been reified in its frequent articulation (SmithBattle et al., 1997), but is not necessarily reflected in what nurses actually do.

The Surveillance Critique

The surveillance critique, as defined by Nettleton and Bunton (1995), draws from the writings of Foucault (1972, 1975, 1979) and argues that the technologies of health promotion serve to monitor and regulate populations on the one hand, and on the other, to construct new identities. In this situation, the new identity is "the health promoting self." Thus, health promotion is controlling and constraining. The surveillance critique was initially directed at the lifestyle modification focus of early health promotion, and to the extent that this form of health promotion remains in existence, the critique holds. Bunton (1992) argues, however, that even the post-Ottawa Charter version of health promotion is a new form of social regulation and control. Health promotion is not just the process by which health is improved, but also the process by which the new health bureaucracies take control of our lives.

Surveillance technologies include those by which populations are monitored, assessed, and profiled to document health status for the purpose of developing population-based interventions (Lupton, 1995; Nettleton & Bunton, 1995). Although surveillance has always been important in modern health systems, it is now directed at ever-expanding populations and aspects of everyday life. The Ottawa Charter says that health is created and lived by people *in the settings of everyday life.* It is this increasing surveillance of these aspects of living that raises concerns, because these individual actions were previously uncharted and unmonitored. Examples of the types of surveillance activities that raise concerns include monitoring the sexual activities of gay people in the interest of controlling the human immunodeficiency virus or workplace monitoring of employee drug use.

In these examples, it is easy to see the possibilities for threats to civil liberty and privacy. But many of these new forms of surveillance are not, on the face of it, overtly oppressing or controlling. Instead, Foucault might argue that through the discourses of health promotion and the application of health promotion technologies, a subtle coercion takes place as individuals internalize rules of behavior. The power in this internalization is that it results in a form of self-censorship and self-regulation, thus eliminating the need for governments to censor and regulate (Poland, 1992). It is the construction of a new identity, the health promoting self, that is the implicit, perhaps even unintended aim of the new health promotion technologies. Thus, the construction of an "appropriate" social identity then becomes a critical element of social regulation.

The surveillance critique cautions nurses to be alert for potential adverse consequences of our caring health promotion technologies (Nettleton & Bunton, 1995). The assumption in health promotion is that our humanistic practices are not coercive, and are better than more traditional authoritarian practices. In fact, those health promotion techniques that would have us listen to the views of our clients and come to know their perspectives require that we "penetrate into the lives and minds" (p. 47) of those people. This may not be without ill effect. It is possible that such egalitarian sharing may make it more difficult for someone to challenge or reject what we, as practitioners are interpreting as a negotiated course of action. The end result is that an apparently supportive and caring practice ends up being more coercive than the authoritarian regime we seek to replace. In fact, this authoritarian regime may be much easier for clients to challenge and reject (Nettleton & Bunton, 1995).

Population Health: An Emerging Era in Health Promotion?

There may now be a new era emerging in health promotion, the era of population health, although the relationship of population health to health promotion is not entirely clear. What is clear, however, is that the next chapter in the historical development of health promotion will have to account in some way for the emerging discourse on population health. A full discussion of this issue is beyond the scope of this chapter, in part because it constitutes a larger story than we have the space to tell, and in part because the history is still in the making. The following provides an overview of the introduction of population health into the ongoing dialogue on health promotion.

A few years ago, Coburn and Poland (1996) pointed out that a population health discourse in Canada, led by the Canadian Institute of Advanced Research (CIAR) (Evans, Barer, & Marmor, 1994) was competing with or might even be replacing health promotion as a way of understanding the determinants of health. But what is population health? How is it related to health promotion? Dunn and Hayes (1999) point out that there is considerable confusion about what population health means. They distinguish "population health" in its literal sense from a "population health perspective," a "population health framework," and a "population health approach." In 1994, the Federal/Provincial/Territorial Advisory Committee on Population Health published a document entitled *Strategies for Population Health: Investing in the Health of Canadians* that described the CIAR population health framework and proposed strategies for acting on the determinants of health. In a later press release by the same committee, population health was defined as:

. . . the health of a population as measured by health status indicators and as influenced by social, economic and physical environments, personal health practices, individual capacity and coping skills, human biology, early childhood development, and health services. (Federal/Provincial/Territorial Advisory Committee on Population Health, 1997)

A population health approach is an approach to public policy that focuses on taking action on the interrelated conditions that influence health status, while a population health perspective refers to the population health discourse in its most general sense, and thus is an overarching term (Dunn & Hayes, 1999).

At first, it was difficult to see how population health was different from health promotion because the emphasis on the social determinants of health resonated with the basic thrust of the Ottawa Charter. However, in response to the CIAR population health framework, health promotion advocates raised important concerns about the concept because they feared that the gains made in integrating health promotion into the public health practice of various disciplines would be lost as a result (Bhatti, 1996; Labonte, 1995; Poland, Coburn, Eakin, & Robertson, 1998; Robertson, 1998). In a dialogue between the proponents of both health promotion and population health (see Bhatti, 1996), participants on both sides agreed that they share the intent to improve the health of the population and both are concerned with improving inequalities in health status. Both

have their conceptual basis in the determinants of health and share the goal of a just society (Bhatti, 1996). Where they differ is in terms of focus and method. Population health is more mainstream than health promotion in its political and economic perspectives and while health promotion focuses on addressing inequalities in health experienced by disadvantaged and marginalized groups, population health is more concerned with gradients in health status across all socioeconomic levels. Because of its ecological perspective, health promotion has a more developed understanding of the relationship between human health and ecosystem health than does population health. With respect to method, population health emphasizes quantitative and epidemiological methodologies, whereas health promotion is more likely to use qualitative and social policy approaches (Bhatti, 1996).

To bridge the differences between the two concepts, a population health promotion framework was developed by Health Canada (Hamilton & Bhatti, 1994), *Population Health Promotion: An Integrated Model of Population Health and Health Promotion,* which attempts to integrate ideas from health promotion and population health. This framework has been adopted by some public health nursing departments as a guide for community practice. More recently, Health Canada has published a document entitled *Taking Action on Population Health* (Health Canada, 1998), which clearly defines population health as the guiding focus for the work being done by the Health Promotion and Programs Branch in Health Canada. The document appears to reflect an evolving effort to integrate concepts from the Ottawa Charter and Alma Ata with the CIAR population health model.

Until recently, the debate about the differences between population health and health promotion seems to have been uniquely Canadian, and was not widely reflected in the public health or health promotion literature in other countries. Recently, however, the World Health Organization has published a discussion paper entitled *Population Health—Putting the Concept into Action* (Zöllner & Lessor, 1998). At the same time WHO has sustained its commitment to health promotion as evidenced by their affirmation of the Ottawa Charter's health promotion strategies during the Fourth International Conference on Health Promotion, in Jakarta, Indonesia, in 1997. WHO identified five priorities for health promotion in the 21st century:

1. Promote social responsibility for health
2. Increase investment for health development
3. Consolidate and expand partnerships for health
4. Increase community capacity and empower people
5. Secure an infrastructure for health promotion

To advance these priorities, a global health promotion alliance was endorsed. The following year, at the 51st World Health Assembly, WHO passed a resolution confirming the priorities set at the Jakarta conference. Thus, WHO continues to see health promotion as a global priority. What all of this means for the history of health promotion in nursing is yet to be determined.

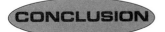

Clearly, health promotion has undergone considerable development both within and outside of nursing in the 25 years since the Lalonde Report was released. This chapter has described two broad historical eras of health promotion, and introduced a third and newly emerging era. Within the first two eras, however, variations in emphasis occurred. Both eras are reflected in the development of health promotion as an interdisciplinary enterprise as well as in nursing, although the development in nursing followed some years behind the interdisciplinary development. Tables 2–1 through 2–4 summarize the key milestones and publications in the history of health promotion in selected countries and for the WHO throughout the eras discussed in this chapter.

The first era of health promotion as lifestyle modification followed the release of the Lalonde Report (Lalonde, 1974) by the Canadian government and the subsequent development of related public health policy in other developed countries. Challenges to the individualistic approaches of this era led to the development of the "new health promotion" or the "new public health" as articulated in the Ottawa Charter for Health Promotion (WHO, 1986). This approach emphasized the importance of taking action on the social determinants of health and illness, social responsibility for health, and collective action.

There is evidence that a shift to the second era of health promotion is underway in nursing, although there are vestiges of health promotion as lifestyle modification still evident in nursing practice and in the recent literature. Much of the development of health promotion concepts in nursing has not necessarily taken place under the rubric of health promotion, but rather as developments in nursing theory in relation to concepts such as empowerment, collaboration, participation, and equity. In addition, foundational concepts in nursing theory have been expanded such that they encompass and are congruent with the philosophy implicit in the Ottawa Charter on Health Promotion. The fact that conceptual development has occurred in nursing, but not been labeled as health promotion, has meant that nursing's contributions to the interdisciplinary development of health promotion have been invisible.

Despite widespread support within and outside of nursing for the new health promotion as defined in the Ottawa Charter, several critiques have emerged. The rhetoric critique challenges that the language, ideals and principles of health promotion are co-opted in practice. The epistemological critique argues that health promotion models that attempt to integrate individual and systems perspectives are trying to merge approaches that are inherently contradictory with the result that differences are glossed over and the radical dimensions are suppressed. The surveillance critique suggests that the technologies of health promotion reflect an agenda for social control by governments and professionals.

Although recent nursing research provides some evidence challenging the relevance of some of these criticisms, there remain several barriers to health promotion practice in many settings where nurses work, particularly in hospitals and institutional settings. In one study exploring health promotion practice in hospital nursing, several barriers to implementation were identified, including: nurses' traditional task orientation, lack of authority in decision making, and lack of resources (Berland, Whyte, & Maxwell, 1995). Latter (1998) also found that nursing educators were ill-prepared to teach health promotion, lacking the knowledge and education in this area themselves. Another barrier was the lack of clarity about health promotion in relation to the meaning of concepts, different underlying ideologies, and the role of nurses in health promotion. Challenges to future progress in health promotion have also been discussed, including: the lack of role models in practice, the incongruence of nursing models that run counter to the new paradigm in health promotion, the organization of nursing work, and the fact of nurses being a disempowered group in their organizations (Latter, 1998). Robinson and Hill (1995) suggest that the wider social context supports a narrowly focused biomedical view of health, which makes a health promotion perspective difficult to realize in practice. They also observe that students have not experienced empowerment in their nursing education and that this presents a very challenging obstacle to health promotion in practice. It is evident that we still have work to do to bring clarity of meaning to the concept of health promotion, and to find ways to actualize it in practice. At the same time, in Canada at least, nurses must also come to terms with the meaning of population health for their practice, given the shift in policy focus toward a population health approach.

✳ Reflective Questions

1. What does health promotion mean to you? Which of the perspectives presented in this chapter reflect your understanding of health promotion? Is your own perspective different in any way from the perspectives reflected here?
2. Now that you have learned about the different critiques of health promotion, do any of these reflect your own experience of health promotion in the practice setting? In what way?
3. What are the implications of these critiques for your own nursing practice?
4. What barriers to health promotion have you experienced yourself in practice? How have you handled these? What might you do differently next time?
5. Can you describe a situation from your practice experience that exemplifies a health promotion perspective as articulated in the Ottawa Charter definition?
6. What does the concept population health mean to you? How do you think it differs from health promotion? What might be the implications of the shift toward population health for nursing practice?

REFERENCES

Alberta Association of Registered Nurses. (1989). *Position statement on health promotion.* Edmonton: Author.

Allison, K. (1982). Health education: Self-responsibility vs. blaming the victim. *Health Education,* Spring, 11–24.

Anderson, E. T., & McFarlane, J. M. (1995). *Community as partner: Theory and practice in nursing.* Philadelphia: J. B. Lippincott.

Badgley, R. F. (1978). Health promotion and social change in the health of Canadians. *Proceedings of the Seminar on Health Education and Behaviour Modification Programs,* September 15–18. Ottawa: Health and Welfare Canada.

Bandura, A. (1986). *Social foundations of thought and action. A social cognitive theory.* Englewood Cliffs, NJ: Prentice Hall.

Baum, F. (1990). The new public health: Force for change or reaction? *Health Promotion International, 5,* 145–150.

Baum, F., & Sanders, D. (1995). Can health promotion and primary health care achieve health for all without a return to their more radical agenda? *Health Promotion International, 10*(2), 149–160.

Berland, A., Whyte, N. B., & Maxwell, L. (1995). Hospital nurses and health promotion. *Canadian Journal of Nursing Research, 27*(4), 13–31.

Becker, M. (1986). The tyranny of health promotion. *Public Health Review, 14,* 15–23.

Bent, K. (1999). The ecologies of community caring. *Advances in Nursing Science, 21*(4), 29–36.

Bhatti, T. (1996). *Report of the roundtable on population health and health promotion.* Ottawa: Health Canada, Health Promotion Development Division.

Bright, J. S. (1997). *Health promotion in clinical practice: Targeting the health of the nation.* London: Balliére Tindall.

Brown, E. R., & Margo, G. E. (1978). Health education: Can the reformers be reformed? *International Journal of Health Services, 8,* 3–26.

Brown, P. A., & Piper, S. M. (1997). Nursing and the health of the nation: Schism or symbiosis? *Journal of Advanced Nursing, 15,* 297–301.

Brubaker, B. H. (1983). Health promotion: A linguistic analysis. *Advances in Nursing Science,* April, 1–14.

Brunt, J. H., Lindsey, E., & Hopkinson, J. (1997). Health promotion in the Hutterite community and the ethnocentricity of empowerment. *Canadian Journal of Nursing Research, 29*(1), 17–28.

Bunton, R. (1992). More than a wooly jumper: Health promotion as social regulation. *Critical Public Health, 3*(2), 4–11.

Bunton, R., & Burrows, R. (1995). Consumption and health in the 'epidemiological' clinic of late modern medicine. In R. Bunton, S. Nettleton, & R. Burrows (Eds.), *The sociology of health promotion: Critical analyses of consumption, lifestyle and risk* (pp. 206–222). London: Routledge.

Butterfield, P. G. (1990). Thinking upstream: Nurturing a conceptual understanding of the societal context of health behavior. *Advances in Nursing Science, 12*(2), 1–8.

Canadian Nurses Association. (1988). *Health for all Canadians: A call for health care reform.* Ottawa: Author.

Canadian Nurses Association. (1992). *Policy statement on health promotion.* Ottawa: Author.

Canadian Public Health Association. (1990). *Community health~public health nursing in Canada: Preparation and practice.* Ottawa: Author.

Canadian Public Health Association. (1996). *Action statement on health promotion in Canada.* Ottawa: Author.

Caraher, M. (1994). Nursing and health promotion practice: the creation of victims and winners in a political context. *Journal of Advanced Nursing, 19,* 465–468.

Chalmers, K., & Kristjanson, L. (1989). The theoretical basis for nursing at the community level: A comparison of three models. *Journal of Advanced Nursing, 14,* 569–574.

Chopoorian, T. J. (1986). Reconceptualizing the environment. In P. Moccia (Ed.), *New approaches to theory development* (pp. 39–54). New York: National League for Nursing.

Clarke, H., & Mass, H. (1998). Comox Valley Nursing Centre: From collaboration to empowerment. *Public Health Nursing, 15*(3), 216–224.

Coburn, D., & Poland, B. (1996). The CIAR vision of the determinants of health: A critique. *Canadian Journal of Public Health, 87*(5), 308–310.

Coreil, J., & Levin, J. S. (1984). A critique of the lifestyle concept in public health education. *International Quarterly of Community Health and Education, 5*(2), 103–114.

Courtney, R., Ballard, E., Fauver, S., Gariota, M., & Holland, L. (1996). The partnership model: Working with individuals, families and communities toward a new vision of health. *Public Health Nursing, 13*(3), 177–186.

Crawford, R. (1977). You are dangerous to your health: The ideology and politics of victim blaming. *International Journal of Health Services, 7*(4), 663–680.

Davies, S. (1991). *The historical origins of health fascism.* London: Forest.

Daykin, N., & Naidoo, J. (1994). Feminist critiques of health promotion. In R. Bunton, S. Nettleton, & R. Burrows (Eds.), *The sociology of health promotion: Critical analyses of consumption, lifestyle and risk.* (pp. 59–77). London: Routledge.

Department of Health and Social Security. (1976). *Prevention and health: Everybody's business.* London: HMSO.

Department of Health and Social Security. (1981). *Care in Action: A handbook of policies and priorities for the Health and Personal Social Services in England.* London: HMSO.

Department of Health and Social Security. (1986). *Primary health care: An agenda for discussion.* London: HMSO.

Department of Health and Social Security. (1992). *The Health of the nation.* London: HMSO.

Department of Health and Social Security. (1992). *The Health of the nation . . . and you.* London: HMSO.

Diekemper, M., SmithBattle, L., & Drake, M. A. (1999). Bringing the population into focus: A natural development in community health nursing practice. Part 1. *Public Health Nursing, 16*(1), 3–10.

Donahue, J. M., & McGuire, M. (1995). The political economy of responsibility in health and illness. *Social Science and Medicine, 40*(1), 47–53.

Dreher, M. C. (1982). The conflict of conservatism in public health nursing education. *Nursing Outlook, 30*(6), 504–509.

Duncan, S. M. (1996). Empowerment strategies in nursing education: A foundation for population focused clinical studies. *Public Health Nursing, 13*(5), 311–317.

Dunn, J., & Hayes, M. V. (1999). Toward a lexicon of population health. *Canadian Journal of Public Health, 90*(Suppl. 1), S7–S10.

Edwards, N., & Craig, D. (1987). *Does nursing education reflect the goals of primary health care?* Hamilton, Ontario: McMaster University.

Epp, J. (1986). *Achieving health for all: A framework for health promotion.* Ottawa: Health and Welfare Canada.

Evans, R. G., Barer, M. L., & Marmor, T. R. (Eds.). (1994). *Why are some people healthy and some people not?* New York: Aldine de Gruyter.

Feather, N. T. (1982). *Expectations and actions: Expectancy-value models in psychology.* Hillsdale, NJ: Erlbaum.

Federal/Provincial/Territorial Advisory Committee on Population Health. (1994). *Strategies for population health: Investing in the health of Canadians.* Ottawa: Minister of Supply and Services Canada.

Federal/Provincial/Territorial Advisory Committee on Population Health. (1997, January). *Press release on population health.* January. Ottawa: Health Canada.

Foucault, M. (1972). *The archeology of knowledge.* New York: Random House.

Foucault, M. (1975). *The birth of the clinic: An archeology of medical perception.* New York: Random House.

Foucault, M. (1979). *Discipline and punish: The birth of the prison.* New York: Vantage.

Frank, J. (1995). Why 'population health'? *Canadian Journal of Public Health, 86*(3), 162–164.

Frohlich, K. L., & Potvin, L. (1999). Collective lifestyles as the target for health promotion. *Canadian Journal of Public Health, 90*(Suppl. 1), S11–S14.

Gibson, C. H. (1991). A concept analysis of empowerment. *Journal of Advanced Nursing, 16*(3), 354–361.

Gottleib, L. (1992). Nurses not heard in the health promotion movement. *Canadian Journal of Nursing Research, 24*(4), 1–2.

Green, L. W. (1994). Health promotion in Canada: An outsider's view from the inside. In A. Pederson, M. O'Neill, & I. Rootman (Eds.), *Health promotion in Canada: Provincial, national and international perspectives* (pp. 314–326). Toronto: W. B. Saunders.

Green, L. W., Richard, L., & Potvin, L. (1996). Ecological foundations of health promotion. *American Journal of Health Promotion, 10*(4), 270–281.

Green, L. W. (1999). Health education's contributions to public health in the twentieth century: A glimpse through health promotion's rear-view mirror. *Annual Review of Public Health, 20,* 67–88.

Green, L. W., & Raeburn, J. M. (1988). Health promotion. What is it? What will it become? *Health Promotion (International), 3*(2),151–159.

Green, L. W., & Kreuter, M. W. (1993). Are community organization and health promotion one process or two? *American Journal of Health Promotion, 7*(3), 221.

Hagan, L., O'Neill, M., & Dallaire, C. (1995). Linking health promotion and community health nursing: Conceptual and practical issues. In M. Stewart (Ed.), *Community nursing: Promoting Canadians' health* (pp. 413–429). Toronto: W. B. Saunders.

Hamilton, N., & Bhatti, T. (1996). *Population health promotion: An integrated model of population health and health promotion.* Ottawa: Health Canada, Health Promotion and Development Division.

Hancock, T. (1985). Beyond health care: From public health policy to healthy public policy. *Canadian Journal of Public Health, 76*(3, Suppl. 1), 9–11.

Health Canada. (1998). Health promotion in Canada—A case study. *Health Promotion International, 13*(1), 7–26.

Health Canada. (1998). *Taking action on population health.* Ottawa: Population Health Development Division.

Hills, M. D., & Lindsey, E. (1996). Health promotion: A viable curriculum framework for nursing education. *Nursing Outlook, 42*(4), 158–162.

Hills, M. (1998). Student experiences of nursing health promotion practice in hospital settings. *Nursing Inquiry, 5,* 164–173.

Hitchcock, J. E., Schubert, P. E., & Thomas, S. A. (1999). *Community health nursing: Caring in action.* Albany, NY: Delmar.

Hudson-Rodd, N. (1994). Public health: People participating in the creation of healthy places. *Public Health Nursing, 11*(2), 119–126.

Jewell, S. E. (1994). Patient participation: What does it mean to nurses? *Journal of Advanced Nursing, 19,* 433–438.

Jones, P. S., & Meleis, A. I. (1993). Health is empowerment. *Advances in Nursing Science, 15*(3), 1–14.

Kelly, M. P., & Charleton, B. (1995). The modern and the postmodern in health promotion. In R. Bunton, S. Nettleton, & R. Burrows (Eds.), *The sociology of health promotion: Critical analyses of consumption, lifestyle and risk* (pp. 78–90). London: Routledge.

Kendall, J. (1992). Fighting back: Promoting emancipatory nursing actions. *Advances in Nursing Science, 15*(2), 1–15.

Kickbush, I. (1989). Back to the future: Moving public health into the '90s. In P. Wolczuk, J. McDowell, & K. Ainslie (Eds.), *Proceedings from the national symposium on health promotion.* Victoria: British Columbia Ministry of Health.

Kickbush, I. (1994). Introduction: Tell me a story. In A. Pederson, M. O'Neill, & I. Rootman (Eds.), *Health promotion in Canada: Provincial, national and international perspectives* (pp. 8–17). Toronto: W. B. Saunders.

Kleffel, D. (1991). Rethinking the environment as a domain of nursing knowledge. *Advances in Nursing Science, 14*(1), 40–51.

Kulbok, P., Laffrey, S. C., & Goeppenger, J. (1995). Community health promotion: A multilevel framework for practice. In M. Stanhope & J. Lancaster (Eds.), *Community health nursing: Promoting the health of aggregates, families and individuals* (pp. 265–283). St. Louis: Mosby.

Kulbok, P., Baldwin, J. H., Cox, C. L., & Duffy, R. (1997). Advancing discourse on health promotion: Beyond mainstream thinking. *Advances in Nursing Science, 20*(1), 12–20.

Labonte, R., & Penfold, S. (1981). Canadian perspectives in health promotion: A critique. *Health Education, 19*(3/4), 4–9.

Labonte, R. (1993). *Health promotion and empowerment: Practice frameworks.* Toronto: Participaction and the Centre for Health Promotion.

Labonte, R. (1994). Death of program, birth of metaphor: The development of health promotion in Canada. In A. Pederson, M. O'Neill, & I. Rootman (Eds.), *Health promotion in Canada: Provincial, national and international perspectives* (pp. 72–90). Toronto: W. B. Saunders.

Labonte, R. (1995). Population health and health promotion: What do they have to say to each other? *Canadian Journal of Public Health, 86*(3), 165–168.

Lalonde, M. (1974). *A new perspective on the health of Canadians.* Ottawa: Health and Welfare Canada.

Latter, S. (1998). Nursing, health education, and health promotion: Lessons learned, progress made, and challenges ahead. *Health Education Research, 13*(2), i–iv.

Little, S., & Labonte, R. (1992). *Determinants of health: Empowering strategies for nursing practice.* Vancouver: Registered Nurses Association of British Columbia.

Lowenburg, J. S. (1995). Health promotion and the 'ideology of choice.' *Public Health Nursing, 12*(5), 319–323.

Lupton, D. (1995). *The imperative of health: Public health and the regulated body.* London: Sage.

Maben, J., & MacLeod Clark, J. (1995). Health promotion: A concept analysis. *Journal of Advanced Nursing, 22,* 1158–1165.

MacLeod Clark, J. (1993). From sick nursing to health nursing: evolution or revolution? In J. Wilson-Barnett & J. MacLeod Clark (Eds.), *Research in health promotion and nursing* (pp. 256–270). Basingstoke, England: MacMillan.

Maglacas, A. M. (1988). Health for all: Nursing's role. *Nursing Outlook, 36*(2), 66–71.

McKnight, J., & VanDover, L. (1994). Community as client: A challenge for nursing education. *Public Health Nursing, 11*(1), 12–16.

Minkler, M. (1989). Health education, health promotion and the open society: An historical perspective. *Health Education Quarterly, 16*(1), 17–30.

Moccia, P. (1988). At the faultline: Social activism and caring. *Nursing Outlook, 36*(1), 30–33.

Nettleton, S., & Bunton, R. (1995). Sociological critiques of health promotion. In R. Bunton, S. Nettleton, & R. Burrows (Eds.), *The sociology of health promotion: Critical analyses of consumption, lifestyle and risk* (pp. 41–58). London: Routledge.

Norton, L. (1998). Health promotion and health education: What role should nurses adopt in practice? *Journal of Advanced Nursing, 28*(6), 1269–1275.

Novak, J. (1988). The social mandate and historical basis for nursing's role in health promotion. *Journal of Professional Nursing, 4*(2), 80–87.

O'Brien, M. (1994). The managed heart revisited: Health and social control. *Sociological Review, 42*(3), 395–413.

O'Brien, M. (1995). Health and lifestyle—a critical mess? Notes on the dedifferentiation of health. In R. Bunton, S. Nettleton, & R. Burrows (Eds.). *The sociology of health promotion: Critical analyses of consumption, lifestyle and risk* (pp. 191–205). London: Routledge.

O'Neill, M. (1997). Health promotion: Issues for the year 2000. *Canadian Journal of Nursing Research, 29*(1), 71–77.

Parish, R. (1995). Health promotion: Rhetoric and reality. In R. Bunton, S. Nettleton, & R. Burrows (Eds.), *The sociology of health promotion: Critical analyses of consumption, lifestyle and risk* (pp.13–37). London: Routledge.

Pender, N. (1982). *Health promotion in nursing practice.* Norwalk, CT: Appleton-Century-Crofts.

Pender, N. (1996). *Health promotion in nursing practice.* (3rd edition). Stamford, CT: Appleton & Lange.

Pinder, L. (1994). The federal role in health promotion: Art of the possible. In A. Pederson, M. O'Neill, & I. Rootman (Eds.), *Health promotion in Canada: Provincial, national and international perspectives* (pp. 92–106). Toronto: W. B. Saunders.

Poland, B. (1992). Learning to walk our talk: The implications of sociological theory for research methodologies in health promotion. *Canadian Journal of Public Health, 83*(Suppl. 1), S31–S46.

Poland, B., Coburn, D., Eakin, J., & Robertson, A. (1998). Wealth, equity and health care: A critique of a 'population health' perspective on the determinants of health. *Social Science and Medicine, 46,* 85–98.

Raeburn, J. (1994). The view from down under: The impact of Canadian health promotion on developments in New Zealand. In A. Pederson, M. O'Neill, & I. Rootman (Eds.), *Health promotion in Canada: Provincial, national and international perspectives* (pp. 327–334). Toronto: W. B. Saunders.

Rafael, A.R.F. (1999). The politics of health promotion: Influences on public health promoting nursing practice in Ontario, Canada from Nightingale to the Nineties. *Advances in Nursing Science, 22*(1), 23–39.

Registered Nurses Association of British Columbia. (1990). *Primary health care: A discussion document.* Vancouver: Author.

Ritchie, L., Boutell, B., Buchan, C., Foster, P., & St. Aubrey, M. (1995). Practicing what we preach. *Nursing BC,* November–December, 14–16.

Robertson, A. (1998). Shifting discourses on health in Canada: From health promotion to population health. *Health Promotion International, 13*(2), 155–166.

Robertson, A., & Minkler, M. (1994). New health promotion movement: A critical examination. *Health Education Quarterly, 21*(3), 295–312.

Robinson, S., & Hill, Y. (1995). Miracles take a little longer: Project 2000 and the health-promoting nurse. *International Journal of Nursing Studies, 432*(6), 568–579.

Rodwell, C. M. (1996). An analysis of the concept of empowerment. *Journal of Advanced Nursing, 23,* 305–313.

Roger, G., & Gallagher, S. (1995). The move toward primary health care in Canada: Community health nursing from 1985 to 1995. In M. Stewart (Ed.), *Community nursing: Promoting Canadians' health* (pp. 37–58). Toronto: W. B. Saunders.

Rush, K. (1997). Health promotion ideology and nursing education. *Journal of Advanced Nursing, 25,* 1292–1298.

Ryan, W. (1971). *Blaming the victim.* New York: Pantheon.

Schoultz, J., & Hatcher, P. A. (1997). Looking beyond primary care to primary health care: An approach to community-based action. *Nursing Outlook, 45,* 23–26.

Schultz, P. R. (1987). When client means more than one: Extending the foundational concept of person. *Advances in Nursing Science, 10*(1), 71–86.

Seedhouse, D. (1997). *Health promotion: Philosophy, prejudice and practice.* Chichester, England: Wiley.

Sherwin, S. (1992). *No longer patient: Feminist ethics and health care.* Philadelphia: Temple University Press.

Sills, G. M., & Goeppinger, J. (1985). The community as a field of inquiry in nursing. *Annual Review of Nursing, 3,* 3–23.

Skelton, R. (1994). Nursing and empowerment: Concepts and strategies. *Journal of Advanced Nursing, 19,* 415–423.

Skrabanek, P. (1992). Politics and ideology of health promotion. *Medical Audit News, 2*(6), 82–83.

Smith, J. A. (1981). The idea of health: A philosophical inquiry. *Advances in Nursing Science, 3*(3), 43–50.

Smith, M. C. (1990). Nursing's unique focus on health promotion. *Nursing Science Quarterly, 3*(1), 105–106.

SmithBattle, L., Drake, M. A., & Diekemper, M. (1997.). The responsive use of self in community health nursing. *Advances in Nursing Science, 20*(2), 75–89.

Starzomski, R., & Rodney, P. (1997). Nursing inquiry for the common good. In S. E. Thorne & V. Hayes (Eds.), *Nursing praxis: Knowledge and action* (pp. 219–236). Thousand Oaks, CA: Sage.

Stevens, P. E. (1989). A critical social reconceptualization of environment in nursing: Implications for methodology. *Advances in Nursing Science, 11*(4), 56–68.

Stevens, P. E., & Hall, J. (1992). Applying critical theories to nursing in communities. *Public Health Nursing, 9*(1), 2–9.

Stevenson, H. M., & Burke, M. (1992). Bureaucratic logic in new social movement clothing: The limits of health promotion research. *Canadian Journal of Public Health, 83*(Suppl. 1), S47–S53.

Stokols, D. (1992). Establishing and maintaining healthy environments: Toward a social ecology of health promotion. *American Psychologist, 41,* 141–168.

Styles, M. (1994). Empowerment: A vision for nursing. *International Journal of Nursing Studies, 41*(3), 77–80.

Task Force Report on Health Promotion and Consumer Health Education (1976). *Preventive Medicine USA.* New York: Prodist.

Terris, M. (1976). The epidemiological revolution, national health insurance, and the role of health departments. *American Journal of Public Health, 66,* 1155–1164.

Thorne, S., Canam, C., Dahinten, S., Hall, W., Henderson, A., & Reimer, S. (1998). Nursing's metaparadigm concepts: Disimpacting the debates. *Journal of Advanced Nursing, 27,* 1257–1268.

U.S. Department of Health, Education and Welfare. (1976). *Forward plan for health, FY 1978–82.* (DHEW Publication No. OS 76–50046). Washington, DC: U.S. Public Health Service.

U.S. Department of Health, Education and Welfare. (1979). *Healthy people: The Surgeon General's report on health promotion and disease prevention.* (DHEW Publication No. 79–55071). Washington, DC: U.S. Government Printing Office.

U.S. Department of Health, Education and Welfare. (1980). *Promoting health/preventing disease: Objectives for the nation.* Washington, DC: U.S. Government Printing Office.

U.S. Department of Health, Education and Welfare. (1986). *1990 Objectives for the Nation: A midcourse review.* Washington, DC: U.S. Government Printing Office.

U.S. Department of Health, Education and Welfare. (1990). *Healthy people 2000: National health promotion and disease prevention objectives* (DHHS Publication No. PHS 91–50213). Washington, DC: U.S. Government Printing Office.

Veal, A. J. (1993). The concept of lifestyle: A review. *Leisure Studies, 12,* 233–252.

Watson, J. (1990). The moral failure of the patriarchy. *Nursing Outlook, 38*(2), 62–66.

Weber, M. (1948). Class, status and party. In H. Gerth & C. W. Mills (Eds.), *From Max Weber* (pp. 180–195). New York: Oxford University Press.

Whitelaw, S., McKeown, K., & Williams, J. (1997). Global health promotion models: Enlightenment or entrapment. *Health Education Research, 12*(4), 479–490.

Wikler, D. (1978). Persuasion and coercion for health: Ethical issues in government efforts to change life-styles. *Millbank Memorial Fund Quarterly/Health and Society, 56*(3), 303–338.

Williams, D. M. (1989). Political theory and individualistic health promotion. *Advances in Nursing Science, 12*(1), 14–25.

World Health Organization (1977). *Health for All by the Year 2000.* Geneva: Author.

World Health Organization. (1978a). *Primary health care: Report of the international conference on primary health care.* Alma-Ata, USSR. Geneva: Author.

World Health Organization. (1978b). The Alma-Ata conference on primary health care. *WHO Chronicle, 32*(11), 409–430.

World Health Organization. (1981). *Regional strategy for attaining health for all by the year 2000.* Copenhagen: Author.

World Health Organization. (1984). *Health promotion: A discussion document on the concepts and principles.* Copenhagen: WHO Regional Office for Europe.

World Health Organization. (1985). *Targets for health for all.* Copenhagen: WHO Regional Office for Europe.

World Health Organization (1986). *Ottawa Charter for health promotion.* Ottawa: Canadian Public Health Association & Health and Welfare Canada.

Zöllner, H., & Lessor, S. (1998). *Population health— Putting concepts into action.* Copenhagen: WHO Regional Office for Europe.

SECTION TWO

Key Concepts for Transforming Health Promotion Practice

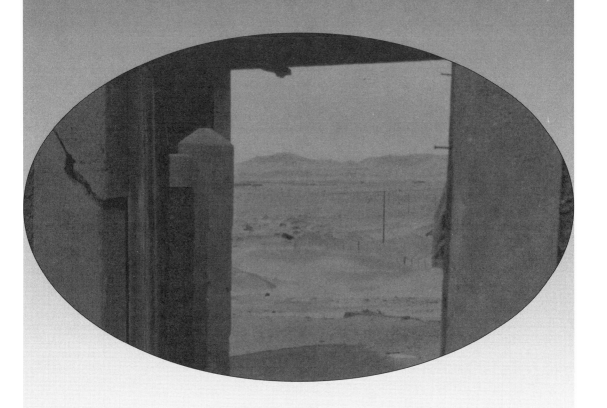

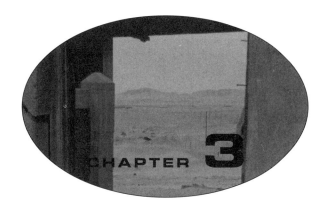

Beyond Interpersonal Communication: The Significance of Relationship in Health Promoting Practice

GWEN HARTRICK

A few years ago I attended a forum focused on improving communication between women with breast cancer and their health care providers. The opening speaker, who was a physician, began by showing two slides. The first was a microscopic view of breast cancer cells. As we observed this first slide the speaker commented that if he were to ask the physicians in the room about how this breast cancer might best be treated, the responses would in all likelihood be fairly similar. Although there might be slight variations, there were relatively standard treatment protocols and interventions for the type of breast cancer shown on the slide. The second slide was of a woman standing in a garden of flowers. Her smile was as radiant as the sun that was shining on her. As the speaker projected this second slide on the screen, he looked up at the audience and stated, "This is the woman whose breast cancer you just saw—and this is where the difference in treatment begins."

For me, this distinction cuts to the core of the matter. Governed by an ethic of cure, "health" care has all too often focused on the treatment and cure of physical disease, while the people living those diseases have gone unacknowledged. Standard treatments have been "applied" and "prescribed," and there has been little room for people and their uniqueness. Fortunately, times are changing. Our expanded understand-

ing of health has led to the recognition that disease-treatment models of care are limited in the promotion of health and healing. It is now understood that people's experiences of health go far beyond the absence of disease (World Health Organization, 1986). Health is an experience constructed through relationships with others and a shared repertoire of intersubjective meanings (Labonte, 1993). Health is a resource for living and encompasses choice, the ability to realize aspirations, and to exercise control in one's life (WHO, 1986).

This broader view of health has had profound implications for health practitioners. Defining health as encompassing far more than the absence of disease means that methods of practice that have been appropriate for disease care may not be viable (Barr & Cochran, 1992; Bopp, 1989; Choi, 1985; Cochran, 1990; Epp, 1986; Hartrick, 1997a; Labonte, 1989; Lord & Farlow, 1990; Maglacas, 1988; McKnight, 1989; WHO, 1986). As the opening example highlights, treating disease does not address people's meaningful experience and the effect that experience has on their overall health. Consequently, health practitioners are being required to transform their conventional ways of thinking and behaving (Bopp, 1989; Hartrick, Lindsey, & Hills, 1994; Lindsey & Hartrick, 1996). Although this transformative process has been underway for sometime, in observing the everyday practice of health practitioners the dominance of disease-treatment perspective is, at times, still apparent. One particular place where I have observed this dominance of the disease-care perspective is in the domain of relational practice. Although we have begun emphasizing "collaborative" and "power-with" client-practitioner relationships, assumptions underlying relational practice often comply with a disease-treatment perspective.

In this chapter I wish to challenge some of these assumptions that currently dominate relational practice. I define relational practice as a humanely involved process of respectful, compassionate, and authentically interested inquiry into people's experiences. Relational practice involves a way of being with people that is mutual and collaborative. My intent in highlighting relational practice within discussions of health promotion is to encourage readers to look beyond the disease-care legacy that may be constraining their relational practices. In moving beyond the disease-care legacy, it becomes possible to examine how relational practice might be reconstituted to be more in keeping with a philosophy of **health promotion**.

Health Promoting Practice: A Relational Ontology

To become more health promoting, Labonte (1989) contends that health professionals need to relate to, and abide by, a philosophy of health promotion rather than a specific process or method. According to Labonte, a philosophy of health promotion serves as the driving force behind any decision making and any action. Hartrick and associates (1994) summarize the central beliefs found within the health promotion literature that serve as a foundation for a health promoting philosophy. In discussing these beliefs, Hartrick and colleagues highlight that a health promoting philosophy emphasizes the ontological foundation of practice. At the core of health promotion is a "way-of-being" that is relational.

In essence, a philosophy of health promotion gives birth to a relational ontology. This relational way-of-being transforms the nature of client-practitioner relationships. The conventional disease-treatment relationship of expert practitioner and compliant patient is

supplanted with a more egalitarian, participatory form of alliance. However, in following a philosophy of health promotion, practitioners do not just *act* collaboratively, they *become* collaborators.

Although a philosophy of health promotion decrees a relational way-of-being, further examination of the qualities and attributes of a health promoting relational way-of-being is required. Up to this point discussions of relational practice in health promotion have tended to focus on the *role* health practitioners play. The *constitution* of relational practice in health promotion has received less attention. Given the significance of "relational being" in the philosophy and practice of health promotion, further examination of the beliefs and assumptions that shape our understanding of (1) what constitutes a relational way-of-being, and (2) the nature and purpose of relational practice in health promotion is warranted.

Re-examining Our Assumptions of Relational Practice

> ### ✳ Reflective Questions
>
> Take a piece of paper and write down what you have learned or believe about client-practitioner relationships. For example:
>
> **1.** What does a positive relationship look like?
> **2.** What knowledge or ability do health practitioners need to be able to form positive relationships with clients?
> **3.** What is the purpose in forming those relationships?
> **4.** Why are relationships important in health promotion?

As I have taught health practitioners about relational practice, I have found that the beliefs and assumptions people bring to their practice shape the way they *are* in relationships. I have found that there are certain fundamental assumptions about relational "being/practice" that shape people's practices. In particular, there are three assumptions that emerge from the disease-treatment perspective that continue to flourish and at the same time profoundly hinder people's ability to move beyond disease care relationships to health promoting ones. These hindering assumptions include:

1. Practitioners engage in relationships as a "means to an end."
2. Relationships are helpful but not absolutely essential to the health care process.
3. Communication skills are the foundation for relational practice.

Let us examine each of these assumptions on the basis of what we know about health promotion.

Assumption 1: Relationships Are a "Means to An End"

As a result of our disease-treatment legacy, many people continue to assume that health care relationships between clients and health practitioners are a "means to an end." This assumption is also still present in many of the educational textbooks and in some professional literature. Relationships are conceptualized, and talked about, as tools or mediums that can be used in the daily work of health practitioners to improve their care of clients. Novice health practitioners learn that relationships and good communication can facilitate health care assessment, intervention and treatment, and health care outcomes. Relationships and good communication are valued for what they can provide or ultimately produce (e.g., less psychological distress, more information for assessment, and so forth).

In considering this assumption in light of what we have come to understand about health promotion, the incongruities quickly become apparent. Although in disease care the health practitioner is the chief actor engaged in assessment, diagnosis, and treatment, and might therefore "use" communication and relationship to strategically support their "expert" intervention, in health promotion people are the chief actors and at the center of any health initiative (Choi, 1985; Labonte, 1993; Lindsey & Hartrick, 1996). This means that health practitioners are no longer the ones in charge of and "doing" the relating. Rather, health promotion involves a mutual process of client-practitioner engagement. Con-

tinuing to think of relationships as being under the power of health practitioners obscures the essential mutuality of health promoting relationships.

Because relationships are not wielded or controlled by health practitioners, they no longer serve as a "means to an end"; that is, relating is no longer the property of the expert practitioner. Relationships do not provide a "tool" or "strategy" for achieving a particular outcome. Moreover, conceiving of relationship as a means to an end may well hinder the mutual process of inquiry and action that health promoting relational practice *is.* Continuing to value relationships because they provide a means to an end conceals the inherent experiential worth of relationship. The relational experience is, in and of itself, health promoting. That is, our understanding of the empowerment process has underscored the potentially humanizing value in even brief and task-focused relational connections. As Jordan (1997a) describes, the deepest sense of one self is formed in relation with others. Human experience is relational. Although relationships may well promote certain outcomes, *their most significant value is the intrinsic connectedness people experience when they are in-relation.*

Assumption 2: Relationship Is Not Essential to the Health Care Process

Just as people have not been included as an essential part of the disease-treatment process, if one listens to the way some health practitioners and educators talk, one can often hear an underlying assumption that health care can occur without a relationship. Although often not spoken directly, the assumption that it is possible to provide care without relationally engaging with the person is played out everyday by health practitioners who may describe themselves as "too busy" and having "no time" to meaningfully engage with the people they care for. The emergency room nurse who has numerous other tasks that need completing and hurriedly goes in to assess "the abdominal pain in bed two" or the community health nurse with a heavy caseload who focuses on the postnatal visit checklist and never really stops to determine if that checklist is what is relevant to the woman or mother she is visiting provide a couple of examples.

It is not difficult to see how this assumption, and the subsequent practice it fosters, have been supported within a disease-treatment model of care (e.g., it might seem possible to treat malignant cells, diagnose appendicitis, or check for engorged breasts without being "in-relation"). However, in assuming that relational practice is dispensable, health practitioners often ignore the relational flow that is occurring. As a result, they fail to see the influence relationship is having on health and health promotion.

An example of the power of relationship and the short time the meaningful relational connection may take is exemplified in an example provided to me by a former student. This emergency room nurse described how she had found that taking a couple of seconds to relationally connect with someone as they were being wheeled into the department from an ambulance seemed to make a difference to what transpired for both the person and herself. The meaningful connection they both experienced in those few seconds transformed the emergency experience. For example, she said that when she willed herself to relationally connect even for a few seconds (regardless of how busy she was), many of the people she cared for seemed less anxious or less affected by the noise and busyness of the department. In addition, the overall time patients needed her actually seemed to decrease. Overall, her relational experience had convinced her that her ability to provide responsive and meaningful care to people living through an emergency experience was profoundly enhanced by a seemingly minor relational connection.

Willed or Not, Health Promoting Practice Is Relational

Whether practitioners are aware or not, relationship is operating in all situations, spontaneously weaving between people (Perlman, 1979; Robinson, 1996). Relationship may be ignored or it may be recognized and responded to, but it is always present and influential. As such, relationships can have an empowering or disempowering influence on people and health, just as in the emergency room nurse's example, where the nurse's choice to be-in-relation affected people's capacity to live in the chaos and stress of a busy emergency department.

Assumption 3: Communication Skills Are the Foundation for Relational Relating

Just as people have been objectified and reduced to a disease or problem, relational practice has been objectified (taken out of human experience) and reduced to discrete, externally applied communication skills (Hartrick, 1997b, Hartrick, 1999). Many people assume that learning and using particular behaviors lead to good relationships. However, the attributes of human relating extend far deeper into human experience than behavioral skills (Arndt, 1992; Gadow, 1985; Hartrick, 1997b; Montgomery, 1993; Watson, 1988). *Human relating* is a caring process that involves values, intent, knowledge, commitment, and actions (Watson, 1988). The emergency room nurse did not focus on using behavioral skills, but rather intentionally chose to be-in-relation with the people she cared for. Although communication skills may aid the development of relationship, the ability to be in "caring-relation" requires far more than the refinement of behavioral communication skills. It *requires an appreciation of people's connectedness, the development of relational awareness, and an interest in the movement of relationship* (Jordan, 1989). As such, I suggest that health promotion requires that we move beyond thinking of human relating as the behavior that separate people engage in. Since health promotion involves relationship and the relational flow of connection, to speak of "interpersonal" practice is no longer viable. In health promotion, interpersonal practice is reconstituted as relational practice.

Reconstituting Relational Practice: *Being* Health Promoting

As we analyze the taken-for-granted assumptions that continue to govern relational practice and reveal the disease care vestiges that continue to be embedded within them, the need to reconstitute our practice to be relational becomes clear. Whether or not practitioners are aware of the relational experience, health promotion is a relational process. Moreover, health promoting relational practice requires us to let go of our expert emphasis on trusty tools and techniques and open ourselves up to a "relational way-of-being" that is health promoting.

Our quest to reconstitute our relational way-of-being may be aided by letting go of the behavioral models of relationship that emphasize communication skills. These models of relationship continue to constrain our understanding of relational practice (Jordan, 1997b; Miller, 1986). Turning to theoretical perspectives that emphasize the relational nature of "being" may foster the development of more relational practices.

Quantum physics (Capra, 1976; Gleick, 1987) and complexity theory (Prigogine & Stenger, 1984) may be of particular significance during our reconstituting process. Complexity theory *is* a theory of relationship. The fundamental idea in complexity theory is that all things in nature are interrelated. This "new science" provides a foundation for a clearer understanding of the universe as interdependent and relational, where the observer cannot be separated from the observed. "In the quantum world, relationships are not just interesting; to many physicists, they are *all* there is to reality" (Wheatley, 1994). Similarly, in health promotion, relationships are not just helpful, they are its essence.

Learning From the "New Science"

Discoveries and theories within the "new science" have called into question many of the fundamental assumptions that have governed our understandings of "the way things are." Emerging from the fields of physics, mathematics, and engineering, complexity theory has been used to challenge taken-for-granted perspectives within the social sciences and humanities as well as the physical sciences. Although we do not want to repeat our original mistake of using the theory derived from the physical sciences as a foundation for developing human and social science practices, complexity theory can be helpful as we attempt to move beyond the assumptions that currently dominate relational practice in health promotion.

In particular, considering complexity theory within the context of relational practice may help us step out of our linear thinking about relationships and generate questions that might help us re-envision health promoting relational practice. For example, in nursing, Ray (1994) contends that reexamination of nursing practice within the "new science theory" promises to revolutionize nursing science. Ray contends that concepts advanced in complexity science are consistent with concepts presented in the nursing literature including relationality, belongingness, holism, value, purpose, and choice. Similarly, in psychology the work of the Stone Center (Jordan, 1997b), which has served to challenge the dualistic perspective of the autonomous self and the subject-object relationship, is complementary to concepts within complexity theory. Jordan contends that the Stone Center's new relational theory is similar to the new physics in that it "emphasizes the contextual, approximate, responsive and process factors in experience" (p. 15).

While I do not intend to present a discussion of complexity theory (many others have provided full discussions (e.g., Capra, 1976; Chopra, 1989; Gleick, 1987; Mark, 1994; Prigogine & Stenger, 1984; Ray, 1994; Wheatley, 1994; Zohar, 1990), I wish to highlight certain ideas or principles within complexity theory that might be helpful to contemplate as we begin to reconstitute our relational practices. I present these ideas as "food for thought." It is not my goal to present a reconstituted model of health promoting relational practice. I believe the reconstituting process must be a personal one that occurs as practitioners inquire into their own relational practices. Rather, my intent in highlighting ideas from complexity theory is to "push the envelope" of our thinking about relational practice so we may see beyond the disease-care assumptions that limit us.

In essence, I present the meaning *I* have made of ideas within this theoretical perspective. It is not meant to be representative of complexity theory; my description of the ideas is a reconstruction that does not do justice to the intricacies of the theory itself. I have reconstituted the ideas to have relevance for my health promoting relational practice. I encourage readers to engage with the ideas as they may be pertinent to their own relational practices. However, for knowledge of complexity theory you will no doubt want to read elsewhere.

Complexity Theory: Some Transforming Ideas

In discussing the significance of complexity theory for health promoting relational practice, I will discuss four ideas or assertions emerging from complexity theory that seem particularly relevant: (1) relationship is it, (2) people always act in relationship to something else, (3) relationships are seamless fabrics, and (4) relationships evoke a potential that is already present.

Relationship Is It

Pause for a moment and try to think of a time when you are not in-relation. Although you can probably think of many solitary activities, further scrutiny will reveal that in each of these activities you are still in-relation with something or someone. For example, during a solitary walk in the forest you are in-relation with nature, while reading a book you are in-relation with the text, even during meditation you are living in-relation with larger forces of energy.

This relational nature of life is one of the central premises of complexity theory. Complexity theory asserts that nothing exists independent of its relationship to something else. According to complexity theory, the influence of this relational connection may be subtle or more profoundly felt. A well-known example from complexity theory that demonstrates the significance of relationship is the "butterfly effect." Complexity theory posits that the beat of a butterfly's wing could trigger a breath of breeze that eventually, through a series of initially minute and unforeseeable changes, could become a tornado (Vicenzi, White, & Begun, 1997). The path and force of this "breath-tornado" is determined by a complex number of variables. Minute changes to the initial conditions of one or more of the variables could dramatically change the path and force of the breeze. The actual "outcome" of the beat of the butterfly's wing is ultimately determined by an infinite number of variables and their relational interactions.

The butterfly effect reflects the sensitivity of living systems to other living systems. In addition, it emphasizes the unpredictability and nonlinearity of cause and effect. One small fluctuation in one variable can dramatically change the outcome of something else. Yet, the variables are so many, and the complexity of interactions so great, that the subsequent outcomes can never be fully known or predicted.

As I have thought about this "butterfly effect" within the context of people's experiences of health and health promotion, many thoughts have occurred. First, I have been reminded of the World Health Organization's (1986) emphasis on the social determinants of health. For me, it underscores how people's experiences of health are interrelated, and affected by, everything else in their living world. Second, the butterfly effect highlights the natural relational connection between people. As Buber (1958) has described, we are "relational beings." Although we cannot predict the effect one person will have on another, people live in constant relation and are continuously affected by those relationships. However, the effect of those relationships may not be recognized or known.

A third aspect that has resonated with my experience in health promoting relationships is the idea that the effect of one person's action may not be in proportion to the effect on the other. That is, the butterfly effect tells us that the smallest action of one may have dramatic effects on the other, whereas seemingly greater actions may have relatively little effect. Because the response is determined by a multitude of complex variables, the same relational connection may also have different effects at different times.

As I read complexity theory and think about past experiences with clients, I realize that I have observed this "butterfly effect" many times in my practice. There have been times when my deeply concerted actions have had little effect, and other times when I have seen a seemingly brief connection have a transforming effect on someone else. Although there has seemed to be "little relationship" between how I have been or what I have done and the outcome for the person, I now realize that perhaps it was not a matter of the degree of relationship. Rather, I was assuming a predictable, linear cause-and-effect outcome. Predictably, if I do "this," then "that" should occur.

Realizing that relationships are not linear or predictable has highlighted the subtlety and potential of relational practice. In realizing that "relationship is it," as a health promoting practitioner I have developed a heightened sensitivity to relationship, paying close attention to my relational responsiveness. I do not act to effect a certain outcome, but instead consciously focus on the relational flow between myself and others.

I have also approached my practice with new questions in mind. I invite the readers to consider some of the questions I have pondered.

✺ Reflective Questions

1. How might I honor the relational nature of people's health and healing experiences?
2. How might I better support the complexity of health experiences and the patterns of connection that foster them?
3. If I cannot effectively predict and control the outcomes, how might I *be* health promoting?

Overall, as I have become clearer in my belief that "relationship is it," I have moved beyond wanting to "use" relationships. My intent as a health promoting practitioner has transformed: I now seek to join with people to *become* part of the power and potential of the relational flow of health.

People Act in Relationship to Something Else

Complexity theory informs us that we live in a participative universe; that is, people always act in relationship to something else (Zohar, 1990). Consequently, each person presents different aspects of herself or himself in different places and in different relationships. This does not mean people are inauthentic; they are merely quantum (Wheatley, 1994). Take a minute to think about this idea within your own life. For example, have you found that you are different in different situations or with different people?

Because we always act in relationship to something else, it follows that our acts of observation are always in relation to that which we are observing; that is, we influence and in some way determine what we observe. Put in quantum theory terms, quantum matter develops a relationship with the observer, and matter is changed in the process of observation. This means that although we do not create reality, we are essential to what reality is drawn forth.

This participatory nature of being and observing has highlighted the influence *I* have on the health promotion process and on what *I* experience. I have come to understand that what I observe in others is profoundly influenced by me. Similarly, others draw forth differing aspects of me. In recognizing that I can influence what is drawn forth, I have become more conscious in my observations and in my interpretations. Specifically, I have begun to envision health promotion as a relational process that seeks to "draw forth health." For example, when I work with a family to develop an allergen-free environment for their child with asthma, I look to see how they are promoting a more healthful environment rather than looking at what they are not doing. In essence, through my observations I draw forth and highlight their capacity. At the same time, I attempt to build on that already existing capacity.

In this drawing-forth process, I see myself as comparable to a traveling companion on an uncertain journey (Spreen Parker, 1990). Wheatley's metaphor of playing jazz music helped me image my health promoting relational practice. Like the jazz musician, I—as a health practitioner—am in-relation with each and *take part* in selecting the melody, setting the tempo, establishing the key and inviting other players. After that, the music is not something I can direct; it is a unique sound created through the unified relational whole.

As a public health nurse who wants to prevent a measles outbreak, I might offer an information session for parents to provide information about measles, immunization, and its effects. However, parents will choose individually whether they will attend. In addition, each parent who attends will hear and interpret the information somewhat differently. Different parents will find different information relevant, confusing, informative, and so forth. On the basis of what each parent "draws forth" and what I and the other parents "draw forth" in each other, different questions will be asked, different examples will be used, the overall meeting will be shorter or longer, and so forth. Because of this relational-way-of-being, each information session I participate in will have a different sound, rhythm, tempo, and so forth. Furthermore, the results of the information session cannot be predicted or controlled. For example, parents will make decisions about immunization in relation with everything else in their world and lives.

Relationships Are Seamless Fabrics

Because "relationship is all there is" (Wheatley, 1994), the focus of science (and health practice) shifts from description and explanation, prediction and control, to supporting dynamic connectedness. As Jantsch (1980) declares, in life the issue is not control, but dynamic connectedness. These two words "dynamic connectedness" are key to the way relationship is conceptualized; that is, within complexity theory relationships are considered process structures that connect. These structures maintain form over time, yet have no rigidity; rather, they are dynamic and ever-changing. The flow of relationship is like a seamless fabric, where boundaries are elusive and ever-changing.

As I have thought about relationship as a seamless fabric and taken this idea into relational health promotion, I have found myself looking more at the whole. For example, while I might be listening to an individual describe a health concern, I find myself listening beyond the separateness of the individual. In so doing, I find I hear (draw forth) the larger life experience. I begin to hear of the interrelatedness of people's experiences—how their health concern is related to their personal aspirations, life patterns, and life challenges. Using the example of working with a family to create an allergen-free environment, I listen for how the changes necessary to create this environment will have an impact on their life overall. Do they have the financial resources to make the changes? What will the extra housework required to maintain a dust-free environment mean given their busy family and work life? How does their relational connection to the larger community influence the situation? Overall, in understanding relationship as a seamless fabric, I no longer see separate individuals with health concerns. Instead, I see people and health experiences as part of a coherent whole. My relational field of vision (Wheatley, 1994) draws forth a more holistic view, helps me let go of goals and preselected destinations (that I realize I cannot control or predict anyway),

and simultaneously provides a clarity of purpose. Because people are received as the relational beings they are, a clarity of purpose and direction for health promotion emerges.

Relationships Evoke a Potential That Is Already Present

Complexity theory speaks of power as the capacity generated through relationships. According to Wheatley (1994), power is an energy that can come into existence only through relationships. In essence, relationship is a catalyst in the support, nurturance, and freeing of people's energies (Perlman, 1979). Relationships may be brief, transitory, even one time. What gives power its charge (negative or positive) is the quality of relationships (Wheatley, 1994). Relationships of respect and openness create a positive energy and serve as potent sources of power.

Complexity theory's emphasis on the pivotal force of relationship in the generation of energy and power has underscored the importance of relationship to my health promoting practice. With empowerment being a fundamental element in the promotion of health (RNABC, 1992), I strive to foster opportunities for people to feel and become more empowered in their life and health experiences. Complexity theory reminds me that empowerment occurs through relationships, and that the potential for empowerment lies within respectful, authentic relationships. Through these relationships people and their experiences of health are transformed. "Connections of different kinds alternate or overlap or combine and thereby determine the texture of the whole" (Heisenberg, 1958, p. 107).

Overall, complexity theory has clarified the tension between "going with the flow of relationship" and "mandating for change." Although I have always believed that being in-relation to receive people as they are is the most powerful way in which change is promoted, at times I find myself pulled into "changing" actions.

In reading complexity theory, it has become clearer to me that what I have difficulty with is letting go of the "predictability" that is assumed in advocating for change. When one sets oneself up as a change agent, there is an embedded assumption that change is controllable and predictable; that is, if I set out as a change agent, it is likely that something will change. In contrast, if I do not set out to change something, nothing will change. Complexity theory informs me that the power for change does not lie within *me*, but in the relationships between others and myself. Furthermore, there is no predictability to change, nor can change be controlled. As I have come to recognize the complexity of change, and the relational nature of the change process, I have gradually moved beyond looking toward "change." I have shifted my focus away from predictability toward *potential*. In practice I now question how I might foster the power and energy that potentially lies within people as they *are* in health promoting relation.

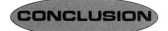

CONCLUSION

Complexity theory reveals that we are relational beings living in a relational world. The whole of the earth rests in relations of deep interdependency (Jardine, 1990). As we live in our participative universe of relationships our experiences of health flow out of a dynamic connectedness with our living world. This dynamic connectedness highlights the power and potential of relationships in the flow of health. As we let go of the disease-care assumptions that have constrained our ability to practice relationally and move beyond a fragmented view of relational practice, we can begin to see that relationships are far more than "means to an end." Realizing the potential of "relational being" fosters our ability to *become* more health promoting in our practice and to enhance the creative health promoting process that *is* relational.

REFERENCES

Arndt, M. J. (1992). Caring as everydayness. *Journal of Holistic Nursing, 10*(4), 285–293.

Barr, D., & Cochran, M. (1992). Understanding and supporting empowerment: Redefining the professional role. *Networking Bulletin Empowerment and Family Support, 2*(3), 1–9.

Bopp, M. (1989, March). Spiritual barriers to health promotion. *Proceedings of the National Symposium on Health Promotion and Disease Prevention*, Victoria, B.C. (pp. 91–96).

Buber, M. (1958). *I and thou*. New York: Scribner.

Capra, F. (1976). *The tao of physics*. New York: Bantam.

Cartwright, T. J. (1991, winter). Planning and chaos theory. *American Psychological Association Journal*, 44–56.

Chopra, D. (1989). *Quantum healing: Exploring the frontiers of mind and body science*. New York: Bantam.

Choi, M. W. (1985). Preamble to a new paradigm for women's health care. *Image: The Journal of Nursing Scholarship, 17*(1), 14–16.

Cochran, M. (1990). *Empowerment and family support*. Speech given to the Mayor's Task Force on Children and Families. Victoria, B.C.

Doll, W. E. (1993). *The post-modern perspective on curriculum*. New York: Teachers College Press.

Epp, J. (1986). *Achieving health for all: A framework for health promotion*. Ottawa: Minister of Supply and Services.

Gadow, S. (1985). Nurse and patient: The caring relationship. In A. H. Bishop & J. R. Scudder (Eds.), *Caring, curing, coping* (pp. 31–43). Tuscaloosa, Alabama: University of Alabama Press.

Gleick, J. (1987). *Chaos: Making a new science*. New York: Viking.

Gribbin, J. (1984). *In search of Schroedinger's cat: Quantum physics and reality*. New York: Bantam.

Hartrick, G. A. (1999). Transcending Behaviorism in Communication Education. *Journal of Nursing Education, 38*(1), 17–22.

Hartrick, G. A. (1997a). Beyond a service model of care: Health promotion and the enhancement of family capacity. *Journal of Family Nursing, 3*(1), 36–56.

Hartrick, G. A. (1997b). Relational capacity: The foundation for interpersonal nursing practice. *Journal of Advanced Nursing, 26*, 523–528.

Hartrick, G. A., Lindsey, A. E., & Hills, M. (1994). Family nursing assessment: Meeting the challenge of health promotion. *Journal of Advanced Nursing, 20*, 85–91.

Heisenberg, W. (1958). *Physics and philosophy*. New York: Harper Torchbooks.

Jantsch, E. (1980). *The self-organizing universe*. Oxford: Pergamon.

Jardine, D. (1990). To dwell with a boundless heart: On the integrated curriculum and the recovery of the earth. *Journal of Curriculum and Supervision, 5*(2), 107–119.

Jordan, J. (1989). *Relational development: Therapeutic implications of empathy and shame*. Wellesley, MA: Stone Center.

Jordan, J. (1997a). A relational perspective for understanding women's development. In J. Jordan (Ed.), *Women's growth in diversity. More writings from the Stone Center*. New York: Guilford Press.

Jordan, J. (1997b). *Women's growth in diversity. More writings from the Stone Center*. New York: Guilford Press.

Labonte, R. (1989). *Health promotion and empowerment: Practice frameworks*. Toronto: Centre for Health Promotion, University of Toronto.

Labonte, R. (1993). *Health promotion and empowerment: Practice frameworks* (Issues in Health Promotion

Series #3). Toronto: Centre for Health Promotion, University of Toronto.

Lindsey, A. E., & Hartrick, G. (1996). Health promoting nursing practice: The demise of the nursing process. *Journal of Advanced Nursing, 23*, 106–112.

Lord, J., & Farlow, D. A. (1990). A study of personal empowerment: Implications for health promotion. *Health Promotion, 10*, 2–8.

Maglacas, A. M. (1988). Health for all: Nursing's role. *Nursing Outlook, 36*(2), 66–71.

Mark, B. (1994). Chaos theory and nursing systems research. *Theoretic and Applied Chaos in Nursing, 1*(1), 7–14.

McKnight, J. (1989). Do no harm: Policy options that meet human needs. *Social Policy, 20*(1), 5–15.

Miller, J. B. (1986). *What do we mean by relationships?* (Work in Progress No. 22) Wellesley, MA: Stone Center Working Paper Series.

Montgomery, C. L. (1993). *Healing through communication. The practice of caring.* Newbury Park, CA: Sage.

Perlman, H. (1979). *Relationships: The heart of helping people.* Chicago: University of Chicago Press.

Prigogine, I., & Stenger, I. (1984). *Order out of chaos.* Toronto: Bantam.

Ray, M. (1994). Complex caring dynamics: A unifying model of nursing inquiry. *Theoretic and Applied Chaos in Nursing, 1*(1), 7–14.

Registered Nurses Association of British Columbia. (1992). *Determinants of health: Empowering strategies for nursing practice* (A background paper). Vancouver, B.C.: Author.

Robinson, C. (1996). Health care relationships revisited. *Journal of Family Nursing, 2*(2), 152–173.

Spreen Parker, R. (1990). Nurses' stories: The search for a relational ethic of care. *Advances in Nursing Science, 13*(1), 31–40.

Vicenzi, A., White, K., & Begun, J. (1997). Chaos in nursing: Make it work for you. *American Journal of Nursing, 97*(10), 26–32.

Watson, J. (1988). *Nursing: Human Science and Human Care.* New York: National League for Nursing.

Wheatley, M. J. (1994). *Leadership and the new science.* San Francisco: Berrett-Koehler.

World Health Organization. (1986). *Ottawa Charter for health promotion.* Ottawa: Health and Welfare, Canada.

Zohar, D. (1990). *The quantum self: Human nature and consciousness defined by the new physics.* New York: William Morrow.

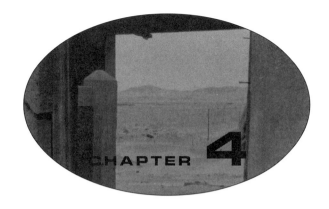

CHAPTER 4

Health Promoting Interactions: Insights from the Chronic Illness Experience

SALLY E. THORNE

It's funny, you know. All these people are smarter than you are at some particular thing, but there's not one person who is smarter than me about me. And so it's always tricky, because there's a certain area where they have more knowledge, and more expertise. But they don't see the whole as much as you do, and you have to make your own decisions.

Reflective Consumer

Although much of the current focus in health promotion literature is legitimately directed toward increasing the health of populations at a social and health policy level, the concept of health promotion is equally relevant in the day-to-day interactions that all health care professionals have with their clients (Mechanic, 1999). No longer considered neutral channels through which health services are accessed and information imparted, health care professionals are better understood today as active agents of a social ideology that defines what counts as a health issue, what interpretations of health matters are sufficiently important to warrant allocation of scarce resources, and which aspects of health and well-being are an appropriate focus for promotion efforts.

From a consumer perspective, health care professionals are the human face of a system of ideas that is of critical importance in accessing knowledge, making effective decisions, and obtaining the supports and resources necessary to attain the highest level of health possible (Wells, 1998). For the patient on the receiving end of a

new diagnosis, prognosis, or treatment plan, the care and concern expressed verbally and nonverbally by the health care professional may communicate the difference between hope and despair, between optimism and defeat. Thus, analysis of the actions and motivations of health care professionals in a health promotion context is relevant to the development of practical theory that will help us better appreciate how people interact with their health in a social context.

It seems self-evident that skilled communication between professionals and their clients involves a complex interaction between substance and process, what we communicate, and how we do it. When the health care professional engages in interaction with any client, the values, beliefs, and assumptions conveyed to the client become the context within which information exchange occurs, understandings of the situation are reconciled, and problems are identified and solved. Thus the role of these human exchanges in controlling the discourses around health promotion and in constructing the ideological positions that will be privileged is a fruitful element of health promotion development.

This chapter explores the face of health promotion interaction using insights obtained from accounts of those with a particular interest in health promotion—persons living with ongoing health challenges. My interest in this field grew out of an extensive program of insider research into the experience of those with chronic illness or cancer. Because they have explicit health challenges, persons with chronic illness tend to be highly attuned to matters of their own health, strongly motivated to acquire the resources and supports they need in order to live as well as possible, and acutely sensitive to any barriers within the health care system that interfere with their ability to shape the lifestyle they understand as most conducive to their uniquely defined overall health and well-being.[1] Consequently, they are often leaders in consumer advocacy about issues that have subsequently become popularized within the mainstream of society. In a sense, they collectively become the voice of expertise about what it is like to be on the receiving end of health care services in our society today. The patterns and themes within their accounts of helpful and unhelpful health care professional attitudes and actions consequently reveal much about the subtle human dimension of what does and does not promote health in the health care interaction.

Chronic Illness as Context

To better appreciate the relevance of their perspectives, it is important to place the experience of persons living with chronic illness in a larger social context. Despite the emphasis in health care professional education on acute and critical care, chronic illnesses actually account for the vast majority of health care costs, productivity loss, and burden on families (De Ridder, Depla, Severens, & Malsch, 1997). Further, much acute and critical care involves individuals who have a preexisting chronic illness or will have one once the acute episode is over. Because diagnostic criteria and processes for most chronic diseases are embedded in socially constructed negotiations, it is not really possible to generate exact figures for how many people within a society

---

[1]Although chronic mental illness is traditionally differentiated from chronic physical illness as conceptually and experientially distinct phenomena, there is considerable reason to believe that many of the same elements of health care structure, process, and interaction are applicable regardless of the specific chronic disease (Thorne, 1999). Because the social image of chronic mental illness complicates our assumptions about the meaning and validity of consumer insights, the ideas in this paper are drawn from the specific context of physical illness, recognizing that there will be many similarities with the circumstances of those who have primary or comorbid chronic mental illnesses.

actually live with chronic illness. It is generally agreed, however, that the chronically ill are by far the largest health care consumer population in industrialized countries (Kuh & Ben-Shlomo, 1997; Thorne, 1993).

By definition, an illness is chronic if it is not self-limiting, or if there is no known cure. Because health care professionals and the consumers of health services alike experience chronic illness as a departure from the dominant ideology of a curative system, individuals and families who live with chronic conditions encounter significant frustrations in negotiating health care (Royer, 1998). They understand that they are not conforming to the expected social role of patients (that is, they are not getting cured). Because of this failure to conform to the "patient role," they often become the target of frustrations within the system and may feel implicit blame for diverting increasingly scarce health care resources away from those who truly deserve them (Thorne, 1993).

When persons with chronic illness seek alternative or self-care solutions to the particular challenges that their chronic disease entails, they are understood not to be engaging in health promotion, but to be searching for "miracle cures." When they seek additional supports or resources within the traditional health care system, they are labeled as "demanding." Thus, because the socially sanctioned "health care system" turns out to be inadequate in meeting the health needs of a great many people who face illness in their lives, it becomes a logical target of analysis for those who try to make sense of their chronic illness experience. Increasingly, individuals who have experienced various diseases and health challenges network with each other through such mechanisms as support groups, nonprofit societies, political action initiatives, or Internet discussion groups. These mechanisms catalyze their interpretations into a shared sociopolitical discourse.

These common experiences, documented by many researchers engaged in interpreting the experience of chronic illness in western society (such as Charmaz, 1991; Royer, 1998; Thorne, 1993), tell us a lot about the ideological culture of our health care system. Whether or not they are inclined to be social critics, people with a chronic illness are often thrust into a health care system that has evolved to reveal certain priorities and to ignore other health-related matters. Thus, consumer insights about how and why our systems and services are structured as they are, and the motivations underlying our behavior as health care professionals, help us understand our own ideological underpinnings and challenge us anew to re-examine and deconstruct them.

Unfettered by the logic that we professionals might use to justify some of our more irrational bureaucratic decisions and policies, consumer analyses offer us new ways of recognizing the values and truths we hold about health and illness, the assumptions we make about the roles formal and informal health care systems play in the health of individual people and, perhaps most important, the limits of traditional biomedical science for addressing matters of health and well-being. Embedded in these analyses is a complex and disconcerting understanding of how we as health care professionals enact the ideological positions of this dominant health care system in all aspects of our practice, including our communications with recipients of our service.

On the basis of an extended program of research into various aspects of chronic illness experience from an insider perspective, I have become convinced that this consumer analysis from the chronic illness perspective offers us insights that extend beyond our explicit hegemonic role in chronic illness care. It can be quite sobering to consider the opinion of many consumers that professionals strategically construct barriers that reduce their access to services and resources, and thereby reduce the load on the formal health care system. It is disconcerting to hear their accounts about being considered less valuable recipients of health services than are those with acute or episodic health problems. Analyses of how the health care system and the professionals within it operate, reveals troubling evidence of a common discourse within health care that discounts and discredits this chronic illness perspective as a psychological manifestation of disease rather than a legitimate analysis of society.

Synthesizing insights from the interpretations of consumer research into chronic illness experience, it becomes possible to identify themes within health care interactions that explicitly support or detract from health promotion at the individual level. By documenting and interpreting these patterns, we can begin to appreciate that values relevant to the health promotion enterprise operate strongly at the interface between individual professionals and individual consumers. Further, if we pay attention to generalized health promotion strategies at a societal level, but do not strengthen the health promotion potential within routine health care interactions, we will have missed an integral aspect of the health promotion process.

This chapter represents an attempt to draw on the consumer perspective, as it has been documented in insider research about chronic illness experience, to strengthen the health promoting aspects of health care interactions, and to challenge and reconfigure those that are health defeating.

✳ Reflective Questions

1. What is the relationship between health promotion at the societal-community level and health promotion at the individual level?

2. How is a health promotion approach to interacting with clients different from a more typical health care or health education approach?

3. What can we learn from persons on the receiving end of health care that might help us understand how to promote health more effectively?

Health Defeating Patterns in Health Care Interactions

Accounts of consumers with chronic illness reveal a number of common problems in health care communications. By examining themes and patterns within those problems, it is possible to detect important patterns of health care professional behavior that frustrate or complicate consumer efforts at promoting their own health. In this discussion, the health defeating patterns in health care interactions include: fighting over who ought to have authority in illness management decisions, discrediting the various options that consumers consider relevant, attempting to control noncompliant behaviors, and controlling the definition of what counts as a relevant outcome.

Fighting over Authority

Among the most common patterns that persons with chronic illness report in relation to health care is the matter of who ought to control what happens to the patient[2] (Ainsworth-Vaughn, 1995). Although most people would happily defer to the authority of an expert clinician when they encounter a health challenge for the first time, or have an illness experience that is unfamiliar to them, those who have to live with their chronic illness day in and day out almost always become the real experts on their own situation. While the professionals may have generalized ("textbook") knowledge, the person who feels the sensations, struggles with the limitations, and tries to figure out how to manage living with illness becomes the legitimate authority on how the disease is affecting his or her life. Although some professionals recognize that anatomical knowledge and biochemical information constitute only a limited amount of information about what is really happening to the patient, many seem incapable of dealing with information outside those parameters. For example, they may pay more attention to what monitors and machines tell them about function than what the patient says helps or hinders the condition.

Even though few patients consider themselves more expert than their professionals in *all* matters related to their disease, most come to recognize that they do become the experts in some aspects. In fact, an increasing number of consumers actively seek information and become remarkably astute at critically interpreting its quality and utility. However, persons with chronic illness frequently encounter health care professionals who are unwilling or unable to recognize any meaningful patient expertise, and who expect their own interpretations to trump any opinion the patient has about the disease or its proper management. Complicating matters, these clinicians represent a long tradition within medicine in which communicating uncertainty is to be avoided, and therefore authoritative statements are understood as helpful (Royer, 1998).

Discrediting Options

One problematic point of contention that is increasingly apparent in our society is the conflict that patients and practitioners have in relation to complementary/alternative therapies.[3] Although most people with chronic illness intuitively recognize that eating well, sleeping well, reducing stress, exercising their bodies, balancing their energies, engaging in comfort measures, tending to their spirit, and sustaining a positive attitude are inherently beneficial, and many augment these with specific therapeutic strategies derived from non-Western traditions, they are routinely faced with health care professionals who cannot accept the value of any action that is "unproven." What has been subjected to rigorous testing throughout the history of western biomedical science includes only that subset of strategies that directly relate to surgical manipulation, technological interventions of some kind, or biochemical alteration (medications). Although kindness, gentle touch, support, reassurance, and caring are among those measures that are unquestionably important to anyone who has suffered any bodily malfunction, they are not amenable to single-causation testing, isolation from the context in which they occur, or reduction to mathematical quantification. Unfortunately, too many health care professionals assume that

---

[2]The term *patient* is strategically used here, since persons who live with chronic illness are well aware that their status shifts when they come under the authority of a health care professional. Although they may think of themselves as *persons with chronic illness* or *consumers of health care* when they are in the public domain, they typically understand the health care interaction as a context in which their social role is highly circumscribed by the ideologies and structures of the health care system. Interestingly, persons with chronic illness typically slip comfortably between one language and the other, and therefore I prefer not to force a *politically correct* language onto the dialogue, but instead try to appreciate what they mean when they use the various terms.

[3]The term *complementary/alternative therapies* is used to designate those remedies or strategies that are sometimes considered *unproven* or that derive from folk or popular medicine rather than allopathic tradition or conventional (Western) biomedical science. A great deal of what people engage in to promote their health can be reframed as unproven methods, despite the probability that most health and healing is a result of *all* of the various things people do in their daily lives to manage symptoms, maintain well-being, and sustain health.

the only things that matter are those that can be scientifically proven (Wellard, 1998).

Over recent years, with increasing demands to justify health care expenditures in a corporate context, the pressure toward "evidence-based practice" has accelerated. However, consumer perspectives on what counts as evidence may be radically different from the scientific norm. As rational sensate beings, most persons with chronic illness learn subtle ways to detect what helps them and what hinders them in the functional and health-related matters that are relevant to their chronic illness management. Because living well is typically a far higher priority than is conforming to conventional logic, they are much more likely to take a course of action that works for them, as far as they can judge, than they are to adhere to professional advice merely because it is offered by an authority figure. Researchers who study chronic illness from the perspective of those who live with it invariably discover that patients modify and manipulate their "medical orders"[4] (Charmaz, 1991; Royer, 1998). They work out theories as to why one way of doing things helps while another does not, and often recognize that although their theories may not make logical sense, they are the best explanation that they have at the moment. Such theorizing by persons with chronic illness is often fluid and "in process." Some people find it quite helpful to have some sort of explanation for why something works, even though they may recognize that it sounds completely irrational from the perspective of conventional health care professional science.

Controlling Noncompliance

The pervasiveness of the discrepancy between professional and patient perspectives with regard to what is effective and what is not becomes apparent when one reviews the abundant literature on why patients refuse to comply[5] with medical prescription (Thorne, 1990; Wellard, 1998). From an epidemiological perspective, it is quite possible to demonstrate that populations that take one course of action in dealing with a common condition tend to do better than do populations that follow another course. Scientists establish this by approximating "uncontaminated" laboratory conditions as much as possible, and conducting randomized controlled trials to measure one remedy against another on some quantifiable outcome measure. However, in their enthusiasm for applying evidence to practice, health care professionals may fail to recognize that population generalizations can never predict what will actually work for any one individual.

For example, among individuals who become expert in self-care decision making about their long-standing Type I diabetes, it is commonly recognized that simply adhering to prescribed insulin levels is inconsistent with maintaining glycemic balance and adjusting to a range of unpredictable conditions (Paterson & Thorne, in press). Because of this, the individual who complies too rigidly cannot engage in the experimentation required to become sufficiently skilled to cope with real life challenges. Thus, while the rationality of mathematical probability guides the professional opinion, the empirical logic of testing and sensing drives the patient perspective.

Over the years, in their attempts to predict who will be compliant and create strategies to increase compliance, researchers have discovered that noncompliance with medication errors cannot be explained by intelligence, education, gender, social status, ethnicity, or personality characteristics (Thorne, 1990). Rather, it is a widespread phenomenon among all those whose living well depends on fine-

[4]The term *medical orders* is used here to denote the very common pattern of authoritative prescription by professionals (nurses as well as doctors) in contrast to the equally common phenomenon of *noncompliance*. To order something connotes an imbalance in power and privilege, a situation that is encountered by most persons with chronic illness at some point in their experience with health care professionals.

[5]The term *noncompliance* implies that an order has been given and the patient has failed to follow through in the prescribed manner. Because it is such a loaded term, many nurses use the term *nonadherence* in an effort to suggest more respect for the patient's decision making. From my work with persons with chronic illness, however, I have discovered that the terminological distinction matters not to those so labeled and indeed, many patients strategically self-identify as *noncompliant* to signify their active resistance against what they deem to be inappropriate authority over their lives.

tuning the balance between medical orders and their own sense of what is required. The research typically assumes that the professional logic is the "correct" one, and so there is no comparable body of literature on characteristics of professionals who are unable to consider options beyond the standard prescription.

Despite the probability that many of those who fail to follow prescribed medical orders precisely are making active and meaningful choices about their own lives, many health care professionals interpret their social obligation as enforcing compliance with a vengeance. Because of this, many people with chronic illness report experiences in which health care professionals have used "scare tactics" to frighten them into compliance with accounts of the worst complications that might occur, and stern lectures in which they feel infantilized and humiliated in relation to their choices (Hess, 1996; Roberson, 1992). This "critical parent" dynamic is widespread within health care, and although many health care professionals would never engage in this kind of interaction, most persons with chronic illness have encountered it in the real world (Thorne, 1993). Such interactions are often highly disturbing to the individual on the receiving end. While these kinds of interactions on the part of health care professionals rarely produce any constructive change in client health behaviors, they often trigger a fascination for what motivates health care professionals to behave in such a manner.

Defining Relevant Outcomes

Beyond the conflicts associated with differing perspectives on how one ought to manage or live with a chronic condition, many patients encounter important differences of opinion about the intended outcome of health care for a chronic illness (Kleinman, 1992). Most commonly, they discover that much of medical care is organized into body system functions, so the cardiologist is interested in their heart and circulatory systems, whereas the nephrologist may be concerned only with their kidneys and urinary function. Not surprisingly, a great many chronic illnesses involve multiple organ systems and require the involvement of more than one specialist, discipline, or service. Typically, each aspect of the health care system

has its own set of assumptions about what the goal of treatment ought to be. The dietitian may be concerned with caloric intake, the gastroenterologist with colon irritability, and the psychologist with identity.

The patient, however, is concerned about how to live as well as possible with inflammatory bowel disease. Rarely do patients find that specialists appreciate the world of the patient beyond the boundaries of their particular professional aspect of interest. Where they do acknowledge "quality of life" as a relevant outcome, they typically define it according to general population norms as opposed to what has meaning for each individual patient. Thus, persons with chronic illness commonly encounter diametrically opposite recommendations from specialists of different orientations or disciplines (even within the conventional health care system), and begin to recognize that each specialty within the health care system has a distinct vision of what it is that the patient is supposed to attain.

Perhaps the most problematic conflictual interactions are over the differences between cure and care. Although it is undoubtedly true that most people initially search for ways to rid themselves of the chronic conditions with which they are diagnosed, many come to recognize that cure is not foreseeable (they rarely abandon all hope), and begin to identify alternative objectives, such as better functional ability, more energy, less discomfort, and so on. Often these alternative objectives are highly individualized and reflect valued activities or experiences, such as managing a part-time job, maintaining a particular golf score, or helping diaper the new grandchild. Much of their experimentation with prescribed treatments and alternative therapies is directed toward discovering ways to obtain even minor improvements in their quality of living.

When they encounter disparaging attitudes toward these efforts from their health care professionals, and when their own empirical evidence that some treatment or remedy does improve their life a little, they begin to doubt that the health care professional cares as much for their quality of life than for their lab tests or organ function measures. Thus, they are often placed in a "Catch-22" situation by the attitudes of health care professionals. If they comply with medical remedies that have no possibility of symptom improvement, they are seen as adjusting well to their illness; if they seek options outside the traditional health care system, they are seen as irrationally seeking cure and living with false hope. Although hope may well be among the most important elements that a patient requires in order to experience a life of high quality, some health care professionals interpret hope as expectation, and try to thwart it. To meet the expectations of health care professionals about how they ought to accept and adjust to their disease, patients must abandon the search for ways to promote their own self-defined health status.

As many persons with chronic illness will tell us, life's quality is derived from factors much more complex and mysterious than physiological functioning and bodily comfort (Charmaz, 1991). Pure bliss may not be a normal characteristic of the human condition; indeed, struggling against adversity may well represent the more universal thread of what makes us uniquely human. Thus persons with chronic illnesses are faced with the challenge of configuring their disease and its management into contexts and lives filled with searching, interacting, accomplishing, understanding. They may not wish to spend any more time and energy than is absolutely necessary attending to the demands of their disease; rather, their priorities at various times may be their family dynamics, their work stress, their spiritual health (Royer, 1998; Ternulf Nyhlin, 1991). When health care professionals insist on disease-related measurables as outcome measures, they lose their grasp on what life is all about for their patients (Bergsma, 1997; Wellard, 1998).

From my work with persons affected by chronic disease, it has become apparent to me that communications with health care professionals are a powerful influence on the lives of those who must interact with them to obtain the services they need to live as well as possible. Although certainly not universal, the patterns of health defeating behaviors described here are all too common, and most persons who have extended contact with the health care system encounter them regularly. They can demoralize, frustrate, and inhibit the confidence people require to actively pursue their own health promotion. Even more important, they can place people in the terrible bind of having to sacrifice the ways they would like to pursue health in order to placate the professionals and obtain services.

✳ Reflective Questions

1. Think about your own interactions with clients in your practice. In what ways might you inadvertently detract from their efforts at health promotion?

2. How can a health care professional work toward reducing the health defeating patterns described above?

Health Promoting Patterns in Health Care Interactions

Fortunately, many persons with chronic illness also encounter some health care professionals capable of rising above these common patterns and who effectively engage in health promoting interactions. Often, they describe these kinds of relationships as exceptions from the norm, and understand that they occur when health care professionals are willing to operate from a different set of assumptions than they would in acute or episodic care (Thorne & Robinson, 1988, 1989). By articulating the patterns and themes apparent in health promoting interactions from their perspective, we can begin to see the possibilities for improving health care practice more globally. The patterns that will be discussed here include: understanding the larger context in which the chronic illness is experienced, engaging in partnerships characterized by adaptability and flexibility, recognizing the inherent limits of scientific knowledge in relation to health promotion, and working toward effecting change within the health care system.

Understanding the Larger Context

Diseases happen to people who are not merely biological organisms but who are part of a larger social context—as members of families, communities, and other social structures. It is only under unusual circumstances that people's lives focus on only one priority, and such is the case for those who live with chronic illness. Except during those special instances in which they must focus their attention acutely on their bodily manifestations, disease management tends to take its place among a dynamic and fluid set of priorities and processes.

When health care professionals show appreciation for the lives of those they encounter, and in particular, when they accept that disease management may not be the highest priority most of the time, their patients feel acknowledged and valued as unique individuals. Although our traditional logic tells us that this kind of mutual respect is only possible in the context of long-standing health care relationships developed over time, persons with chronic illness report that it is fully evident in even brief and episodic communications. They tell us that this appreciation for the larger context of their lives is a matter of attitude rather than relationship, and that it evokes their capacity for trust and confidence.

The other aspect of context that consumers often recognize is those determinants of health beyond their immediate consciousness. Even though epidemiological analysis of population data is well beyond their focus of attention most of the time, they do understand that opportunities for health care are not equally distributed and that resource allocation is not always a matter of justice. Although most health care professionals enjoy some measure of middle-class privilege within society, many of their clients do not. The correlation between relative poverty and almost all diseases within a society is well recognized (for example, Mechanic, 1999). Thus, apparently simple disease management strategies appropriate for persons with some privilege might be entirely unthinkable to those whose daily struggle for survival dominates living. For example, some people with rheumatoid arthritis might be able to travel to warmer climates for symptom relief during a cold Canadian winter, but many others would have no recourse to such advantages.

Health care professionals who recognize the complex dynamics inherent in the relationship between social and economic determinants and health are more attuned to spotting inequities, predicting access problems, and offering nonjudgmental support. They appreciate that, especially among the most vulnerable segment of society, every health care interaction represents an opportunity to begin to reduce those larger inequities by helping people feel comfortable with their rights, helping them understand the processes, and supporting them in finding effective ways to meet their health care needs. By creating relationships in which people feel valued and respected, they increase the individual's options for appropriate engagement in health care processes and thereby promote health.

Engaging in Flexible Partnerships

In contrast to the traditional authority relationships expected of health care provider–consumer relationships, and the technical expertise required of many acute illness contexts, effective chronic illness care demands a considerable degree of flexibility and balance. As has been explained, persons with chronic illness typically become the genuine experts in their own bodily manifestations of disease, in the social context in which they live it, and in the interactions between these factors. The health care professional has access to complex and ever-changing bodies of general knowledge that may be highly relevant to the consumer, but that may not affect disease management decisions in any significant manner. Chronic illness care tends to involve experimentation with various approaches, monitoring relief of symptoms or progression of disease indicators, and specific symptom management. A number of the necessary requisites to living well with many chronic illnesses involve controlled access on the basis of professional advice and referral. Thus, regardless of a patient's confidence in the professional's orientation to the problem, he or she may feel obliged to interact effectively with health care professionals in order to obtain prescription medicines, referrals for therapies, disability benefits, or necessary treatments.

When health care professionals acknowledge and respect the expertise of persons with chronic illness, they empower their clients to make decisions about those matters that affect their lives and openly negotiate appropriate resource requirements to facilitate living as normally as possible despite the disease. In recent years, it has become popular to suggest that enlightened clinicians should encourage all patients to take active control of their self-care management (Cahill, 1996; Lott, Blazey, & West, 1992).

However, it is apparent to those who study a range of chronic illness experiences that this perspective is also problematic (Thorne & Paterson, 1998). First, there are times and occasions in the lives of even the most assertive and competent patients during which the burden of decision making is too demanding and professional control over decisions may be warranted (such as during times of family crisis, acute illness, and so on). Second, the intentionality of permitting consumers to dictate their own course of action can backfire, leading them to feel blamed when their decisions result in disease progression or complications. And finally, there are many times within the course of any chronic disease trajectory at which even the most informed and independent individual may not recognize what is happening and what the options are.

Professional expertise, when exercised judiciously and in the context of respectful relationships, can sometimes facilitate health promotion far better than would simply assuming that patients always know what is in their own best interests. Among the many examples of such effective intervention I have heard from patients are stories of situations in which nurses or other health care professionals carefully but purposefully steered them toward a course of action they later considered the single most important factor in their ability to live well. This might include shifting from a walker to a wheelchair for a patient with multiple sclerosis, defying rigid feeding schedules for a parent of a child with a long-term gastrostomy, or beginning to experiment with insulin doses for a young adult with Type 1 diabetes. What made these intervention decisions so effective was not that they were "right," but rather that they were made on the basis of an understanding of the patient, the specific elements of context, and the general patterns that emerge in relation to illness experience. Thus, according to persons with chronic illness, effective partnerships are not constituted in any one singular framework; rather they must be sufficiently flexible to allow genuine sharing of authority and the exercise of expertise by both participants.

Recognizing the Limits of Science

As was evident from the earlier discussion of conflicting views about alternative/complementary therapies, health promotion in chronic illness must include recognition of the inherent limits of biomedical science in supporting daily living. Most individuals with chronic illness (indeed a majority of the public overall) explore unconventional or folk remedies and therapeutics in their effort to manage symptoms and live as well as possible (Jonas, 1998; Kelner & Wellman, 1997). When they encounter curiosity or enthusiasm from their health care providers with regard to a range of possible options, scientifically proven or otherwise, they respond by being more open in reporting what they experiment with and what effect they believe it has on their illness or daily living. Health care professionals who profess concern for the everyday lives of their clients will naturally be delighted when they find something that helps, and will participate in supportive education and monitoring as appropriate. To achieve such attitudes, health care professionals do need an understanding that science is only one among a great many forms of evidence that will be relevant to the self-care choices made by patients.

When we consider the reasons that persons with chronic illness fail to comply with prescribed treatments, especially medications, we often discover that noxious side effects outweigh the anticipated benefit that can be obtained from the treatment. Because they often come to recognize that healthful living habits are consistent with feeling as well as possible, especially with a chronic illness, many people come to recognize the adverse effects of chemotherapeutic agents as threatening to their general health. Many persons with chronic illness have been leaders in advocating for more natural products, avoidance of toxic substances in the environment, and the intuitive wisdom of creating the conditions under which the body has the best chance to heal itself naturally (remember Florence Nightingale?). Thus, health promoting interactions in health care recognize the complex reasons why people make the choices that they do, and respect a range of possible strategies toward dealing with chronic health challenges.

Working Toward System Change

Finally, a characteristic of all truly health promoting interactions in health care is that they are predicated on the views of professionals who are willing to critically analyze and challenge the status quo in health care. As has long been recognized by many in the field, health care services have been set up and structured to meet the needs of professionals and to serve the demands of acute care rather than chronic illness (Royer, 1998; Strauss, et al., 1984; Thorne, 1993). Rules, structures, and bureaucracies intended to restrict access to and control services invariably serve some client situations well and others very badly. Therefore, health care professionals whose allegiance to the system takes precedence over their concern for appropriate care cannot be truly effective practitioners in the chronic illness context.

From the accounts of persons with chronic illness, it becomes apparent that the most respected health care professionals are those who can share their outrage when patients are unjustly denied resources, who believe patients when they report unreasonable barriers to access, and who can appreciate the amount of energy and work that is required to negotiate for appropriate services. By validating the patient's expert knowledge about his or her unique responses to illness, by listening to the patient's perspective on the available options, and by accepting the inherent limitations of anything medical science can offer, a professional creates a context for trust and open communication. Within such a context, risks can be evaluated (and sometimes supported), probable outcomes can be honestly discussed, and patients can be empowered at the same time as they are protected. Strauss and colleagues, in 1984, called for a health care system that was much more responsive to the needs of the chronically ill. When they recognize how far we are even now from realizing that change, health care professionals interested in promoting health understand that they must become part of a change process.

✳ Reflective Questions

1. Which of these health promoting patterns of interaction are possible in your clinical practice area?

2. What barriers or challenges make it difficult to engage in interactions characterized by a health promotion orientation?

3. What professional or personal values do you hold that might conflict with the kinds of interaction strategies described above?

Implications for Nursing

Nursing is ideally placed to play a prominent role in health promotion, particularly in the context of chronic illness care (Corbin, 1998). As is clear from the accounts of those who engage in health care interactions because of chronic illness, effecting a health promotion ideal requires that nurses challenge many of the traditional notions underlying professional practice norms (McWilliam, Stewart, Brown, Desai, & Coderre, 1996; Wellard, 1998). To create the conditions under which health promotion can be optimized, the traditional concept of "expertise" must be sufficiently broadened as to allow a fluid and respectful interpretation of the knowledge and skills that both the nurse and client bring to the exchange.

Similarly, the basic ideal of evidence-based practice will require a critically reflective perspective on what counts as evidence for both general applications and specific individual situations. Nurses will require an understanding not only of the advantages of empirical science, but also of its limitations in providing all of the knowledge that will be required to guide and support people as they sort out how to achieve the highest level of health that is possible within the context of their diseases. Following on these challenges, nurses will also have to reconsider their responsibilities regarding patient autonomy, safety, and security, since an authentic exchange will sometimes reveal health-seeking strategies that violate the science or the logic of mainstream thought.

Beyond these general insights about the implications of health promotion in chronic illness, the interactional skills of nurses may well determine the degree to which integration of complex health promotion actions, attitudes, and skills may or may not be achievable for clients confronting an ongoing health challenge. From the patterns and themes health care consumers reveal in their accounts of such interactions, it seems clear that the requisite professional communication skills for enhancing rather than frustrating health promotion can be learned and developed. Thus, it seems apparent that the larger aims of health promotion must be grounded within the human interactional context so that nurses can effectively enact them in their practice. In examining the health promoting and health defeating interactions in health care from the perspective of persons living with chronic illness, we begin to understand that health promotion is indeed a fundamentally human enterprise.

I think empowering people to make their own choices is a big part of what's necessary. It's a little bit more than *giving permission, but it's giving them the knowledge that they need to make those decisions as well.*

Reflective Consumer

BOX 4–1

CASE ILLUSTRATION

Your client, a 23-year-old man with a 12-year history of inflammatory bowel disease, reveals to you that he experiments with a wide range of substances (such as marijuana), diets (such as high protein), alternative therapies (such as herbal remedies and acupuncture), and self-care strategies (such as occasional fasting and mindful meditation) to reduce the impact of his chronic disease on his ability to live a "normal everyday life." Consider the following questions:

- How do you determine which of the strategies he experiments with should be encouraged and which should be discouraged? Consider what you currently know, what experts in the field might know, and what is currently unknowable?
- How would you decide which messages to give this client with regard to his coping options? How would you determine the appropriate role of your own beliefs and opinions in communicating with this client?
- What would be the predictable impact if you communicate negative value judgements to your client about his choices? What might be the predictable impact of trying to convey support for strategies that cause you considerable concern? How can you articulate what you consider to be legitimate concerns without coming across as judgmental?
- In what ways might you and your client work together to discover ways to determine which self-management strategies work for him, which might require modification, and which might incur unacceptable risks?
- How would you ultimately evaluate whether your interactions with your client had been health promoting or health defeating?

REFERENCES

Ainsworth-Vaughn, N. (1995). Claiming power in the medical encounter: The whirlpool discourse. *Qualitative Health Research, 5,* 270–291.

Bergsma, J. (1997). *Doctors and patients: Strategies in long-term illness.* Dordrecht, Netherlands: Kluwer.

Cahill, J. (1996). Patient participation: A concept analysis. *Journal of Advanced Nursing, 24,* 561–571.

Charmaz, K. (1991). *Good days, bad days: The self in chronic illness and time.* New Brunswick, NJ: Rutgers University Press.

Corbin, J. M. (1998). The Corbin and Strauss chronic illness trajectory model: An update. *Scholarly Inquiry for Nursing Practice, 12*(1), 33–41.

De Ridder, D., Depla, M., Severens, P., & Malsch, M. (1997). Beliefs on coping with illness: A consumer's perspective. *Social Science & Medicine, 44,* 553–559.

Hess, J. D. (1996). The ethics of compliance: A dialectic. *Advances in Nursing Science, 19*(1), 18–27.

Jonas, W. (1998). Alternative medicine: Learning from the past, examining the present, advancing to the future. *Journal of the American Medical Association, 280,* 1616–1617.

Kelner, M., & Wellman, B. (1997). Health and consumer choice: Medical and alternative therapies. *Social Science & Medicine, 45,* 203–212.

Kleinman, A. (1992). Pain and resistance: The delegitimation and relegitimation of local worlds. In M. D. Good, P. E. Baldwin, B. J. Good, & A. Kleinman (Eds.), *Pain as a human experience: An anthropological perspective* (pp. 169–197). Berkeley, CA: University of California Press.

Kuh, D., & Ben-Shlomo, Y. (1997). Introduction: A life course approach to the aetiology of adult chronic disease. In D. Kuh & Y. Ben-Shlomo (Eds.), *A life course approach to chronic disease epidemiology* (pp. 3–14). Oxford: Oxford University Press.

Lott, T. F., Blazey, M. E., & West, M. G. (1992). Patient participation in health care: An unused resource. *Nursing Clinics of North America, 27*(1), 61–75.

McWilliam, C. L., Stewart, M., Brown, J. B., Desai, K., & Coderre, P. (1996). Creating health within chronic illness. *Advances in Nursing Science, 18*(3), 1–15.

Mechanic, D. (1999). Issues in promoting health. *Social Science & Medicine, 48,* 711–718.

Paterson, B., & Thorne, S. (in press). Expert decision-making in relation to unexpected blood glucose levels. *Research in Nursing & Health.*

Roberson, M.H.B. (1992). The meaning of compliance: Patient perspectives. *Qualitative Health Research, 2,* 7–26.

Royer, A. (1998). *Life with chronic illness: Social and psychological dimensions.* Westport, CT: Praeger.

Strauss, A. L., Corbin, J., Fagerhaugh, S., Glaser, B., Maines, D., Suczek, B., & Wiener, C. (1984). *Chronic illness and the quality of life* (2nd ed.). St. Louis: Mosby.

Ternulf Nyhlin, K. (1991). Patients' experiences of managing diabetes mellitus: A fine balancing act. *Scandinavian Journal of Caring Sciences, 5*(4), 187–194.

Thorne, S. E. (1990). Constructive non-compliance in chronic illness. *Holistic Nursing Practice, 5*(1), 62–69.

Thorne, S. E. (1993). *Negotiating health care: The social context of chronic illness.* Newbury Park, CA: Sage.

Thorne, S. E. (1999). Rethinking the problem of non-compliance in chronic illness. In J. Guimòn, W. Fischer, & N. Sartorius (Eds.), *The image of madness: The public facing mental illness and psychiatric treatment* (pp. 231–238). Basel: Karger.

Thorne, S., & Paterson, B. (1998). Shifting images of chronic illness. *Image: Journal for Nursing Scholarship, 30,* 173–178.

Thorne, S. E., & Robinson, C. A. (1988). Health care relationships: The chronic illness perspective. *Research in Nursing and Health, 11,* 293–300.

Thorne, S. E., & Robinson, C. A. (1989). Guarded alliance: Health care relationships in chronic illness. *Image: The Journal of Nursing Scholarship, 21*(3), 153–157.

Wellard, S. (1998). Constructions of chronic illness. *International Journal of Nursing Studies, 35,* 49–55.

Wells, S. M. (1998). *A delicate balance: Living successfully with chronic illness.* New York: Plenum.

CHAPTER 5

Listening to Multiple Voices: Public Participation in Health Care Decision Making

ROSALIE C. STARZOMSKI

The following scenarios illustrate some of the concerns, issues, and challenges surrounding public participation in health care decision making. Please read the scenarios and reflect on the questions that follow.

Scenario A: A Community Diabetes Education Program

A group of educators is interested in developing a local health promotion program to disseminate information about the risk factors associated with diabetes. The educators are aware that this is a problem in many communities, but are particularly concerned with the alarming increase of diabetes in aboriginal communities. They are interested in establishing an advisory group, which would include consumers and health care providers, to help them with their project. The educators know several health care providers who might be suitable, but do not have a plan to determine who from the public should be involved. They want to make sure their group is representative of the public and they want to include clients who have diabetes, particularly clients from aboriginal communities.

> ✳ **Reflective Questions**
>
> 1. Is this a topic that you think would be important to the public?
> 2. How will the educators go about selecting individuals to be involved in their advisory group?
> 3. What should they consider when determining group membership?
> 4. What are some of the issues the educators should consider when selecting members of the public to be part of their advisory group?
> 5. How will the educators ensure they have the right mix of people involved (for example, members of the health care provider community, representatives from aboriginal communities, etc.)?

Scenario B: School Safety— A Safe Walk Program

A regional health board and a school board want to establish a "safe walk" program for the elementary students in their area. The boards are concerned about the number of students being driven to school by parents. Not only are students getting less exercise by being driven to school, but there are also major traffic problems in the area with the influx of cars dropping children off and picking them up. The boards want to include all stakeholders in the development of a new program, but are unsure how to develop a plan for public involvement.

※ Reflective Questions

1. What do you think the boards should consider when attempting to involve stakeholders?
2. Who are the stakeholders?
3. Who should be involved in the planning of such a program?
4. How will the group make certain the people involved are representative of the community?

Scenario C: Xenotransplant Clinical Trials

The federal government is considering the possibility of allowing xenotransplantation (transplanting animal organs into humans) clinical trials. Before making a decision, several major concerns must be considered, one of which is the possibility of transmitting animal viruses to humans. Some people fear that this will potentially cause an outbreak of disease similar to the acquired immunodeficiency syndrome (AIDS) epidemic. The federal government wants to hear public perspectives on xenotransplantation prior to developing policy about clinical trials.

※ Reflective Questions

1. How can public input be obtained about this important issue?
2. What are some of the specific strategies that might be used to obtain this public input?
3. What are some of the problems in obtaining public input on issues that are national in scope?

As we proceed through this new millennium, there is increasing emphasis on moving to a col-

laborative model of decision making in order to make good decisions about health care. Important challenges confront societal groups in ensuring that health care needs are identified and met, and that health care resources are distributed in a fair and equitable manner. At all levels of the health care system, it is believed that planning for health care services and resolving health care dilemmas requires consideration of many sources of information by a variety of societal groups (Roy, Williams, & Dickens, 1994). There is growing support for the idea that to identify societal health care needs, and to resolve resource allocation dilemmas, a partnership of consumers and health care providers is required (Note: the terms "consumers" and "the public" are used interchangeably in this chapter). Furthermore, there is a great need for health care providers and members of the public to recognize the importance of a patient/client–focused approach to health care and to speak out together to ensure that health care choices are made that are beneficial to the common good (Saul, 1995; Starzomski & Rodney, 1997).

Many believe that, by including consumer voices in health care decision making, decisions will be enriched and there will be more opportunity to meet the needs of individuals, families, and groups (B.C. Ministry of Health, 1993; Bracht, 1990; Charles & DeMaio, 1993; Eyles, 1993; Gordon, 1990; National Forum on Health, 1997; Ottawa Charter for Health Promotion, 1986). It is believed that decision making will be enhanced if consumers are involved in determining the need for changes in health promoting behaviors at the micro (individual) level of the health care system, developing health promotion programs at the meso (institutional/agency) level, and expanding programs at the macro (societal) level that focus on health promotion for populations. In the Ottawa Charter, great importance is given to strengthening community action: "Health promotion works through concrete and effective community action in setting priorities, making decisions, planning strategies, and implementing them to achieve better health. At the heart of this process is the empowerment of communities, their leadership, and control of their own endeavors and destinies."

Although the idea of public participation in health care decision making is thought to be desirable, congruent with the basic tenet of democracy—government by the people, for the people (Kymlicka, 1990)—it is not clear what the goals of public participation are or ought to be. The question of whether public participation is a means to an end, an end in itself, or both, has been raised by several authors (Charles & DeMaio, 1993; Center for Health Economics and Policy Analysis (CHEPA), 1991; Hurley, Birch, & Eyles, 1992; Starzomski, 1997).

Who is the public? Why should the public be more involved in health care decision making today than in the past? How do we ensure that members of the public—consisting of many ethnocultural groups with different values, beliefs, and concerns—get included in the discussions about health and health care that have an impact on them? Is public involvement required in order to capitalize on the expertise of the lay public that health care providers lack? Do members of the public have a right to be involved in health care decisions because they are the ones who pay for health care? Does the public believe they have a duty to be involved in the discussions about the fair allocation of resources as part of their obligation as members of society? Or, is public participation merely a "politically correct" way to attempt to reform the system? These are some of the questions that have been raised in the current discussion about public involvement in heath care decision making.

My purpose in this chapter is to review research and literature about public involvement in health care decision making and to provide a critical review of the role of consumers in this area. Initially, the historical background regarding the involvement of consumers will be presented and the argument advanced that consumer participation in health care decision making is neither well conceptualized nor defined. The benefits and concerns related to involving consumers in health care decision making will be identified and, finally, research regarding consumer involvement in health care decision making will be reviewed.

Historical Overview

The concept of consumer participation in health care, the emerging issues, and the areas requiring further study are best understood by exploring the history and the development of consumerism in health care. Consumerism in health care had its roots in the civil and human rights movements that arose in North America in the 1960s. Efforts by consumer advocates, such as Ralph Nader, highlighted consumer rights and the role of the public in lobbying for services that met their needs. Nader was a leader in the consumer movement, investigating automobile safety and encouraging the public to articulate their concerns to automobile manufacturers. Automobiles were made safer as a result of Nader's interventions.

This consumer momentum extended to health care as the public became more informed about health care issues, their rights within the health care system, and the benefits and potential power they, as consumers, had within the system (Checkoway, 1981; CHEPA, 1991; Rosen, Metsch, & Levey, 1977). During this period, consumers became disillusioned with a health care system they saw dominated by providers, particularly physicians, where their voices as consumers were not being heard (Crichton & Hsu, 1990; Illich, 1975; Starr, 1982). Many consumers perceived physicians as arrogant, unwilling to cooperate on an equal basis with other allied health professionals and patients, too oriented to medical technology, and unwilling to listen to the social needs of consumers (Crichton & Hsu, 1990, p. 243).

Concerns were raised about the asymmetrical power structures in health care and the inability of consumers and allied health professionals to have a voice in decision making (Illich, 1975). Illich highlighted the need for teamwork in health care, acknowledging the requirement for greater recognition of the contributions of allied health professionals, such as nurses, in improving patient outcomes. Moreover, he emphasized the important role of the consumer in the health care system, believing that the consumer needed more control and decision-making authority in what he saw as a professionally dominated system (Starzomski, 1997).

The move toward healthy public policy and a change in focus in health care from elimination of disease (cure) to promotion of health, prevention of illness, maintenance of function, and chronic symptom management (care) spurred the consumer movement on its way as more people became active participants in their health care (Bracht, 1990; Hall, 1980; Milio, 1985; Ottawa Charter, 1986; Pederson, Edwards, Kelner, Marshall, & Allison, 1989; Thorne, 1993). Furthermore, the influence of the women's movement had a profound effect on the health care system as feminists attempted to redefine women's health issues, began to reorganize reproductive and maternity services, and suggested that a different voice needed to be heard in the health care arena (CHEPA, 1991; Gordon, 1990; Schwartz & Biederman, 1987). As a result of these changes, a variety of **self-help** and self-care groups emerged as consumers responded to their own health care needs and attempted to gain control over their care in a professionally dominated health care system (Checkoway, 1981; Schwartz & Biederman, 1987; Starzomski, 1997).

Although the involvement of the lay public in decision making about health care and governance of health care organizations have not occurred in a major way, there have been strides achieved by lay health groups. For example, self-help volunteer groups dealing with women's health issues such as less intervention in childbirth, organizations that represent the disabled, and groups advocating for less medical intervention for the dying have gained a place in the health care system (Coburn, D'Arcy, Torrance, & New, 1987). In addition, health charities were created to address the pressing health needs of the consumers they represented. Advocacy groups, working on behalf of individuals with, for instance, AIDS, breast cancer, prostate cancer, and kidney disease are highlighting the needs of consumers with these health conditions (Starzomski, 1997; Wachter, 1992). When discussing the rise and the encouragement by government of volunteer organizations in Canada, Crichton & Hsu (1990) state, "individual electors have not been happy about the bureaucratic centralization of power in welfare states, so the public has tried to preserve traditional structures [health charities] for involving consumers when all else has failed" (p. 245).

Although many groups are beginning to be included in discussions about health care decision making, there are those who have been excluded. These groups include the poor, the elderly, aboriginal people, and new immigrants who historically have not had a major voice in ensuring that their health care needs have been articulated or met.

In a review of national and international trends in health care, Siler-Wells (1987) predicted that there would be a move beyond the patient role to a more egalitarian and empowered partnership role for consumers. This trend is a major theme in government reviews of health care systems (Canadian Nurses Association, 1992; National Forum on Health, 1997).

In addition to the consumer movement, there is now considerable dialogue in the political arena, as well as a growing discussion by authors in a wide body of literature, about involving the public in health policy development and instilling public values in decisions regarding health care resource allocation. This discussion is evident in the literature of health care practitioners as well as in the health policy, health promotion, health economics, health care ethics, technology assessment and outcome evaluation literature (Charles & DeMaio, 1993; Crooks, 1985; Drummond, 1987; Evans, 1984; Goodman, 1992; Hadorn, 1991a; Starzomski, 1997).

In addition, contemporary literature about societal trends anticipated in the 21st century focuses on the growing importance of the consumer movement. Morrison (1996), in describing the major changes influencing society today and in the future, highlights the need to include consumers in all facets of societal development. He underscores the importance of responsiveness to consumer needs and outlines the value of technology in aiding consumers to access information quickly, thereby enhancing their decision-making ability. Indeed, one only has to reflect on the rise of the Internet and the prolific use of the World Wide Web to see how quickly many consumers have embraced technology to access information, thereby increasing their knowledge and ability to be involved in decision making about issues that are important to them.

Current Interest in Public Involvement

Current interest in consumer participation in health care stems from two major ethical factors: (1) a growing recognition that patient preferences ought to be incorporated into decision making involving individual treatment choices, and (2) the desire to increase public accountability for health care resource allocation decisions in order to make providers more accountable to the communities they serve (Charles & DeMaio, 1993). On an individual level, this includes the view that the expertise of professionals is no longer sufficient to ensure a responsive health care system, and that individual preferences become important as people make decisions about specific treatment options. These consumer values influence the goals for health care as well as the evaluation of treatment costs and benefits (Blue, Keyserlingk, Rodney, & Starzomski, 1999; CHEPA, 1991; Starzomski, 1986). On a community level, the limitation of professional expertise is recognized because health is defined as broader than health care. Hence, the public is demanding that the system be capable of responding to an extensive array of community-defined needs, and not simply the needs defined by health care "experts" (Charles & DeMaio, 1993; CHEPA, 1991; Reiser, 1992). Yeo (1996) suggests that "the best rationale for public participation is one solidly grounded in community autonomy, or community empowerment" (p. 51).

Governments are also emphasizing the importance of the involvement and accountability of consumers as health care becomes more complex, costs rise, and decisions about health care priorities are required (Emson, 1991; Manga & Weller, 1991). Consumer involvement in health care decision making is supported by the public's perception that governments are now less competent, trustworthy, and useful than they were in the past (Eyles, 1993). As a result, consumers are demanding involvement in decisions related to their own health care as well as in decisions about how health care will be delivered in their communities (CHEPA, 1991; Garland & Hasnain, 1990a; Garovitz, 1985; Hill, 1990).

Most reports dealing with public participation propose that it is beneficial and leads to better decision making; however, there is virtually no research evidence to support this claim (Charles & DeMaio, 1993; Lomas & Veenstra, 1995). Charles and DeMaio propose one reason for the lack of research in this area is the conceptual confusion around the issues. For example, there is little consensus and a lack of conceptual clarity about what the terms "lay," "consumer," "community," "public," or "consumer participation" actually mean (Arnstein, 1969; Charles & DeMaio, 1993; Eyles, 1993; Feingold, 1977). These authors also acknowledge the need for more research in the area of consumer participation in decision making. Furthermore, although there is widespread support for the move to a decentralized decision-making approach with increased consumer involvement in health care (B.C. Ministry of Health, 1991, 1993; Bruce, 1992; CHEPA, 1991; Nova Scotia Gov-

ernment, 1989), there is little evidence that the models of devolution and decentralization, where health care decision making by consumers is encouraged, actually work (Hurley et al., 1992; Lomas & Veenstra, 1995).

There are a few examples in the literature where attempts have been made to involve consumers in health care decision making. In the United States, particularly in Oregon, discussions at the grassroots level have examined how health care resources should be allocated (Colbert, 1990; Crawshaw, 1990; Crawshaw, Garland, Hines, & Lobitz, 1985; Dougherty, 1991; Hadorn, 1991b, 1991c; Hines, 1986; Jennings, 1988, 1990a, 1990b; Sipes-Metzler, 1991; Wallace-Brodeur, 1990). In Canada, some grassroots discussions have taken place during Royal Commissions on health care and during the 1997 National Forum on Health. In most provinces, such as Quebec, Saskatchewan, Nova Scotia, and British Columbia, there have been efforts to include consumers in a consultation process as those provinces reform their health care systems (B.C. Ministry of Health, 1991, 1993; Blue, Keyserlingk, Rodney, & Starzomski, 1999; CHEPA, 1991; Hurley, Lomas, & Bhatia, 1993; Lomas, 1996; National Forum on Health, 1997; Nova Scotia Government, 1989, 1994). There have also been several attempts in countries outside North America, such as Great Britain and New Zealand, to include more consumers in health care decision making (Bowling, 1996; Ham, 1993; Klein, 1993).

Some authors are critical of what they call "rhetoric" in regard to public inclusion in health care decision making. In many situations, they believe public involvement in health care is token, with providers still occupying the dominant roles within the system where they make the important decisions (Emson, 1991; Manga & Weller, 1991; Yeo, 1996). Moreover, because of the vertical, **hierarchical** decision-making systems prevalent in society, it is not readily apparent how consumer voices will be heard, nor how they will receive the information they need to be involved (Checkoway, 1981; Gordon, 1990; Reiser, 1992; Riddick, Cordes, Eisele, & Montgomery, 1984, Yeo, 1996).

For example, Woodward and Stoddart (1989) point out that the public needs to be more aware of the expected costs and benefits of various types of investigations and procedures in order to become involved in the debate about who should be offered various types or intensities of care. Further, they suggest that one of the challenges facing the health care system is to achieve an informed social consensus regarding the level of health care spending, a project that requires a cooperative effort on the part of all members of society. Crawshaw and associates (1989) support this claim, stating:

The role of the expert is clear and necessary in describing what is possible, but the expert cannot and should not be expected to present the limiting, broad policy values that inform a just democracy. Only legislators, supported by a courageous constituency, can establish the moral yardstick that must decide which "life and death" health benefits should be pursued under existing conditions. (p. 363)

The level of resource commitment to common goods, such as health care, is considered to be ultimately a matter of societal choice, with some authors proposing that members of the public ought to be involved in developing policies about the use of technology and the allocation of finite resources that are reflective of ethical principles and societal values (Pellegrino, Sieglar, & Singer, 1991). Winner (1993) further develops this idea and points out that there is no moral community or public space in which technological issues are topics for deliberation and common action. He states:

As we ponder issues of this kind [technological issues that require social choices], it is not always clear which principles, policies, or forms of moral reasoning are suited to the choices at hand. The vacuum is a social as well as an intellectual one. Often there are no persons or organizations with clear authority to make the decisions that matter. In fact, there may be no clearly defined social channels in which important moral issues can be addressed at all. Typically, what happens in such cases is that, as time passes, a mixture of corporate plans, market choices, interest group activities, lawsuits, government legislation takes shape to produce jerrybuilt policies. But given the number of points at which technologies generate significant stress and conflict, this familiar pattern is increasingly unsatisfactory. (p. 47)

Technology development and the decisions about how to use technology have been largely under the control of experts and have been

highly politicized (Fox & Swazey, 1992; Rettig, 1989; Winner, 1993), hence, the need for more public involvement in future discussions about allocation of resources to ensure that the interests of the public are well met. Winner (1993) supports public involvement in discussions about allocation of resources, suggesting that further work is required to examine how the public can be involved. He states:

Rather than continue the technocratic pattern in which philosophers advise a narrowly defined set of decision makers about ethical subtleties, today's thinkers would do better to re-examine the role of the public at this time. Unfortunately, the Western tradition of moral and political philosophy has little to recommend on this score, [and] almost nothing to say about the way in which persons in their roles as citizens might be involved in making choices about the development, deployment, and use of new technology. (p. 49)

From Turf Mentality to Team (Together Everyone Achieves More) Mentality

Compounding the problem of a lack of consumer voice in health care decision making is the additional concern that not all voices of health care providers are being heard in discussions. When discussing the best ways to make decisions about health care and develop healthy public policy, it has been noted that there is a need to move away from "turf mentality" to "team mentality," with more emphasis on collaboration among health care providers and consumers (Cull, 1992).

To develop collaborative partnerships between consumers and health care providers, it has been suggested that traditional hierarchical, vertical decision-making structures, where only some groups have power, need to be changed (Knaus, Draper, Wagner, & Zimmerman, 1986; Mitchell, Armstrong, Simpson, & Lentz, 1989). This change is necessary to allow consumers, and indeed some health care providers, to have an active voice in health care decision making (Starzomski, 1997). In the move to focus on this collaborative approach, there has been considerable attention given to the power imbalances between health care professionals and patients/clients of health care services (see also Chapter 4 in this volume by Sally Thorne).

Collaboration among health care team members leads to better decision making and positive patient outcomes (Baggs, Ryan, Phelps, Richeson, & Johnson, 1992; Knaus et al., 1986; Koerner, Cohen, & Armstrong, 1985; Mitchell et al., 1989). Yet, communication, collaboration, and effective decision making among health care providers are fraught with concerns about asymmetrical relationships, "turf wars," who has power in the system, vertical versus shared decision-making models, lack of respect for contributions of some health professionals, the physician in the traditional "captain of the ship" role not encouraging team functioning, and institutional constraints that block the ability of teams to function in a manner to facilitate positive outcomes (Mariano, 1989; Rodney & Starzomski, 1993; Schattschneider, 1990; Starzomski, 1997, 1998). Some authors believe that the reasons these issues have not been resolved may be related to the differences in values, moral reasoning, and philosophical perspectives of different health care provider groups (Campbell-Heider & Pollock, 1987; Canadian Medical Association, 1996; Grundstein-Amado, 1992; Stein, Watts, & Howell, 1990), although this has not been studied extensively.

Exposing asymmetrical relationships and power imbalances has been facilitated by employing critical social theory in analyses and in practice. Critical social theory emerged from Marxist philosophy and was developed by theorists such as Habermas (1989) and Freire (1989). These critical theories have been embraced by investigators in health care and nursing (Allen, Benner, & Diekleman, 1986; Campbell & Bunting, 1991; Hedin, 1986; Kendall, 1992; Stevens, 1989).

In critical theory, the purpose of knowledge is to release individuals from domination (emancipation), thus studies and practice informed by **critical theory** are designed to expose hidden power imbalances and enlighten agents about how they ought to act rationally to realize their own best interests (Campbell & Bunting, 1990; Schwandt, 1990). Critical theory is useful because it offers an approach to inquiry and practice that advocates emancipation, freedom from oppression, action, and ultimately direction for change (Bronner & Kellner, 1989; Campbell & Bunting, 1991)—the key constituents to enabling consumers and health care pro-

viders to be meaningful participants in health care decision making (Starzomski, 1997).

A premise on which the involvement of consumers in health care is based is that consumers hold different values and ideas about health care than do providers and so-called experts (Crawshaw, Garland, Hines, & Anderson, 1990), although there have been few studies that support this claim. The studies that have been conducted thus far tend to focus generally on attitudes of health care providers and consumers, without exploring these attitudes in depth (Lee, Penner, & Cox, 1991; Todres, Guillemin, Grodin, & Batten, 1988). Furthermore, there is little research examining whether the public (as well as the various groups that comprise "the public") and health care providers differ in their reasoning and choices about issues such as the allocation of resources for health care. A recent study by Starzomski (1997) suggests that consumers and health care providers actually make moral decisions in very similar ways, using comparable styles of moral reasoning. In fact, the results of this study provide some evidence that consumer and health care providers have more in common than once thought, including a shared belief that sound health care decisions require input from both groups.

Challenges and Opportunities

Some authors support the inclusion of consumer values into health care decision making and differentiate the contributions that consumers and health care providers can make to good decision making. For example, it is suggested that technical decisions about health care are those based on the application and extrapolation of scientific information and are, therefore, within the domain of experts (Eyles, 1993). Eyles notes, on the other hand, that there are value-based decisions concerned with resolving important societal issues where consumers are seen as those best qualified to resolve disputes over goals and directions of health care. Hurley and associates (1992) suggest that one of the challenges involved in allocating resources efficiently in the health care sector is combining expert knowledge about the effectiveness of medical treatments and the structure and financing of the system with information about the needs, values, preferences, and local circumstances of communities (p. 3). The crux of the problem is that, although providers possess better knowledge about the expected effectiveness of health care in improving health status, individuals are the best judges of how these improvements affect their well-being (Evans, 1984). Reiser (1992) states: "experts and consumers can benefit from a view of health care that emphasizes human diversity and focuses on particularistic solutions bearing the mark of the individuals whom illness affects" (p. 1515).

It is acknowledged that "good" health care decisions are not possible until the layperson or public supplies the value framework to be used (Caws, 1991; Jennings, 1991; Veatch, 1985a, 1991a; Veatch & Moreno, 1991). Veatch (1985b) suggests that value systems drawn from cultural, religious, and philosophical ideological systems are central to planning health care directions. He posits that value systems provide a framework for choosing among policy alternatives, who the policy-makers will be, and whether there is any possibility for cooperation among the various stakeholders in the policy arena. Pellegrino (1985) suggests that a nation's or community's health policy is its strategy for controlling and optimizing the social uses of its knowledge and resources. Human values, he concludes, are the guides and justifications people use for choosing the goals, priorities, and means that make up a strategy.

According to Pellegrino, ethics act as the bridge between health policy and values by examining the moral validity of the choices that must be made as well as seeking to resolve the conflicts between the values that inevitably occur in making these choices. He goes on to describe health policy as reflecting the fundamental beliefs and commitments that tie a nation most closely to its identity and integrity as a human community. These commitments, he states, are society's human values, allowing communities to exert their influence over the momentum of technological advance through expression in the choices and priorities of their health policies. Furthermore, according to Veatch (1985b), there is a need for persons to discover whether they share a tradition of values about health care that would help them define the package of health care services that best serves the community. Veatch (1985a) proposes that the role of the public in ethical decision making is an essential one, and this includes roles related to making policy decisions about the allocation of resources (Starzomski, 1997).

Many potential benefits to the health care system have been suggested as a result of consumer involvement in health care. These benefits include defining the needs of the community, developing effective ways to meet those needs, as well as fostering a sense of civic responsibility, and a sense of belonging to a community. Furthermore, there is potential for an enhanced level of concern for fellow consumers, a greater sensitivity to the social causes of many health problems and sensitivity to the needs of different ethnocultural groups (Blue et al., 1999; Charles & DeMaio, 1993; Checkoway, 1981; CHEPA, 1991; Eyles, 1993; Starzomski, 1997; Wachter, 1992).

Concerns have been raised about consumer involvement in health care decision making. As mentioned earlier, there is no clarity about what the goals of consumer participation are or ought to be, or whether consumer participation is a means to an end, an end itself, or both (Charles & DeMaio, 1993; CHEPA, 1991; Hurley et al., 1992). In addition, there is little consensus about what the terms "lay" or "consumer participation" mean, leading to conceptual confusion about where and how consumers would actually be involved in the system. Such concerns have led to the development of analytic frameworks describing public participation by discussing different stages and levels. These frameworks help to reinforce the notion that consumer participation is not a homogenous concept (Arnstein, 1969; Charles & DeMaio, 1993; Feingold, 1977; MacKean & Thurston, 1996). For example, MacKean and Thurston expand on Arnstein's ladder of citizen participation and discuss various stages of public involvement in decision making. At the bottom rung of the ladder is nonparticipation. The next phase is information exchange and consists of informing, consultation, and advising. Finally, the top rung of the ladder is made up of partnership, delegated power, and citizen control.

Other concerns about consumer involvement in health care decision making center on the potential emphasis on individual responsibility, and an undervaluing of the expertise of health care providers. Stated in another way, lay involvement may encourage interest group politics and decision making based on emotional or personal responses rather than on facts and input from those with expertise. Health care providers and bureaucrats who prefer to retain centralized power are worried that their power base may be eroded (Crichton & Hsu, 1990). On the other hand, there are concerns that, in some cases, consumer participation may consolidate the power of bureaucrats rather than the community groups they are charged to represent (O'Neill, 1992). Furthermore, there may be a move to emphasize majoritarian decision making to the detriment of small disenfranchised groups, and there may be opportunities for regional disparities to emerge (Boisaubin, 1988; Wachter, 1992). Finally, some writers have suggested that the process of decision making may be slower if there is public consultation in decision making about health care issues (Blue et al., 1999; Charles & DeMaio, 1993; Checkoway, 1981; CHEPA, 1991; Eyles, 1993; Starzomski, 1997).

Interestingly, discussions about including consumers and their values in health care parallels discussions in the forestry literature (Tanz & Howard, 1991) and environmental movement (Wiseman, Vanderkop, & Nef, 1991), where at one time, consumers were involved only as part of radical special-interest groups. There is a growing desire to have consumers, experts, government, and industry working closer together to help resolve some of the problems related to forestry practices and the environment. In these areas, consumer participation has developed to become more of an accepted part of responsible citizenship, a notion not yet embraced wholeheartedly in health care.

Promises and Pitfalls

A review by policy analysts of more than 35 major commissions and health care task forces conducted in Canada over the past few decades revealed three common goals: a greater emphasis on disease prevention and health promotion, a move to community-based care alternatives, and the need to increase the importance of accountability among the stakeholders (Canadian Nurses Association, 1992). The importance of the concept of accountability and community involvement was re-inforced in the Prime Minister's 1997 National Forum on Health. Recommendations were made suggesting that decisions about health care delivery and resource allocation ought to be made as close to the community level as possible, allowing local people to shape their own system of delivery (National Forum on Health, 1997). In addition, decentralization and devolution of health care services was seen as a key component of efforts to empower both individuals and communities, restoring the balance in a system perceived by many to have been co-opted by experts (Hurley et al., 1992, p. 2).

It is not enough to merely state that consumers should be involved in health care decision making. Several conditions have been proposed for meaningful public participation in decision making, including assuring that consumers have adequate information, that there are a majority of consumers in the group, that there is a strong mandate from the community with formal and informal access to constituents, and that people selected to represent communities have strong personalities so as not to be intimidated or dominated by the so-called experts within the group (O'Neill, 1992).

Restructuring of health care services is leading to proposals where, in some places, there is potential for public and provider dialogue about health care decision making (Hurley et al., 1993). For example, in the United States and Canada there have been several examples of consultation with the public to determine public opinion and community values about health care priorities and allocation of resources (Charles & DeMaio, 1993; CHEPA, 1991; Emson, 1991). The best examples in Canada have been Royal Commissions on health care issues, such as the Royal Commission on New Reproductive Technologies (Proceed with Care, 1993). More recently, there has been the National Forum on Health Care (1997) directed by the Prime Minister to collect information nationwide from different public and provider groups about the health care system, and to make recommendations about the future of health care in Canada. It is interesting to note, however, that there has been very little formal research in the area of public participation in health care, although it is an area that is generating considerable debate among many societal groups.

The Oregon Plan

In the United States, the "social experiment" that occurred in Oregon, although not designed as a formal research study, illuminated a number of areas reviewed earlier in this chapter related to consumer involvement in health care decision making (Dixon & Welch, 1991; Oregon Department of Human Resources, 1992). A phenomenal amount of attention and debate were directed at Oregon's effort to reform certain pieces of health care legislation, a debate that came to be known as the "Oregon Experiment" (Nelson & Drought, 1992). As a way of dealing with the rationing questions that were plaguing the state, elected officials, community leaders, consumers, and health care professionals attempted to define an adequate, minimum standard of health care for their consumers (Daniels, 1991; Eddy, 1991a, 1991c). Fox and Leichter (1991) suggest that this was a process where Oregonians sought to discover whether they shared a tradition of values about health care that would help them define the package of health services that constituted the common good. Fox and Leichter added, "if one was looking (searching) for a classic exercise of American democracy in the sunlight, it is Oregon's debate" (1991, p. 7).

The Oregon program became a focal point for debate on virtually every aspect of U.S. health policy: access, cost effectiveness, rationing, and basic care (Eddy, 1991b; Garland, 1992; Garland & Hasnain, 1990b). The plan sparked a major debate surrounding the complexities and ethics related to resource allocation and involvement of consumers in developing health policy (Golenski & Thompson, 1991; Menzel, 1992a, 1992b). Eddy (1991b) pointed out that the plan provided "a focus for national debate, a target to shoot at, a starting point for improvement" (p. 2135). Proponents of the plan praised its boldness and suggested that it would bring discussions of appropriate care to the forefront so that the issues could be debated in the public arena (McPherson, 1991).

Opponents suggested that the plan discriminated against poor women and children and illustrated many of the problems that arise when using quality of life indicators as a means of determining how resources should be allocated (Fox & Leichter, 1991; Goodman, 1991; Gore, 1990; Veatch, 1991b). Another criticism was levied at the process used for collecting some of the necessary information. Town hall meetings were held, but those in attendance were primarily affluent health care providers and not the disadvantaged for whom the plan was being designed (Blue et al., 1999; Starzomski, 1997).

The Oregon social experiment illustrates that the task of prioritizing health services involves a judgement composed of facts and values. Hence, it becomes essential to incorporate citizen values about what they wish to see in a health care system, with ethical, economic, and outcome approaches to policy decision making, in order to make the best possible societal decisions (Blue et al., 1999). Moreover, Hadorn (1993) suggests that, despite the efforts of many researchers, there are still uncertainties about how society might use outcome data to set priorities in the health care system. He says that, although the idea of determining the health outcomes associated with different treatments, determining how people feel about those outcomes, then giving priority to treatments that produce more preferred outcomes may sound simple, it is fraught with complications, not least of which is discrimination against some individuals (Hadorn, 1991b, 1992).

Hadorn (1993) when speaking about the Oregon attempt to involve consumers and providers in an outcome and preference based effort to set priorities says:

Unfortunately, although the Oregon project provided a wealth of experience on one possible approach to estimating and dovetailing preferences, the result of that project—a priority list containing 688 condition-treatment pairs—is of questionable utility. Because of the wide range of procedures and indications contained within each "line item" on the list, substantial additional specification will be needed before the list can be applied to actual patients. (p. 2)

He continues:

An important unresolved issue in the field of resource allocation is whether people's preferences differ significantly based on demographic characteristics or, particularly, on whether they have experienced (or are experiencing) medical conditions or disabilities. Concern over such differences was the stated reason for the initial denial of the waiver needed by the State of Oregon to implement its much-discussed effort to set health care priorities in its Medicaid program. (p. 5)

Public and Health Care Provider Roles in the Allocation of Resources

Recent research has examined perceptions of the public and of health care providers about the roles they desire in health care decision making. For instance, Starzomski (1997) conducted 34 focus groups with a variety of consumer and health care provider groups to determine the level of involvement they believed they should have in resource allocation decision making for organ transplantation. The results of the study showed that there was a great deal of support for better health care planning that would include collaboration among all stakeholder groups. At the macro level of the system, focus group participants indicated a desire to include more participants, other than government, in decisions about health care. There was also a call for more transparent decision making throughout the system.

Consumers, in particular, wanted to ensure that the values they held about health care were integrated into a discussion about resource allocation. They saw this occurring to some extent at the level of regional boards and community health councils, but also believed that more innovative ways of obtaining their input was required. Many consumers believed that macro level decisions should be left up to the "experts," and although they wanted input, they did not see a role for themselves in making choices at this level.

Most health care providers saw a role for themselves in macro-level decision making, with physicians indicating that there was a need for more involvement by members of their profession. Other professional groups supported roles for health care providers, as well their own group, in having input into decisions about how resources should be allocated. Interestingly, some staff nurses in the focus groups had difficulty articulating a role for themselves at any level in the system, a problem that may be related to a sense of lack

of power and decision making in their roles (Rodney & Starzomski, 1993). It was at the meso and micro level of the system that many participants recognized a need for change from the current process of making decisions (Starzomski, 1997).

Participants identified a role for more consumers at both levels of the system, although some health care providers had difficulty envisioning a role for consumers when they discussed this idea in their focus groups. In particular, transplant patients wanted a role on boards of organizations and selection committees that governed organ transplantation, roles that have been predominantly held by health care professionals. Most health care provider groups supported this role for consumers and also saw roles for themselves. For instance, critical care nurses saw a role in becoming more involved in recipient selection and criteria development for transplantation. Consumers and many of the providers wanted the transplant process to be a more transparent one and saw expanded consumer involvement as a beginning step.

Some authors have suggested that there is little opportunity for the public to be involved in macro level health care decision making, nonetheless, it is a value espoused by many (Eyles, 1993). Given that communities are naturally heterogeneous, the challenge lies in determining who ought to be involved and how they should be involved. Abelson and colleagues (1995) discovered that when they polled 280 citizens in Ontario, Canada, from a variety of potential decision-making groups (randomly selected consumers, attendees at town hall meetings, appointees to district health councils, elected officials, and experts in health care and social services) and asked their opinion about their willingness to be involved in devolved decision making, there were varying responses. Elected officials were most willing and thought their group best suited to this role, whereas "average" citizens were least willing and thought their group least suited. These results challenge the assumptions that communities (or potential decision-makers) all want to be *involved* in decision making. This finding is consistent with Starzomski's (1997) study, in which consumers wanted to ensure that they had input into some macro-level decisions, but did not want necessarily to be making the decisions. In other words, consumers wanted a voice but not necessarily a choice (Abelson et al., 1995). Given the new structures in many areas of Canada and the U.S. of regional health boards, community health councils, and advisory committees to these groups, there are more opportunities than ever before to ensure that the public and health care providers have the opportunity to at least exercise such voice.

A macro level attempt to solicit public feedback about health care was undertaken by the National Health Forum (1997). Discussion groups were organized throughout the country to obtain some consensus about the values Canadians hold regarding health care. An important recommendation by the Forum was prefaced with comments that the present ad hoc approach in Canada of linking values with health policy issues is not acceptable, and that more attention is needed on obtaining citizen input prior to developing health policy. The Forum members suggested that, as an inaugural attempt to enhance the process of ethical reflection in Canada, the Federal Minister of Health should take the lead in discussing with provincial/territorial counterparts, and key groups with a substantial interest in ethics, ways to establish permanent linkages among ethics networks and bodies. The Forum members saw this as a first step in establishing a national body to provide ethical direction, and they cautioned that, "a 'just in-time' method of creating working groups and committees to address ethical dilemmas that society debates is no longer acceptable" (pp. 21–24). In other words, it is essential that ethical reflection and debate occur well in advance of policy decision making that determines resource allocation.

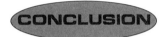

CONCLUSION

In summary, public involvement in health care decision making is multifaceted. There is no consensus about how to include the public in meaningful ways in the development of healthy public policy, although there is agreement by many that public participation in health care decision making is desirable. There is a clear need to be sensitive to the contexts where public participation is being recommended. This is an area where definitely, "one size does not fit all." As Hurley and associates (1992) point out:

it is very difficult to design a decision making structure that represents community interests and values fairly and which integrates them with expert knowledge in a balanced fashion. Designing such structures is perhaps the most formidable challenge facing those who truly wish to develop decentralized systems that are responsive to the needs, values and preferences of the communities they serve through decision-making processes that reflect their values. (p. 18)

This review of consumer involvement in health care decision making points to the need for further research about the role of the consumer in health care to determine at what level of the system consumers ought be involved and how they ought to be involved. There is no doubt, however, that decisions required in health care will continue to demand the involvement of consumers and health care providers in the decision-making processes. These decisions will be complex and difficult, such that no one set of voices or one societal group will be adequate to make the choices that are needed. A collaborative effort will provide the best method to ensure that wise choices are made. Indeed, it is hoped that together everyone can achieve more when it comes to making decisions about our health and health care for the future.

REFERENCES

Abelson, J., Lomas, J., Eyles, S., Birch, S., & Veenstra, G. (1995). Does the community want devolved authority? Results from deliberative polling in Ontario. *Canadian Medical Association Journal, 153,* 403–412.

Allen, D., Benner, P., & Diekelmann, N. (1986). Three paradigms for nursing research: Methodological implications. In P. L. Chinn (Ed.), *Nursing research methodology: Issues and implications* (pp. 23–38). Rockville, MD: Aspen.

Arnstein, S. (1969). A ladder of citizen participation. *Journal of the American Institute of Planners, 25,* 216–224.

British Columbia Ministry of Health. (1991). *Closer to home—The report of the British Columbia Royal Commission on Health Care and Costs.* Victoria, B.C.: Author.

British Columbia Ministry of Health. (1993). *New directions for a healthy British Columbia.* Victoria, B.C.: Author.

Baggs, J., Ryan, S., Phelps, C., Richeson, J., & Johnson, J. (1992). The association between interdisciplinary collaboration and patient outcomes in a medical intensive care unit. *Heart & Lung, 21*(1), 18–24.

Blue, A., Keyserlingk, T., Rodney, P., & Starzomski, R. (1999). A critical review of North American health policy. In H. Coward & P. Ratanakul (Eds.), *An intercultural dialogue on health care ethics* (pp. 215–225). Waterloo, Ontario: Wilfrid Laurier.

Boisaubin, E. (1988). Charity, the media, and limited medical resources. *Journal of the American Medical Association, 259,* 1375–1376.

Bowling, A. (1996). Health care rationing: The public's debate. *British Medical Journal, 312,* 670–674.

Bracht, N. (1990). *Health promotion at the community level.* Newbury Park, CA: Sage.

Bronner, S., & Kellner, D. (1989). Introduction. In S. Bronner & D. Kellner (Eds.), *Critical theory and society: A reader* (pp. 1–21). New York: Routledge.

Bruce, T. (1992). Defining the cost of health care. *Nursing BC, 24*(1), 1–4.

Campbell, J., & Bunting, S. (1991). Voices and paradigms: Perspectives on critical and feminist theory in nursing. *Advances in Nursing Science, 13*(3), 1–15.

Campbell-Heider, N., & Pollock, D. (1987). Barriers to physician-nurse collegiality: An anthropological perspective. *Social Science & Medicine, 25*(5), 421–425.

Canadian Medical Association. (1996). *Working together: A joint CNA/CMA collaborative practice project.* Ottawa: Author.

Canadian Nurses Association. (1992). HEAL unveils proposals for health care reform. *CNA Today—The National News In Nursing, 2*(1), 3.

Caws, P. (1991). Committees and consensus: How many heads are better than one? *Journal of Medicine and Philosophy, 16*(4), 375–391.

Center for Health Economics and Policy Analysis (CHEPA). (1991). *Summary Report—Health care and the public: Roles, expectations and contributions.* Fourth Annual Health Policy Conference, McMaster University—Center for Health Economics and Policy Analysis, Hamilton, Canada.

Charles, C., & DeMaio, S. (1993). Lay participation in health care decision making: A conceptual framework. *Journal of Health Politics, Policy and Law, 18*(4), 883–904.

Checkoway, B. (1981). *Citizens and health care: Participation and planning for social change.* Toronto: Pergamon.

Coburn, D., D'Arcy, C., Torrance, G., & New, P. (1987). Health and Canadian society—Trends, issues and research. In D. Coburn, C. D'Arcy, G. Torrance, & P. New, *Health and Canadian society—Sociological perspectives* (pp. 649–668). Markham, Ontario: Fitzhenry & Whiteside.

Colbert, T. (1990). Public input into health care policy: Controversy and contribution in California. *Hastings Center Report, 20*(5), 21–22.

Crawshaw, R. (1990). A vision of the health decisions movement. *Hastings Center Report, 20*(5), 21–22.

Crawshaw, R., Garland, M., & Hines, B. (1989). Organ transplants: A search for health policy at the state level. *Western Journal of Medicine, 150,* 361–363.

Crawshaw, R., Garland, M., Hines, B., & Anderson, B. (1990). Developing principles for prudent health care allocation—The continuing Oregon experiment. *Western Journal of Medicine, 152,* 441–446.

Crawshaw, R., Garland, M., Hines, B., & Lobitz, C. (1985). Oregon health decisions: An experiment with informed community consent. *Journal of the American Medical Association, 254,* 3213–3216.

Crichton, A., & Hsu, D. (1990). *Canada's health care system: Its funding and organization.* Ottawa: Canadian Hospital Association Press.

Crooks, G. M. (1985). Health policy making in America: The process of building consensus. In Z. Bankowski & J. H. Bryant (Eds.), *Health policy, ethics and human values—An international dialogue.* Geneva: Council for International Organizations of Medical Sciences.

Cull, E. (1992). *Opening address.* Toward a Better Understanding of the Broader Determinants of Health: Economic and Policy Implications Conference. Center for Health Services and Policy Research Day, Vancouver, B.C.

Daniels, N. (1991). Is the Oregon rationing plan fair? *Journal of the American Medical Association, 265,* 2232–2235.

Dixon, J., & Welch, H. (1991). Priority setting: Lessons from Oregon. *The Lancet, 337,* 891–894.

Dougherty, C. J. (1991). Setting health care priorities: Oregon's next steps. *Hastings Center Report, 21*(3), 1–10.

Drummond, M. (1987). Resource allocation decisions in health care: A role for quality of life assessments? *Journal of Chronic Disease, 40,* 605–616.

Eddy, D. (1991a). What's going on in Oregon? *Journal of the American Medical Association, 266,* 4117–4120.

Eddy, D. (1991b). Oregon's methods: Did cost-effectiveness analysis fail? *Journal of the American Medical Association, 266,* 2135–2141.

Eddy, D. (1991c). Oregon's plan: Should it be approved? *Journal of the American Medical Association, 266,* 2439–2445.

Emson, H. (1991). Down the Oregon trail—The way for Canada? *Canadian Medical Association Journal, 145,* 1441–1443.

Evans, R. (1984). *Strained mercy: The economics of Canadian health care.* Toronto: Butterworth.

Eyles, J. (1993). *The role of the citizen in health care decision making* (Policy Commentary C93–1). Toronto: McMaster University Centre for Health Economics and Policy Analysis.

Feingold, E. (1977). Citizen participation. A review of the issues. In H. Rosen, J. Metsch, & S. Levey (Eds.), *The consumer and the health care system: Social and managerial perspectives*. New York: Spectrum.

Fox, D., & Leichter, H. (1991). Rationing care in Oregon: The new accountability. *Health Affairs, 10*(2), 7–27.

Fox, R., & Swazey, J. (1992). Leaving the field. *Hastings Center Report, 22*(5), 9–15.

Freire, P. (1989). *Pedagogy of the oppressed*. New York: Continuum.

Garland, M., & Hasnain, R. (1990a). Community responsibility and the development of Oregon's health care priorities. *Business & Professional Ethics Journal, 9*(3 & 4), 183–200.

Garland, M., & Hasnain, R. (1990b). Health care in common: Setting priorities in Oregon. *Hastings Center Report, 20*(5), 16–18.

Garland, M. (1992). Justice, politics and community: Expanding access and rationing health services in Oregon. *Law, Medicine & Health Care, 20*(1–2), 67–81.

Garovitz, S. (1985). An integration of societal values. In Z. Bankowski & J. H. Bryant (Eds.), *Health policy, ethics and human values—An international dialogue*. Geneva: Council for International Organizations of Medical Sciences.

Golenski, J., & Thompson, S. (1991). A history of Oregon's basic health services act: An insider's account. *QRB, 17*(5), 144–149.

Goodman, C. (1992). It's time to rethink health care technology assessment. *International Journal of Technology Assessment in Health Care, 8*(2), 335–358.

Goodman, N. (1991). Resource allocation: Idealism, realism, pragmatism, openness. *Journal of Medical Ethics, 17*(4), 179–180.

Gordon, C. (1990). A consumer's perspective on health care. Unpublished manuscript , Medical-Legal Society Forum, Vancouver, B.C.

Gore, A. (1990). Oregon's bold mistake. *Academic Medicine, 65*, 634–635.

Grundstein-Amado, R. (1992). Differences in ethical decision making processes among nurses and doctors. *Journal of Advanced Nursing, 17*(2), 129–137.

Habermas, J. (1989). The tasks of a critical theory of society. In S. Bronner & D. Kellner (Eds.), *Critical theory and society: A reader* (T. McCarthy, Trans., pp. 292–312). New York: Routledge.

Hadorn, D. (1991a). The role of public values in setting health care priorities. *Social Science & Medicine, 32*, 773–781.

Hadorn, D. (1991b). Setting health care priorities in Oregon: Cost effectiveness meets the rule of rescue. *Journal of the American Medical Association, 265*, 2218–2225.

Hadorn, D. (1991c). The Oregon priority-setting exercise: Quality of life and public policy. *Hastings Center Report, 21*(3), 11–16.

Hadorn, D. (1992). The problem of discrimination in health care priority setting. *Journal of the American Medical Association, 268*, 1454–1459.

Hadorn, D. (1993). *Outcomes management and resource allocation: How should quality of life be measured?* Health Policy Research Unit Discussion Paper Series (HPRU 93:7D). Vancouver: University of British Columbia.

Hall, E. M. (Special Commissioner) (1980). *Canada's national-provincial health program for the 1980's. A commitment for renewal*. Saskatoon: Croft Litho.

Ham, C. (1993). Priority setting in the NHS: Reports from six districts. *British Medical Journal, 307*, 435–438.

Hedin, B. (1986). Nursing, education, and emancipation: Applying the critical theoretical approach to nursing research. In P. Chinn (Ed.), *Nursing research methodology: Issues and implementation* (pp. 133–146). Rockville, MD: Aspen.

Hill, T. (1990). Giving voice to the pragmatic majority in New Jersey. *Hastings Center Report, 20*(5), 20.

Hines, B. (1986). Health policy on the town meeting agenda. *Hastings Center Report, 16*(2), 5–7.

Hurley, J., Birch, S., & Eyles, J. (1992). *Information, efficiency, and decentralization within health care systems* (CHEPA Working Paper #92–21). Hamilton: McMaster University.

Hurley, J., Lomas, J. & Bhatia, V. (1993). *Is the wolf finally at the door? Provincial reform to manage health-care resources* (CHEPA Working Paper #93–12). Hamilton: McMaster University.

Illich, I. (1975). *Medical nemesis*. Toronto: McLelland and Stewart.

Jennings, B. (1988). A grassroots movement in bioethics. *Hastings Center Report, 18*(3, Suppl.), 1–16.

Jennings, B. (1990a). Democracy and justice in health policy. *Hastings Center Report, 20*(5), 22.

Jennings, B. (1990b). Grassroots bioethics revisited: Health care priorities and community values. *Hastings Center Report, 20*(5), 16.

Jennings, B. (1991). Possibilities of consensus: Toward democratic moral discourse. *Journal of Medicine and Philosophy, 16*(4), 447–463.

Kendall, J. (1992). Fighting back: Promoting emancipatory nursing actions. *Advances in Nursing Science, 15*(2), 1–15.

Klein, R. (1993). Dimensions of rationing: Who should do what? *British Medical Journal, 307*, 309–311.

Knaus, W., Draper, E., Wagner, D., & Zimmerman, J. (1986). An evaluation of outcome from intensive care in major medical centers. *Annals of Internal Medicine, 104*, 410–418.

Koerner, B., Cohen, J., & Armstrong, D. (1985). Collaborative practice and patient satisfaction: Impact and selected outcomes. *Evaluation & the Health Professionals, 8*(3), 299–321.

Kymlicka, W. (1990). *Contemporary political philosophy*. New York: Oxford University Press.

Lee, S., Penner, P., & Cox, M. (1991). Comparison of the attitudes of health care professionals and parents toward active treatment of very low birth weight infants. *Pediatrics, 88*, 110–114.

Lomas, J., & Veenstra, G. (1995). If you build it, who will come? Governments, consultation and biased publics. *Policy Options, November,* 37–40.

Lomas, J. (1996). Devolved authority in Canada—The new site of health care system conflict? In J. Dorland & S. M. Davis (Eds.), *How many roads . . . Decentralization of health care in Canada* (pp. 25–34). Kingston, Ontario: Queen's School of Policy Studies.

MacKean, G., & Thurston, W. (1996). A Canadian model of public participation in health care planning and decision making. In M. Stingl & D. Wilson (Eds.), *Efficiency vs. equality: Health reform in Canada* (pp. 55–69). Halifax: Fernwood Publishing Co. Ltd.

Manga, P., & Weller, G. (1991). Health policy under conservative governments in Canada. In C. Altenstetter & S. Haywood (Eds.), *Comparative health policy and the new right: From rhetoric to reality.* New York: St. Martin's Press.

Mariano, C. (1989). The case for interdisciplinary collaboration. *Nursing Outlook, 37*(8), 285–288.

McPherson, A. (1991). The Oregon plan: Rationing in a rational society. *Canadian Medical Association Journal, 145,* 1444–1445.

Menzel, P. (1992a). Oregon's denial: Disabilities and quality of life. *Hastings Center Report, 22*(6), 21–25.

Menzel, P. (1992b). Some ethical costs of rationing. *Law, Medicine & Health Care, 20*(1–2), 57–66.

Milio, N. (1985). Healthy nations: Creating a new ecology of public policy for health. *Canadian Journal of Public Health, 76*(Suppl. 1), 79–87.

Mitchell, P., Armstrong, S., Simpson, T., & Lentz, M. (1989). American Association of Critical-Care Nurses Demonstration Project: Profile of excellence in critical care nursing. *Heart & Lung, 18*(3), 219–237.

Morrison, I. (1996). *The second curve: How to command new technologies, new consumers and new markets.* New York: Ballantine Books.

National Forum on Health. (1997). *Canada health action: Building on the legacy* (Vols. 1 & 2). Ottawa: Author.

Nelson, R., & Drought, T. (1992). Justice and the moral acceptability of rationing medical care: The Oregon experiment. *Journal of Medicine and Philosophy, 17*(1), 97–117.

Nova Scotia Government (1989). *Towards a new strategy—The report of the Nova Scotia Royal Commission on Health Care.* Halifax, Nova Scotia: Author.

Nova Scotia Government (1994). *Nova Scotia's blueprint for health care reform.* Halifax, Nova Scotia: Author.

O'Neill, M. (1992). Community participation in Quebec's health system: A strategy to curtail community empowerment. *International Journal of Health Services, 22*(2), 287–301.

Oregon Department of Human Resources. (1992). *The Oregon health plan.* Salem, Oregon: Author.

Ottawa Charter for Health Promotion. (1986). First International Conference on Health Promotion, Ottawa.

Pederson, A., Edwards, R., Kelner, M., Marshall, V., & Allison, K. (1989). *Coordinating healthy public policy—An analytic literature review and bibliography.* Paper prepared for the Health Promotion Directorate/National Health Research and Development Program Working Group on Priorities for Health Promotion/Disease Prevention Research. Ottawa: Minister of Supply and Services Canada.

Pellegrino, E. (1985). Health policy, ethics and human values. In Z. Bankowski & J. H. Bryant (Eds.), *Health policy, ethics and human values—An international dialogue.* Geneva: Council for International Organizations of Medical Sciences.

Pellegrino, E., Sieglar, M., & Singer, P. (1991). Future directions in clinical ethics. *Journal of Clinical Ethics, 2*(1), 5–9.

Proceed with Care. (1993). Final report of the Royal Commission on New Reproductive Technologies. Canada: Minister of Government Services.

Reiser, S. (1992). Consumer competence and the reform of American health care. *Journal of the American Medical Association, 267,* 1511–1515.

Rettig, R. (1989). The politics of organ transplantation: A parable of our time. *Journal of Health Politics, Policy and Law, 14*(1), 191–227.

Riddick, C., Cordes, S., Eisele, T., & Montgomery, A. (1984). The health planning process: Are consumers really in control? *Health Policy, 4,*117–127.

Rodney, P., & Starzomski, R. (1993). Constraints on the moral agency of nurses. *The Canadian Nurse, 89*(9), 23–26.

Rosen, H., Metsch, J., & Levey, S. (1977). *The consumer and the health care system: Social and managerial perspectives.* Toronto: Spectrum.

Roy, D., Williams, J., & Dickens, B. (1994). *Bioethics in Canada.* Scarborough, Canada: Prentice Hall.

Saul, J. R. (1995). *The unconscious civilization.* Concord, Ontario: ANANSI.

Schattschneider, H. (1990). Power relationships between physician and nurse. *Humane Medicine, 6*(3), 197–201.

Schwandt, T. (1990). Paths to inquiry in the social disciplines: Scientific, constructivist, and critical theory methodologies. In E. G. Guba (Ed.), *The paradigm dialog* (pp. 258–276). Newbury Park, CA: Sage.

Schwartz, H. D., & Biederman, I. S. (1987). Lay initiatives in the consumption of health care. In H. D. Schwartz (Eds.), *Dominant issues in medical sociology* (2nd ed.). New York: Random House.

Siler-Wells, G. (1987). *Changing priorities for Canada's health care system.* Executive Brief Series. Ottawa: Canadian Hospital Association.

Sipes-Metzler, P. (1991). Oregon update. *Hastings Center Report, 21*(6), 13.

Starr, P. (1982). *The social transformation of American medicine.* New York: Basic Books.

Starzomski, R. (1986). Patient and staff involvement in decisions for ESRD treatment. *American Nephrology Nurses Association Journal, 13*(6), 325–329.

Starzomski, R. (1997). *Resource allocation for solid organ transplantation: Toward public and health care provider dialogue.* Unpublished doctoral dissertation, University of British Columbia, Vancouver.

Starzomski, R., & Rodney, P. (1997). Nursing inquiry for the common good. In S. Thorne & V. Hayes (Eds.), *Nursing praxis: Knowledge and action* (pp. 219–236). Newbury Park, CA: Sage.

Starzomski, R. (1998). Ethics in nephrology nursing. In J. Parker (Ed.), *Nephrology nursing—A comprehensive textbook* (pp. 83–109). Pitman, NJ: American Nephrology Nurses Association.

Stein, L., Watts, D., & Howell, T. (1990). The doctor-nurse game revisited. *New England Journal of Medicine, 322,* 546–549.

Stevens, P. (1989). A critical social reconceptualization of environment in nursing: Implications for methodology. *Advances in Nursing Science, 11*(4), 56–68.

Tanz, J., & Howard, A. (1991). Meaningful public participation in the planning and management of publicly owned forests. *The Forestry Chronicle, 67*(2), 125–130.

Thorne, S. (1993). *Negotiating health care: The social context of chronic illness.* Newbury Park, CA: Sage.

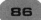

Todres, I., Guillemin, J., Grodin, M., & Batten, D. (1988). Life saving therapy for newborns: A questionnaire survey in the State of Massachusetts. *Pediatrics, 81,* 643–649.

Veatch, R., & Moreno, J. (1991). Consensus in panels and committees: Conceptual and ethical issues. *Journal of Medicine and Philosophy, 16*(4), 371–373.

Veatch, R. (1985a). Lay medical ethics. *Journal of Medicine & Philosophy, 10*(1),1–5.

Veatch, R. (1985b). Value systems: Their role in shaping health policy. In Z. Bankowski & J. Bryant (Eds.), *Health policy, ethics and human values—An international dialogue.* Geneva: Council for International Organizations of Medical Sciences.

Veatch, R. (1991a). Consensus of expertise: The role of consensus of experts in formulating public policy and estimating facts. *Journal of Medicine and Philosophy, 16*(4), 429–445.

Veatch, R. (1991b). Should basic care get priority? Doubts about rationing the Oregon way. *Kennedy Institute of Ethics Journal, 1*(3), 187–206.

Wachter, R. (1992). AIDS, activism, and the politics of health. *The New England Journal of Medicine, 326*(7), 128–133.

Wallace-Brodeur, P. (1990). Community values in Vermont health planning. *Hastings Center Report, 20*(5), 18–19.

Winner, L. (1993). Citizen virtues in a technological order. In E. Winkler & J. Coombs (Eds.), *Applied ethics—A reader* (pp. 46–69). Cambridge: Blackwell.

Wiseman, H., Vanderkop, J., & Nef, J. (1991). Ethics and technology: Across the great divide. In H. Wiseman, J. Vanderkop, & J. Nef (Eds.), *Critical choices: Ethics, science and technology* (pp. x–xiv). Toronto: Thompson Educational Publishing.

Woodward, C., & Stoddart, G. (1989). *Is the Canadian health care system suffering from abuse?* (CHEPA Working Paper #19) Hamilton, Ontario: McMaster University.

Yeo, M. (1996). The ethics of public participation. In M. Stingl & D. Wilson (Eds.), *Efficiency vs. equality: Health reform in Canada* (pp. 39–54). University of Lethbridge, Alberta: Fernwood.

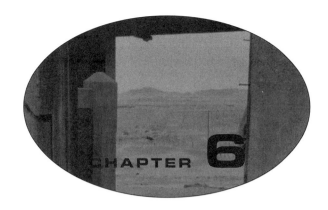

CHAPTER 6

Emancipatory Politics and Health Promotion Practice: The Health Professional As Social Activist

MADINE VANDERPLAAT

✳ Reflective Questions

Imagine that you have been offered a nursing position in a clinic located in a community characterized by low income, low levels of education, and a high percentage of single parents. As part of your duties you are required to establish a resource center for the women and families who visit your clinic. What are your thoughts?

1. List some of the steps you would take in planning for this center.
2. What do you anticipate the major needs to be?
3. How might these needs best be addressed?
4. How do you envision your role in the process?

Social interventions and social programming have been a central feature of Western societies since the 1960s. The social welfare and health sectors have been particularly aggressive in implementing programs designed to improve the human condition, especially among those populations whose living circumstances are considered to be problematic. Over the last 40 years there has been a sustained belief that as educators, researchers, and practitioners we can make a difference—that we have the capacity to bring about social change. Originally, this confidence was closely tied to the belief that science and the application of scientifically generated knowledge and techniques could unravel the complexities of human life and provide solutions to societal ills. By viewing the social world from the perspective of cause-and-effect relationships, the roots of societal ills could be exposed and addressed. The "expertise" of health professionals, social scientists, and educators rested in their ability to translate human behavior and social relationships into categories that could be scientifically measured and manipulated. By the 1970s the emphasis on science, technique, and expertise had come under considerable attack. The social sciences had not demonstrated any significant capacity to reduce poverty or improve the well-being of marginalized populations. The role of the expert intervener was criticized and rejected increasingly by social thinkers, particularly those engaged in feminist research, community development, and critical education. By the 1980s, practitioners and activists within the health, education, and social welfare sectors were looking to these more emancipatory social movements to guide their interventionary strategies. Empowerment emerged as the defining theme both in terms of process and outcome. Social intervention thus developed a blatantly political as well as instrumental dimension. Professionals and academics were encouraged to exercise their skills and knowledge in the name of social justice and with the express purpose of eradicating social inequalities. A considerable body of literature, as well as controversy, was generated as theorists, researchers, and practitioners tried to find a politically correct location for their interventionary interests.

The purpose of this chapter is to examine these developments from the perspective of the health promotion professional, in particular, the nursing practitioner. In doing so, I want to move beyond the rhetoric of emancipatory politics (political activities focusing on social change) and instead explore how emancipatory interests are and can be implemented and where the health professional can locate herself or himself in these practices. Specifically, the chapter includes the following:

- A brief history of the emergence of an emancipatory approach to health promotion and the philosophical differences between this approach and traditional interventionary strategies
- An exploration of the linkages between emancipatory politics and empowerment-oriented programming and evaluation practices
- An examination of the roles of practitioners and researchers within an emancipatory model
- A discussion of two key concepts for defining the role of the health professional as social activist

While the chapter seeks to provide readers with a clear understanding of emancipatory approaches to health promotion, its primary intent is to challenge health professionals to see themselves as potential activists who can contribute in a very significant way to meaningful societal change and social justice.

Throughout the discussion, and for illustration purposes, I will be referring to two large-scale Canadian health promotion programs—*The Nobody's Perfect Parenting Program* and *The Community Action Program for Children (CAPC)*. These two programs exemplify the changes that have taken place over the last decade in our understanding of what it means to be empowerment-oriented in our programming and evaluation strategies. They also represent excellent examples of some of the ways in which academics, health promotion professionals, and social activists have had to rethink their positions and roles within an empowerment-oriented interventionary strategy.

My own involvement with these two programs has been as an evaluator. In this capacity, I have had the privilege of collaborating with a dynamic group of individuals in Health Canada, provincial departments of health and social services, and community-based agencies. Our collective experience with these programs is illustrative of the struggle to find an ethically defensible location for ourselves in the interventionary process.

Traditional Approaches to Intervention

Empowerment-oriented social programming emerged during the 1980s. Prior to this time, interventions in the fields of health, education, and social welfare had been strongly influenced by the dominant positivist perspectives in the social sciences. This type of social program assumed that individuals who were marginalized from mainstream society were so because of the social or educational deficits they possessed. The assumption ensured that most social programs assumed a treatment-oriented approach whereby the populations in question were exposed to and instructed in the knowledge and skills identified as appropriate for alleviating their particular social problem. Projects were thus deemed effective if participants demonstrated the required behavioral changes. The role of the academic and the professional in this type of intervention was to specify the behaviors and attitudes that contributed to a particular social problem, to identify the characteristics of the at-risk or target population, to design remedial strategies, and to ensure that the prescribed knowledge and skills were transmitted in an appropriate manner. The role of the evaluator was to develop appropriate instruments for measuring whether or not the desired behavioral and attitudinal changes had taken place.

By the mid-1970s, this type of social programming was being heavily criticized on a number of fronts. Many theorists and practitioners argued against the idea that the resolution to social problems was in fact a technical one—that all one had to do was identify the gaps or deficits in people's knowledge and life skills and to provide the appropriate instrumental learning experiences (Habermas, 1987). Equally forceful criticisms came from those who argued against a program philosophy that promoted blaming the victim—the assumption inherent in the technical approach was that marginalized populations were to blame for their marginalized state (Ryan, 1971). As the debates over the effectiveness of social interventions wore on, more and more practitioners began to look at alternative philosophies to underscore their interventionary efforts. In particular, one began to see the language of emancipatory politics emerging in the literature.

Empowerment-Oriented Interventions

Research and actions guided by the principles of emancipatory politics are those that aim to liberate or free people from oppressive social structures and relations. Originally developed in the margins of the social sciences, by the 1970s and 1980s this work was rapidly gaining ground in fields related to the human services. Heavily influenced by the writings of critical adult educators (Freire, 1970; Fay, 1987; Giroux, 1988; Collins, 1991), feminist educational theorists (Hart, 1989; Lather, 1991), and social action researchers (Hall, 1981; Maguire, 1987), this body of literature presents a drastic alternative to traditional ways of thinking about social intervention.

The term emancipatory politics actually covers a wide range of political positions and, in practice, has produced a diverse array of philosophies and purposes. However, a number of key principles underscore most emancipatory interests and distinguish them from traditional approaches to social intervention. First, social action informed by emancipatory politics rejects the individual deficit concept implicit in traditional social programs. Theorists and practitioners whose work is guided by an emancipatory interest argue for an approach to intervention that recognizes that people's lives and life chances (the opportunities they have available to them) are profoundly affected by their social, cultural, economic, and political circumstances. These circumstances are seen as inherent in the social system and not the product of individual weakness or deficit.

Second, emancipatory interests also reject the aspiration to manipulate behavioral changes through the direct transfer of technical knowledge and skills. An emancipatory approach recognizes that social change must be structural as well as behavioral. People cannot move out of their marginalized positions if the social systems and relations that keep them there are not drastically altered.

Knowledge is acquired to not simply change oneself but to also change the social circumstances in which people find themselves. As such, intervention develops a political potential as well as an instrumental one. In doing so, the emphasis moves away from the individual and toward the group or collective as the driving force behind social change.

Third, and perhaps the principle that distinguishes this discourse most clearly from its predecessors, is the acknowledgment and deep respect for all people's capacity to create knowledge about their own experiences and the resolutions to problems arising from these experiences. Traditional approaches have always relied on the "expert" to identify the problems experienced by a population and to recommend the most feasible solutions. From an emancipatory perspective, the only valid knowledge from which to initiate social change comes from the everyday understandings and experiences of those involved rather than the annals of the social scientific community.

The activity usually identified with emancipatory interests is commonly understood to involve some construct of empowerment. A review of the health, education, and social welfare literature reveals considerable diversity in definitions of empowerment, ranging from the simple acquisition of specific skills to politically motivated consciousness raising. How the term is used and the meanings attached to it are embedded in the context and discipline in which it is found. The answer to Simon's (1987) query "empowerment for what?" is situation specific. In general, the use of the term implies some understanding of increasing one's capacity to act rather than to be acted upon. Whether this is individual or collective action depends on the context. There is also a general assumption that empowerment results in some form of social change. Further, whether this is perceived as individual or structural depends on the discipline or field.

How the academic and professional fit into this discourse has been the subject of considerable debate (Barr & Cochran, 1992; Ellsworth, 1989; Fine, 1994; Lather, 1991). At a philosophical level, the arguments have centered on what role we should play in an empowering practice. The controversy rages around the issue of *privilege*. If we are committed to a philosophy that promotes the capacity of the marginalized to act for and on their own behalf and that values the language of lived experience over the language of the "expert," where do we with our degrees, credentials, middle-class lifestyles, and (in most cases) whiteness locate ourselves?

Most critical theorists and community activists reject a blatant "vanguard" approach, whereby those of us with privilege lead the way, as it were, for those who have been marginalized. We have become self-conscious enough of our privilege to recognize the paternalistic and consequently disempowering implications of such a stance. However, most disciplines still adhere to the belief that the role of the academic and professional is to empower. In the family and community development literature, for example, the task of those in the field is talked about in terms of empowering less powerful people (Dominelli, 1992; Whitmore, 1991). Other theorists, who are uncomfortable with using the word "empowerment," with its connotations of acting on or for another, prefer to use the term *enablement*, which they define as working to create empowering opportunities (Collins, 1991; Giroux, 1988; Simon, 1987).

It is important to recognize that, regardless of the term used, in both situations the practitioner is the source of the power in empowerment whereas the program participants are its recipients. The problem that many theorists and practitioners have with this position is that it suggests that power, or the opportunity to acquire or realize power, cannot only be given, granted, and shared, it can also be taken back, withheld, and controlled. From this perspective, those with power determine how others will be empowered, which means they can also limit or determine the extent to which people should be empowered. This is clearly inconsistent with an emancipatory ethic. As the following quote from the management sciences illustrates, empowerment is a term that all too readily can be stripped of its emancipatory potential. "Although we have focused on the positive effects of empowerment, it is conceivable that such management practices may have negative effects. Specifically, empowerment may lead to over-confidence and, in turn, misjudgments on the part of subordinates" (Conger & Kanungo, 1988, p. 480).

The philosophical objections to the concept "to empower" have led other thinkers—most notably Rappaport (1985) and Zimmerman (1990) in the field of psychology, and Lather (1991) in the area of critical pedagogy—to reject outright any notion of empowerment that has as its root the transmission of power from an agent to a subject. Rappaport argues that empowerment is not a process of giving; empowerment is taking power or retaking power over one's life. For Zimmerman and Rappaport, to be empowered is "to gain psychological control over oneself, to extend a positive influence to others and the larger community" (Rappaport, 1985, p.18). To be empowered is to be able to do things for oneself and others. "Empowerment is not something that can be given; it must be taken. What those who have it and want to share it can do is to provide the conditions and the language and beliefs that make it possible to be taken by those who are in need of it" (Rappaport, 1985, p.18). This notion of internalizing power or taking control is also evident in family therapy definitions of an empowering process. "The person who is the learner, client, etc. must attribute behavior change to his or her own actions if one is to acquire a sense of control" (Dunst & Trivette, 1987, p. 445).

Likewise, Lather (1991) states that "empowerment is a process one undertakes for oneself: it is not something to be done 'to' or 'for' someone" (p. 4). In opposition to much of the psychological literature, Lather denies all concepts of empowerment that relate exclusively to individual self-assertion and to the psychological experience of feeling powerful. For Lather, empowerment involves "analyzing ideas about the causes of powerlessness, recognizing systemic oppressive forces, and acting individually and collectively to change the conditions of our lives" (Lather, 1991, p. 4). Likewise Tronto (1992) argues that a feminist description of empowerment sees the concept as an "act by individuals and groups as they come to understand themselves as actors capable of acting" (p. 103). The problem with these articulations of the concept is that it becomes increasingly difficult to see where the professional and academic should fit in. As we will discuss later, the challenge has been to find an ethically defensible position for our involvement with marginalized communities.

Roles of Practitioners

There is of course a considerable gap between how emancipatory interests and philosophies of empowerment are expressed in principle and how they are actually carried out in practice. Likewise, the emphasis that academic theorists have placed on debating the ethics of empowerment may not have as much prominence in the minds of those who actually practice in the field. Although by no means a perfect reflection of emancipatory principles, Health Canada's public health strategies are illustrative of how elements of emancipatory principles have been incorporated into health policy and the implications this has had for practitioners.

In 1986 Health Canada, in association with The World Health Organization (WHO), produced the *Ottawa Charter* (WHO, 1986). In addition to the usual emphasis on personal resources and lifestyles, the *Charter* also emphasized the importance of community development, empowerment, and action in the pursuit of health promotion. The new programming strategy recognized that health was profoundly affected by people's social context and by societal factors such as economic conditions, employment, and housing. In the *Charter*'s words: "The fundamental conditions and resources for health are peace, shelter, education, food, income, a stable ecosystem, sustainable resources, social justice, and equity" (WHO, 1986, p. iii).

In recognizing these basic prerequisites to health, the *Charter* called for social action geared toward building healthy public policy, creating supportive environments, strengthening community action, developing personal skills, and reorienting health services to the needs of the individual as a whole person. These action strategies are underscored by a commitment to the development of knowledge and resources, increased public participation, and network/coalition building (Epp, 1986).

In elaborating the key principles that emerge from the *Ottawa Charter,* Raeburn (1987) notes that under the new policy "projects are to be owned, controlled, and determined by the people whom they are intended to benefit" (p. 2). In addition, "the leaders of projects should come from the population of interest [and] the style of working is 'empowering'" (Raeburn,

p. 2). Regardless of specific health promotion goals, all projects were to encourage participants to develop strong social supports, life skills, and self-esteem (Epp, 1986; Raeburn, 1987). Within this model, the role of experts and professionals was envisioned as "consultants, advisors, and supports to people who are trying to act on their own initiative" (Raeburn, p. 2). The principles underscoring the *Ottawa Charter* were later developed more fully in Health Canada's *population health* strategy (Health Canada, 1994). This model focuses more specifically on the factors that determine health as objects of policy and program intervention. These determinants of health include: income and social status, social support networks, education, employment and working conditions, physical environment, biology and genetic endowment, personal health practices and coping skills, and healthy child development and health services.

One of the first programs to seriously attempt to put the principles of the *Ottawa Charter* into practice was the *Nobody's Perfect Parenting* program. The *Nobody's Perfect* program is an educational health promotion program for parents of children from birth to age five. Specifically, the program is designed for "low-income, single, young, socially or geographically isolated parents or parents with limited formal education" (Health and Welfare Canada, 1988, p. 6). The overall intent of the program is "to give parents access to accurate, up-to-date information on their children's health, safety, development, and behavior (and) to encourage confidence in a parent's ability to be a good parent" (p. 6). In doing so, the program acknowledges that "Health problems must be viewed both in terms of individual and social factors" (p. 9).

The *Nobody's Perfect* program was a unique departure from conventional health promotion programming in a number of ways. It recognized the value of parents' traditional knowledge and sought to build on this knowledge rather than replace or ignore it. The program allowed parents to decide what topics they would like to discuss. Further, it incorporated the principles of adult education that value the knowledge students bring to learning rather than relying on traditional modes of instruction that solely value the knowledge held by the teacher. Likewise, the program was organized and delivered through a "facilitator" rather than an instructor. Facilitators were often public health nurses or community development workers; however, in some provinces, former *Nobody's Perfect* participants were trained as facilitators, a significant step in the move away from privileging the "expert" skills of the professional. Probably the most significant contribution that *Nobody's Perfect* made to future empowerment-oriented endeavors was its emphasis on the importance of mutual support as a key component of an empowering process.

Although by today's standards *Nobody's Perfect* constitutes a relatively conservative approach to empowerment, a decade ago it signaled a major shift in health promotion thinking and practice. For the first time, the role of the intervener came under scrutiny. Program facilitators were trained not only in program content but also in the empowerment-oriented philosophy underscoring the program. Those of us who worked in the management of the program or its evaluation also tried to make our practices consistent with this philosophy. Our attempts to translate the idea of empowerment into our everyday practices focused on developing more respectful relationships with program participants. What that meant in reality was a conscious attempt to avoid the use of impositional or intrusive methods in our dealings with the *Nobody's Perfect* community. So, for example, even though program materials did cover a select number of topics, the program did not have a structured curriculum; parents were encouraged to focus on areas that were of particular interest to them.

Likewise, as evaluators we did not use rigid behavioral indices or scales to measure the effects of the program on participants. Instead, we relied on more **qualitative** or naturalistic approaches to gather information from parents. Our initial efforts to be empowering retained its technical or instrumental approach by focusing almost exclusively on methods and techniques. We concentrated on modifying data collection instruments and interviewing styles just as program facilitators focused on educational techniques. We did not challenge our own position of privilege, let alone even question it. Likewise, we were quite comfortable with our role as "empowerers." Looking back, it is obvious that we had taken only a few hesitant steps outside the safe parameters of traditional interventionary and evaluation practices. However,

at the time, even these tentative efforts were greeted with considerable criticism from the more conventional health and evaluation communities.

Community Action Program for Children

A decade later a number of us who had worked with *Nobody's Perfect* had the opportunity to collaborate on the Atlantic Regional Evaluation of the *Community Action Program for Children (CAPC).*[1] *CAPC* is designed to improve the health and well-being of children and their families, particularly those who live in poverty or social isolation. *CAPC* projects can take numerous different forms but usually involve some sort of community family resource center that offers a variety of different programs and activities for both children and parents. *CAPC* reflects the Health Canada's Population Health model (Health Canada, 1994), which builds on the *Ottawa Charter*'s (1986) emphasis on broad-based community support and participation. Projects are developed through community partnerships and are designed to be user-driven in the sense that participants are the ones who decide how the project will be run, what programs they will access, and how resources will be allocated. Project coordinators, who are often well-educated professionals, tend to see themselves as social activists first and foremost. They, and the *CAPC* community in general, are consciously political. In keeping with the participatory, collaborative nature of the program, the evaluation strategy used was based on a **participatory action research** model that required the community, Health Canada personnel, and the evaluators who were university based to work together as a team. It also dictated that the direction and content of the evaluation would be determined by the *CAPC* community.

Those of us involved in the management and research components of the evaluation started out only slightly more politically conscious than we had been during the *Nobody's Perfect* evaluation. Parents and staff participated in all aspects of the evaluation from design to analysis to interpretation. This time

[1]CAPC program information available at www.hc-sc. gc.ca/hppb/childhood-youth/cbp/capc/

there was an open acknowledgment of the *CAPC* community as equal stakeholders in the research process. It was also our collective understanding that as long as we did not impose our expertise or dictate the direction and content of the evaluation we were being "empowering" without pretensions to empower. Little thought was given to what participatory meant in terms of our own activities. The concept of participation was worked out only as it applied to program participants. It soon became evident that this reasoning was seriously jeopardizing the successful completion of the evaluation.

Although a detailed discussion of the events that led to this realization is beyond the scope of this chapter, it is enough to say here that our (the management and research team's) commitment to producing a realistic and meaningful picture of the *CAPC* experience was being undermined by our attempt to carve out a nonpolitical space for ourselves. We were quite willing to say what we would not be or do but we had not confronted the difficult task of determining what our role *should* be. By not doing so we had in effect severely limited the "empowering" or political capacity of the *CAPC* evaluation. We had created the circumstances that enabled parents to establish the criteria by which the effectiveness of *CAPC* would be measured by privileging their experiences with the program over a predetermined set of objectives created by specialists. We had not, however, created the circumstances that allowed this voice to be carried much beyond the actual *CAPC* experience and into the communities and social systems within which *CAPC* exists. In other words, we had focused on the promotion of human agency without addressing the social structures that shape and constrain that agency. By limiting our interest in empowerment to parent's ability to parent rather than examining how the knowledge produced by parents and the *CAPC* community could be used to challenge existing social policies and practices, we had once again reduced the idea of social change to mean behavioral change.

Our collective struggle to come to a new understanding of our role was and is an ongoing process. Many of the insights gained and discussed here emerged slowly over the course of the evaluation and in subsequent discussions among members of the management and research team. Some of what we came to understand was incorporated into the evaluation and our relationship with program participants (O'Hanlon & VanderPlaat, 1997). Other insights emerged after the completion of the evaluation when we began to document our experiences for conference papers and journal articles.

Two Key Concepts

One of the most important understandings that emerged from our collective reflections was the realization that an emancipatory approach to intervention is meaningless without a commitment to the assumption of *mutuality* and the practice of **reflexivity**. These two concepts, both of which come from the feminist literature, provide considerable guidance to those of us "who presume to want to make a difference, who are so bold or arrogant as to assume we might" (Fine, 1994, p. 80).

Mutuality

Feminist psychologists at the Stone Center, Wellesley College, Massachusetts, have been working with the concept of mutuality or mutual empowerment, which offers an understanding of empowerment that is very useful for those of us whose activities are guided by an emancipatory ethic. Although the term was originally developed to facilitate individual psychological growth, the concept of mutuality has much to offer the social activist. Rather than seeing empowerment in either/or terms, that is, in terms of either giving power to someone else or taking power for oneself, theorists and practitioners associated with the Stone Center suggest that we think about empowerment both in terms of a capacity to move into action and as an ability to be moved into action (Surrey, 1987; Fedele & Harrington, 1990). As such, power is not given or taken but emerges through interaction with "the other" (Jordan, 1986).

From this perspective, empowerment becomes a relational process whereby the direction of our academic and professional activities is acquired through relationship and connection with others. At the very heart of the concept is the principle that one can never be just an empowerer or a person in need of empowerment. In a mutual approach to empowerment, everyone involved, regardless of position of power and privilege, recognizes that she or he is both agent and subject in the empowerment process. In other words, our ability to be empowering or to support someone else's capacity to be empowering grows out of the mutual recognition that we all have much to offer, that we all have much to learn, and that in a truly empowering process everyone changes. Empowerment is always mutual.

In order to incorporate a sense of mutuality into our interventions, we first need to locate ourselves. Rather than assuming we are apolitical and objective (as in detached), we have to acknowledge where we fit into the social structure and how our relationship with program participants is defined. As professionals working for universities, governments, and community agencies, we need to be forthright about our role as systemic agents. As program managers, evaluators, and academics, we are part of the expert and bureaucratic system that defines and explains the circumstances of people's lives. Social scientists articulate the nature of our social problems, program managers and educators design interventionary solutions, and evaluators give public expression to what a program looks like and how its effectiveness will be judged.

In essence, we help to create and maintain the social relationships and structures within which we all live. By pretending to be apolitical or outside of these systemic structures, we are, in effect, supporting the status quo. By doing nothing, we allow existing social, political, and economic constraints to go unchallenged. We give program participants the message that we want them to change and to become empowered, but that this empowerment must take place within social structures that do not require change. We use the language of emancipatory politics to legitimize our quest for behavioral changes in a population we see as being "at-risk" or problematic. We see empowerment as a technique to get program participants to improve themselves in characteristics we wish to see changed or to value as different, and to feel some sort of responsibility and ownership for that process. In essence we understand empowerment to have a therapeutic function, not a political one. Alternatively, we can pay lip service to the debilitating effects of systemic forces but tell participants that, by virtue of our objec-

tivity and participatory research ethic, any attempts at structural social change must be entirely up to them (LaCompte & de Marrais, 1992). We cannot impose. We cannot (and will not) put our privilege and expertise and reputations to work on their behalf.

Mutuality demands that we as academics and professionals place ourselves firmly in the center of the empowerment process—not *instead* of program participants but *with* them. Mutuality requires that those of us with privilege recognize this power and take responsibility for the systems and social structures that contribute to people's disempowerment, and which we help to maintain. A commitment to mutual empowerment opens the way for program participants to teach us about the realities of their lives so that we, in turn, can base our practices on these experiences. In doing so, participants become empowered subjects who create the discourses we work with rather than being the subjects of these discourses (Brodkey & Fine, 1991).

Likewise, program participants can avail themselves of the resources and knowledge we have acquired for use on their own behalf. For example, in the evaluation of *CAPC*, I had to learn to listen—really listen—to the *CAPC* community to ensure that the design of the evaluation and the methodologies used did not in and of themselves disempower *CAPC* parents, distort the *CAPC* experience (through methodological "blindness"), or reduce the impacts of the program to simple behavior management. Likewise, those on the management team had to be willing to open their practices to the scrutiny of the *CAPC* community. Conversely, program participants learned to use evaluation research as a tool not only to improve their own projects but also to establish the legitimacy of *CAPC* in the broader community.

The concept of mutuality is not, of course, restricted to the relationship between professionals, academics, and program participants. A commitment to mutual empowerment must also exist among professionals and academics. There is an unfortunate tendency, especially within the academic and activist community, to see some positions as being more legitimate than others. For example, activists working "in the field" generally see themselves as being more political and having greater political potential than those working in universities. In turn they, along with feminist academics, question the extent to which professionals working for governments can truly reconcile a commitment to activism with their bureaucratic location. In addition, community workers, academics, and public servants have often seen their efforts come to a grinding halt due to *turfism*—the politics of who owns which social problem and how it should be addressed (VanderPlaat, 1997). Considerable energy is expended arguing over whether the objectives and effects of programs like *Nobody's Perfect* and *CAPC* are best articulated through the disciplinary lens of developmental psychology, sociology, early childhood education, or community development. As we learned from our experiences with *CAPC,* a much needed and more productive approach would be to recognize and work through the multiple locations of social activism (Felski, 1989; Strong-Boag, 1994).

Reflexivity

The activity and practice that best corresponds with a commitment to mutuality is that of *reflexivity.* The term is frequently used by feminist researchers and refers to the need to "reflect upon, examine critically, and explore analytically" the nature of our practices (Fonow & Cook, 1991, p. 2). Likewise, it requires that we enhance our critical awareness "of whom and what the knowledge one produces serves in society" (Benhabib, 1986, p. 281). Reflexivity takes the focus away from the behavior of marginalized populations and looks at our own in terms of how we contribute to marginalization. Unless we are intentionally disempowering (or hypocritical), we usually do not realize how our practices can be debilitating. The process of reflexivity emerges from our interactions with a program community as it is here that we learn the experiential consequences of our actions. For example, in the *CAPC* evaluation, the management and research team fostered the notion of *transparency* in their management and evaluation practices. Members of the *CAPC* community were consulted and invited to respond to every decision made whether it is a management issue or one pertaining to the evaluation. Consequently, a decision that had the potential to be disempowering could be quickly revealed and addressed.

The empowering potential of a reflexive concern with our practices is well illustrated by the evaluation and management team's struggle with language. When the first draft of the *CAPC* evaluation was distributed to the *CAPC* community, there was considerable reaction to the way we evaluators had portrayed the program participants. Despite our best intentions to be respectful and participatory (for example, we had refrained from using terms like "at-risk" and "target population,"), we had still employed the language of traditional evaluation (and intervention) to talk about the relationship between parents and the program. By speaking in terms of impacts and effects, we had objectified parents as people who had things done to them. By looking at how parents had "improved," we had once again focused on behavior as the only criteria for program effectiveness and slipped back into a language that constructed this particular population as being needy, passive, incapable of action, and deficit driven. We needed to make fundamental changes in how we wrote about the *CAPC* community. For example, rather than using the phrase "*CAPC* gives parents . . ." we learned to think in terms of how "parents use CAPC to . . ."; instead of "parents get help with . . ." we focused on how "parents access resources related to . . ."; and we now came to see "parents building on existing skills" rather than "learning skills."

The re-examination of how we wrote about parents also forced us to examine the analytical framework for the evaluation. By seeing parents as active users of an intervention rather than its "target," we could now look at the effectiveness of *CAPC* in terms of what parents could do with the program, rather what it had done to them. As a result, we were able to move from behavioral measures of effectiveness to demonstrating how parents' use of *CAPC* as a resource contributed to the overall goals of the Population Health model (Health Canada, 1994).

It is important to note that while the management and research team had not been intentionally disempowering in their use of language, they did not immediately "get it" as far as the general issue was concerned. At first there was considerable resistance to what most of us saw as a nit-picky or overly politicized point. The language being used was not our language but the language of our professions and disciplines, and our first reaction was to hide behind this credentialism. Through our interactions with the *CAPC* community, we gradually came to understand the political implications of using terms such as "poor women" who "have problems" (as opposed to "women living in poverty" who "meet challenges"). In this sense, we needed the *CAPC* community to provide us with the insights to challenge the constraints imposed by our expert cultures.

The Challenge

Much of the evaluators' and management team's reflexive thinking took place after the completion of the *CAPC* evaluation. In starting to understand our role in the empowerment process we began to look more carefully and critically at our own disciplines and practices. Individually and collectively we have started to write papers and articles (including this chapter) that challenge our traditional roles as interveners (Bernard, Rivard, Samson, VanderPlaat, & Vivian Book, 1998a, 1998b, 1999; VanderPlaat, 1997, 1998a, 1998b). We use the *CAPC* evaluation as an illustration of what it taught us about empowerment-oriented intervention rather than focusing exclusively on what the program taught parents.

Our experience with *CAPC* gave us a number of insights into what implications an active commitment to emancipatory politics has for the professional. Reconciling one's activist interests with one's profession is not an easy task. As a nursing student, for example, you are being socialized into a discipline that is guided by a specific discourse—a way of looking at the world and defining what is important, legitimate, and ethical. This discourse gives you a certain authority or privilege in your dealings with your patients and provides the basis of how you, as a nurse, are assessed by other people in the health professions. Our disciplines and the discourses associated with them provide us with a safe and familiar location from which to practice. It is, therefore, much easier to learn the discourse, and to learn it well, than to challenge its assumptions, values, and beliefs.

A common criticism against professionals who have committed themselves to social activism is the charge that they have lost their objectivity, that they are somehow biased in their approach to intervention and research. In responding to this critique, it is important to remember that the concept of "objectivity" as it refers to being disinterested or apolitical is itself a myth. As professionals and academics, our way of looking at the world is a product of our personal histories combined with training and socialization in a particular discipline. What we see and how we understand it is constructed within a specific perspective. There is no way of stepping outside that perspective and seeing things from nowhere or finding a "God's eye view" for oneself (Haraway, 1988).

The field of health promotion is particularly influenced by disciplines that hide behind "method" and "rigor" in their claim to objectivity. For example, many parent and child welfare programs rely heavily on behavioral indices to establish the effectiveness of a program. It is generally assumed that these indices are a more "objective" measure of what the program actually does than the subjective assessments of parents. In reality these indices are politically loaded. They carry a number of assumptions that cannot possibly be interpreted as disinterested or unbiased. The privileging of quantitative over qualitative data is a bias in that it assumes that only social phenomenon that can be reduced to numbers can be treated as fact. Assuming that parents cannot accurately speak for themselves and that their behavior must be tested is a strong and biased statement about how we perceive the integrity of program participants.

The not too implicit message is that as "experts" we know the signs of a good parent and that these behaviors can be "measured." We do not trust parents, especially those who are young, female, unsupported, or living in poverty, to be able to establish the context within which their parenting experiences can be understood. In some cases evaluators have gone as far as to allow only "observable" data to establish the existence and appropriateness of parenting skills. The rationale is that the women in question cannot be counted on to give a truthful or accurate account of their parenting situations. Likewise, the criteria against which parents' behavior is assessed is heavily biased in favor of a psychological perspective on the world, which, as noted earlier, is but one way of understanding social life. In addition, the indices are painfully middle-class in the values they reflect with no consideration given to cultural differences.

The professional/activist's response to the charge of bias can, therefore, easily point out that the pretense to objectivity is not only a political stance in itself but a highly disempowering one as well. We do not deny our bias or interest but we must also be careful to articulate this interest in terms of an ethical position rather than an uncritical defense of empowerment-oriented social programming. A commitment to emancipatory politics does not preclude good research or practice. An intervention's claims to being empowerment-oriented does not necessarily make it so.

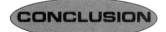
CONCLUSION

The purpose of this chapter is to challenge the nursing student/practitioner to see herself or himself as a potential social activist. Whether one works as a public health nurse, or in a community clinic or a hospital, all nurses, as do all of us who are engaged in the human services, have the capacity to contribute to a more equitable and just society. To this end, we need to recognize that we can shape our disciplines and practices as well as be shaped by them. Central to this challenge is the idea that "empowerment" is not a term that should be applied and thought out only in terms of "the other." To achieve meaningful social change those of us who are committed to an emancipatory ethic must become active participants in the empowering process. This involves not only examining how our own privilege may disempower others. It also requires that we use this privilege to challenge the disciplinary and institutional barriers that stand in the way of meaningful social change.

✸ Reflective Questions

1. How are issues of power and privilege played out in your nursing program? In what type of situations are you aware of your power/privilege? Discuss a situation where you have felt disempowered.

2. Look at the answers you gave to the questions at the beginning of the chapter. In light of the previous discussion, what changes would you make to your responses? What challenges do you think you might face if you did assume a more activist role in this type of scenario?

REFERENCES

Barr, D., & Cochran, M. (1992). Understanding and supporting empowerment: Redefining the professional role. *Networking Bulletin: Empowerment and Family Support, 2*(3), 2–8.

Benhabib, S. (1986). *Critique, norm and Utopia: A study of the foundation of critical theory.* New York: Columbia University Press.

Bernard, N., Raven, P., Rivard, M., Samson, Y., VanderPlaat, M., & Vivian Book, L. (1998a, November 7). *The role of the evaluator in a participatory action research evaluation.* Paper presented at the American Evaluation Association Conference, Chicago, IL.

Bernard, N., Raven, P., Rivard, M., Samson, Y., VanderPlaat, M., & Vivian Book, L. (1998b, June 5). *Empowerment evaluation in practice: Lessons from the Atlantic Regional Evaluation of CAPC.* Paper presented at the Canadian Evaluation Conference, St. John's.

Bernard, N., Raven, P., Rivard, M., Samson, Y., VanderPlaat, M., & Vivian Book, L. (1999, April 9). *Learning to listen: What program participants can teach us about empowerment.* Paper presented to the 5th International Qualitative Health Research Conference, Newcastle, Australia.

Brodkey, L., & Fine, M. (1991). Presence of mind in the absence of body. In H.A. Giroux (Ed.), *Postmodernism,*

feminism, and cultural politics (pp. 100–118). New York: State University of New York Press.

Collins, M. (1991). *Adult education as vocation.* New York: Routledge.

Conger, J. A., & Kanungo, R. N. (1988). The empowerment process: Integrating theory and practice. *Academy of Management Review, 15,* 471–482.

Dominelli, L. (1992). More than a method: Feminist social work. In K. Campbell (Ed.), *Feminist criticism: Argument in the disciplines* (pp. 83–106). Buckingham, UK: Open University Press.

Dunst, C. J., & Trivette, C. M. (1987). Enabling and empowering families: Conceptual and intervention issues. *School Psychology Review, 16,* 443–456.

Ellsworth, E. (1989). Why doesn't this feel empowering? Working through the repressive myths of critical pedagogy. *Harvard Educational Review, 59,* 297–324.

Epp, J. (1986). *Achieving health for all: A framework for health promotion.* Ottawa: Health and Welfare Canada.

Fay, B. (1987). *Critical social science.* Ithaca, NY: Cornell University Press.

Fedele, N. M., & Harrington, E. (1990). Women's groups: How connections heal. *Work in Progress No. 47.* Wellesley, MA: Stone Center Working Paper Series.

Felski, R. (1989). *Beyond feminist aesthetics: Feminist literature and social change*. London: Radius.

Fine, M. (1994). Working the hyphens: Reinventing self and other in qualitative research. In N. Denzin & Y. Lincoln (Eds.), *Handbook of qualitative research* (pp.70–82). Newbury Park, CA: Sage.

Fonow, M. M. & Cook, J. A. (1991). Back to the Future. In M. M. Fonow & J. A. Cook (Eds.). *Beyond Methodology: Feminist Scholarship As Lived Research* (pp. 1–15). Indianapolis: Indiana University Press.

Freire, P. (1970). *Pedagogy of the oppressed*. New York: Seabury Press.

Giroux, H. A. (1988). Literacy and the pedagogy of voice and political empowerment. *Educational Theory, 38,* 61–75.

Gore, J. (1992). What we can do for you! What can "we" do for "you"? Struggling over empowerment in critical and feminist pedagogy. In C. Luke & J. Gore (Eds.), *Feminisms and critical pedagogy* (pp. 55–73). New York: Routledge, Chapman and Hall.

Habermas, J. (1987). *The philosophical discourse of modernity*. Cambridge, MA: MIT Press.

Hall, B. L. (1981). Participatory research, popular knowledge, and power: A personal reflection. *Convergence, 14,* 6–19.

Haraway, D. (1988). Situated knowledges: The science question in feminism and the privilege of partial perspective. *Feminist Studies, 14,* 575–599.

Hart, M. (1989). Critical theory and beyond: Further perspectives on emancipatory education. *Adult Education Quarterly, 40,* 125–138.

Health Canada. (1994). *Strategies for population health: Investing in the health of Canadians*. Ottawa: Health Canada Communications Directorate.

Health and Welfare Canada. (1988). *Nobody's Perfect Administration Manual*. Ottawa: Supply and Services Canada.

Jordan, J. V. (1986). The meaning of mutuality. *Work in Progress No. 17*. Wellesley, MA: Stone Center Working Paper Series.

LaCompte, M. D., & de Marrais, K. B. (1992). The disempowering of empowerment: Out of the revolution and into the classroom. *Educational Foundations, 6,* 5–31.

Lather, P. (1991). *Getting smart: Feminist research and pedagogy with/in the postmodern*. New York: Routledge.

Lincoln, Y. S., & Guba, E. G. (1985). *Naturalistic inquiry*. Beverly Hills, CA: Sage.

Maguire, P. (1987). *Doing participatory research: A feminist approach*. Amherst, MA: Center for International Education.

O'Hanlon, A., & VanderPlaat, M. (1997). *The Atlantic Regional Evaluation of the Community Action Program for Children*. Halifax: Health Promotion Directorate, Health Canada.

Raeburn, J. (1987). People projects: Planning and evaluation in a new era. *Health Promotion, 27*(2), 2–13.

Rappaport, J. (1985). The power of empowerment language. *Social Policy, 16,*15–21.

Ryan, W. (1971). *Blaming the victim*. New York: Pantheon Books.

Simon, R. (1987). Empowerment as a pedagogy of possibility. *Language Arts, 64,* 370–382.

Strong-Boag, V. (1994, June 13). *Too much and not enough: The paradox of power for feminist academics working with community feminists on issues related to violence*. Paper presented to the Social Science Federation of Canada Symposium, University of Calgary.

Surrey, J. L. (1987). Relationship and empowerment. *Work in Progress No. 30*. Wellesley, MA: Stone Center Working Paper Series.

Tronto, J. C. (1992). Politics and revision: The feminist project to change the boundaries of American political science. In S. R. Zalk, & J. G. Kelter (Eds.), *Revolutions in knowledge: Feminism in the social sciences* (pp. 91–111). Boulder, CO: Westview Press.

VanderPlaat, M. (1997). Emancipatory politics, critical evaluation and government policy. *Canadian Journal of Program Evaluation, 12,* 143–162.

VanderPlaat, M. (1998a). Empowerment, emancipation and health promotion policy. *Canadian Journal of Sociology, 23,* 71–90.

VanderPlaat, M. (1998b, August 22). *Health Canada: Negotiating relationships among and within academia, government and community*. Paper presented at The Society for the Study of Social Problems, 48th Annual Meeting, San Francisco.

Whitmore, E. (1991). Evaluation and empowerment: It's the process that counts. *Networking Bulletin: Empowerment and Family Support, 2*(2), 1–7.

World Health Organization. (1986). Ottawa Charter for health promotion. *Health promotion (International), 1*(4), iii–v.

Zimmerman, M. (1990). Toward a theory of learned hopefulness: A structural model analysis of participation and empowerment. *Journal of Research in Personality, 24,* 71–86.

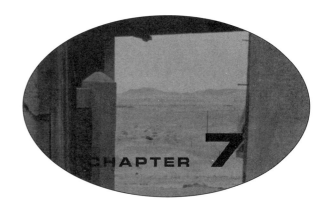

CHAPTER 7

Transformational Leadership for a Health Promotion Practice

GAIL CAMERON

"Come to the edge," he said.
They said, "We are afraid."
"Come to the edge," he said.
They came. He pushed them . . . and they flew.

Guiollaume Apollinaire

Health care restructuring, organizational change, reduced resources, increased technology, and policy changes are only a few of the trends that create a work environment where nurses feel they are working on "the edge." Within this contextual turbulence, nurse leaders are challenged to invite others with whom they work to "come to the edge and fly," or to make creative changes in how they practice. "Flying" in the face of turbulence takes an enormous amount of commitment and trust for all nurses—whether they are leaders or followers.

Today's nurse leaders help others "to fly" by creating opportunities for them to make sense of the changes that are occurring and by motivating them in participatory decision making, collaborative practice models, and excellence in practice—all with limited resources. This style of leadership, referred to as transformational leadership, is neither "top-down" nor "bottom-up"; it combines leading and learning with all employees during organizational change.

Transformational leadership is responsive rather than reactive to shifting health care demands and is accomplished by influencing individuals to perform beyond expectations by fostering a sense of commitment to a vision. It is described as an effective style to accomplish radical change within organizational work teams and committees (Binney & Williams, 1995; Mariner-Tomey, 1993; Senge, 1994).

Transformational leadership uses a health promotion approach and strategies. The central tenets of both transformational leadership and health promotion are empowerment, collaboration, and advocacy (Maben & McLeod Clarke, 1995; Wallerstein, 1992). Current literature on leadership suggests that the biggest challenge for nurses who want to integrate a health promotion approach into a transformational leadership style is "to be" health promoting—that is, to use a leadership approach that is consistent with the philosophical beliefs and principles of health promotion. All nurses, even student nurses, fill leadership roles in everyday situations, and all can benefit from applying health promotional skills and developing a transformational leadership style to ensure that the work environment is healthy for nurses.

The intention of this chapter is not to provide an exhaustive list of details about leadership attributes and successful leadership strategies—these can be found in numerous books on leadership. Rather, the intention is to provide a view of leadership from the perspective of health promotion and to provide reflective questions to help you make meaning of the concepts.

The chapter has two sections. The first presents the philosophical beliefs and principles of health promotion as they apply to transformational leadership. This includes the concepts of power as it relates to empowerment, collaboration, and advocacy, all of which are concepts central to transformational leadership. The second section is a more general discussion about how health promotion principles are applied by transformational leaders. At the end of each section, there are questions that invite you to reflect on your own practice. These questions might trigger you to consider different ways of 'being' in your role as a transformational leader.

Philosophical Perspectives on Health Promotion

The philosophy of health promotion is based on a number of beliefs and values that form the foundation and driving force behind any action that reduces power inequities (Ministry of Skills Training and Labor, 1995). Health promotion encompasses equalizing power relationships and moving decision making to the people who are affected by those decisions as opposed to the leader making all the decisions. "Defined in patriarchal terms, power is the capacity to impose one's will on others, accompanied by a willingness to apply negative sanctions against those who oppose that will" (Chinn, 1995, p. 8). Stevens and Hall (1992) claim that power, whatever the source, is valued in hierarchical systems, is taken for granted, and operates without much notice. This section looks at the concepts of power, empowerment, collaboration, and advocacy.

Power

A discussion of power is needed to understand the concepts of empowerment, collaboration, and advocacy. Two different paradigmatic approaches to the use of power are based on perspectives of *scarcity* and *synergy*.

The traditional approach, found in most organizations, is the scarcity **paradigm**. This professes that all resources, including human resources, are scarce and that people and groups must compete for them. The adversarial nature of this competition leads to the development of institutional bureaucracies to justify why one group of people should have some resources over others. Over time, these justifications lead to a masking of reality and to legitimizing frozen and lawlike authority structures. As the **hierarchy** expands and

groups become more self-serving in their attempts to gain access to resources, there is resistance within the group toward sharing or helping others. Unequal relationships develop between oppressor and the oppressed. These unequal relationships become even more established when the oppressed begin to believe the myths concerning their own unequal status, thus legitimizing their own domination (Katz, 1984; Kendall, 1992).

An alternative view to the scarcity paradigm is synergy. Synergy is a pattern by which individuals relate to each other, where human activities and intentions are intrinsically expanding and renewable, and need not be viewed as scarce. Synergy requires an attitude that guarantees that resources are shared equitably among members of a work community, and that the whole is greater than the sum of its parts. Central to the experience of synergy among members of a community is that awareness of the working together increases. This encourages further exchanges of responses, which generates further renewable resources (Kendall, 1992).

Transformational leaders create learning environments that encourage team members to reflect on their practice, make meaning of what they do, and then identify changes that can be made in their practice. This can happen individually or as a work team or committee.

Chinn (1995), a nurse leader whose writings focus on building communities that are respectful and value diversity and equality, describes "power with" in contrast to "power over'" strategies; "power with" strategies are consistent with the synergy paradigm. There are several "power with" strategies that transformational leaders can use together to create a collective future; some examples of these strategies include:

- power of collectivity—personal power of each individual is important for the well-being of the group;
- power of unity—shared decision making;
- power of sharing—leadership according to talent, interest, ability, or skill;
- power of distribution—sharing equitably according to need; and,
- power of diversity—encourages creativity, values alternative views, and flexibility.

Transformational leaders are committed to using these "power with" strategies with staff members and colleagues, and frequently provide a buffer between the hierarchical "power over" approach used by organization administration and the staff for whom they are responsible.

This health promotion philosophy creates learning environments that facilitate individual and organizational change. Such a philosophy is a prerequisite to building relational work communities. Nurses who experience a "power with" philosophy explore new ways to collaborate with each other and clients. Team or committee members find their voice and fully engage in a process of exploration, critical thinking, and dialogue. The staff has a shared vision and values and uses mutual problem solving, and there is equitable resource allocation and improved efficiency (Eng, Salmon, & Mullan, 1992). The related health promotion concepts of empowerment, collaboration, and advocacy are consistent with a "power with" approach and synergy.

Empowerment

Although empowerment is the "raison d'être" of health promotion, it has also been a misunderstood term as many authors describe situations without appearing to consider what empowerment means or entails (Labonte, 1990; Rissel, 1994). Although differences about the meaning of empowerment exist, the following attributes of empowerment are most consistent with how it is used in health promotion and employed by transformational leaders.

Empowerment is a multilevel concept and is both a process and an outcome (Clarke & Mass, 1998; Drevdahl, 1995; Rissel, 1994). It focuses on individuals (micro level), and organizations (macro level). As a process, empowerment "is the process by which individuals and work communities are enabled to predict, control, and participate in their own environment" (Eng, Salmon, & Mullan, 1992, p. 5). As an outcome, individual empowerment results in increased feelings of self-determination and self-worth, and autonomous decision making (Carlson-Catalano, 1992; Gibson, 1991; Wallerstein, 1992).

Organizational empowerment results in a raised level of psychological well-being among members, decision making favorable to the

group(s) in question (Rissel, 1994), relief from oppressive conditions, increased knowledge and skills through activism and praxis, group cohesion (Yeitch & Levine, 1992), greater equality in accessing resources and status, and achieving authority (Ministry of Skills Training and Labor, 1995).

Studies of individuals in the work place have focused on what happens when workers perceive that they lack control over their own destinies. There is evidence that individuals who work in high-demand situations, and who lack adequate resources, supports, or abilities to exert control in their lives are susceptible to ill health (Labonte, 1990; Wallerstein, 1992). Yeitch and Levine (1992) point out that empowerment is not about helping individuals adapt to existing organizational structures that lay responsibility for personal failures on the workers (who are expected to change their personal characteristics that supposedly cause these failures); rather, empowerment recognizes the role of social, economic, and political forces that cause contextual problems.

Health promotion advocates need to understand power and power dynamics, address contextual problems, and bring about system changes that will enable nurses' control over their own destiny. Through challenging structural and physical risk factors in a collective setting, nurses come to believe that they can control their worlds, recognize their ability to work together to acquire resources, and affect an actual transformation of sociopolitical conditions (Wallerstein, 1992). Empowerment is embodied within "power with" strategies, and is foundational to creating more respectful and productive work environments.

Collaboration

Collaboration is a "power with" strategy that is characteristic of a health promotion approach used by transformational leaders, and is analyzed by Henneman, Lee, and Cohen (1995). They identify the following five attributes of collaboration:

1. Two or more individuals participate in a joint venture.
2. Participants willingly cooperate and share in planning and decision making.
3. Participants view themselves as members of a team contributing to a common goal.

4. Participants offer expertise and share responsibility for the outcomes.
5. Relationships between participants are non-hierarchical and power is shared, based on individual's knowledge and expertise versus their role or title.

As a result of collaboration, issues and solutions can be seen differently, new choices emerge, and action for change is supported. Collaboration is a process and an outcome of a "power with" approach.

Advocacy

Advocacy in health promotion can be defined as the securing of necessary resources to support autonomous nursing practice and ensuring access to nursing services for clients. Advocacy is a health promotion principle and a system-level strategy transformational leaders use to create empowering environments on behalf of nurses, clients, or others for whom they are responsible. Attributes of an empowering system that advocates for interventions aimed at the system, structure, program, and individual levels have been listed in detail by Vogt and Murrel (1990) in *Empowering Organizations*. Table 7–1 contains an adaptation of their advocacy interventions that managers can use to empower at individual and organizational levels.

Successful advocacy for staff and patients requires understanding the needs of both groups as well as recognizing the power dynamics within the organization. Leaders must "walk the line" between strongly advocating for empowering practices, while simultaneously negotiating rule-driven systems without alienating those in authority. Strategies used for advocacy include negotiation, conflict resolution, and divergent and innovative thinking.

Leaders recognize successful advocacy when work teams or committee members obtain resources that satisfy their stated desires. This is different from influencing workers' behavior to achieve the leader's own goals. For example, one transformational leader provided the nurses on a psychiatric unit with a glucometer so the nurses could do blood glucose screenings for patients with diabetes instead of requiring the nurses to call the laboratory staff to come and do the screening. The leader was respond-

ing to the nurses' desire to provide total patient care on the psych unit like nurses provide on all other units in the hospital. The leader provided the resources that allowed the nurses to meet their goals instead of meeting the institutional goal of saving money by having the lab staff perform the screening function.

Binney and Williams (1995) claim that both "top-down" and "bottom-up" approaches to organizational change are flawed. They suggest an alternative approach where individuals at all levels of the organization can be involved in shaping radical change by combining leading and learning. They describe how leadership for change is everybody's responsibility requiring individuals to have a genuine shared understanding of current reality—both internal and external. This shared understanding assists the work team in creating synergistic energy for personal and organizational change, such as defining goals, developing action plans for addressing problems, and then mobilizing resources. All of these are health promotion principles.

Changing the way things are done is best accomplished when leaders and members share a vision and are committed to health promotion principles. This means leaders let go of the need to be the "expert," believe in the capacities of the team or committee members, are less directive, and empower individuals and organizations. The focus is on facilitating staff and colleagues to change their practice as necessary, rather than on controlling the actions of staff to fit with the leader's agenda. This approach involves using "power with" strategies such as shared decision making and building consensus whenever possible.

Transformational leadership is the leadership style that is best suited to meet these challenges.

✳ Reflective Questions

1. What do I do that encourages empowerment in my colleagues and team members?
2. How do I secure resources needed to support the teams' best practice?
3. What process could I use to develop agency or committee goals, values, and action plans?

TABLE 7-1

EMPOWERING STRATEGIES FOR THE TRANSFORMATIONAL LEADER

Transformational leaders:

- model empowerment behaviors and attitudes.
- continually assess progress toward empowerment of self, group, system.
- coach and mentor.
- offer timely assistance and help to others.
- demonstrate patience, recognizing that both personal and system changes take time.
- recognize and value individual differences, and also appreciate good work.
- practice nonjudgmental reactions.
- are scrupulous in dealing with private information.
- accept mistakes of self and others and work to correct them.
- facilitate open communication by listening actively to others.
- articulate their ideas clearly.
- focus on developing effective work teams.
- encourage others to participate and assume more responsibility, power, and work.
- involve the team in collaborative decision making and problem solving.
- collaboratively set goals, visions, and norms for group work.
- cultivate an encouraging manner to help "bring people out."
- verbalize support and optimism for others' actions and ideas, and offer praise appropriately.
- are open and willing to connect, sharing themselves appropriately.
- improve interpersonal skills by being willing to give, receive, and request feedback.
- are willing to confront and explore issues and conflicts, using conflict-resolution skills for conflicts between self and others and between or among individuals and groups.
- accept ambiguity as a step toward clarification and help others deal with it.
- distinguish between the role and the person and humanize both.
- recognize stress and develop coping skills.
- reflect personal values in their actions, and encourage others to act on theirs.
- set their own values and maintain them, even in unfavorable environments.
- ensure individuals' rights to disagree and be different.
- provide nonthreatening opportunities for self-assessment and support ways to improve.
- recognize conflict and collaboration as neutral, and use them positively.
- establish regular information sharing to achieve mutually beneficial results.
- encourage bridge building and networking.
- clarify expectations, including task assignment, for all employees.
- identify relevant experiences with each person being flexible about special needs.
- improve resource availability.
- are personally trusting and trustworthy.
- create safe environments for taking risks and assume responsibility.
- make use of experience as well as formal expertise, and validate their own and others' experiences.
- recognize and respect people's needs and feelings.
- possess technical/organizational/system competence.
- reinforce others' creativity.
- implement synergistic strategies.

Source: Adapted from Vogt, J. F., & Murrel, K. L. (1990). *Empowerment in organizations: How to spark exceptional performance* (pp. 105–107). San Diego, CA: Pfeiffer, with permission.

Transformational Leadership

Burns (1978) was the first author to describe transformational leadership, and draw a distinction between it and transactional leadership. Transformational leadership is a complex process of leadership that motivates members to transcend their own self-interest for a shared vision that reflects higher goals. Transformational leaders serve as change agents within organizations by effectively engaging the emotional and spiritual energy of the members, then challenging this energy to make desirable

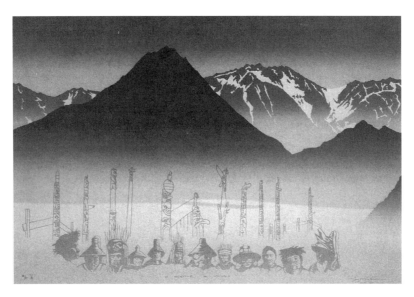

"A Meeting of Chiefs," by Roy Henry Vickers. Reproduced with permission of the artist, Eagle Dance Enterprises, Ltd., 1164 Stelly's Cross Road, Brentwood Bay, BC V8M 1H3, Canada.

personal and organizational changes. "Such leadership occurs when one or more persons engage with others in such a way that leaders and members raise one another to higher levels of motivation and morality. The motives of the leader and members become identical through this transforming process" (Manley McDaniel, 1993, p. 22).

An example of higher-level morality and a shift from self-interest occurred on one hospital unit. The unit manager, a transformational leader, had created an environment where nurses were encouraged to do collaborative problem solving and decision making related to practice issues. To accommodate a backlog of surgeries, the nurses, who did their own scheduling, willingly decided to take turns working evenings and weekends to keep the Post Anesthetic Room open (with no additional monetary benefits).

In contrast, transactional leadership, a more traditional form of leadership, evolves from the motivations of the leader and team or committee members. "Transactional leadership is motivated by the self interests of members and occurs when the leader rewards the members' efforts in exchange for their performance. Interaction between leader and members is limited to the exchange transaction. The effects of transactional leadership are episodic and short-lived" (Manley McDaniel, 1993, p. 22).

When transactional leadership exists, some front-line nurses are less likely to be invited to participate in envisioning how to meet the challenges of internal or external demands to their work. Nonparticipation in the "big picture" problem solving can result in insular thinking, resulting in a desire to "maintain the status quo" and an attitude of "that's not my job can become the norm." This makes it difficult to find nurses willing to do anything not clearly outlined in the job description or the union contract, such as volunteering to work on committees or serving as preceptors for nursing students.

Transformational leadership involves shifting values and understandings from a traditional hierarchical approach or way of "being" to a health promotion approach—it is health promotion in action. Leaders' competence as transformational leaders depends on the dynamic interaction of their personal skills, knowledge, and attitudes as they reflect health promotion principles and philosophy.

In their development of a health promotion curriculum, Beddome, Budgen, Hills, Lindsey, Manchester Duval, and Szalay (1995) used a classification system of nurses' attributes. The attributes were categorized into ontology, epistemology, and praxis, in other words, what nurses need "to be," "to know," and "to do."

In reality, the distinction between "being," "knowing," and "doing" looks arbitrary. "Being" relates to how the action or "doing" is performed; it is derived from a value of caring and is about being in relationship (Sheilds

& Lindsey, 1998). Knowledge informs both "being" and "doing." The essence of transformational leadership from a health promotion perspective is more about "being," or the approach, than it is about "doing." The attributes of transformational leaders are reflected by the question, "Is what is being done, being done in a health promotion way?"

Being

Freire (1970/1993) proposed a dialogic or collaborative approach that transformational leaders use for health promotion with team or committee members in the work place. Even though the approach contains elements of "being," "knowing," and "doing," it is presented here to illustrate how transformational leaders relate to others. The listening-dialogue-action model that Friere suggests includes *listening* to understand the issue or problems, *talking* about them, and *taking the action* envisioned during the dialogue.

Listening

"Listening [the first step of the Freire model] exceeds a needs assessment; it is a participatory and continuing process which uncovers issues of emotional and social significance for those involved" (Wallerstein, 1992, p. 203).

The problems encountered when shifting from an "expert" practice to a "health promotion" practice are described in two research studies that focused on three British Columbia agencies.

In the first study, Cameron and Mah Wren (1999) described a participatory process by which staff, clients, and agency personnel were involved in stating their different perspectives about whether staff "walked their talk" according to the organization's health promotion values. This process was used during reconstruction of the organizational culture, and involved "listening" through surveys, meetings, individual interviews, and telephone calls.

In the second study, Hartrick (1998) "listened" to staff from a community agency and an acute care hospital, using an educative research process consisting of ongoing cycles of analysis, dialogue, action, and reflection. The staff participants analyzed their current practices, assumptions underlying those practices, and contradictions of tension between es-

poused values and values-in-use in their practices. In both cases, listening to health care workers describe their perceptions about health promotion practice created an environment where they felt valued and were willing to further explore issues that resulted in action.

Talking

Transformational leaders also engage in collaborative dialogue, the second step in Friere's model, with all staff or committee members. The emphasis is on understanding their multiple perspectives—as illustrated in the previous examples. There are no experts and recipients of knowledge, but equal partners in an exploratory process to identify issues. The intention during the dialogue phase is to discuss and interpret the issues together by questioning assumptions that have been used previously to address the problem. This participatory process encourages all members to enhance their understanding of the root cause of the issue (Wallerstein, 1992).

Identifying issues involves seeking out the ideas of others, even if an idea seems flawed. It is imperative that leaders believe that those closest to the job and the client are in the best position to identify issues and make improvements. Developing a shared view of the issues and opportunities is a powerful way to begin developing energy for change.

Some helpful questions to aid issue identification include: "What is important? Whose views have been heard? Whose views have not been heard? What issues are not important at this time? What are the parts of the issue? Why does the issue exist?" (Budgen & Cameron, 1999, p. 288).

For example, before merging two departments within an organization, a transformational leader could invite all staff members of the two departments to a meeting. If it is not possible for all members to attend, then representatives from each group, such as full-time, part-time, and casual staff, nurses, physio/occupational therapists, social workers, and support staff could be invited.

At the meeting, after being informed about the merger, the entire staff could be invited to use a **nominal group process** of building consensus by first brainstorming the issues—such as new roles, job descriptions, and communication protocols expected to emerge. Then, staff members could prioritize the issues according to their importance by voting or gaining agreement through participatory dialogue (Delbecq, VandeVen, Gustafson, 1975).

During this process, it will become clear that key stakeholders—such as specific physicians—who are not in attendance, may need to be invited to subsequent meetings; that some issues, such as conference room facilities, are not relevant at this time; and involving the entire staff in the planning and implementation of the merger creates an atmosphere of trust and commitment to the change process.

Acting

Before action is taken, team members envision successful outcomes and set goals. The leader then supports the team members in taking responsibility for turning their ideas into action. The leader assumes the role of resource provider, coach, barrier-breaker, and cheerleader—not the person who "does the doing." This is not a linear process, but rather a cyclical, iterative process; it involves clarifying, making sense, building consensus, and evaluating outcomes of actions. The real sense of team satisfaction and job empowerment comes not just from being listened to, but from playing an instrumental role in making things happen (Wilson, George, Wellins, & Byham, 1994).

"Walking the Talk"

Transformational leaders recognize the importance of practicing their health promotion values, or "walking their talk." They take responsibility for effecting change within themselves and the organization. Through reflection and self-examination, for example, they determine whether they will hold themselves accountable if something goes wrong. They choose to learn from mistakes and overcome deficiencies. To raise their own self-awareness, they seek feedback from team or committee members, from peers, from reports, and from clients. Self-awareness can result in positive self-regard, which can then be extended to positive regard for others. Positive regard for others enables them to reach their full potential.

When leaders "walk their talk" they enhance their credibility and win respect, trust,

and faith—difficult to achieve and easy to violate. To gain and maintain trust, leaders must truly believe that team members will make the right decisions and want to give it their best. Leaders must be trustworthy and demonstrate a willingness to disclose information. It is disturbing to staff when they sense their leaders are not telling them what they really think or feel. When one unit manager informed the staff they would soon be responsible for discharge planning on the weekends, the staff freely voiced their concerns about their lack of time to do an adequate job. They feared some patients could end up being readmitted because the required home supports may not be in place quickly enough. The leader listened to their concerns, agreed with them, and then invited them to problem solve how to address the issues. This created a bond of trust between the leader and staff (Wilson, et al., 1994).

Some transformational leaders have been described as being charismatic with extraordinary abilities to inspire others (Manley McDaniel, 1993). Charismatic leaders can excite members with enthusiasm and optimism to envisage a different and more challenging future. These leaders are capable of moving members to achieve extraordinary levels of accomplishment both in terms of performance as well as in their own development.

Manley McDaniel claims that transformational leaders use language rich with metaphors and symbols to heighten team members' awareness of what is required to accomplish a shared goal. One leader, for example, reviewed the year's activities and projected the future using a diagram of the "yellow brick road" from the *Wizard of Oz*. Manley McDaniel goes on to say that leaders articulate the importance of the vision and communicate confidence in members' abilities. This elevates members to a level of autonomous self-regulation and motivates them to perform beyond their original expectations. They make decisions that reflect shared organizational values, not mandated rules.

Motivated work teams become self-directed, accepting responsibility for the quality of their work and sharing responsibilities that formerly resided solely with their supervisors and managers. For example, team members might hire new employees, handle conflict, schedule their own work, or develop their own plans and budgets. They also develop a sense of ownership and pride, and trust is high among team members and between the teams and their leaders. Transformational leaders provide mentorship along with motivation so that the staff develops skills to accomplish various responsibilities.

Mentoring

Mentoring is linked to empowerment and occurs between leaders and team or committee members, or experienced and inexperienced nurses. It involves seeing value in people so clearly that they come to see it in themselves (Watson, 1988), and encourages the development of each member as a unique individual. Leaders mentor by first understanding each individual's level of maturity and capacities, and then coaching them to achieve the desired skills. Mentoring is achieved by:

1. Listening to team members
2. Providing constructive feedback regularly, not just during performance appraisals
3. Talking about ways in which team members need to prepare themselves for the future
4. Discussing ways in which employees can grow in their current jobs, not only through promotions or lateral moves
5. Promoting networking with staff in other parts of the organization

Outcomes for individuals are the development of skills, self-knowledge, self-control, and readiness for self-motivation, within a social context (Angelini, 1998). Outcomes at the group level include greater readiness for cooperation and less competition among members.

> ✹ **Reflective Questions**
>
> **1.** What values are observable through my actions?
> **2.** How often do I encourage/praise others? Is there anybody whom I do not encourage?
> **3.** How much of the time do I spend talking versus listening?
> **4.** Do I accept each person's ideas? How do I demonstrate my acceptance?
> **5.** Do I include all the people in the decision-making process who are affected by the decision?
> **6.** Who is left out and why?

Knowing

Transformational leaders' ways of "knowing" begin with their personal commitment to life-long learning. They have knowledge of current internal and external trends and realities, as well as an understanding of power dynamics, politics, change theory, group process, verbal and written communication, negotiation, conflict resolution, team building, and shared decision making (Hein, 1998). They define the "job to be done," and engage in doing the "right work" rather than just "working right." The former results in effectiveness, whereas the latter results in efficiency. Although both are needed, efficiency without effectiveness will not move the organization forward. Being effective gains leaders' operational credibility with their managers and respect from staff and clients.

However, during periods of rapid organizational change, there are times when leaders are not aware of all the changes that are happening and are as confused as everyone else. Being comfortable with ambiguity is essential for leaders and team members alike. During these times, leaders need to recognize the limits of what they can do, and not challenge the impossible, but focus their efforts where they can succeed. This is when leaders can support team or committee members to work things out for themselves, to clarify the issue, and to review and learn from what they have done.

> ✹ **Reflective Questions**
>
> **1.** How do my colleagues and team members demonstrate their discomfort with ambiguity around issues? Who shows the most discomfort? How can I support them?
> **2.** How do colleagues and team members experience me when I am stressed?
> **3.** What resources can I access to help me solve problems?

Doing

Transformational leaders' values are made visible in their praxis, or what they "do." Chinn (1995) states that there is a link between values and action, and refers to "knowing what you do, and doing what you know" (p. xvi).

Transformational leaders role-model the values embedded in a health promotion approach to engage staff in the creation of organizational visions and goals that reflect a health promotion philosophy.

A vision is an end goal that helps paint a picture of where we want to go, whereas values help define the approach we use to achieve the vision. The emphasis is on "we" in this statement. Visions that are imposed on team or committee members, at best, command compliance—not commitment. Involving all team or committee members in establishing visions, goals, and norms is beneficial to gain their sense of ownership and shared meaning. If people have been involved in developing the goals and norms, this shared sense of direction is a powerful motivating force. It inspires people for two reasons—it values their efforts and contributions from the past, and it recognizes their aspiration and hopes for the future. Together these create a powerful stimulus for change" (Senge, 1994, p. 206).

Finally, shared visions change peoples' relationship with the organization; it is no longer "their agency." It becomes "our agency," "our issue," and "our solution." Leaders and staff or committee members, then, need to keep the organization's vision and values in the forefront of every team or committee decision and action. "Vision and values, not policy manuals, must be the beacons that guide day-to-day team behavior" (Wilson, et al., 1994, p. 74). They also provide the focus and energy for learning. "While adaptive learning is possible without vision, generative learning [or creating new ideas] occurs only when people are striving to accomplish something that matters deeply to them" (Senge, 1994, p. 206).

Creating Learning Environments

Creating learning environments to facilitate individual and organizational change is central to the health promotion approach transformational leaders use. Learning environments evolve from the belief that knowledge is not discovered, but rather is created, and that learning by doing will most likely bring personal and organizational change. Learning by doing involves taking time to reflect, and reflecting while doing produces learning.

To facilitate learning, leaders can also provide training programs and resources at the point when people can apply them. This avoids the situation where everyone learns the same things, regardless of their capability, interest, or preparedness to apply the ideas. If work teams learn together, individual and organizational development can powerfully reinforce one another, and a strong team develops as they confront challenges through shared experience. This shared experience results in a great release of energy as people begin to believe in the team and in what it can do.

A supportive learning environment facilitates the effective functioning of a relational community. Likewise, a relational community will likely ensure the creation of a learning environment. In their discussion about relational communities, Shields and Lindsey (1998) point out that the focus is on relationships and power. This community concept has meaning for power relations within work teams and committees. Based on the work of McMillan and Chavis (1986), Shields and Lindsey outline four requirements for a relational community, which are:

Membership, influence, integration and fulfillment of needs, and shared emotional connection. Membership implies the feeling of belonging or sharing. It may include such aspects as boundaries, emotional safety, a sense of belonging and identification, personal investment, and a common symbol system. Influence describes both being attracted to a community people that they want to be part of, and having influence over what occurs within the community. . . . The third element of integration and fulfillment of needs suggests member's needs . . . will be met with the resources of the community or group. . . . Shared emotional connection, the final element, attends to the importance of closeness and interaction between group members. This element may encompass shared history, culture, and spiritual bonds. (p. 27)

Working in a relational team or committee means working cooperatively with people, and seeking their welfare as well as our own. People working together multiply their abilities in ways that are not explained. Members of a relational team fill in for each other when a member goes home sick, they pick up information at meetings for missing members, they band together if a member is dealt with unfairly, they prefer each others' company in the cafeteria, and they help each other to get the work done. Relational teams and committees experience synergistic energy, are highly productive, and their morale is good—evidence of health promotion in action.

✳ Reflective Questions

1. What do I know about staff morale? How much sick time is there on my unit?
2. How are team or committee members' contributions recognized?
3. What new roles/tasks have team or committee members assumed this past year?

CONCLUSION

This chapter has discussed a promising and preferred form of leadership in the context of nursing. The concepts that underpin transformational leadership are similar to, and in fact a direct extension of, health promotion beliefs and principles. The current rapidity of change in health care agencies and organizations requires leaders who are not only personally responsive to change, but who can share their vision with team and committee members, see others' views and visions, are responsive to change, and can motivate team members to take action.

This approach has potential to create a work environment for nurses that is congruent with the tenets of health promotion. Such congruence will go some way to support nurses in their health promotion practice.

As nursing enters a new millennium, we will continue to be at "the edge"—there may be even greater visions, opportunities, and challenges. As nurses, we can "be afraid," or we can navigate the turbulence by experiencing the synergistic energy that emanates from working with self-assured team members in an empowering environment. As transformational leaders who use a health promotion approach we can "push ourselves to fly" by working collaboratively toward formulated goals that represent personal and organizational values, needs, and expectations (Marriner-Tomey, 1993).

The scenario in Box 7–1 illustrates how one transformational leader created a vision to change the organizational culture and then supported the staff to make the changes. The details of the organizational change process within this community agency in British Columbia are available in a publication by Cameron and Mah Wren (1999).

✳ Reflective Questions

1. Use the list in Table 7–1 to identify the strategies the transformational leader described in Box 7–1 (on page 110) used. How many can you identify?
2. Do I have opportunities to apply similar strategies? What are they?

BOX 7-1

TRANSFORMATIONAL LEADERSHIP IN ACTION

"We must be the change we wish to see in the world."
Gandhi

The manager of a Community Health Care program used strategies of transformational leadership to facilitate the reconstruction of the organizational culture. Her staff members, share a history and enjoy a relational community. They deliver in-home services in health care in three communities (Cameron, 1998). With restructuring, new relational communities had to be forged. There was ambiguity around roles, accountability, and recording systems all within the context of scarce resources. The manager was a visionary leader with an ability to articulate the direction of health care—even when it seemed to change every day. Over time, the staff and the external health care community gained trust in the manager as a transformational leader.

Although the context of the Community Health Care program was within a traditional hierarchical system, the manager was committed to encouraging the staff and the organization to use a health promotion approach with clients, agency personnel with whom they interacted, and with one other. This meant letting go of their "expert" role, sharing power, and increasing collaboration. While the staff had always provided client-centered care, there was a new emphasis on including clients and their families in more of the decision making related to their care.

The manager, using a transformational leadership style, motivated the staff by modeling a health promotion approach, and proactively sharing her vision and the need for change with the management team and the entire staff at a series of meetings. She used metaphors such as "the yellow brick road" to illustrate the path the staff had journeyed on, their accomplishments along the way, and their future course.

The entire staff was invited to participate in setting organizational goals and values. The manager demonstrated her trust in them by listening, challenging them to "think outside the box," and communicating her confidence in their ability to do so. The staff brainstormed and provided exemplars to illustrate organizational values. The opinions of all staff were invited and valued.

These discussions resulted in reflections on whether the staff was consistently delivering service to clients and interacting with agency personnel according to their espoused values. In other words, "were they walking their talk?" The management team listened to the discussion, participated in the dialogue, and then facilitated the development of an action plan to survey the clients and agency personnel with whom they worked. The Community Health Care staff wanted to get clients' and agency personnel's perceptions about whether they "walked their talk."

A learning environment had existed within the Community Health Care organization for years. The staff was well equipped to open their boundaries and invite agency personnel and clients to participate in ad hoc committees with them, make decisions about survey designs, data collection and analysis methods, and devise action plans to address the findings. Mistakes were viewed as learning opportunities, and some plans and strategies were changed. The manager provided the project with staff, transportation, and material resources.

During all the collaborative interactions there was an attempt to use "power with" relations. Diversity was assured by inviting personnel from all agencies with whom the staff interacted to participate in ad hoc committees or to serve as survey participants; sharing was accomplished by inviting front-line personnel, rather than relying on supervisors to represent them. The manager kept the staff informed about changes through meetings, memos, and e-mail. Staff members responded by assuming some leadership roles and acting as change agents within the organization and with external committees.

The manager's ability to view her staff members as individuals and to inspire them made the transition to a health promotion culture, using a "power with," approach an empowering experience for this Community Health Care staff.

REFERENCES

Angelini, D. J. (1998). Mentoring in the career development of hospital staff nurses: Models and strategies. In E. C. Hein (Ed.), *Contemporary leadership behavior: Selected readings* (5th ed., pp. 143–154). Philadelphia: Lippincott.

Beddome, G. (Cameron), Budgen, C., Hills, M. D., Lindsey, A. E., Manchester Duval, P., & Szalay, L. (1995). Education and practice collaboration: A strategy for curriculum development. *Journal of Nursing Education, 34,* 11–15.

Binney, G., & Williams, C. (1995). *Leaning in the future: Changing the way people change organizations.* Naperville, IL: Nicholas Brealey.

Budgen, C., & Cameron, G. (1999). Program planning, implementation, and evaluation. In J. E. Hitchcock, P. E. Schubert, & S. A. Thomas (Eds.), *Community health nursing: Caring in action* (pp. 267–300). Albany, NY: Delmar.

Burns, J. M. (1978). *Leadership.* New York: Harper & Row.

Cameron, G. (1998). Transformational leadership: A strategy for organizational change. *Journal of Nursing Administration, 28*(10), 3.

Cameron, G., & Mah Wren, A. (1999). Reconstructing organizational culture: A process using multiple perspectives. *Public Health Nursing, 16,* 96–101.

Carlson-Catalano, J. (1992). Empowering nurses for professional practice. *Nursing Outlook, 40,* 139–142.

Chinn, P. L. (1995). *Peace & power: Building communities for the future* (4th ed.). New York: National League for Nursing.

Clarke, H. F., & Mass, H. (1998). Comox Valley nursing center: From collaboration to empowerment. *Public Health Nursing, 15,* 216–224.

Delbecq, A. L., VandeVen, A. H. & Gustafson, D. H. (1975). *Group techniques for program planning: a guide to nominal group process and Delphi technique.* (Management applications series.) Glenview, Ill: Scott, Foresman.

Drevdahl, D. (1995). Coming to voice: The power of emancipatory community interventions. *Advances in Nursing Science, 18*(2), 13–24.

Eng, E., Salmon, M. E., & Mullan, F. (1992). Community empowerment: The critical base for primary health care. *Family and Community Health, 15,* 1–12.

Freire, P. (1970/1993). *Pedagogy of the oppressed* (20th anniversary ed.), trans. M. B. Ramus. New York: Continuum.

Gibson, C. H. (1991). A concept analysis of empowerment. *Journal of Advanced Nursing, 16,* 354–361.

Hartrick, G. (1998). Developing health promoting practices: A transformative process. *Nursing Outlook, 46,* 219–225.

Hein, E. C. (1998). *Contemporary leadership behavior* (5th ed.). Philadelphia: Lippincott.

Henneman, E. A., Lee, J. L., & Cohen, J. I. (1995). Collaboration: A concept analysis. *Journal of Advanced Nursing, 21,* 103–109.

Katz, R. (1984). *Empowerment and synergy: Expanding the community's healing resources.* New York: Hayworth.

Kendall, J. (1992). Fighting back: Promoting emancipatory nursing actions. *Advances in Nursing Science, 15*(2), 1–15.

Labonte, R. (1990). Empowerment: Notes on professional and community dimensions. *Canadian Review of Social Policy, 26,* 64–75.

Maben, J., & McLeod Clarke, J. (1995). Health promotion: A concept analysis. *Journal of Advanced Nursing, 22,* 1158–1165.

Manley McDaniel, A. M. (1993). Beyond charisma: Transformational leadership. In A. Marriner-Tomey (Ed.), *Transformation leadership in nursing* (pp. 17–32). St Louis, MO: Mosby Year Book.

Marriner-Tomey, A. (1993). *Transformation leadership in nursing.* St Louis, MO: Mosby Year Book.

McMillan, D. W., & Chavis, D. (1986). Sense of community: A definition and theory. *Journal of Community Psychology, 14,* 6–23.

Ministry of Skills Training and Labor. (1995). *Collaborative nursing curriculum.* Unpublished curriculum. Okanagan University College, Kelowna, B.C.: Author.

Rissel, C. (1994). Empowerment: The holy grail of health promotion? *Health Promotion International, 9,* 39–47.

Senge, P. M. (1994). *The fifth discipline: The art and practice of the learning organization.* Toronto, ON: Doubleday.

Sheilds, L. E., & Lindsey, A. E. (1998). Community health promotion nursing practice. *Advances in Nursing Science, 20*(4), 23–36.

Stevens, P. E., & Hall, J. M. (1992). Applying critical theories to nursing in communities. *Public Health Nursing, 9,* 2–9.

Vogt, J. F., & Murrel, K. L. (1990). *Empowerment in organizations: How to spark exceptional performance* (pp. 99–124). San Diego, CA: Pfeiffer.

Wallerstein, N. (1992). Powerlessness, empowerment, and health: Implications for health promotion programs. *American Journal of Health Promotion, 6,* 197–205.

Watson, J. (1988). *Nursing: Human science and human care: A theory of nursing.* New York: National League for Nursing.

Wilson, J. M., George, J., Wellins, R. S., & Byham, W. C. (Eds). (1994). From commander to coach: A model for the evolving role of the leader. In *Leadership Trapeze: Strategies for leadership in team-based organization* (pp. 57–75). San Francisco: Jossey-Bass.

Yeitch, S., & Levine, R. (1992). Participatory research's contribution to a conceptualization of empowerment. *Journal of Applied Social Psychology, 22,* 1894–1908.

Zimmerman, M. A., & Rapport, J. (1988). Citizen participation, perceived control, and psychological empowerment. *American Journal of Community Psychology, 16,* 725–743.

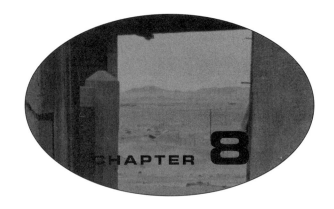

CHAPTER 8

Nurses Influencing Health Care Policy: International Perspectives

NORA B. WHYTE

Kathmandu, Nepal

A Canadian nursing consultant finds herself in the midst of a most remarkable scene on International Women's Day, a national holiday in Nepal. She enters a city square—bordered by temples, statues, and a royal palace—to see hundreds of people gathered for the official launch of a national campaign on safe motherhood. On a platform in front of one of the buildings, the Minister of Health and representatives from international organizations are assembled to proclaim a major initiative to reduce maternal mortality and promote infant health. Following the speeches, the crowd is treated to a play on the theme of safe motherhood.

After the formalities, people mingle and visit display booths set up around the square. Organizations promoting breast-feeding, family planning, and immunization are displaying posters and pamphlets for the public. One display in particular captures this visitor's attention. Five nursing students are in charge of a tabletop display they had developed as a group project for health teaching in the villages. They had constructed two small models of typical village scenes: one depicting the environment for a safe home delivery, the other showing unsafe conditions. These are colorful scenes complete with thatched houses, families, animals, and even vegetables growing in a kitchen garden for good prenatal nutrition. The students' project is a simple yet powerful way to communicate their health promotion message to local people. The whole event is impressive both for the strategies used to reach the public and the

demonstration of collaboration among government and voluntary groups. Nursing leaders and the group of students are making an important contribution to the start of Nepal's safe motherhood campaign.

For many years nurses have been encouraged to play a more active role in health policy. In particular, the International Council of Nurses (ICN) and national nursing associations have urged members to assume greater leadership in primary health care and health system reform (Baumgart, 1993; CNA, 1995; ICN, 1988; Oulton, 1996). Although position statements issued by nursing organizations and editorials in journals advocate greater involvement by nurses in reorienting health systems, there are few concrete examples of what nurses are actually doing to influence the direction of those reforms.

This chapter highlights practical strategies used by nurses in three countries in their health policy initiatives. Nurses are actively engaged in influencing change in a variety of ways within diverse situations and cultures, as illustrated by the students promoting safe motherhood in Nepal, and by the action of individual nurses and nursing associations throughout the world. The selected examples are presented against a backdrop of global health reform and a renewed interest in primary health care.

When nursing organizations talk about influencing health care policy, what do they mean? Health policy is "the set of rules by which decisions affecting health status or outcomes are made in a given society" (Baumgart, 1993, p. 167). Health policy includes all the legislation related to a nation's health system, reflecting that society's values about issues of universal access to services and distribution of resources. Baumgart notes that if nurses are to influence health policy in the public interest, they must consider issues of accessibility, resource allocation, and standards of health care delivery. For the purposes of this chapter, health care policy refers to both the formal structures guiding health systems at national or state/provincial levels as well as the more informal aspects of planning, delivering, and evaluating services at local levels.

The Global Context: Primary Health Care

Common challenges have prompted health reform worldwide. In its new *Health for All* policy, the World Health Organization (WHO, 1997) outlines major forces shaping health and health care today. These include demographic changes, inequities within and among countries, environmental issues, urbanization, and global economic factors. Establishing flexible, responsive, and accessible health care remains a challenge in most countries, according to WHO. Reorienting health care delivery to community-based services is still hindered by lack of support for prevention and health promotion. The principles of primary health care, as articulated in the Alma Ata Declaration (WHO, 1978), have been poorly understood. The full scope of primary health care was rarely put into practice; rather, most countries opted for selective reforms that had little effect on creating more responsive health care.

What is the full scope of **primary health care** and why should nurses continue to push for its adoption? Primary health care is considered to be both a philosophy of health care and a practical approach to providing a range of health services at the community level. According to the Canadian Nurses Association (CNA), "primary health care is essential care (promotive, preventive, curative, rehabilitative, and supportive) that is focused on preventing illness and promoting health" (CNA, 1995, p. 1). The original concept of primary health care as a global strategy to achieve health for all by the year 2000 (WHO, 1978) also called on national govern-

ments to ensure that people everywhere had the basic prerequisites for good health: safe water, sanitation, food security, economic development, and quality of life.

The principles of primary health care are accessibility, public participation, health promotion, appropriate technology, and intersectoral cooperation (WHO, 1978). On the whole, these principles mean that people should be engaged in decisions about their own health and the overall health of their community. Health services are developed with public involvement to determine the most appropriate and accessible methods of delivery. In many countries around the world, these principles are implemented through community health centers that offer accessible, interdisciplinary services at the local level and provide linkages to other parts of the system (hospitals and specialty services). These centers provide basic medical care to individuals and families, along with prevention and health promotion activities, encompassing a range of programs that might include immunization, parenting education, support groups for people living with chronic illnesses, seniors' fitness programs, and youth clinics.

These community health centers often have an outreach component, such as home visiting by nurses or health education in schools, and frequently become the focal point for advocacy and community action on local issues. Partnerships with other sectors might involve the health center staff working with service clubs, churches, and police on a violence prevention project or with an environmental group on a community garden. In keeping with primary health care principles, community health centers are usually governed by an elected board of community representatives or have other ways of encouraging public involvement in decision making through advisory groups and community meetings.

Primary health care is a good fit with nursing. In its policy statement on the role of the nurse in primary health care, the Canadian Nurses Association (1995) views it as "natural extension of nursing practice" and emphasizes that all nurses have a vital role to play in implementing primary health care (p. 1). Over the years, nursing leaders have worked at various levels, both within governments and through their professional organizations, to advance the primary health care movement.

In their study of chief nursing officer positions in national governments, Splane and Splane (1994) document the ways in which nursing's policy efforts have been enhanced by having an effective nursing presence in health ministries, supported by strong national and international associations with shared values. They note also how these nursing leaders had "welcomed primary health care as being in close harmony with their longstanding approach to health" (p. 196).

In her keynote address at the International Council of Nurses Quadrennial Congress in 1997, Dame June Clark reinforced this strong connection between nursing and primary health care:

Primary health care is about making health care accessible and acceptable to all people, whatever the social, economic or political circumstances of their country. It is about attitudes towards health and approaches to health care delivery. It is about working in partnership with people—individuals, families, communities, populations—to achieve the shared goals of health for all. That is why it is nursing. (p. 149)

Primary health care is closely related to this book's theme of health promotion. Health promotion practice uses a variety of approaches and strategies, all designed to enhance people's capacity for health, whether at the individual level or in families, groups, populations, and communities. The underlying principles are similar and the terms are often used interchangeably. In the context of global health reform, primary health care merits particular attention because of the urgency for cost-effective, accessible service delivery. Primary health care as characterized by community health centers should be the foundation of a country's health system.

This chapter illustrates—in three different contexts—how nurses influence health system reform. Selected exemplars from Japan, Nepal, and South Africa provide details of actual strategies used by groups of nurses to facilitate changes in nursing and health care at many levels, from their local neighborhoods to subnational and national levels. Although the circumstances are different in each country, nurses experience common challenges worldwide and draw upon similar competencies as they participate in initiatives for change.

The content of these scenarios is based on the author's observations from the vantage point of an outsider during short-term consultations to nursing associations in these countries. It is not meant to be a comprehensive review of international nursing policy development. Rather, it will give you a flavor of practical approaches to influencing changes in health services and health promotion. The Japanese scenario provides more detail because it chronicles a five-year policy project with a variety of layers and strategies.

Why should nurses and nursing organizations concern themselves with broad issues of health care policy? Is there any point in attempting to change health care systems? If so, what can nurses contribute? In another keynote address at the ICN Congress, Smith (1997) presented clear answers to these questions when she spoke of the nursing role in mobilizing community capacity for health:

Nurses' leadership in health care is essential because . . . the health care system and the health of people are dependent upon the nurse as on no other professional, particularly for the advancement of primary health care internationally . . . and nurses have the resourcefulness, flexibility and critical thinking skills to discover and mobilize rich resources often overlooked by others. (p. 107)

Ways in which nursing associations, and their individual members, are learning to assert their leadership are illustrated in the following situations. Our "virtual world tour" begins in Japan.

Japan: Lessons in Health Promotion Leadership

During the past decade, nursing leaders in Japan have recognized serious challenges facing their health system and the profession. Although Japan ranks highly in most population health status indicators (Wilkinson, 1996; WHO, 1996), recent economic and demographic factors are creating pressure on health and social services. Between 1993 and 1997 the Japanese Nursing Association (JNA) carried out a major policy project to influence the development of community-based health care throughout Japan. JNA is the professional organization for the country's registered nurses, assistant nurses, and midwives and is a longstanding member of ICN. The project provides an instructive exemplar because of the multifaceted approach that the nursing association developed. Some of the strategies are described in detail to illustrate the ways in which a policy initiative can make a difference at local, regional, and national levels.

Context

During the 1990s, nursing in Japan went through a period of unprecedented change in response to major economic and social changes in the country. Changing demographics (more than half the population live longer than 80 years), coupled with public pressure for improvements in services, such as home nursing care and home support, posed challenges to the health care system (Murashima, Hatono, Whyte, & Asahara, 1999). Developing comprehensive systems for community-based care for the elderly became a national priority for the government and for the professions.

In the early 1990s, the National Ministry of Health and Welfare and JNA held discussions about ways to transform health care and nursing to meet these changing demands. Nursing leaders had already recognized that a new type of education was required to prepare nurses for changing practice environments, particularly for community-based care and clinical specialization in areas of chronic illness and gerontological nursing. Through a major curriculum reform, nursing education was reoriented to prepare graduates with competencies for a wider range of roles to meet the changing social context (Mitoh, 1997). The number of baccalaureate programs in the country rose from 11 in 1990 to 65 in 1998 (JNA, 1998). As well, many new graduate programs were established during this period.

Project Background

In 1993, the government provided JNA with a substantial grant to embark on a project that would examine new roles for nurses in community-oriented care and assist with the development of policy for health reform. JNA formed a committee to oversee the project; most committee members had been active in

the JNA and were leaders in nursing education, research, and community health practice. They met several times per year over the course of the project with individual members taking on specific responsibilities as the project progressed. The executive director and national headquarters' staff provided operational support as needed. The overall purpose of the project was "to promote more effective health services suitable to the changes of an aging society" (JNA, 1994). Following the first year, JNA sent a report to the government documenting its activities and results along with a proposal for another phase of the project to build on the work it had begun. This proved to be a strategic tactic, and was repeated successfully every year for five years.

Information Gathering

Early in the project, the committee embarked on a series of study visits to collect information about health care reforms and community health nursing in other countries. The committee turned these study tours into an educational and leadership development opportunity by inviting JNA members to participate. Groups of seven to twelve nurses—with a committee member as tour coordinator and mentor—visited Denmark, Sweden, England, Canada, and Australia. Upon their return, each group prepared an extensive report on these health care systems including descriptions of current issues in health reform, nursing roles, and nursing education. Group members came from many parts of Japan; this helped in disseminating information throughout the country because they shared their experiences with colleagues in their local nursing associations and workplaces. JNA also collected information from other countries and used its connections within ICN to learn about international trends. This initial phase took about a year, during which time the committee developed ideas about themes to pursue in subsequent phases of the project and planned strategies to achieve its goals. The links with nurses in other countries were maintained through follow-up visits by committee members and by bringing Danish and Canadian consultants to Japan at various points in the project. Of particular interest to the government and JNA in the mid-1990s were the innovations in home care evident in

Denmark and the emphasis on health promotion that they had observed in both Australia and Canada.

Education of Members

In the year following the international study tours, considerable work was carried out to educate JNA members about leadership for health promotion. The visits had highlighted the value of political action by nurses in shifting practice to having greater emphasis on health promotion. They had been impressed, also, by situations in other countries where nurses had initiated community-based demonstration projects and were practicing from a health promotion perspective, such as a nursing center in British Columbia, Canada (Registered Nurses Association of British Columbia, 1996). Through its branches in 46 prefectures (states), JNA invited nurses to apply as participants in a four-day seminar in Tokyo on the topic of health promotion. The project grant enabled JNA to pay the nurses' travel expenses and other costs associated with organizing the event. The seminar was attended by 25 nurses representing many parts of the country and different areas of nursing practice. These participants were selected on the basis of demonstrated leadership in their agency or nursing association and application letters in which they expressed goals for developing a health promotion project in their respective workplaces. Most were practicing nurses from hospitals, while some worked in occupational health, nursing education, and community nursing.

The committee members and senior staff from JNA and a Canadian consultant (the author) were also involved in the seminar. During the four days, participants were engaged in plenary sessions and small-group work in which they discussed key concepts of health promotion and analyzed case studies from Japan and Canada. By the end of the seminar, each nurse described her ideas for a small demonstration project or a change that she would hope to implement in the coming year. Ideas for proposed projects included: developing better links between a hospital and community services, planning a hospice program, carrying out a community needs assessment, facilitating a support group, and

working with the public on a "healthy community" project. Seminar participants offered practical suggestions to one another about ways to get started on these projects. Several committee members offered their assistance with the projects (e.g., helping with proposal writing or going to a nurse's community for follow-up).

Another learning opportunity hosted by JNA was a lecture and networking event held at the conclusion of the seminar to extend the content to a wider nursing audience. Two hundred nurses from the Tokyo area attended this gathering where highlights from the seminar were shared and a presentation was given on "nurses influencing change."

Skill Development

At the 1995 seminar, participants had raised numerous questions about how they could work more closely with the public to identify local health concerns and mobilize community members in creating healthy communities. Promoting citizen participation in the health system, as exemplified in the international healthy cities/healthy communities movement, was a relatively new idea in Japan at the time. Consequently, the JNA committee decided that the next phase of their project should focus on skill development for public health nurses in the area of community health promotion. They decided to try a different method this time, using a participatory workshop to give nurses hands-on experience with a community meeting.

One public health nurse, who had attended the 1995 seminar, volunteered her city as a site for the 1996 workshop and generated support from her colleagues to host and organize the event in Miura. Miura is a coastal city of 52,000 people serving as the main center of an agricultural area in Kanagawa prefecture. Located 50 kilometers from Tokyo, it was a convenient site for JNA's workshop. There are about 12 public health nurses (PHNs) in the area, mainly involved in maternal-child health, school programs, and public health protection activities. Most PHNs are employed by the city health department, but a few are part of the prefectural health system serving the surrounding rural communities. Some of these PHNs had begun support groups for new parents, had learned from their group members how keen people were for information about health services, and had developed ideas for programs that were needed in their community. They were aware that community members would like an opportunity to meet with health professionals to share their opinions.

The JNA committee worked with the nurses in Miura to plan the workshop. A three-day program was envisioned, beginning with a day for the PHNs to prepare for the community meeting and to discuss principles of community health promotion. In addition to the PHNs from Miura, JNA invited about 10 PHNs from other parts of the country (some of whom had been at the previous seminar and had initiated projects as a result). Meanwhile, the Miura PHNs began talking with community members and other interested health providers (e.g., hospital staff, a community social worker, and the district medical health officer) about their plans for the community meeting and what they hoped to achieve by increasing public participation in local health care decision making. The community meeting was scheduled for the second day with the final day earmarked for time to reflect on the process and to plan follow-up activities. The same Canadian consultant was invited to return to Japan as a resource person for the workshop. Planning for the workshop was going well until a few months before the event, when the city administrator (with responsibility for all the public health programs) told the chief PHN that organizing and participating in a community workshop was not a suitable public health nursing activity. He and his senior civic officials could not endorse a public meeting of this kind nor would they "allow" any staff to attend.

On hearing this shocking news, the JNA committee members and executive director drew upon their diplomacy skills and political acumen to salvage their plans. They made an appointment with the mayor and senior staff and decided on a constructive strategy to present their position. The JNA representatives used the meeting to educate the mayor and his officials about the rationale for community meetings and emphasized the benefits to Miura, namely, positive publicity and recognition for its leadership in community health promotion. Further, JNA promised that some funds would be available to the public health department to finance future meet-

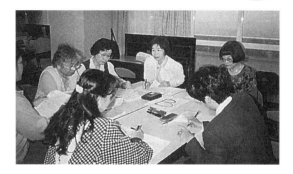

FIG. 8–1. Community members and public health nurses conduct a meeting in Miura City, Japan. *(Photo: Nora Whyte.)*

ings or demonstration projects. The meeting concluded with the mayor's assurance of the city's utmost support for this "worthwhile endeavor."

Considering these initial struggles for support, the actual community meeting (a day-long session with 40 participants) was a great success. Community members and public health staff soon became comfortable with working and learning together. Participants took turns with the roles of small-group facilitators and recorders (Fig. 8–1). At first, some community members were hesitant to contribute to group discussions and they may have wondered what it was all about. Before long, everyone was engaged in lively brainstorming and thoughtful discussions, and by day's end, several community members were standing at the front of the room presenting reports on behalf of their groups, who cheered them on in case of anxiety.

The day was filled with humor, honest sharing of concerns, and creative ideas for ways to improve health in Miura. In commenting on the day, one woman from a mothers' group said: "This is the first time that health professionals have asked for my opinion. . . . I really felt they listened to what I had to say." A delightful comment from another young woman received nods and laughter from others: "I was very nervous when I arrived this morning, not knowing what to expect in a community meeting. I had planned to leave at lunch-time because my husband was home with the children. By noon, I was enjoying it so much that I phoned him to say I'm not coming home until it's over!" Most of the workshop participants returned for a public lecture given on the final day and were on hand to greet the mayor who was the guest of honor at a lavish JNA reception at the end of the workshop. They shared their enthusiasm with him and volunteered to serve on committees to move the workshop's ideas forward. There were photo opportunities galore and health promotion moved up on the civic agenda.

Some of the known outcomes of this event are: that it led to acceptance of public meetings for discussion of health issues in this community, that some of ideas presented (e.g., the need for more parenting education and support groups) were incorporated into public health programs in Miura following the initial workshop, and that this strategy was applied in other communities. JNA published a guidebook for holding public meetings, using the Miura workshop (complete with photographs taken that day) as an example of a how to begin the process and how to engage community members in a health planning project (JNA, 1996).

Documentation

The guidebook mentioned previously is just one of many publications resulting from JNA's policy project. JNA leaders paid special attention to careful documentation of its research into other health systems and distributed these materials widely. Funds were used to record and publish seminar proceedings and special lectures throughout the five years of the project. They also used their journals and newsletters to publicize aspects of the project. Another strategy to make international health promotion concepts more accessible to Japanese nurses was the translation of key documents from English into Japanese. These included such documents as the *Ottawa Charter for Health Promotion* (World Health Organization, Health and Welfare Canada, & Canadian Public Health Association, 1986), *Achieving Health for All: A Framework for Health Promotion* (Epp, 1986), and *Action Statement for Health Promotion in Canada* (Canadian Public Health Association, 1996). Prior to JNA's policy project and its efforts to disseminate ideas about health promotion, most Japanese nurses had little exposure to the broad notions of health promotion articulated in these statements.

Unique Challenges

It remains a challenge for Japanese nurses to be recognized as equal partners within the health team, traditionally dominated by physicians and administrators (Tierney & Tierney, 1994). Similarly, establishing partnerships with community members is a slow process given Japan's long history of social boundaries separating professionals from ordinary citizens. This makes the need for success stories, however small, even more pressing.

Recent reforms in nursing education throughout Japan mean that today's nursing graduates have beginning competencies in health promotion, including community development and advocacy skills (Murashima et al., 1999). This is a new phenomenon, however, and it will be some years until these competencies are the norm among Japanese nurses. JNA's work to assist the current workforce to develop knowledge, skills, and attitudes consistent with health promotion principles is commendable.

Reflecting on this complex five-year experience, it is clear that JNA carried out a comprehensive policy project with concrete results (JNA, 1999). The project evolved from one focused on improving care to an aging population to a broad-reaching program aimed to position nurses as leaders in local and national arenas. Through the project, JNA provided education to groups of nursing leaders so that they could contribute more effectively to change within their communities. Nurses gained skills in planning and facilitating community meetings, learned how to write proposals, and participated in demonstration projects. The Japanese Nursing Association created a high profile for the project within Japan by disseminating reports to nurses, other professions, and government. Through study tours and consultations, the project also established international linkages with nursing organizations in other countries.

Finally, it is worth pointing out that other groups and sectors in Japan are taking greater interest in health promotion and public participation, and are seeking nursing's expertise in these areas. Increasingly, people are becoming involved in decisions about health issues and services in their neighborhoods, towns, and cities. Healthy cities and communities projects—often involving local people, health professionals, and municipal officials taking action on locally identified issues—are now being recognized with national awards (Iwanaga, 1996).

Nepal: Strengthening Nursing to Improve Health Care

In marked contrast to the affluence and status of Japan in the world community, Nepal is among the most socioeconomically disadvantaged nations in the world. Its population health status indicators, such as maternal mortality, and other measures of social development (e.g., literacy), place Nepal near the bottom of the world development index (WHO, 1996). The Nursing Association of Nepal (NAN), with about 1,800 members, faces the dual challenges of developing the nursing profession and contributing to the health care system.

Although the government of Nepal has adopted a primary health care approach to its long-range health plan, Nepal continues to have a major problem with funding for and delivery of basic health services to remote areas of the country, compromising rural citizens' access to health care. Health professionals are reluctant to work outside the main cities. NAN is taking leadership on this issue in two ways. One is through policy work at the national level. This includes having NAN representatives appointed to government committees dealing with issues such as training of local primary health workers and overall health system planning.

As the nursing association became better organized during the 1990s, its president and other leaders were asked to serve on national committees. During 1996, for example, NAN was involved in a series of activities related to a national campaign on safe motherhood. Through the association, nurses have developed good relationships with many international nongovernmental organizations, including Save the Children Fund and UNICEF. Several times each year, NAN hosts workshops on topics of common interest to which these organizations are invited. Through these collaborations the nursing profession extends its reach to

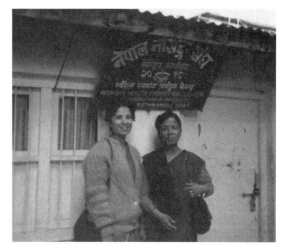

FIG. 8–2. Two nurses at the Women's Health Promotion Center in Kathmandu, Nepal. *(Photo: Nora Whyte.)*

vulnerable groups, such as rural populations, urban women, and refugees.

A second type of influence comes from role modeling different approaches to health service delivery for specific underserved populations. A visible example was NAN's three-year operation of a health center known as the "Women's Health Promotion Center" on the grounds of its Kathmandu headquarters (Fig. 8–2). Funds donated by the Norwegian Nursing Association provided staffing and supplies for a drop-in health promotion and disease prevention service to low-income women and their children. The center was a converted house, which provided a comfortable atmosphere for counseling and health education activities. Services included family planning, treatment of common health problems, promotion of breast-feeding, teaching self-care, and immunization. These women and their families, many of whom were migrants from rural areas, had previously had no access to preventive and promotive health care. Nurses living in Kathmandu assisted at the center on a voluntary basis. NAN members attending committee meetings at the office would help out when the center was busy and the presence of families coming and going during the day added liveliness to the NAN headquarters. During the period of its operation, this center provided a valuable community-based health service and was a clear indication that NAN was not solely concerned with nurses' self-interest.

Looking back on her time working at the health center, one Nepali nurse recalled how an encounter with a young woman had influenced her career. A mother of three young children arrived at the center from a rural village; the nurse was concerned about her presenting symptoms and quickly arranged for a hospital admission where a diagnosis of advanced cervical cancer was made. The nurse spent time with the woman during the last month of her life and made arrangements for family members to assume care of the children. This sad situation prompted the nurse to do something about cancer screening for women; she went to Australia for a graduate program through which she gained experience in cancer prevention and screening. She collected ideas from similar programs in other countries and eventually returned to Nepal to initiate an outreach program through the national cancer hospital.

Another example of leadership comes from the activities of the branches of NAN in the rural areas of Nepal. Using a similar approach to that of the Women's Health Promotion Center, some rural branches have developed local service projects. In the district of Pokhara, for example, a NAN member donated land for the branch to establish a primary health care clinic that would focus on maternal-child health services for local families. The nurses were already doing voluntary educational events for women and had determined that having an easily accessible health center would be of great benefit to the community. By 1996, fund raising for the center was underway. In another district about two hours' drive from Kathmandu, a small group of nurses and physicians from the national university provided Saturday clinics in a small village as part of their community service (Fig. 8–3). Their ongoing visits to the village also gave moral support to the local community development workers and created a profile for health activities. The local member of parliament had become a champion for health programs and was instrumental in establishing a community health center, which was the focal point for health education, literacy and skill development, and treatment.

NAN is an organization still going through its initial stages of capacity building for nursing. Formal, long-term evaluation would be necessary to monitor changes using health outcome indicators. However, the previous examples offer a glimpse of the role of a professional association as a catalyst for change. NAN's modeling of primary health care work, as seen in its outreach to vulnerable populations and collaboration with the voluntary sector, may set the stage for improvements in

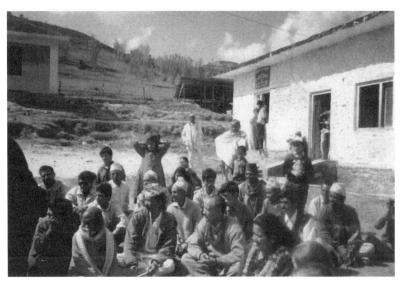

FIG. 8–3. Health education session conducted by volunteer nurses in rural Nepal. *(Photo: Nora Whyte.)*

the national health system. The role played by NAN leaders in these model projects may inspire other nurses to consider working in primary health care.

Quality of health care remains a concern in Nepal. Hospitals and health centers do not have resources for continuing education. NAN has been a major source of continuing education for nurses, in areas including management skills, family planning, communications, and HIV/AIDS prevention. NAN's leadership in continuing education is being recognized, particularly after it initiated the country's first-ever survey of nurses' continuing education needs (conducted as part of a Canadian Nurses Association project in 1995). An intensive series of continuing education events, using a **train-the-trainer** approach was carried out with funding from the Canadian Nurses Association.

There are numerous efforts being made to improve Nepal's health care infrastructure. Concentrating on strengthening the nursing profession has been strategic in the case of NAN. Over a period of about 10 years, outside support from other nursing organizations helped to create a critical mass of articulate nurses who would have otherwise not come together with a common focus on improving their health system. Through its years of partnership with the Canadian Nurses Association, for example, NAN learned to establish mechanisms for member participation, manage its organization, promote regulation of nursing practice, gain ideas for fund raising and sustainability, and develop its capacity to influence health policy. As a result, the combined knowledge and skills of 1,800 nurses has created a powerful resource for the health system and, ultimately, the population's health.

South Africa: Nursing in a New Society

South Africa is considered to be one of the pioneers of primary health care, having introduced community-oriented primary care through model health centers in the 1940s (Starfield, 1998). Fifty years later, the government is placing renewed emphasis on primary health care as part of its strategy for health reform (Department of Health, South Africa, 1997). Nurses are involved in what has become known as the "progressive primary health care movement" and are contributing to change as health care is becoming more accessible to the whole population. A South African-Canadian partnership project that is indicative of these changes is a nursing initiative to promote primary health care in rural areas by training nurses and by involving lay women, traditional birth attendants, and traditional healers in a participatory educational process.

An educational program has been developed to train rural women to be involved in their own and their children's health, and to improve their access to health and social services in their communities. This initiative is underway in the province of KwaZulu-Natal with the long-term goal of reaching remote and rural populations throughout the country. The project partners—University of Natal, the Nursing Section of the KwaZulu-Natal Primary Health Care Service (provincial health department), and Canada's McMaster University—are committed to evaluating the outcomes of the project.

That South Africa's nurses are in a position to contribute to national health reform through their professional organization is a remarkable feat, considering the divisions of past decades when membership in nursing associations mirrored the government's policy of apartheid (Marks, 1994). One of the significant developments since the change of government in 1994 is the unification of the 14 disparate nursing organizations throughout South Africa. Fragmented by their historical divisions, nursing leaders worked on bringing their respective groups together through a negotiation process. By 1996, following several years of serious negotiation and planning, South African nurses disbanded all their existing associations and formed a racially integrated professional association and union, the Democratic Nurses Organization of South Africa (DENOSA). As Thembeka Gwagwa, DENOSA's first executive director, stated, "We were all driven apart during the apartheid years. Now we share a common vision of the profession" (CNA, 1998).

The nursing profession received attention from other professions and the South African government for its leadership in being the first profession to unify (Fig. 8–4). DENOSA was also recognized by the international nursing community in 1997, through its admission to both the Commonwealth Nursing Federation and the International Council of Nurses. Recently, three South African nurses participated in ICN's *Leadership for Change Project,* designed to help nursing leaders prepare for new roles in a period of rapid change in health systems and nursing (Shaw, 1999). The South Africans attended workshops in Zambia with their counterparts from other countries in Eastern and Southern Africa to share experiences and develop new leadership skills. Networking and mentoring were identified as critical supports for emerging leaders in order for them to contribute more fully to policy development in their countries and to help other nurses assume decision-making roles. Increasingly, South African nurses are forming new international connections through their participation in organizations, projects, and conferences. Based on her experience at home and abroad, Thembeka Gwagwa (personal communication, January 25, 2000) noted that contributing to policy formation is one of the greatest challenges facing nurses of this world. As a unified body of nurses with a wealth of political expertise, DENOSA is well positioned to influence national health policy and to share its knowledge with the international nursing community.

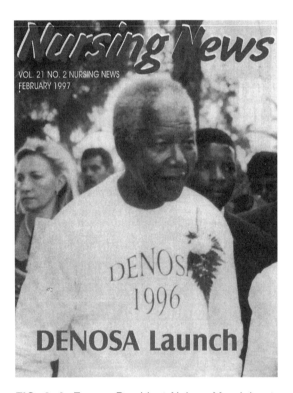

FIG. 8–4. Former President Nelson Mandela attends the opening ceremonies to launch DENOSA in Pretoria, December 1996. *(Photo: Daleen van Manen,* courtesy of DENOSA.*)*

✳ Reflective Questions

Before moving on to the chapter's final section, readers may want to take time to reflect on these exemplars and the following questions.

1. What strategies were used to involve "grassroots" nurses?
2. Identify some of the gender, cultural, economic, and political factors that influenced these situations. What factors would affect similar projects in your country?
3. What were the strengths of the projects undertaken by these nursing associations?
4. What limitations were evident in these situations?
5. How well did these nursing organizations balance self-interest with the public good?
6. Consider the activities of nursing organizations (unions and professional associations) in your own country, state, or province. What are they doing to influence changes in health care in your context? Do they have position statements on health promotion and primary health care?
7. How might you apply the lessons learned from any of these countries to bring about a change in your practice area or community?

Leadership in Reorienting Health Care

Increasingly, nurses are learning to influence health care policy toward the ideals expressed in the primary health care and health promotion literature. As highlighted in these exemplars, leadership by national nursing organizations can make a difference in building the profession's credibility and capacity to influence policy. Nursing groups in all three countries have benefited from international partnerships with counterpart organizations; in turn, they contributed to advancing nursing and health care reform beyond their borders. Long-term partnerships between nursing organizations, characterized by mutual exchange and learning, are becoming more common today. Such partnerships begin by developing joint objectives for a project and are sustained through collaboration in implementing and evaluating the project. Being part of an international project helps to raise the profile of nursing in a country such as Nepal and increases the profession's influence.

As described in this chapter, nurses were successful in initiating major changes in their health systems when they adopted multiple strategies to achieve their goals. Nursing associations do have a role to play in educating members about the broad issues of health reform and in reorienting their national health systems to encompass health promotion perspectives and strategies. Morgan and Marsh (1998) note that nurses can "demonstrate leadership in health promotion by moving beyond the individual perspective that has dominated health promotion nursing research and practice" (p. 382). Grounded in a solid understanding of the principles of primary health care, nurses are establishing partnerships with other sectors, mounting demonstration projects, contributing to health policy decisions, and becoming more active in local and national politics.

Steps to Success

There is no magic formula for this process nor is it possible to list "10 easy steps to success." We can, however, learn from these examples and consider how these lessons might apply to other contexts. Some basic ideas are outlined below:

- Become knowledgeable about the organization of your health care system and analyze where and how it needs to change. This is often difficult during periods of rapid change, such as following a change of government or when restructuring is occurring. Gathering as much background information as possible and keeping up with current developments are key aspects of doing one's "homework."
- Focus on a specific aspect of health care where a service gap exists and where your efforts will have a reasonable chance of success. The Japanese nurses recognized serious gaps in community-based services for elders and made this their cause during the first phase of their project.
- Use a wide range of strategies for carrying out a policy project including: developing position statements, forming coalitions with other organizations, establishing a demonstration site to test and model the desired change, disseminating information during the project (e.g., through newsletters, meetings, and a project Website), and documenting and transmitting your successes.
- Involve nurses from different practice settings and with various backgrounds useful to your project. The work of the Nursing Association of Nepal has been advanced by having educators and practitioners working together on its various project committees.
- Take risks when you see an opportunity and find ways to overcome barriers. Nursing leaders in South Africa have honed their political action skills through some difficult times and are now able to share those skills with others.

As illustrated by these examples from other countries and by accounts in the international nursing literature, nurses are taking on leadership roles in their workplaces, communities, states, and nations. These activities range from serving on local committees to becoming active in a nursing organization to running for public office. Indeed, developing political skills through one's nursing association has helped launch the political careers of international nursing leaders including Syringa Marshall-Burnett, President of the Jamaican Senate, and Mo-Im Kim, South Korea's Minister of Health (Hewitt, 1998; Kim, 1998). Inspirational leaders and stories exist in every country; this chapter has highlighted a few of these stories to illustrate that nurses can and do influence changes in health care policy through their knowledge, leadership, and perseverance.

Acknowledgments

The author acknowledges, with gratitude, the cooperation of the nursing organizations featured in this chapter: the Japanese Nursing Association, the Nursing Association of Nepal, and the Democratic Nurses Organization of South Africa. The inspirational nurses involved in launching and carrying out these projects are to be commended for their dedication and vision. The Canadian Nurses Association also deserves acknowledgment for its commitment to international partnership projects with national nursing associations. For their kind assistance in providing current information about national and local activities, special thanks are extended to Thembeka Gwagwa, Jabu Makhanya, Akio Kitayama, Junko Takano, Basanti Majumdar, Bishnu Rai, and June Webber. For their ongoing support and insights into international health and nursing, the author thanks her colleagues in the Vancouver International Nurses Network.

REFERENCES

Baumgart, A. J. (1993). Quality through health policy: The Canadian example. *International Nursing Review, 40,* 167–170.

Canadian Nurses Association. (1995). *Policy statement on the role of the nurse in primary health care.* Ottawa: Author.

Canadian Nurses Association. (1998). *The Canadian Nurses Association overseas development programme annual report to the Canadian International Development Agency (April 1997–March 1998).* Ottawa: Author.

Canadian Public Health Association. (1996). *Action statement for health promotion in Canada.* Ottawa: Author.

Clark, J. (1997). The unique function of the nurse. *International Nursing Review, 44,* 144–152.

Department of Health, South Africa. (1997). *White paper for the transformation of the health system of South Africa.* Pretoria: Author.

Epp, J. (1986). *Achieving health for all: A framework for health promotion.* Ottawa: Health and Welfare Canada.

Hewitt, H. H. (1998). Imaging the worlds we wish for. *Reflections, 24,* 8–13.

International Council of Nurses. (1988). *Nursing and primary health care: A unified force.* Geneva: Author.

Iwanaga, T. (1996). *Manual for health promotion through creating a healthy community.* Tokyo: Igaku-Shoin.

Japanese Nursing Association. (1994). *A project for the further development of community health nursing services.* Tokyo: Author.

Japanese Nursing Association. (1996). *Guidebook for a community meeting.* Tokyo: Author.

Japanese Nursing Association. (1998). Nursing colleges set to reach 65. *JNA News, 25.*

Japanese Nursing Association. (1999). *New community health nursing activities toward the 21st century: Results and recommendations of the 5-year project.* Tokyo: Author.

Kim, M-I. (1998). Breaking tradition: A personal reflection by Mo-Im Kim. *Reflections, 24,* 14–17.

Marks, S. (1994). *Divided sisterhood: Race, class and gender in the South African nursing profession.* Johannesburg: Witwatersrand University Press.

Mitoh, T. (1997). Preparing Japanese nurses for the 21st century. *International Nursing Review, 44,* 62.

Morgan, I. S., & Marsh, G. W. (1998). Historic and future health promotion contexts for nursing. *Image: Journal of Nursing Scholarship, 30,* 379–383.

Murashima, S., Hatono, Y., Whyte, N., & Asahara, K. (1999). Public health nursing in Japan: New opportunities for health promotion. *Public Health Nursing, 16,* 133–139.

Oulton, J. A. (1996). Change brings opportunities. *International Nursing Review, 43,* 96.

Registered Nurses Association of British Columbia. (1996). *The Comox Valley nursing center: A report on a demonstration project initiated by the Registered Nurses Association of British Columbia.* Vancouver: Author.

Shaw, S. (1999). Preparing nurse leaders for the new millennium: The ICN Leadership for Change project. *International Nursing Review, 46,* 140–145.

Smith, G. R. (1997). Creating community power in health care. *International Nursing Review, 44,* 105–109.

Splane, R. B., & Splane, V. H. (1994). *Chief nursing officer positions in national ministries of health: Focal points for nursing leadership.* San Francisco: University of California Press.

Starfield, B. (1998). *Primary care: Balancing health needs, services, and technology.* Oxford: Oxford University Press.

Tierney, M. J., & Tierney, L. M. (1994). Nursing in Japan. *Nursing Outlook, 42,* 210–213.

Wilkinson, R. G. (1996). *Unhealthy societies: The afflictions of inequality.* London: Routledge.

World Health Organization. (1978). *Alma Ata 1978. Primary health care: Report of the International Conference on Primary Health Care.* Geneva: Author.

World Health Organization. (1996). *The world health report 1996: fighting disease, fostering development.* Geneva: Author.

World Health Organization. (1997). *Health for all in the 21st century.* Geneva: Author.

World Health Organization, Health and Welfare Canada, and Canadian Public Health Association. (1986). *Ottawa Charter for health promotion.* Ottawa: Author.

Challenges and Controversies

Revisiting and Re-Creating Knowledge for Transformative Health Promotion Practice

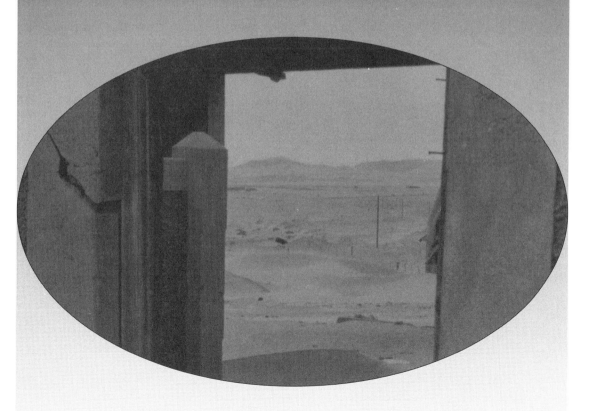

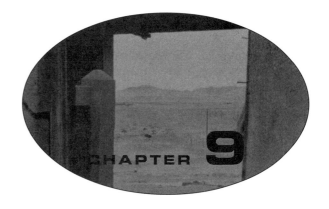

CHAPTER 9

Self-Care: Re-examining the Myth*

DEBORAH THOUN NORTHRUP

A short time ago, I attended a physician-sponsored forum designed to hear concerns from an invited and select public represented by community health care leaders. The forum also was designed to address the precarious status of Canada's Health Care System in general and the autonomy and well-being of medicine in particular. Although varied, comments reflected a consistent theme of individual responsibility as integral to "fixing" health care. Whether people were supposed to lobby government and/or march on Parliament Hill, advocate for oneself or loved ones, or investigate alternate therapists/healers and associated remedies, assuming more responsibility for health care presented itself as the prescription for a failing system.

A particularly noteworthy comment by an influential member of the community that captured the essence of the discussion was that "people needed to be taught to be more fully engaged in **self-care** if Canada's Health Care System was to survive." Although I found this declaration to be somewhat alarming, I was struck by the contradiction between an industry demanding that people take care of themselves to ease strain on the system and the simultaneous adoption by the same industry of expert language, theories, and practices intended to advance an endless pursuit of professionally guided or managed self-care.

Clearly, such modification of doctrine marks a shift of emphasis related to interventions, that is, bio-medical duties versus educational-moral du-

ties, but fails to embrace a radical transformation of attitude or orientation to health care that sets a new direction or invigorates its sustainability. Certainly, the persistent commitment to some version of interventions influenced by an agenda of corporate *objectives* or *ends* must be at odds with notions of progress. Indeed, this sacrosanct measure calls for individuals and families to accommodate themselves to the demands and claims of the health care marketplace and enables government and health care providers alike to shirk responsibility for the fundamental reconstitution of a health care system. Indeed, within Canada, self-care is considered to be "one of the pillars of health promotion and health care reform" (Health Canada, 1999, p. 1).

As the call for endorsement and promotion of self-care as a "pillar of health care reform" amasses strength and support, nurses must be prepared to explore and critically examine such practice and draw attention to its problematic features. It is my hope that the reflections presented here will prepare the ground for you to address the contradictions, implications, and consequences of supporting self-care and to take stock of its central assumptions.

Within nursing, there is widespread interest in and encouragement for the practice of self-care (Chin, 1985; Gaffney & Moore, 1996; Geden & Taylor, 1999; Orem, 1985, 1995; Orem & Vardiman, 1995; Smith, 1989; Taylor, 1988, 1989, 1991). The taken-for-granted assumption guiding this present practice is that self-care exemplifies a shift from an authoritative medical model orientation to a therapeutic mode of social control located within the individual (Lasch, 1984). Identifying or

*An earlier version of this paper was published in *Advances in Nursing Science* 15(3), 59–66 as Self-care myth reconsidered.

naming the assumptions that make individual control possible, however, must derive from a program of exploration and research, as well as an examination of current values.

Such exploration initiates a process of self-reflection within nursing that is consistent with the assertion that we are a distinct field of study. Thus far, self-care philosophy and theory in nursing have been little challenged. The particularly strong emphasis on the ethic of self-care that pervades society and consequently influences knowledge development in nursing and the practice that ensues serves to support a competitive **individualism** and reinforce entrepreneurial thinking in health care. It follows that an understanding of the self-care ideology currently being articulated and developed within the discipline of nursing and its effect on achieving the overall goals of health policy warrant attention. I believe that recognition of the sociohistoric limitations undergirding contemporary self-care theory demystifies it and renders unconditional acceptance less attractive.

To acquaint readers with the many dimensions and features of self-care, this chapter begins with a brief overview of the historic roots of self-care as well as selected self-care perspectives. Attention is then paid to contemporary interest in and issues related to self-care. Next, the implications of self-care on future health and sick care delivery are explored. Finally, as I am particularly concerned with the influence of self-care ideology on practice, I conclude by posing questions that are intended to help us examine the limitations and possibilities that exist within our current notions of self-care practice.

Historic Roots

Historically, the widespread practice of non-professional health care can be traced to ancient Greece (Sehnert, 1978). Ordinary citizens, having limited access to highly paid physicians, maintained their health through various forms of self-care and reliance on friends, family, neighbors, and lay healers found in the market square. Although the early Greek culture valued health, it provided one of the earliest examples of a society in which health maintenance was associated with affluence (Williamson & Danaher, 1978). Even though accounts of lay health practices have changed somewhat over time, they remain reasonably consistent in various cultures prior to the 19th century.

In discussion of self-care history in America spanning the years 1880 to 1950, Cassedy (1977) observes:

Whenever people have been able to obtain their own medicines, or have read books about hygiene, or have had relatives, neighbors or travellers to suggest remedies, they have been ready in large numbers to rely on such sources and on their own judgements rather than resort to physicians even with serious ailments. (p. 96)

According to Norris (1979), the relinquishing of self-care by society to health care professionals began with the advent of early diagnosis, elective surgery, scientific pharmacology, and complex technology. Sehnert (1978) adds that higher incomes, health insurance coverage, and a wide variety of medico-technical advances brought about after World War II led to further reliance on professionals to solve health problems. Consequently, medicine emerged as a strong and compelling institution for health care in industrialized society that was nourished by a proliferation of expert knowledge and activities. Reflecting on the growing impact of medical practices, science, and technology, Illich (1976) argues that the institution of medicine fosters dependency, limits individuals' capacities for self-care, and undermines peoples' perceptions of their own competence in wellness and illness.

Ironically, the shift taking place in the causes of disease and the treatment of disabilities began fuelling a growing disaffection toward medicine. The counterculture and human potential movements of the 1960s "expressed rebellion against many traditional forms of authority in North American society" (Sirott & Waitzkin, 1984, p. 252). One manifestation of this rebellion was the development of self-care as an alternative form of living and healing. In particular, the women's health movement and the self-help movement begun by Downer in 1971 emerged out of dissatisfaction with health care services for women (Rodriguez-Trias, 1984). Disillusionment with the claims of modern medicine continues to surface through the growth of litigation related to negligence, through the burgeoning industry of alternate therapies and patient advocacy groups, and through the inability of biomedical research to address and arrest the incidence and prevalence of viruses such as HIV and Ebola and bacteria such as necrotizing fasciitis (Williams, Gabe, & Kelleher, 1994). Although a historical account of self-care indicates that self-care ideology has deep roots in the populace and in the values of self-control and self-determination (Levin, 1976), it is suggested here that the appeal and endorsement of contemporary self-care practice are misguided and erroneously conferred by professionals and laypersons alike.

Self-Care Perspectives

A review of the literature reveals that the meaning of self-care differs both between and among laypersons and professionals. Levin, Katz, and Holst (1979) suggest that this diversity of self-care conceptualizations is a function of the definer's discipline, special interests, professional goals, and political orientation. In concert with this diversity, Williamson (1977) contends that the economic and political implications of self-care make the proposition of simple definition impossible and single definition nonsensical. Problems arising from such confusion are complicated further by lay and professional cultures that generally are ignorant of the myriad ways in which other groups define self-care (Stern & Harris, 1986). Hence, recognition and understanding of differing self-care perspectives are essential.

A general theme found in the medical, sociological, and nursing literature is that self-care is giving care to oneself that *ideally* should be given by health care professionals. Within medicine, Fry (1980) identifies self-care as one of four levels of care found *within* all health systems and outlines four roles that are central to self-care: health maintenance; disease prevention; self-diagnosis, self-medication, and self-treatment; and, patient participation in health care services. Levin (1978), considered by many to be the "father" of self-care, defines self-care as "a process whereby a layperson can function on his/her own behalf in health promotion and prevention and in disease detection and treatment" (p. 11).

More recently, Health Canada (1999) defines self-care as "the decisions and actions taken by someone who is facing a health problem in order to cope with it and improve his or her health" (p. 1). The emphasis on the actions of the individual found here requires that the individual participate in a range of practices that demonstrate a breadth of knowledge and skill and employ technologies central to notions of health, and informed and responsible citizenry (Peterson & Lupton, 1996). Clearly, the self-care actions derived from this particular medicalization of the concept of self-care are related to the roles of people within, not outside of, the health care system. The practical intent of self-care is thus achieved only when medical control and supervision are operative.

From a social science perspective, Williamson and Danaher (1978) claim that self-care, while taking place outside the framework of health care, remains influenced by existing social institutions of care and the context of economic, social, and political structures. Closely aligned with this perspective, Butler, Gertman, Oberlander, and Schindler (1979–1980) propose that self-care "encompasses formal consumer health education programs and patient education efforts designed to teach self-care knowledge and skills" (p. 96). Accordingly, education is considered pivotal to self-care. In addition, these authors introduce the notion of the self-care consumer that is variously defined as the ultimate user of a commodity (Webster's Handy College Dictionary, 1981) or the purchaser of goods and services (Sikes, 1982). Thus, we can infer that the consumer of self-care purchases health care in the guise of taking care of oneself. As for the services available for purchase, it should not be surprising that such services tend to align with dominant economic models and thus support the status quo rather than offering a truly innovative approach (Cant & Sharma, 1998). As such, society re-creates itself through the normal functioning of social relations found within the health care delivery system (Fay, 1987). Given the maintenance of this order, self-care conceptualizations found within the medical and social sciences suppose a degree of built-in deformity that acts to endorse and reproduce dominant health care knowledge and practice. In other words, relations of power and knowledge, often hidden in apparently "emancipatory" strategies, are instilled and nourished. An example of such nourishment is present in the strong positive association between self-care and such terms as empowerment, individual control, self-determination, and liberation.

Can nursing, committed to and enamoured by the contemporary popularity of self-care, claim to be different? An illumination of the social conditions that play a role in creating and sustaining self-care doctrine within nursing is offered as one means of uncovering and addressing the ontology that self-care presupposes. This form of critique, derived from Marx, aims to demonstrate the ways in which the self-understandings of a group of people may be distorted by social conditions (Easton & Guddat, 1967). In this vein Marx states:

We do not anticipate the world dogmatically, but rather wish to find the new world through criticism of the old; . . . even though the construction of the future and its completion for all times is not our task, what we have to accomplish at this time is all the more clear: relentless criticism of all existing conditions, relentless in the sense that the criticism is not afraid of its findings and just as little afraid of conflict with the powers that be. (p. 112)

Contemporary Issues

Over the past two decades, the nursing profession has witnessed a growing public interest in and popularity of self-care. Katz and Levin (1980) account for this social phenomenon by suggesting that self-care represents a spontaneous reaction to dissatisfaction with the present health care system. Underlying the phenomenon, however, is a plurality of motives (social, cultural, and behavioral) and ideologies (individualism, humanitarianism, **liberalism**). The most pervasive ideological component of the self-care movement found within these motives is that of individual responsibility for, and control over, the conditions that affect one's life (Crawford, 1980). As such, the contemporary self-care movement contains ideological remnants of "the more narcissistic orientation of the past two decades" (Sirott & Waitzkin, 1984, p. 254) with its emphasis on self rather than societal interests. Consistent with this narcissistic preoccupation with the self, Katz and Levin (1980) contend that the self-care movement "represents a way of overcoming anomie, and of establishing independence and identity even in a mass society" (p. 331). The clinical

thrust of the self-care movement from this perspective is against the dehumanization and medicalization of everyday life, as well as the limits of medicine (Crawford, 1980; Green, Werlin, Schauffler, & Avery, 1977; Illich, 1976; Levin, 1976, 1978; Williamson, 1977).

Laid out in this way, self-care is proffered as a solution to the problems of alienation, dependence, and identity confusion, such as "eye drops are sold to solve the problems of air pollution" (Manders, 1978, p. 61). The suggestion here is that the contemporary self-care movement within North America occurs within a context of individualism in urban industrial capitalism implying ideals such as equality, tolerance, and concern for individuals as well as the environment. This position, although plausible, seems to deny the existence of power relations within Western thinking and fails to explain the social trends that have created the present popularity of self-care. Consequently, the connections between social and economic changes and changes in cultural and personal life are not addressed.

From a critical social perspective, Lasch (1984) argues that the contemporary health care system is part of a larger pattern of dependence, disorientation, and loss of control. He claims that narcissism is a reflection of a growing deterioration of social relationships under advanced capitalism, identifying capitalism as a system of mass production sustained by a culture of mass consumption (i.e., two sides of the same process). As a culture of consumption, capitalism has had to discourage people from providing for their own wants. Moreover, consumerism and the promotion of commodities are dependent on individuals who no longer rely on their own resources or trust their own judgements (Lasch, 1984). Consequently, products are produced in ways that signal to consumers that they cannot provide for their own needs and therefore must consume what others—that is, experts—produce for them.

Lasch (1984) refers to the propaganda surrounding self-care as seductive advertising of wish fulfillment, specifically the wish for self-control and individual problem solving. In addition, such advertising seeks to create the illusion of variety and to present self-care as a personal achievement and intellectual discovery. Several authors suggest that the consumption of this self-care fantasy brings a sense of "belonging" and "a way of being" in the world (Crawford, 1980; Lasch, 1984; Manders, 1978). If critical theorists are correct, it can be assumed that proponents of self-care have a tendency to confuse self-determinism with the exercise of consumer choices.

The health care delivery system has had great success in getting people to buy the massive output of commodities it produces. This has resulted in spiralling health care costs, maldistribution of personnel, physician overload, and discontent of society with health care services (Illich, 1976; Levin, Katz, & Holst, 1979; Sehnert, 1978; Williamson, 1977). Thus, it comes as no surprise that self-care is regarded increasingly as an integral part of the health care sector and a solution to the problems and challenges of dwindling health care resources. Given this situation, the present concern of capitalism has turned to the stimulation of self-care consumption often evident in advertising aimed at persuading people to invest more and more of themselves in the pursuit of controlling, monitoring, and improving their health. Using critical social spectacles then, the self-care alternative has the capacity to contain and dissipate widespread feelings of powerlessness and victimization while acting as a mechanism of social control aimed at preserving a social order.

The proliferation of health education professionals provides the most obvious example of interference in individuals' attempts to gain control over their lives. Self-care practices, formerly assigned to private life, are allegedly too obtuse and technical for popular understanding. Hence, self-care activities are assimilated into the demands of the marketplace and subsequently found under the control of experts (Illich, 1977) who operate within systems of expert knowledge. Levin (1978) ties the growth of a whole education industry to marketplace demands and provides a reflective description of a health care system concerned with the rational reconstruction of society and the maintenance of power relationships. He writes:

Patient education is becoming an attractive interest in terms of its income-producing potential and, even more significant, its potential for bending patient behavior to accommodate the needs of the system. . . . as long as patient education does not interfere with the control inherent in the caregiver's role it is a safe and appealing undertaking. (p. 170)

In addition to the notions of expert control and domination, Rockhill (1985), a sociologist/anthropologist, claims that the institutionalization and professionalization of health education acts to sever working-class education from social movements. Indeed, there is a glaring absence of the empowerment programs that fuelled the reform movements of the 1960s (Boshier, 1986). Consequently, the self-care movement, transformed into the self-care commodity, has lost its potential as a strategy for fundamental structural transformation.

The advent and proliferation of contemporary self-care doctrine within the nursing literature occurred during the sociopolitical context of the 1970s described earlier. Fuelled by the political, ecological, and feminist movements of this period, nursing, like other professions, experienced an expansion of personal as well as social consciousness. Accordingly, this period surfaced radical questioning of authority, particularly patriarchal authority, and concern about the autonomy of the discipline that engendered a rapid drive within nursing "to escape intellectual bondage from medicine" (Moody, 1990, p. 60). Hence, knowledge of self-care developed as a basis for more human forms of action and as one means of disciplining the profession. Not surprisingly, there has been wide agreement that the impact of the era was seen in the movement toward professionalism in which nursing was engaged (Chinn & Jacobs, 1987; Fawcett, 1989; Moody, 1990). Even though it can be said that the establishment of nursing as a science distinct from medicine was enhanced by the development of self-care deficit theory (Orem, 1971), the idea that self-care theories are closely articulated or deeply connected with the social context of the 1970s is indisputable.

The abundant use of self-care rhetoric and the liberal adoption of self-care practices in health care delivery strongly suggest that self-care has assumed the status of "goods and resources" within the commodity economy of health care. When seen as an object of exchange with associated value, integration of self-care orientations in health care policy and adoption of self-care practices by health care professionals is more easily understood. Self-care theory, an invention of professionals and not clients (Harris & Stern, 1986), illustrates a seemingly successful attempt at producing another form of expert ready to monopolize the competencies of the lay public (Lasch, 1984).

As such, expert professionals, wittingly or unwittingly, find themselves offering self-care as one more commodity in a market of competing products. Hence, the aforementioned taken-for-granted assumptions of self-care may be false, incoherent, or both. Further, the decline of authority suggested by a shift from an authoritative (medical model) to a therapeutic mode of social control appears illusory. Consistent with this position, Lasch (1984) notes that "the decline of authority is a good example of the kind of change that promotes the appearance of democracy without its substance" (p. 46). Given this line of thinking, one can conclude that the adoption of self-care doctrine within health care can manifest as a particular kind of doing on the part of the professional that masquerades as self-control on the part of the client. Further, Fay (1987) points out that this particular form of practice represents an adherence to unfreedom that sustains dependent relationships and ensures that the correct ideologic line is followed.

In an article exploring seven conceptualizations of health, Meleis (1990) identifies self-care (among other concepts) as the language of the preventive/promotional or anticipatory view of health currently guiding nursing practice. In addition to practice, education, research, and health policy are marked by those who speak the self-care language. Thompson (1987) points out, however, that language is a vehicle for social control and domination. As such, it is incumbent on the social institution of nursing to challenge the undisputed creation of and focus on self-care as a means of structuring nursing knowledge. Our concern during this time of growth as a scientific discipline must involve a critique of the conditions that make our choice of self-care language and self-care actions possible. If we are to stretch beyond our present practice toward new thinking and new boundaries, continuing critical analysis of the hidden, as well as the transparent, is necessary (Fay, 1987).

Future Implications

The issues raised in this chapter portray self-care as a maintenance-oriented solution to the contemporary social and economic woes of society in general and the health care delivery system in particular. This position is presented to provoke thought about the widely held self-understandings related to self-care. The challenge facing all of us is to learn the appropriate additional steps to take in light of this information.

Today, conceptions of health found within nursing literature reflect various worldviews rooted in different assumptions about the human-universe relationship. On one hand, health is viewed as a nonreducible open process of living that can only be defined or described by the person living the life (Newman, 1994; Parse, 1992; Patterson & Zderad, 1988; Rogers, 1970). In contrast, health is variously defined within a summative view of bio-psycho-social-spiritual well-being as determined by societal norms. Currently, the vanguard of health promotion practice is based on this latter view where health is seen to be determined by social, political, and economical structures, frequently referred to as the social determinants of health (Labonte, 1993). Accordingly, nursing practice is increasingly framed within a social model of health that serves to facilitate and nurture human fragmentation and the notion of persons as organized systems and to protect impersonal systems of professional expertise upon which we rely.

A breadth of contemporary theories and models consistent with a self-care orientation are found within the health care literature. Some examples include but are not limited to social learning theory (Bandura, 1977, 1986), coping and social support theories (Bloom, 1990; Stewart, 1993), change theory (Prochaska & DiClemente, 1982, 1985), self-care-deficit theory (Orem,1995), and health promotion and empowerment frameworks (Labonte, 1993). These examples, although not exhaustive, invariably advance a reductionist view of human beings and health. Practice methodologies consistent with this view guide professionals to assess client readiness for change as well as their self-care progress or lack of, to provide and/or direct persons to self-care programs and tools designed to effect change, to support strategies for self-care, to monitor individual commitment to self-care practices, and to measure behavior change and health status.

In addition to the reductionistic quality of these knowledges, the little challenged discourses of self-control, self-awareness, self-monitoring, self-help, self-efficacy, and so on, firmly establish individual responsibility for personal care in particular and the health care system in general. However, neither individuals nor society alone is responsible for the problems confronting health care today. Indeed, this position found within self-care theories, research, and practice only serves further to advance person-environment fragmentation, to perpetuate the separation of the personal from the political, and to transform care of self and others into an individual burden. As Sirott and Waitzkin (1984) and Berliner and Salmon (1980) point out, self-care as currently articulated ignores politics and fails to address the social structural conditions that cause illness and suffering. Such disconnection serves to reinforce the professionalization of self-care and is more likely to set limits on public thinking about how self-care can be used as a vehicle for social transformation and a process of empowerment.

While contemporary self-care doctrine downplays social problems and social solutions, Sirott and Waitzkin (1984) assert that self-care "can encourage greater social responsibility for health and illness when it is linked to wider organizing" (p. 260). Further, they contend that self-care "must aim at the social reconstruction that is a precondition of individuals' caring for themselves" (p. 264). In fact, Reissman (cited in Crawford, 1980) considers self-care to be a symbol of empowerment and possibly one of the few ways that people conceive of themselves as political beings.

The adoption of self-care practices and self-care education within the organization of a country's health care system can be used as one instrument for achieving the overall goals of health policy. Historically however, the empowering process that engages people in critical analysis of root causes as the basis of social action differs from the emphasis on achievement of attainable goals (Wallerstein & Bernstein, 1988). Consequently, self-care and its relation to human life may take many forms. From a critical social perspective, the self-care doctrine currently being articulated in health care must be called into question. The information and analysis presented in this article are intended to shed some light on the social and political constraints that must be brought to bear in this process. Ongoing illumination of the social construction of practice and practice models is needed (Fay, 1987; Thompson, 1987). Thompson (1987) reminds us that such critical scholarship "returns to nursing its voice and its role in the construction of a more fully human world" (p. 37).

✳ Reflective Questions

1. What is the responsibility of the professional in self-care practice?
2. What happens when health education does not produce the desired results, that is, how the professional wants the person to live?
3. How does poverty influence self-care?
4. Who identifies self-care as the goal of practice?
5. When does professional care replace self-care?
6. How do or can professionals implement self-care? Or, what's wrong with this question?
7. How does our social context (Canadian, Provincial) shape the delivery of and responses to self-care?

REFERENCES

Bandura, A. (1977). *Social learning theory*. Englewood Cliffs, NJ: Prentice Hall.

Bandura, A. (1986). *Social foundations of thought and action*. Englewood Cliffs, NJ: Prentice Hall.

Berliner, H., & Salmon, J. (1980). The holistic alternative to scientific medicine: History and analysis. *International Journal of Health Service, 10*(1), 133–147.

Bloom, J. R. (1990). The relationship of social support and health. *Social Service and Medicine 39*, 635–37.

Boshier, R. (1986). Proaction for change: Some guidelines for the future. *International Journal of Lifelong Education, 5*, 15–31.

Butler, R., Gertman, J., Oberlander, D., & Schindler, L. (1979–1980). Self-care, self-help, and the elderly. *International Journal of Aging Human Development, 10*, 95–117.

Cant, S., & Sharma, U. (1998). Reflexivity, ethnography and the professions (complementary medicine): Watching you watch me watching you (and writing about both of us). *The Sociological Review, 46*, 244–263.

Cassedy, J. (1977). Why self-help? Americans alone with their diseases, 1880–1950. In G. Rissi, R. Numbers, & J. Leariff (Eds.), *Medicine without doctors*. New York: Science History.

Chin, S. (1985). Can self-care theories be applied to families? In J. Riehl-Sisca (Ed.), *The Science and Art of self-care*. Norwalk: Appleton-Century-Crofts.

Chinn, P., & Jacobs, M. (1987). *Theory and nursing: A systematic approach* (2nd ed.). St. Louis, MO: Mosby.

Chinn, P., & Kramer, M. (1991). *Theory and nursing: A systematic approach* (3rd ed.). St. Louis, MO: Mosby.

Crawford, R. (1980). Healthism and the medicalization of everyday life. *International Journal of Health Service, 10*, 365–388.

Easton, L. D., & Guddat, K. H. (Eds.). (1967). *Writings of the young Marx on philosophy and society.* New York: Anchor Books.

Fawcett, J. (1989). *Analysis and evaluation of conceptual models of nursing* (2nd ed.). Philadelphia: F. A. Davis.

Fay, B. (1987). *Critical social science.* Ithaca, NY: Cornell University Press.

Fry, J. (1980). *Primary care.* England: William Heinemann Medical Books.

Gaffney, K. F., & Moore, J. B. (1996). Testing Orem's theory of self-care deficit: Dependent care agent performance for children. *Nursing Science Quarterly, 9,* 160–164.

Geden, E., & Taylor, S. G. (1991). Theoretical and empirical description of adult couples' collaborative self-care systems. *Nursing Science Quarterly, 12,* 329–334.

Green, L., Werlin, S., Schauffler, H., & Avery, C. (1977). Research and demonstration issues in self-care: Measuring the decline of medicocentrism. *Health Education Monograph, 5,* 16.

Harris, C. C., & Stern, P. N. (1986). Women's health and the self-care paradox: Case study and analysis. In Stern, P. N. (Ed.), *Women, health, and culture* (pp. 151–164). Washington: Hemisphere.

Health Canada. (1999). *Supporting self-care: The contribution of nurses and physicians* [Online]. Available: http://www.hc-sc.gc/hppb.soinsdesante/pubs/autosoin/viien.htm.

Illich, I. (1976). *Medical nemesis: The expropriation of health.* New York: Pantheon Books.

Illich, I. (1977). *Disabling professions.* London, England: Marion Boyars.

Katz, A., & Levin, L. (1980). Self-care is not a solipsistic trap: A reply to critics. *International Journal of Health Service, 10,* 329–336.

Labonte, R. (1993). Health promotion and empowerment: Practice frameworks. Toronto: Centre for Health Promotion, University of Toronto and participation.

Lasch, C. (1984). *The minimal self: Psychic survival in troubled times.* New York: Harper and Row.

Levin, L. (1976). Self-care: An international perspective. *Social Policy, Sept/Oct,* 70–75.

Levin, L. (1978). Patient education and self-care: How do they differ? *Nursing Outlook, 26,* 170–175.

Levin, L., Katz, A., & Holst, E. (1979). *Self-care: Lay initiatives in health.* New York: Prodist.

Manders, D. (1978). Humanistic pacification and psychic consumption: A critique of the human potential movement. *Social Praxis, 5,* 49–85.

Meleis, A. I. (1990). Being and becoming healthy: The core of nursing knowledge. *Nursing Science Quarterly, 3,* 107–114.

Moody, L. (1990). *Advancing nursing science through research* (Vol. 1). Newbury Park, CA: Sage.

Newman, M. A. (1994). *Health as expanding consciousness* (2nd ed.). New York: National League for Nursing.

Norris, C. (1979). Self-care. *American Journal of Nursing, 79,* 486–489.

Orem, D. E. (1971). *Nursing: Concepts of practice.* New York: McGraw-Hill.

Orem, D. E. (1985). *Nursing: Concepts of practice* (3rd ed.). New York: McGraw-Hill.

Orem, D. E. (1995). *Nursing: Concepts of practice* (5th ed.). St. Louis, MO: Mosby.

Orem, D. E., & Vardiman, E. M. (1995). Orem's nursing theory and positive mental health: Practical considerations. *Nursing Science Quarterly, 8,* 165–173.

Parse, R. R. (1992). Human Becoming: Parse's theory of nursing. *Nursing Science Quarterly, 5,* 35–42.

Paterson, J. E., & Zderad, L. T. (1988). *Humanistic nursing.* New York: National League for Nursing.

Peterson, A., & Lupton, D. (1996). *The new public health: Health and self in the age of risk.* Singapore: South Wind Productions.

Prochaska, J. O., and DiClemente, C. C. (1982). Transtheoretical therapy: Toward a new integrative model of change. *Psychotherapy Theory, Research and Practice 19,* 276–287.

Prochaska, J. O., and DiClemente, C. C. (1985). Common processes of self change in smoking, weight control and psychological distress. In S. Shiffman and T. Wills (Eds.), *Coping and substances use* (pp. 345–364). Orlando: Academic Press.

Rockhill, K. (1985). The construction of professional practice in adult education. *CASAE History Bulletin, May.*

Rodriguez-Trias, H. (1984). The women's health movement: Women take power. In W. Sidel & R. Sidel (Eds.), *Reforming medicine: Lessons of the last quarter century.* New York: Pantheon Books.

Rogers, M. E. (1970). *The theoretical basis of nursing.* Philadelphia: F. A. Davis.

Sehnert, K. W. (1978). Medical self-care: An old remedy recurs. *Virginia Medicine, August,* 565–568.

Sirott, L., & Waitzkin, H. (1984). Holism and self-care: Can the individual succeed where society fails? In W. Sidel & R. Sidel (Eds.), *Reforming medicine: Lessons of the last quarter century.* New York: Pantheon Books.

Smith, M. (1989). An application of Orem's theory in nursing practice. *Nursing Science Quarterly, 2,* 159–161.

Stern, P. N., & Harris, C. C. (1986). Women's health and the self-care paradox: A model to guide self-care readiness. In Stern, P. N. (Ed.), *Women, health, and culture* (pp. 151–164). Washington: Hemisphere.

Stewart, M. J. (1993). *Integrating Social Support in Nursing.* Newbury Park, CA: Gage.

Sykes, J. B. (Ed.). (1982). *The concise Oxford dictionary* (7th ed.). New York: Oxford University Press.

Taylor, S. G. (1988). Nursing theory and nursing process: Orem's theory in practice. *Nursing Science Quarterly, 1,* 111–119.

Taylor, S. G. (1989). An interpretation of family within Orem's general theory of nursing. *Nursing Science Quarterly, 2,* 131–137.

Taylor, S. G. (1991). The structure of nursing diagnosis from Orem's theory. *Nursing Science Quarterly, 4,* 24–32.

Thompson, J. (1987). Critical scholarship: The critique of domination in nursing. *Advances in Nursing Science, 10,* 27–38.

Wallerstein, N., & Bernstein, E. (1988). Empowerment education: Freire's ideas adapted to health education. *Health Education Quarterly, 15* (3), 379–394.

Webster's handy college dictionary. (1981). New York: New American Library.

Williams, G., Gabe, J., & Kelleher, D. (1994). Epilogue: The last days of doctor power. In J. Gabe, D. Kelleher, & G. Williams (Eds.), *Challenging medicine.* London: Routledge.

Williamson, J. (1977). Healthward care. *Social Science Medicine, 11,* 187–190.

Williamson, J., & Danaher, K. (1978). *Self-care in health.* London: Croom Helm.

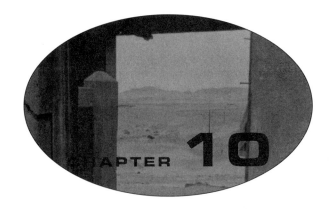

CHAPTER 10

Health Promotion, Moral Harm, and the Moral Aims of Nursing*

JOAN LIASCHENKO

Mrs. A is a 52-year-old professional woman with a master's degree in occupational therapy. She is in good health: Her weight is normal, and she eats well-balanced meals that are low in fat and high in fiber, exercises vigorously four times a week, does not use street drugs, and drinks one glass of wine daily with dinner. She sees her gynecologist yearly for a routine examination, including a PAP smear and mammography, but sees her regular physician only when there is a specific reason. Much of her professional career was spent working in acute care facilities where she saw a variety of patients, including women who were post-mastectomy; thus, she is familiar with breast cancer. Her sister was diagnosed with breast cancer at 43 years of age and was treated by a lumpectomy, radiation therapy, and two courses of chemotherapy. It has been six years since her sister's diagnosis and, other than moderately severe lymphedema, her sister is doing well.

*An earlier version of this paper was published in *Advanced Practice Nursing Quarterly, 4*(2), 1–11, 1998 as Moral evaluation and the concepts of health and health promotion. That version profited much from discussions with colleagues, especially Dr. Marjorie McIntyre of the University of Calgary and from public forums where the ideas were presented. The author gratefully acknowledges Aspen for permission to revise that manuscript and reprint the art and advertising.

The present version has benefited from discussions with Dr. Adeline Falk of the University of Western Ontario, Dr. Stephen Katz of Trent University, the editors, and the reviewers. The author, however, takes full responsibility for the views presented in this chapter.

Mrs. A has fibrocystic disease and despite her knowledge of breast cancer and her risk factors, she does not perform self-breast examination. This is not a knowledge deficit because she has been taught how to do breast self-examination (BSE) several times during her life. Mrs. A always feels a certain dread in going for her yearly gyn exam because she knows that she will be asked if she does BSE.

In the past when providers asked if she did BSE and she said "no," the response was most typically a "lecture" on the importance of BSE—as if she didn't have any knowledge about the relationship between breast cancer detection and BSE. On many occasions she simply told the providers that she did do BSE because it spared her the lectures. On the last occasion, however, she told the nurse practitioner her reasons for not doing BSE. She said she resents the constant surveillance of her body and her breasts. By doing BSE she feels that she is just waiting for her body to betray her and she doesn't want to think of her body like that. She doesn't like the words our culture uses in relation to cancer (war, victim, survivor). She believes that, if she gets cancer, she will cope with it. She may even die from it, but death is part of life. The prevailing attitude in health care that death can be prevented actually frightens her. Upon hearing Mrs. A, the nurse practitioner looks stunned and doesn't respond.

Though not immediately obvious, a strong connection exists between health, health promotion, and morality. Every society faces universal challenges, one of which is the fear of harm, including the harm of disease, and the death that can ensue (Nussbaum, 1988). One societal response to the fear of harm from disease is to contain the danger so that it is more amenable to human intervention (Rosenberg, 1997; Rozin, 1997). As historian Charles Rosenberg notes, "We honor randomness in the abstract but seek to manage it in practice, to constrain misfortune in reassuring frameworks of meaning. We want health to make predictive sense, to be based on coherent relationships between behavior and its consequences" (Rosenberg, 1997, p. 35). The assignment of meaning and the action that follows are efforts at containment, both of disease itself and our fear of it, that have existed throughout history from the ancient world to the present.

Since modern epidemiological techniques have enabled scientists to predict risk factors associated with a variety of diseases, containment in contemporary Western society has become largely a matter of individual responsibility directed at lowering one's risk factors. Strategies of health promotion and disease prevention are used to characterize these behaviors of containment.

Nurses, as well as other health practitioners and people in general, typically think of health promotion as a positive practice but the idea of health promotion is morally troubling for several reasons. One, the concept of health itself is laden with moral meaning but this is rarely acknowledged by nurses or other health practitioners. Two, by making an individual mostly responsible for their own health, the inherent tension between the individual and the group becomes weighted in favor of the group to the disadvantage of the individual. In practical terms, this means that individuals may be penalized by being denied resources to take care of their health. Three, as long as health is viewed primarily as an individual responsibility, other aspects of society, such as corporations and government, are excused of responsibility for health or the conditions of health. Four, society is exonerated from examining how race, class, gender, and poverty contribute to health and health promotion or the lack of it. Five, it leads to an "us-them" mentality that can be unhelpful to patients or clients who seek health-care services. Six, the requirement that people continually monitor their bodies for signs of disease can cause or increase anxiety—as in the case of Mrs. A—and be counterproductive to the achievement of well-being.

These issues are of particular import to nursing because health is central to what nurses understand the aim of their practice to be and they claim health promotion as a prominent feature of their practice. Indeed, as a discipline, nurses are committed to health promotion, viewing health promotion practices as a means to contribute to the patient's well-being. Furthermore, even though several other disciplines are involved in health promotion work, nurses do much of this work directly with individuals, families, and communities.

There is another reason that these issues are significant for nurses. Because of their position in the health care system, nurses can become the means by which the aims of other interests such as third-party payers or institutionalized medicine are actually carried out (Liaschenko, 1995a). That is, although the moral meaning of health and health promotion are the product of society as a whole, nurses—precisely because they define themselves in terms of health promotion and do so much of the work—can unwittingly become instruments of social control. This results in sanctions being levied against those who don't comply with recommended health promotion practices.

This chapter explores the concepts of health and health promotion, not to eliminate it as part of nursing work. Rather, the attempt is to enlarge our thought and imagination so that we may challenge what is morally troubling and seek more moral solutions to the problem of the fear of harm from disease and death.

Health Promotion: What Is It?

As would be expected given the connection between the human desire for control of disease and human behavior, references to health promotion are ancient (Moore & Williamson, 1984). The beginnings of the contemporary health promotion movement are generally given as the 1970s (King, 1994; Woolf, Jonas, & Lawrence, 1996) with the issuance of a Canadian document, *A New Perspective on the Health of Canada* in 1974. This report, most commonly known as the Lalonde Report and named after the Canadian Minister of Health at the time, described what are now familiar as the four influences on health: human biology, environment, access to health care services, and individual behaviors or what we now call lifestyle (Sheinfeld Gorin & Arnold, 1998). Since that time, the idea of health promotion has continued to develop such that there is now a large body of literature including journals of health promotion as well as health professionals who work exclusively in the area of health promotion.

If health promotion is viewed in a general way as strategies directed at improving the four influences on health, it is easy to see how numerous they are and how they might overlap in relation to each other. The United States 1980 document, *Promoting Health—Preventing Disease: Objectives for the Nation,* identified 216 specific health goals in three areas: health promotion, health protection, and disease preventive services (U.S. Office of Disease Prevention and Health Promotion, 1980). This was expanded to include surveillance and data systems in the 1991 report, *Healthy People 2000: National Health Promotion and Disease Prevention Objectives.* Health promotion strategies consist of behaviors related to "individual lifestyle and personal choices . . . that have a powerful influence over one's own health prospects" and include such things as physical activity, the use of tobacco and other drugs, and violent behavior. Health protection strategies are "related to environmental or regulatory measures that confer protection on large population groups" and include such things as occupational health and safety and environmental health. Disease preventive strategies include "counseling, screening, immunization, or chemoprophylactic interventions for individuals in clinical settings" that are directed toward cancer, heart disease, maternal and infant health, and sexually transmitted disease among other things (Pender, 1996, pp. 5–6).

Scholars in the field have continued the attempt to articulate the differences between the categories of health promotion, health protection, and disease prevention (Pender, 1996; Woolf, Jonas, & Lawrence, 1996). For Woolf, Jonas, and Lawrence (1996), disease prevention targets specific disease, whereas health promotion is directed toward reducing risk factors through personal health behaviors or lifestyle patterns. According to Pender (1996), the difference between health promotion, health protection, and disease prevention is motivational. Whereas the motivation for health promotion is positive in the sense of desiring to attain well-being, the motivation for health protection and disease prevention is negative in that one seeks to avoid disease and ill health.

For the purposes of this chapter, however, these distinctions are unimportant, and I refer to all three categories as health promotion. The distinctions are unimportant because regardless of whether individuals are seeking to avoid disease or to attain well-being, a linkage is made between an individual's behavior and whatever state of being is defined as health. This linkage between behavior and the outcome of health is morally problematic because, following this linkage, the individual's behavior is the central location of concern and is submitted to moral judgement by both society and health professionals. Indeed, society may use health professionals as instruments of social control in this way. Thus, as contradictory as it may seem, there exists the possibility of moral harm in our striving for health through the practices of health promotion. We might begin to explore these issues by looking at some definitions of health and how the concept of health is connected to moral evaluation.

Definitions of Health

The practice of defining health as a way to assign meaning, and therefore contain it, is ancient. Plato, for example, defined health as harmony or balance between the four bodily humors and perhaps the body and the soul; he believed disease to be an imbalance between the two:

---

when the soul is dominant, it leads to convulsions and "fills with disorders the whole inner nature of man"; but if the body is dominant, then the soul becomes dull, stupid, and forgetful. (Cohen, 1981, p. 213)

In spite of the ancient tradition, the history of disease and illness has been documented more than that of health. Perhaps this is because health "is a state of being which is absent from consciousness and experienced only in its negation by disease or injury" (van Hooft, 1997a). This negative definition was stated more poetically by French philosopher of biology and medicine, Georges Canguilhem, when he remarked that health was "life lived in the silence of the organs" (Canguilhem, 1989, quoted in Osborne, 1997).

In our scientific age this negative conception is still the most common view of health (Banta & Jonas, 1995). Nonetheless, it was challenged 60 years ago in the early 1940s when the argument was made that health is more than the absence of disease (Payne, 1983), a view officially endorsed in 1945 with the World Health Organization's (WHO) expanded definition of health as total physical, psychological, and social well-being (WHO, 1981). Since that time, there has been considerable theoretical work aimed at articulating health in other than negative ways.

Contemporary conceptualizations include sociological views of health as the "state of optimum capacity of an individual for the effective performance of the roles and tasks for which he has been socialized" (Parsons, 1981, p. 69). According to the philosophical analysis of Caroline Whitbeck, health is a matter of autonomy, understood as a capacity to pursue one's interests, aspirations, and goals. In this view, health requires a certain physical capacity or physical fitness, a realistic view of one's self and others, and the ability to handle stressful situations (Whitbeck, 1981). Some empirical work on understanding health has supported this theory (Haggman-Laitila, 1997).

Van Hooft (1997b), a more recent theorist, views health in a similar way. In his view, health is experienced in four dimensions that are concerned with the most basic physiological functioning of the body related to survival, the success of everyday routines, positive emotional experiences, and a sense of a meaningful life. Even though the first two are similar to Whitbeck's physical capacity or fitness, and the third is similar to her idea of being able to handle stressful situations well, van Hooft's sense of a meaningful life is what follows when one pursues their interests, aspirations, and goals. Central to van Hooft's position is that "health is not just an observable condition of a person's body. It is an experience and a condition of that person's subjectivity" (p. 24) or their sense of themselves as a person, and Whitbeck's theory would support this.

A common view is that health is a state of being describing individuals in relation to what is considered "normal." This concept of normality is not simple and can be used in three ways: pathological, statistical, or evaluative (Susser, 1981). When the concept of normality is pathological, the state of the individual is measured in a dichotomous way, either pathology is altered or it is not, either a disease is present or it is not. For example, there is a "normal" range of white blood cells in the human body and deviations that extend much beyond this range are indicative of pathology. Normality in a statistical sense means that a certain characteristic is dispersed throughout a population in a "normal" distribution, that is, with most cases in the middle and some at the extremes. Characteristics such as height and weight are defined in these ways.

Evaluative refers to values so when the concept of normality is evaluative, the determination of health is being made against certain values that typically reflect the expectations of members of a social group (Susser, 1981). For example, particular social groups have certain values about how to raise children that include, among other things, the type and amount of schooling, the degree of independence encouraged, and the discipline to be used for specific infractions. Violation of these social values can be seen as unhealthy. Another example would be sexual relationships in which anything other than one male and one female who are married to each other is a violation of a group's values and therefore identified as unhealthy. Other examples might be values about work and the use of certain substances such as alcohol and drugs. Conceptions of normality are not static but dynamic, reflecting various social conditions concerning knowledge, beliefs, values, and other social conditions.

Reporting in the nursing literature, Smith (1981) categorized the various conceptualizations of health into one of four models: clinical, role-performance, adaptive, and eudaimonistic or overall well-being. Smith sees these as hierarchically organized with a narrow focus on pathology in the clinical model expanding to include how one functions (role performance model), to how responsive and creative one can be in meeting the demands of the environment (adaptive model), and finally to a sense of overall well-being (eudaimonistic model).

The most recent evolution of the idea of health is that of certain lifestyle behaviors being increasingly seen as under our own control and responsibility (Lupton, 1994). These behaviors include such things as the management of stress, sexual practices, diet, recreation choices, exercise, and use of drugs and alcohol. It is precisely these behaviors that are targeted in health promotion.

Health, Moral Evaluation, and Moral Order

Health is not only a descriptive term about the state of an individual or group but is also a conceptual category. The way we think about health shapes what we describe as healthy or unhealthy as well as those factors that promote or hinder the attainment and maintenance of health. In turn, these concepts lead to actions that have moral significance.

Health is morally significant because it is a social good and can lead to human flourishing (Liaschenko, 1995b). Healthy people, in most cases, are able to pursue projects, goals, aspirations, and lives in ways that are less possible for those who are not healthy or who are less healthy.

Good and bad are moral terms for beneficial and harmful. As a social good, health is morally relevant because people generally feel good when they are healthy and bad when they are not. In this way, health is more than a physical good; it is also a social good. Participating in those projects that give our lives meaning is important to both individuals and society as a whole. To say that health is a social good, however, is not to say that it is morally unproblematic. On the contrary, the concept of health is morally problematic precisely because health is not a neutral term that is devoid of evaluative judgements.

In our contemporary high-tech world, scientific knowledge is the prevailing lens through which we make sense of human life. Although challenged on many fronts, the view that science is neutral regarding moral evaluations is still commonly held, thereby obscuring the moral implications embedded in our understandings of health, health promotion, and disease. Likewise, health is still most commonly thought of as the absence of disease. In this view, health is a technical matter that is reductionistic and limited to narrowly constructed physiological parameters.

Deviations from physiological norms such as blood glucose levels, thyroid hormone levels, and number of white cells lead to the establishment of diagnosis that may include diabetes, Graves' disease, and leukemia. Although such deviations may be interpreted as neutral statements of physiology, judgements are nonetheless made about people with these deviations, and these judgements can have consequences that affect their everyday lives. When people are deemed not healthy, they can be excused from some of their social role obligations or, in some cases, from the responsibility for their actions. Resources can be allocated or recalled and people included in or excluded from membership in certain groups. These consequences show that health is not a neutral term devoid of evaluative statements.

That health is connected to virtues and moral evaluations is an ancient notion that continues to the present. Even though the explicit forms of these evaluations have changed over time, they reflect the common themes of social order, control of the body, and inclusion in or exclusion from a given social group. The significance for nursing turns on the fact that society's system of healing can be used to enact social order by controlling the body and by making pronouncements on the eligibility for inclusion in or the need for expulsion from the group.

In order to arrive at an understanding of the moral implications of contemporary conceptualizations of health, it is useful to explore the long-standing relationship between the conceptualizations of disease and morality. The point I want to convey is that societies discipline—that is, instruct or train—their members into performing those behaviors socially defined as good for health or avoiding those defined as bad for health.

In preliterate times, health and disease were a matter of appeasing the spirits or not, respectively (Janzen, 1981). In the ancient world, "religion, philosophy, and medicine were a single discipline" (Cohen, 1981, p. 211) and because magic or superstition were seen as causative, specific behaviors such as sacrifices or incantations were required to exorcise the evil spirits. In another context (the search for pure knowledge within Western civilization), philosopher Robin Schott notes that there were ancient Greek cults that adopted very ascetic practices in the hopes of attaining immortality (Schott, 1988). Such practices of treating the body in a certain way, for example, fasting, in order to attain something considered a higher good have persisted. Conrad (1994) reported that 19th century health movements did similar things in that proper eating and exercise would lead to purification. Contemporary exercise and dietary regimens reveal similar disciplinary practices in service to the higher good of the cultural ideals of beauty, fitness, and the prevention of disease.

With the advent of Christianity, disease became a matter of punishment for the transgression of God's will, but an interesting transformation took place. With developing Christianity, punishment was seen as directed toward human nature in general rather than toward the individual transgressor. This shift from the individual to human nature allowed for the response of viewing suffering as a means to redemption (Herzlich & Pierrot, 1987) for all and not merely the transgressor. In this way, there is a place and purpose for suffering, an idea still seen today in the notion that suffering can provide meaning to our lives.

Notions of health, disease, and sexuality are particularly intertwined. For example, in his study of biblical ideas of medicine, Levin argues that there is much to recommend the theory that the fall from the Garden of Eden was not about disobedience but about sex, and he asks, "Is original sin original sex?" (Levin, 1970, p. 31). The significance of the renunciation of the body and, in particular, the sexual body in Christianity has been documented by historians and scholars of religion (Brown, 1988; Noble, 1992; Pagels, 1988). The reasons for such control are interesting and complex. For example, Pagels (1988) has argued that renunciation of sex was a way for early Christians to distance themselves from the Romans. In this case, the renunciation was a political act.

All societies control sexual behavior by a variety of means. Of particular interest are the origins of what we would recognize as modern marriage. The practice began approximately 1,000 years ago as a means of controlling inheritance and property rights (Duby, 1983). Marriage was a means of ensuring the identification of progeny so that property would be inherited legitimately. The Church originally wanted nothing to do with these marriages and was only persuaded to bless them after considerable pressure from the state. What in our time is a moral concern with who can engage in sexual behavior had its origin in maintaining a certain social order concerned with wealth. Disease was often viewed as the wages

for violating the social order and this continues to the present in attitudes toward sexual behaviors. This is clearly evident with AIDS, other sexually transmitted diseases, and even children when they are the product of what is considered illicit sex in that they are still viewed by some as the wages of sin.

Moral implications of health and disease also include membership or expulsion from a given group. This is perhaps most obvious with epidemics or plagues as they have been known historically. People with disease were shunned informally at an individual level and ritualistically at the community level. Expulsion can be found in the elaborate rituals of the Middle Ages in which lepers were sent out from the community. The leper was brought to the Church, which had been draped in black for the funeral Mass. Dirt was thrown over the head of the leper, and he or she was led to the lepersaria where they were given the rattle they were required to use to warn others of their approach (Herzlich & Pierrot, 1987). Contemporary instances of this include the social isolation of AIDS patients and the exclusion of those who do not engage in behaviors considered to lower the risk of disease. This exclusion is exercised, among other ways, through the restriction or denial of health coverage.

With the end of the major epidemics, for example, the plague, smallpox, and cholera, understanding illness as a collective event began to be replaced by understanding illness as an individual event. In other words, the experience of illness was no longer a community event, something that would happen to everyone. Instead, with the rise of chronic illness, for example, cardiovascular disease, illness became an individual event with people increasingly seen as having more direct control over their health (Lupton, 1994, 1995). This brings us to consider images of health.

Moral Harms of Health Promotion

The majority of health promotion work nurses engage in focuses on the behavioral patterns of individuals as opposed to the material and social conditions necessary for health. This is understandable in that nurses work within and generally subscribe to a healing system governed by biomedical knowledge whose aim is

BOX 10–1

IMAGES OF HEALTH

Painted in 1615, Peter Paul Rubens' *Hygeia* (see Figure 10–1), the Greek goddess of health, provides us with one view of health. The first thing we notice is the size and strength of the goddess, which conveys her dependability; one can lean against her and be supported. The light comes from above, enabling her to work; Hygeia's gaze is directed downward and is focused unreservedly on her sick charge. She is actively and directly involved with the animal, and there is reciprocity here as, according to legend, the snake revealed the location of an important medicinal herb. Rubens gives us a view of health in which compassion and work are central.

Contrast this with Gustav Klimt's *Hygeia* (see Figure 10–2). Nearly 300 years after Rubens, we see a decided turn of events. Hygeia, although still in contact with the snake, is no longer actively helping and supporting the snake. Reciprocity has weakened as she holds the snake at arms' length and gone is the gaze of concern and attentiveness. Indeed, the gaze of this goddess seems one of condescension. She is beautiful, even alluring, but she does not give, turning her back on suffering, disease, and death. Klimt's *Hygeia* forms the foreground of the painting, which is entitled *Medicine*.

This painting was commissioned, along with one entitled *Jurisprudence* and one entitled *Philosophy,* to adorn the Great Hall at the University of Vienna. Even though all three were quite controversial, *Medicine* was especially so because some interpreters saw Klimt as portraying the impotence of medical science, which angered the Viennese physicians in particular (Whitford, 1993). It may be the case that I am too harsh in my interpretation of Hygeia; rather than condescension, perhaps it is puzzlement and a sense of challenge that she is revealing. True, she is not facing the suffering confronting her par-

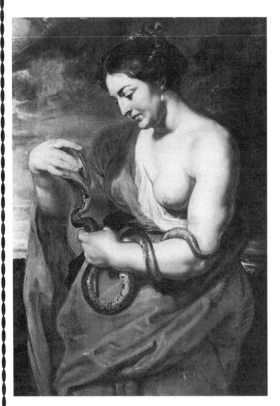 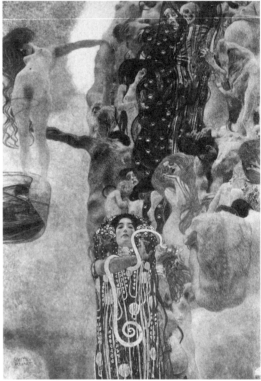

FIG. 10–1. *Hygeia, Goddess of Health* by Peter Paul Rubens. Courtesy of Detroit Institute of Arts Founders Society, Detroit, Michigan.

FIG. 10–2. *Medicine* by Gustav Klimt. Courtesy of Phaidon Press Limited, London, England.

BOX 10 – 1 (cont.)

ticular historical period, a period that witnessed the health of people sacrificed to industrialization under capitalism. Might it be that she is challenged by a vision of a future view of health—one arising from the industrialization and capitalism that produced the present commodity culture (Lupton, 1995) where the contemporary Hygeia makes her home?

A commodity culture is one in which almost any cultural product is endowed with and traded for a monetary value. In such a culture, advertising is central. Lupton (1995) notes that even though advertising "used to give the public details about a commodity or service," now "the primary function of glossy advertising is to create an image around a product which entices consumers to purchase the product and incorporate it into their everyday lives" (p. 121). Not only has advertising been used directly as a health promotion strategy but health itself is being sold—we can experience health if we use the right products and do the right things.

Figure 10–3 depicts the Hygeia of the 1990s and a culture obsessed with health as lifestyle behaviors and personal responsibility. In the 80 plus years since Klimt's *Hygeia,* health has become both a commodity and an isolated pursuit. There is no idea or at least acknowledgment that if health demands personal responsibility then it must have a society that is responsive. The snake has disappeared reflecting a society increasingly eager to exclude those who fail to discipline their bodies according to the prevailing standards of normality. We have transformed the goddess from a visibly strong and powerful presence to a waif-like persona in a beatific pose to the goddess of healthy behaviors and personal responsibility. Hygeia is now an entirely self-absorbed healer and, if she, like anyone else, becomes sick, it will be her own fault. Like anyone else, she will deserve what she gets and what she gets may be substantial blame and little help. Such advertising reinforces the idea that health is solely an individual matter dependent on one's discipline and commitment to a "healthy lifestyle." Standards of normality are thus culturally created and sustained and powerfully linked to economic interests. As one social critic remarked, buying has become a sort of prayer (Savan, 1994). As I understand it, Savan means that the act of buying, like prayer, can have aspects of supplication, even sacrifice. Purchasing certain items will appease the gods of youth, strength, power, beauty, and so forth. Health is no exception, and health promotion is marketed and sold to patients by using techniques of persuasive communication—their behavioral changes must be assured (Stubblefield, 1997).

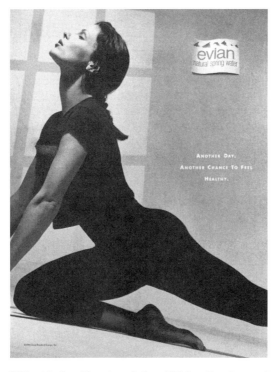

FIG. 10–3. *Hygeia of the 1990s.* Courtesy of Great Brands of Europe, © 1996, San Francisco, California.

to repair a diseased or injured body and not the social fabric in which that body lives. Nurses cannot always directly influence those social factors that impact negatively on health status even when they have identified social conditions such as poverty as a moral concern in their work (Liaschenko, 1997). Even assuming that every nurse was concerned with poverty, unemployment, racism, violence, prisons, and lack of education—in short, social justice—as much as with supporting individual behavioral change, they would be constrained by numerous factors. Most significantly is that the remedies for these problems lie beyond the actions of any one person as well as the resources of any one institution; rather, they require political action that brings together a complex network of multiple social resources. Having said that, there are, nonetheless, moral harms associated with health promotion practices and, therefore, moral harms in which nurses participate.

Do Nurses Inflict Social Harm?

The first moral harm is done by a view of health and health promotion that focuses solely on individual behavior, minimizing those social factors that promote well-being. Even though nurses as individuals or even as part of organized professional work are not able to bring the required resources to bear on the health status of their patients, families, or communities, as citizens, they can support those politicians and programs that are committed to such resources. One could argue that nurses contribute directly to the moral harms that accrue to those individuals who do not have the material resources necessary to health when, as citizens, they do not support a redistribution of those resources. Norton (1997) has argued that unless nurses are actively addressing the factors that affect health, they are not doing health promotion.

The second moral harm concerns the consequences that can come to those who do not follow the virtuous path of the healthy lifestyle. Because disease is increasingly viewed as being under individual control, people who do not engage in health promotion practices and who develop disease increasingly are reprimanded socially. In the extreme, this reprimand becomes punishment in the form of denial of health care coverage, what amounts to an expulsion from the group not unlike the lepers of the Middle Ages minus the ritual of the Mass of separation. People are cast out to fend for themselves and, in this way, are penalized for not meeting the evaluative, cultural standards of normality.

Viewed in this way, health promotion practices become a way to demarcate the medically worthy from the medically unworthy. This was not the original intent of health promotion practices as conceived by those who participated in the discussions that resulted in the Lalonde Report. This demarcation was also not the original intent of health promotion as conceived by nurses. Nursing embraced and initiated a wellness and health promotion agenda as a counterpoint to the narrowly conceived biomedical model but the goals of that agenda have been co-opted within our commodity culture.

Nonetheless, within contemporary society, organized as it is by interacting networks of large institutions, the aims of health-care institutions and the business world supporting them may conflict with the aims of nursing. Although it is not nursing (or other practitioners) that denies coverage but payers, nurses are, nonetheless, one vehicle for the pronouncement. By this I mean that other social institutions, such as insurance companies, make decisions based on assessments done and documented by nurses. People receive priority for jobs, or the reverse, as well as access to or denial of other social goods based on these assessments and documentation. Although nurses have one understanding of what they are doing and why, other social groups are simultaneously enacting their own purposes through the actions of nurses. Complicating this is the fact that the standards of normality are not determined initially by payers but are the product of a medical science that both creates and legitimates the standards. The consequences of denied coverage are enacted by nurses not as individuals but because they are part of a larger system. That the larger health care system is a source of help as well as an instrument of social control can pose a major challenge.

Most nurses work in situations in which they are salaried employees. In such a relationship, nurses sell their labor for monetary remuneration and, although they maintain control over significant domains of their work, it is largely the employing institution that determines how nursing labor will be used. It is health care institutions and not nurses that make decisions about what kind of services they will offer and, obviously, these change over time.

For example, a given health care institution or system may discontinue obstetric services and open ambulatory services, and nurses have virtually no control over these decisions. Such decisions have economic roots and justification to keep an institution solvent or increase revenue, and there is nothing inherently problematic with this. Obviously, institutions cannot lose money continuously or services could not be rendered and nurses would be unemployed. Nonetheless, the aims of health care institutions and the business world supporting them may conflict with the aims of nursing. Consider the following situation.

Suppose that an employer contracted with a group of health care providers to provide a health screening and health promotion program to workers. Nurses would very likely provide these services, and again there is nothing inherently wrong with either the services or providing them. Suppose, however, that the results of these screenings and the monitoring of health promotion activities would be used by employers to deny coverage to employees ("Big Brother Wants You Healthy," *Time*, May 6, 1996, p. 62). Even though it may be in the employer's best interest to restrict or deny coverage, it is clearly not in the workers' best interest. A question for nursing is whether the use of our labor in situations potentially against the best interests of clients alters the morality of the endeavor for nurses and/or nursing.

A third possible moral harm is the anxiety that people may experience in response to health promotion practices, particularly those that monitor the body for signs of disease. Although such practices as cholesterol and blood pressure screening and breast self-examination may mean early detection and increased survival to health practitioners and others, for some people, these practices may mean medical intrusions into their everyday lives, constant reminders that they might fall "victim" in the "war" on disease. Yet, for these people, the emotional energy of the constant vigilance called for in this "war" might be applied more rewardingly to some life project. They may resent and mistrust what they see as the underlying assumption of medical science and

health care—that death can be postponed indefinitely. People who don't follow health promotion guidelines for these reasons are still subject to reprimand and like, Mrs. A from the opening of this chapter, they must either lie or tell the truth and risk being branded eccentric at best or crazy at worst. Should they develop disease, it will be seen as their own choice and, therefore, their fault. In any event, the effect is to be stigmatized like the lepers of an earlier time.

A fourth possible moral harm of health promotion is that it sets up potentially adversarial relationships—us, the morally health righteous, against them, the morally health unrighteous. Society in general and not only nurses and other practitioners can participate in this moral harm. For example, in her research on pregnant women who were trying to stop smoking, Pletsch (1997) reported that these women said their partners, who also smoke, hid cigarettes from them. Such "pointing the finger" instills guilt and perhaps shame for not living up to the cultural expectations for pregnant women. It is difficult to see how this behavior could be helpful—it is as if they live with health police instead of partners.

The danger that nurses can also act as health police is marked. Individual nurses can do so by a matter of temperament and beliefs and nursing, as a discipline, can do so unwittingly because of its place in the social organization of care. Thus, health promotion practices pose moral challenges for nursing.

Moral Challenges for Nursing

I am not advocating for the abandonment of health promotion and I am not claiming that responsibility for one's health by lifestyle habits may not benefit the person in question. Clearly this is not the case. It does so, however, only in the sense that health is "a resource for living" (Barker, 1990) and is neither an end in itself nor a way to save money for third-party payers. The changing social relationships that give rise to our current conceptualizations and practices raise crucial questions for nursing. Within our commodity culture, health is no longer a resource to live a life but is the goal of life itself. Yet if we accept the latter idea of health, then those definitions of health, such as Whitbeck's, that articulate health as the capacity to act in accordance with one's goals and aspirations, seem strangely co-opted. There are nurses who have warned of the dangers of our ideas of health and health promotion and they are to be heeded (Barker, 1990; Caraher, 1997; Herberg, 1989; Lowenberg, 1995). Like Ivan Illich, I believe that "what is wrong with medicine is not its costly but rather picayune procedures, but its concepts and, in particular, health" (1994).

I have no list of pat interventions that can be applied to the moral harms of health promotion. However, resistance begins with thinking that nursing's response to the moral harms of health promotion will turn on how we think about health, health promotion, and the moral aims of our practice as well as how we understand the place of nursing in society. Thinking will require that we ask the following questions. What is the moral aim of nursing? How do these aims relate to ideas of normality, health, and moral order? How do we achieve and maintain our moral aims in a culture where all of us increasingly hold an instrumental relationship to larger social structures and systems of knowledge? What responsibility do we hold for accountability between ourselves as moral agents and the organizations that increasingly structure our lives? Can nursing be a point of resistance to the commodity view of health promotion? Can we offer another vision? Do we want one?

Using our collective imagination and moral wisdom, we can propose and critique courses of action that will seek to preserve what is useful about health promotion and to minimize what is harmful.

REFERENCES

Banta, H. D., & Jonas, S. (1995). Health and health care. In A. Kovner, *Jonas's health care delivery in the United States* (5th ed.) (pp.11–33). New York: Springer Publishing.

Barker, J. (1990). Whose health for all? *Health Visitor, 63*(7), 232–233.

Big brother wants you healthy. (1996, May 6). *Time Magazine,* p. 62.

Brown, P. (1988). *The body and society: Men, women, and sexual renunciation in early Christianity.* New York: Columbia University Press.

Caraher, M. (1997). A sociological approach to health promotion for nurses in an institutional setting. *Journal of Advanced Nursing, 20,* 544–551.

Cohen, H. (1981). The evolution of the concept of disease. In A. Caplan, H. T. Engelhardt, & J. McCarthy (Eds.), *Concepts of health and disease: Interdisciplinary perspectives* (pp. 209–220). Reading, MA: Addison-Wesley.

Conrad, P. (1994). Wellness as virtue: Morality and the pursuit of health. *Culture, Medicine, and Psychiatry, 18* (3), 385–401.

Duby, G. (1983). *The knight, the lady, and the priest: The making of modern marriage in medieval France.* New York: Pantheon.

Haggman-Laitila, A. (1997). Health as an individual's way of existence. *Journal of Advanced Nursing, 25*(1), 45–53.

Healthy People 2000: National health promotion and disease prevention objectives. (1991). (Department of Health and Human Services, U. S. Public Health Services Publication No. 91–50213). Washington, DC: U.S. Government Printing Office.

Herberg, P. (1989). *A critical analysis of the health promotion movement and implications for nursing.* Unpublished doctoral dissertation, University of Utah, Salt Lake City.

Herzlich, C., & Pierrot, J. (1987). *Illness and self in society* (E. Forster, Trans.). Baltimore: Johns Hopkins University Press.

Illich, I. (1994). *Against coping.* Paper presented at the Qualitative Health Research Conference, Hershey, PA, June 11, 1994. Tape #SON 94–2, Conference Recording Service, Berkeley, CA.

Janzen, J. (1981). The need for a taxonomy of health in the study of African therapeutics. *Social Science and Medicine, 15*(8), 185–194.

King, P. (1994). Health promotion: The emerging frontier in nursing. *Journal of Advanced Nursing, 20,* 209–218.

Levin, S. (1970). *Adam's rib: Essays on biblical medicine.* Los Altos, CA: Geron-X.

Liaschenko, J. (1995a). Artificial personhood: Nursing ethics in a medical world. *Nursing Ethics, 2*(3), 185–196.

Liaschenko, J. (1995b). Ethics in the work of acting for patients. *Advances in Nursing Science, 18*(2), 1–12.

Liaschenko, J. (1997). Ethics and the geography of the nurse-patient relationship: Spatial vulnerabilities and gendered space. *Scholarly Inquiry for Nursing Practice: An International Journal, 11*(1), 45–59.

Lowenberg, J. (1995). Health promotion and the "ideology of choice." *Public Health Nursing, 12*(5), 319–323.

Lupton, D. (1994). *Medicine as culture: Illness, disease, and the body in western societies.* London: Sage.

Lupton, D. (1995). *The imperative of health: Public health and the regulated body.* London: Sage.

Moore, P., & Williamson, G. (1984). Health promotion: Evolution of a concept. *Nursing Clinics of North America, 19*(2), 195–206.

Noble, D. (1992). *A world without women: The Christian clerical culture of Western science.* New York: Knopf.

Norton, L. (1997). *Should nurses attempt to change people's health related behavior?* Paper presented at the conference, Philosophy of Nursing—its nature, knowledge and values. September 1997, University of Wales, Swansea, UK.

Nussbaum, M. (1988). Non-relative virtues: An Aristotelian approach. In P. A. French, T. E. Uehling, & H. K. Wettstein (Eds.), *Midwest studies in philosophy, Volume XIII* (pp. 32–53). Notre Dame: University of Notre Dame Press.

Osborne, T. (1997). Of health and statecraft. In A. Petersen & R. Bunton (Eds.), *Foucault, health and medicine* (pp. 173–188). London: Routledge.

Pagels, E. (1988). *Adam, Eve, and the serpent.* New York: Random House.

Parsons, T. (1981). Definitions of health and illness in the light of American values and social structure. In A. Caplan, H. T. Engelhardt, & J. McCarthy (Eds.), *Concepts of health and disease: Interdisciplinary perspectives* (pp. 57–82). Reading, MA: Addison-Wesley.

Payne, L. (1983). Health: A basic concept in nursing theory. *Journal of Advanced Nursing, 8,* 393–395.

Pender, N. (1996). *Health promotion in nursing practice* (3rd ed.). Norwalk, CT: Appleton & Lange.

Pletsch, P. (1997, November 4). *Smoke-free families: A smoking cessation program for urban, pregnant, African-American women.* Paper presented at the School of Nursing, University of Wisconsin, Milwaukee.

Promoting health-preventing disease: Objectives for the nation. (1980). (Office of Disease Prevention and Health Promotion). Washington, DC: U.S. Government Printing Office.

Rosenberg, C. (1997). Banishing risk: Continuity and change in the moral management of disease. In A. Brandt & P. Rozin (Eds.), *Morality and health* (pp. 35–51). New York: Routledge.

Rozin, P. (1997). Moralization. In A. Brandt & P. Rozin (Eds.), *Morality and health* (pp. 379–401). New York: Routledge.

Savan, L. (1994). *The sponsored life: Ads, TV, and American culture.* Philadelphia: Temple University Press.

Schott, R. (1988). *Cognition and eros: A critique of the Kantian Paradigm.* Boston: Beacon.

Sheinfeld Gorin, S., & Arnold, J. (1998). *Health promotion handbook.* St. Louis, MO: Mosby.

Smith, J. (1981). The idea of health: A philosophical inquiry. *Advances in Nursing Science,* 43–50.

Stubblefield, C. (1997). Persuasive communication: Marketing health promotion. *Nursing Outlook, 45* (4), 173–177.

Susser, M. (1981). Ethical components in the definition of health. In A. Caplan, H. T. Engelhardt, & J. McCarthy (Eds.), *Concepts of health and disease: Interdisciplinary perspectives* (pp. 93–106). Reading, MA: Addison-Wesley.

van Hooft, S. (1997a). [Book Review] *Health: An Interdisciplinary Journal for the Social Study of Health, Illness and Medicine, 1,* 245–247.

van Hooft, S. (1997b). Health and subjectivity. *Health: An Interdisciplinary Journal for the Social Study of Health, Illness and Medicine, 1,* 23–36.

Whitbeck, C. (1981). A theory of health. In A. Caplan, H. T. Engelhardt & J. McCarthy (Eds.), *Concepts of health and disease: Interdisciplinary perspectives* (pp. 611–626). Reading, MA: Addison-Wesley.

Whitford, R. (1993). *Gustav Klimt.* New York: Crescent Books.

Woolf, S., Jonas, S., & Lawrence, R. (Eds.). (1996). *Health promotion and disease prevention in clinical practice.* Baltimore: Williams & Wilkins.

World Health Org. (1981). Constitution of the World Health Organization. In A. Caplan, H. T. Engelhardt, & J. McCarthy (Eds.), *Concepts of health and disease: Interdisciplinary perspectives* (pp. 83–84). Reading, MA: Addison-Wesley.

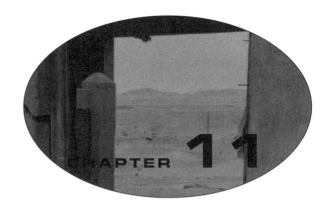

Defining and Managing Health Risk: Snapshots of Women's Strategies Across the Lifespan

MARGARET H. KEARNEY

Health promotion occurs in the context of individual bodies and unique lives. Clients respond to health professionals' recommendations based on their own understandings of who they are, what their bodies need, and what is feasible in their social and cultural contexts (Purkis, 1997; Watson, Cunningham-Burley, Watson, & Milburn, 1996). Moreover, individuals' beliefs about health are not static. As people age and experience illness, physiological changes are accompanied by cognitive learning and attitude changes, all of which are shaped by culture and society. To provide effective care, health professionals must understand the complex interweaving of these personal influences from the client's point of view.

This chapter provides snapshots of events, issues, and problems in women's lives in which they define and evaluate health risks and engage in prevention and self-care activities. The goal is to illustrate how socioeconomic factors and cultural affiliation influence women's abilities to engage in health promoting behaviors. Examples, presented through vignettes, have been taken from **qualitative research** studies, in which researchers seek to portray human experiences from the viewpoint of the study participants themselves.

This chapter focuses on women because they are the major consumers of health care and the main sources of health information for families, yet their voices are often muted in the health care arenas (Lewis & Bernstein, 1996). This silence is especially pronounced on aspects of women's health outside of childbearing and parenting.[1]

The views of women highlighted here are from those whose stories have been given voice and brought within our reach through the work of qualitative researchers. These women's views of health, barriers to health care access, or motivation to seek health care may or may not be representative of the views of women around the world, or even of others from the same ethnic group, age group, or geographic locale.

The images and anecdotes they provide are intended to demonstrate some of the contrasts in world view and life priorities that exist across cultures and communities. Just as these women's situated views are unique, clients served by

[1]Studies of pregnancy and mothering are not discussed in this review, due to the size and complexity of that literature and the comparative adequacy of coverage elsewhere.

health care professionals have their own unique perspectives.

This chapter is designed to expand our horizons of possibility and sensitize us to the range of variation of human health experience.

Views of Health

Seeking Health Care: Why Some Do and Some Don't

The life conditions that create possibilities and constraints for the promotion of clients' health are often invisible to health providers in practice settings. But, before a useful exchange can occur between a professional and a client, the practitioner must understand the clients' views of health and its relative priority, given the life pressures and demands the client experiences. The meaning of health and its origins may vary across cultural and economic contexts.[2]

Barriers to Health Care

To women migrant workers of Mexican origin, for example, health means being relatively free from worries and problems: "To be at peace . . . to be tranquil; if you have problems or many things in your head, you don't feel comfortable, you can't wash dishes comfortably" (Rodriguez, 1993, p. 26).

It's a lot about your state of energy, for me, problems take a lot out of me, not my problems, but my family's, my mother, my mother-in-law, like my mother needed surgery and she's older and I was worried that something could go wrong . . . it affects me, my hair falls out, I get nervous, I can't sleep. (p. 27)

These Mexican women's problems arise from many sources: lack of money, "dealing with the locals" (discrimination from Anglos), and the great stress of living in tran-

---

[2]In this chapter, health, wellness, and well-being are defined situationally, allowing the women in each study to reveal their own definitions and priorities. Health promoting activities are viewed as taking place during self-care as well as being directed by others such as health professionals.

sience, which include risk of accidents and crime during long hours of travel, the pain of separation from extended family, crowding and inadequate facilities in workers' camps, and the need to start over in each location. Participants in this study reported that their husbands do not allow them to have contacts outside the home, created problems by drinking, and did not help with household tasks or parenting. These women believed that behind their husbands' surveillance-related behavior is men's concern about their spouses' interactions with the opposite sex, and this affected women's health-care access:

There's times when they're really sick and they need to go to the doctor, but their husbands just really don't want them to . . . my husband was one of those, he wouldn't let me go because [he thought] I just wanted a man to see me. (pp. 41–42)

Further, their husbands' demands and the women's many other responsibilities severely limited the time available to women to obtain even necessary health care:

You have to wait a long time, you're just sitting there thinking of all the things you have to do when you get home . . . I would take the children to their immunizations, [but] I didn't get my exam for cancer that I needed, I left without my birth control pills . . . It [preventive health care] takes a long time, you lose work time and then you have problems with your husband, he wants to know where you were. (p. 38)

These women reported that personal involvement of health care providers, especially when outreach programs brought nurses into their camps, was a great help and reduced the time women needed to take away from their home responsibilities to meet health needs. This exemplifies how ways of delivering health care can improve access to health care for some groups of women when designed to meet the needs of particular groups.

In another study, African-origin women in the United States, like the Mexican women, reported that they view health as a multidimensional phenomenon, describing the effect of family pressures and life stresses on health and health promotion. Davis (1998) studied mainly single mothers with a variety of income levels, who were told that health and illness were inseparable concepts describing mind, body, and soul. Each component supported the other. For example, hope and perseverance, mind-related qualities, were viewed as complementing health care or the body.

A belief in God and prayer, qualities of the spirit, were viewed as essential to curative processes and to the acceptance of the burdens of illness and stress management. One study participant noted, "I don't get what I want. I have to pray on it . . . When God sees that I'm ready to have certain things, then He puts them things in my life, you know" (p. 36).

In contrast to the Mexican-origin women mentioned earlier, independence from others was valued as a necessary strength. Men were viewed as a necessary burden or a temptation to be overcome. Self-sacrifice and suffering were seen as evidence of strength, and necessary qualities to ensuring that one's children's needs came before one's own. This belief has consequences for the health of these women as evidenced by their report that they ignored the symptoms of health problems as long as possible because they put others' needs first.

Let me take care of my family first and then I'll take care of myself. See, because we've had to be so independent for so long you tend to think of yourself as a Rock of Gibraltar, when indeed, you're not. But you tend to think, "Well, I can go another step further, but this child can't. I can survive, but this person can't." I know if I wait another day or two, I'll get around to it [caring for myself], but it's just a question of putting other folks' feelings and desires and needs first. (p. 37)

Coupled with the priority of caring for others was a mistrust of health care institutions. Friends' and families' opinions were sought and highly regarded when these women were faced with making decisions about acceptable health care. Sharing with other women, "telling it like it is," was an important source of strength and a resource for these African-origin women.

Proactive Health Care

Cultural milieu shaped the views of health for middle-class Indo-Canadian women in particular ways (Choudry, 1998). Close ties among extended family and others in the Indian immigrant community helped women maintain their view of health. Like Mexican- and African-American women, Indo-Canadian women valued health for the sake of being able to care for one's family. However, with their more secure income and greater social support, these women were able to take a more integrated and proactive approach to maintaining health.

For example, they believed that good diet with plenty of vegetables was important, and they had access to financial resources to purchase the ingredients of a healthful diet. Since coming to North America, the women in this study reported that they had begun to observe weight increases. In response, they made attempts to reduce fat intake and reduced their ingestion of fried foods. They believed that eating at regular times of each day was important, and that reducing intake as one aged was an aspect of maintaining good health. Exercise and walking were valued by these women. Rest and prayer were also thought to be important for maintaining a sense of peace, for "just as you get nourishment from food you get strength from prayers" (p. 273). The ultimate definition of health was a thriving family: "What we call being healthy is when your children sit with you and everyone is happy. Then there is no burden on your mind" (p. 272).

In sum, women in these studies found peace and relief from worry when their families flourished and only considered their own health promotion when their families were doing well. Migrant worker women living with discrimination and poverty, and who were separated from their Mexican support systems, faced the greatest obstacles to achieving a sense of peace and well-being. Single African-origin mothers shared support with women in their communities but reported that they were largely alienated from assistance from the men in their lives.

Middle-class Indo-Canadian women in the study reviewed had financial resources and family networks that allowed time for rest, healthful cooking, and exercise.

Other Views of Health and Health Practices

The views of a group of middle-class, European-origin Americans were similar to those of their minority-culture counterparts. Hautman and Harrison (1982) asked a sample of European-origin adults in southern California about their views on health and illness. These economically comfortable, well-educated individuals used biomedical professionals for their health care. Most had private health insurance, yet most shared with the migrant Mexicans and African-origin women cited above their pragmatic view of health as ability to function and the absence of symptoms or discomforts, although peace or freedom from stress was not mentioned. A typical statement about good health was, "I don't wake up with aches and pains every day. I don't have to go to the doctor except for my yearly female physical" (p. 53). They kept themselves healthy in popularly promoted ways:

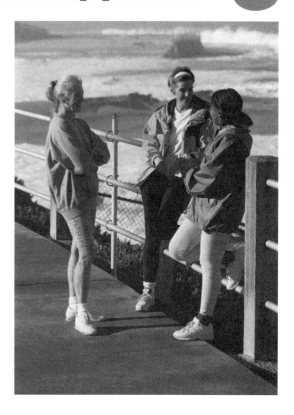

I try to cut out a lot of sugar, white flour, and junk food. I've cut out beef lately, and I've found that I feel better. [I take] multivitamins with minerals because from what I've read I feel I need them. I really don't exercise, but I have been dieting. To me that would seem to help me out a lot toward good health. (p. 57)

However, in addition to these practices, home remedies for ailments were gleaned from books, health magazines, friends, relatives, and media. Some of these included using catnip as a tranquilizer, ginseng or vinegar for blood purification, and garlic for high blood pressure.

In the northwest United States, Woods, Laffrey, Duffy, Lentz, Mitchell, Taylor, and Cowan (1988) asked diverse, mostly middle-class women to describe what being healthy meant to them. Women with the highest levels of education and income described health in holistic terms: optimizing well-being, achieving exuberant self-actualization, and functioning at high levels in all areas of life. Lower-income, older, and less well-educated women were more likely to view health as the Californians did, in terms of the absence of illness or the ability to perform expected social roles.

A follow-up study by Silko (1993) of a smaller group of educated, middle-class midlife women from the same sample revealed that most also held a multidimensional view of health as including physical, mental, and spiritual well-being. They reported that a strong sense of self-worth and knowledge of health promoting practices were the foundations of

their self-care. In contrast to the lower-income women studied and those of Mexican and African origin, these women had a greater range of life choices of career and family roles in which to seek this balance.

Like the other middle-class women described here, including Indo-Canadians, the women Silko studied felt that, at midlife, caring for themselves was as much a cultural mandate as caring for others, and they solicited support from their partners in their self-care. Feeling stressed or out of balance was as legitimate a health problem as were physical symptoms. Their self-care included attending to exercise, diet, and time management; taking control of situations and responsibilities when appropriate; negotiating for time and space for themselves; and caring for others.

The findings of these **grounded theory** studies (Blumer, 1969; Glazer & Strauss, 1967) suggest that women require discretionary time, education, financial stability, and interpersonal support to seek wellness beyond functionality and survival. Women's culture and social majority or minority status also may play a large role in the possibilities in life they view as open to them and the levels of fulfillment they aspire to achieve. Health promotion thus is intertwined with women's self-care and self-development in their complex lives.

In these samples, European-origin women of adequate income were most likely to accept the Western medical expectation to take control of their lives as a route to health. Women from non-European cultural traditions and those without perceived life options were more likely to look to sources of harmony outside themselves, including family tradition and continuity, religion, and unity with the natural world. To promote effective communication between biomedical health institutions and the women they aim to serve, professionals must ask about and work within women's culturally rooted understandings of what it means to be healthy. We can seek to create individualized care plans in which our biomedical goals are used to support rather than invalidate the women's own definitions of health.

Managing Body Changes: Defending against Risk across the Lifespan

In addition to their cultural definitions of health and the resources and support available to achieve them, the physical and interpersonal changes of human development affect women's health priorities and health promoting actions. Women's accounts reveal that their family, social, and cultural environment do not always provide them with the information and support they need to protect themselves from harm. In many cases, dominant sociocultural expectations for their behavior and appearance conflict with the self-care needed to maintain health. In each stage of womanhood, the personal value of health promoting activities is often learned by trial and error.

Young Womanhood: Limiting Sexual Risks

Despite the widespread availability of public health information on contraception and safer sex, several studies have documented that women go through a personal learning process as they test this knowledge in their own lives. In a study of well-educated adolescents and young women, Matteson (1995) found that the women's search for satisfactory contraception required advocating for self. They balanced their views of the risk of pregnancy with the stigma and negative consequences of using birth control. Using birth control required coping with practical and emotional ramifications such as conflict with religious beliefs, concern about effectiveness against pregnancy and sexually transmitted diseases, dealing with inconvenience and remembering to use them, and accepting responsibility for contraceptive use.

As young women, most had used condoms because they were available and known and later branched out to other more controllable or effective methods when situations demanded. Many women had tried a number of methods before arriving at one that suited their current life situations and partners. Statistical evidence of protection against pregnancy was less influential than the woman's personal belief in her method's effectiveness, based on her friends' and her own experiences.

In a markedly different context, women crack cocaine users also described a learning process, although one with greater risk and less satisfactory conclusions (Kearney, Murphy, & Rosenbaum, 1994). The mainly African-origin, low-income women in California in this study described how in the sexual arena as with other life choices, they repeatedly "learned by losing," discovering through failure how to protect themselves. Most of these study participants had become mothers in their teens, which was their first learning experience about their susceptibility to pregnancy.

Many had tried a variety of birth control methods, but successful use was often hampered by lack of understanding of how the methods worked, limited access to health care, ambivalence about pregnancy and mothering, male dominance, and eventually by being high on drugs. Older women had learned over time that the best contraceptive methods were sterilization, condoms, and abstinence. As one said, "I say no a lot" (p. 152). A 28-year-old recalled:

My mother told me to go get an abortion. She said, you know, you're not ready for no kids. Well, I know—I was still in school. But I insisted upon having it, and then after I had her I couldn't take no birth controls . . . because I had high blood pressure . . . And I was a fast breeder . . . About a month after I had her, I got pregnant again, I had an abortion. And the month after that I got pregnant again, I had an abortion. Then a month after that I got pregnant again. Then I had my next daughter. And I got pregnant again after that other abortion . . . So I got my tubes tied, cut, and burned. So I ain't got to worry about it no more. (p. 153)

The violent and oppressive social world of crack cocaine use made it difficult for these women to set limits on sexual risk. Women whose money for drugs had been exhausted sometimes were pressured into providing sex in exchange for drugs. A few had learned the hard way that once they acquiesced, they were relegated to the lowest stratum in the drug world, women who would "do anything for a hit" of crack cocaine: "No woman sets out, well, I don't set out to do it for no hit. But then the men they use you now because of that" (Kearney, et al., 1994, p. 154). In a very difficult context, these crack cocaine users used their hard-earned wisdom to attempt to protect themselves in future encounters.

In a third study of managing sexual risk, Redfern-Vance and Hutchinson (1995) interviewed European- and African-origin women in the United States who had had at least two incidents of sexually transmitted disease (STD) in a two-year period. These women explained their past selves as not thinking and foolishly trusting of men. Some had ignored severe physical symptoms of STDs. They eventually reached turning points when they recognized the personal costs of repeated infections, including health risks, loss of innocence about male protectiveness, and stigmatization for presumed promiscuity. They began to identify patterns in their past experiences that had caused problems, such as giving in too easily to pressures for sex, being swayed by men's claims of monogamy, and being seduced by "slick" men. As they "shed the veils of illusion" (p. 230), they learned, the hard way, to protect themselves. "Every time I started to trust him again, he gave me something else . . . I'm thinking you can't trust anybody" (p. 230).

The authors of this study theorized that once the women began to see their situations more clearly, they developed cognitively-based, rather than emotionally-driven, strategies for self-protection. Such efforts included

staying celibate until they could trust themselves to think clearly; "saying no" to men who might not be monogamous; seeking balance in their lives through increased focus on religion, study, and healthier lifestyles to enhance their sense of self-worth; and taking responsibility for their sexual protection by carrying condoms and insisting that men be tested for disease.

Unwanted sexual attention from strangers is a burden many young women face. In a fourth study of sexual risk management by European-American women who were in their twenties and thirties, Esacove (1998) found that daily experience of being the object of sexual remarks and suggestions eroded these women's self-worth and could lead to feelings of terror. To deter unwanted attention as potential victims, women walked quickly and purposefully; wore a tough facial expression; avoided attracting attention, eye contact, or interaction; took a dog with them; covered their attractive attributes with a hood, sunglasses, or baggy clothing; and avoided places and people linked to sexual encounters. Although the women often felt inadequate or contemptuous of themselves for not stopping the offensive behavior, when they did respond they were equally frustrated by the lack of effect. Some confronted aggressors during the interactions, and others created responses later in their minds, reviewing the experience until some relief of tension was achieved. In the absence of social disapproval for this male behavior or advice on handling unwanted attention, women were left to themselves to discover and deal with this affront to their sense of well-being.

Based on the studies described here of women's experiences of sexual risk, it appears that young women lack guidance and support in dealing with the risks inherent in sexual maturation. Western cultural myths—males' honorable paternalism, their need to sow wild oats, older men protecting younger women, love as conquering danger and fear, and the virtue of women's generosity and forgiveness—continue to place young women and girls at risk of harm. Although comprehensive social change is needed before women will be fully safe and comfortable in relationships and social encounters, health care professionals can bring out and challenge these myths to help women protect themselves against unreasonable sexual demands.

For example, when a young woman states that she does not need to use condoms because her boyfriend has vowed he would never cheat on her, a health professional can inquire about the beliefs and experiences that are behind this claim and work with the client to make a realistic assessment of her risks. Being valued by a health professional and taking the time to think through what is at stake beyond the relationship may give a young woman the support to put her own life ahead of her partner's demands.

Reviewing these studies of young women's efforts to protect themselves against shame and harm in the sexual arena, it is clear that qualitative research on other areas of women's lives is also important. Little has been written in the grounded theory literature about young women's management of other health threats. Sports- and automobile-related injuries, nonsexual infectious disease, mental health problems, and chronic illness also affect women in their teens and twenties. Health professionals should be alert for qualitative studies that can shed light on how young women view and respond to these health issues.

Healthy Lifestyles in Middle Adulthood

Reducing Cardiovascular Risk

Just as the dangers of sexual risk-taking are not immediately apparent to young women, the importance of healthy behaviors is difficult to internalize for women leading busy lives and caring for others. Heart disease is the leading cause of death among women in middle and later age groups (Lewis & Bernstein, 1996), yet it may be felt as a distant threat given the many other demands in women's lives.

In a study of African-American women with a range of employment status, education, and income levels, Keller (1993) found that female kin and religious teachings were the most powerful influences on young black women's perceived risk of heart disease and their actions against it: "My godmother, she was a large woman and to me she was very beautiful and she eats healthy . . . She stay away from salt. She seasons with other foods. She does not like frying foods" (p. 51). It wasn't until a loved one suffered or died from unhealthy behavior that women began to notice small symptoms or changes in themselves, such as headaches or increased blood pressure, and began to accept the links between behavior and health: "I think it is because of their eating habits and patterns, eating all the fatty foods, the fried foods which we are accustomed to when we were growing up" (p. 52). Strong family ties reinforced their desire to avoid causing suffering to their families, to live to raise their children, and to teach them healthier lifestyles. As providers for their loved ones, they wanted to preserve their partners' and children's health as well as their own.

Women in this study who did not change their behavior either believed that they were protected by their genetic makeup or were beset by other more pressing dangers such as violence, unemployment, and poverty (Keller, 1993). The resources available to help them live healthier lifestyles did not seem sufficient to overcome these more pressing obstacles. Some felt their culture acted to sabotage their efforts:

I think the African-American men . . . they may be skinny, but they may like overweight women just because their mothers were overweight, their aunts were overweight, everyone around them was overweight, their sisters were. Exactly, they were all heavy, so they are looking for a meaty woman. I think it has been acceptable because of that. (p. 54)

Even in the face of known risks, lifelong tastes and preferences were difficult to give up, as were the cultural and social traditions of food preparation and appearance.

In a group of culturally diverse U.S. women, perception of cardiovascular risk was explored by Anderson (1992). Women from all ethnic groups found reasons to believe that, even though others were at risk, they themselves were less so. Even those who accepted their risk were not always convinced that behavior change would reduce that risk. One woman noted, "My doctor told me that my blood pressure wasn't the dangerous kind, so I could either take my medicine or not" (p. 97). All placed commitments to others on a higher plane than commitment to their own health. "You're always trying to make sure that everyone else is OK in the family. You're running around to your parents and to your friends and to your kids" (pp. 107–108). These women reported that their stress was heightened by racism and sexism in their daily lives. These pressures not only created obstacles to self-care but also reduced their sense of self-worth and self-confidence.

Other situational or physical barriers to diet and exercise included competing social priorities, fatigue, pain, and discomfort with exercise, poor weather, conflict with other duties and roles, lack of money for checkups, and lack of confidence. When obstacles seemed great, rationalizing and justifying were used to reduce the perception of threat. Women without exercise experience could not judge a reasonable level of fatigue:

I do the Thighmaster when I'm watching TV, but, because I read in the pamphlet and it says, "If you feel tired, do not continue," and when I do the fourth one I feel tired, and I think, "I'd better not do this any more." (Anderson, 1992, p. 110)

Women who were able to find colleagues to exercise or diet with found it more enjoyable and felt more confident. Those who had failed in the past were more uncertain about their likelihood of success than were women who were trying these changes for the first time.

Mexican-origin women's views on reducing cardiovascular risk through diet and exercise were explored by Juarbe (1998) in an American sample. Many of the women in this study did not see themselves as overweight until it was pointed out to them, often in derogatory comments by their spouses. Some husbands verbally expressed acceptance of their heavy wives but demonstrated by their actions (ranging from positive comments about thinner women to infidelity) that they preferred thinner women.

Women engaged in an internal dialogue on how to respond to their excess weight. Those who felt unable to diet or exercise felt that their self-will to change, *la voluntad propria,* was constrained, in some cases by threat of domestic abuse. Any changes these women made were done in secret or disguised, such as exercising while playing with the children. Another major constraint on the will to change was the time demands of their roles as workers and as mothers. Husbands might push for weight loss but did not help with cooking or housework. "Sometimes I have to clean the house, then [go] to work . . . My husband tells me to do exercise . . . but I do not have the time" (p. 775). Change required a strong perceived need and the will to risk destabilizing the family unit.

Quitting cigarette smoking also requires overcoming lack of willpower and obstacles inherent in role demands. In one study, African- and European-origin women in the United States who successfully quit smoking described an increasing commitment to health and personal growth. This commitment grew in response to public health messages, perceived social ostracism in smoke-free environments, pressure from their children, and their own health problems (Thompson, 1995). Eventually they faced an intolerable value conflict between the importance of health and continuing to smoke:

I am watching everything I put on my table to make sure it doesn't have too much fat content, trying to give my kids a decent diet . . . and then I realized I was causing them to have horrible asthma attacks from my smoking, not to say what smoking was doing to me. It was crazy. (p. 73)

Once they determined that smoking was a "disgusting habit" and quitting was essential to health, self-esteem, and family harmony, women were able to make a plan to quit and stick to it. Prayer and affirmations were helpful, particularly to the African-origin women who participated in this study. Pride in their accomplishment increased their self-esteem and their confidence to take on other health promoting changes.

Menopause: Standing at the Crossroads

As with risk perception at younger ages, culture and social context influence women's perceptions of the meaning of menopause and what lies before them for the second half of their lives. Researchers have been particularly interested in menopause, a biophysical process that has been laden with social and emotional implications despite little systematically derived knowledge of women's actual experiences. Quinn (1991) found that a group of middle-class women in the United States who were approaching menopause were unsure about what to expect. Hot flashes were the only symptoms they felt certain as a sign of menopause. Physical changes led some to believe they would be losing part of their identity:

Menopause has to signify the end of a time, a period of my life, when I felt I was very strong and I had a lot of vitality and energy and physical attractiveness. . . . I think there will be a diminishing of that. (p. 28)

Yet, not all participants in this study were discouraged about aging. They expressed determination to view menopause as a natural process that simply signaled letting go of a fading youth and embracing the beginning of a new, differently valuable period. Some felt much wiser and more capable of weathering adversity and change. They looked forward to relief from fear of unwanted or abnormal pregnancy and the hassles of menstruation. To preserve their health and the vitality of their youth, some of the midlife women in Quinn's study began to change their diets, start exercise programs, and take vitamins and calcium. They also began to set aside time for themselves and accommodate times of decreased energy. Simultaneously with the waning of their responsibilities to children, they began to take more control of their time and increase their focus on balancing stressful activities and situations with solitude and time for quiet renewal.

Dickson (1994) also found that African- and European-origin American women who had experienced or were experiencing menopause contrasted social expectations of fragility and resignation with their sense of themselves as strong and self-sufficient.

You're sort of over the hill or pretty close to it, and yet, I feel like I could almost start over. You know, a whole new life. But it's that age in your life when . . . you're supposed to be very settled. It's what people expect of you. (p. 120)

Although the physical symptoms of menopause were viewed as temporary by participating women, their movement into a new phase of life was irreversible. They examined what they had accomplished in relation to their expectations, how they felt about no longer being able to bear children, and what growing old meant to themselves and their families. Along with regret for some, menopause brought freedom, time for themselves, and a shift in priorities toward their own self-development.

Some non-European cultures may provide women with a more positive sense of what to expect after menopause. Filipina-origin women in the United States (Hautman, 1996) described menopause as a marker of changing womanhood, which included changes in the body, the family, and community networks. The women felt it was important to take the physical changes of menopause in stride and had few complaints of hot flashes or other symptoms. More upsetting were emotional changes and forgetfulness that disrupted family and relationships, because they threatened women's self-concept as organized or in control. Changes in roles and relationships were expected and anticipated:

In **Tagalog,** change of life is *ibang buhay.* It is a real change, a change in her demands. When you are in the middle group, you're in the middle and serve both ends, [but later] the Filipina woman collects what is due her. (p. 670)

After menopause, "you transcend into another circle, and that is where you are out and you are demanding" (p. 670). Older women are expected to take on respected roles of authority and wisdom. With their increasing age they were more forthright in expressing their needs. Their careers took on new importance, and they participated in community networks and civic organizations. Their age brought them respect and a new set of responsibilities that were seen as freeing rather than burdensome.

In another cultural contrast, Buck and Gottleib (1991) interviewed First Nations Mohawk women from a Canadian reserve. Like the Filipina women, most of the Mohawk women in this study described midlife as a time of taking stock of their lives, shifting priorities away from meeting the needs of others and toward satisfying their own needs. This shift was seen as a result of children leaving home or as their reward given their age and station as elders. "Time for myself" and meaningful use of time was important. Spending their time meaningfully included doing community work, rearing children, visiting grandchildren, working, and participating in relationships.

In summary, these studies suggest that women with ties to traditional cultures may have access to a clearer "road map" for what to expect after midlife than do many North American women of European origin. They may also have evidence within their social worlds that aging can bring rewards, including discretionary time and authority. Although, at present, European-origin women may live longer than women of color do, the Western cultural focus on attractiveness and mother-hood restricts these women's communication about and preparation for the second half of life. Therefore, the group with the most to gain may have the fewest tools with which to opti-mize their potential in later life.

Health professionals can share with women the evidence from qualitative research that life after menopause is not necessarily fraught with loss of capability and contribution to meaning-ful life. Strategies for working around physical limitations can be developed just as women work around the limitations of mothering and employment responsibilities at younger ages. Health professionals can treat older women with the respect and deference to their self-knowledge that they merit as senior mem-bers of society and can draw on this wisdom to help women develop health promoting strate-gies that fit within their changing life patterns and roles.

Aging: A Wiser Self Coping with a Less Reliable Body

As women grow into their sixties, seventies, and eighties, many notice that while their sense of self persists with vigor, their bodies and surroundings show signs of loss. Physi-cal changes and annoying interruptions of functioning may emerge, such as urinary in-continence, dizziness, and forgetfulness. So-cial networks change, as spouses, relatives, and friends become ill or pass away, children move away and become preoccupied with their own families, and the involvement and satisfactions of their work lives recede. Shift-ing networks and physical capacities can bring changes in women's health priorities and the strategies they use to achieve them.

Adjusting to Functional Losses

Like decline in physical appearance, forgetful-ness decreases women's sense of personal com-petence and social acceptability, and threatens their self-concepts as independent, capable in-dividuals. Cromwell (1994) interviewed older women and one man in the United States who perceived themselves as more forgetful than in previous years. When forgetfulness prevented them from functioning socially or maintain-ing their self-image as competent, it became a concern. "Well, it's sorta like losing a part of yourself, isn't it?" (p. 453). To compensate for forgetfulness, the elders used strategies such as keeping lists and an appointment calen-dar, being sure to replace everything where it belonged, establishing a routine, and double-checking to ensure they had locked doors and turned off the oven, with the goal of pre-empting embarrassment or reminders from others. When the strategies were not effec-tive, it became necessary either to cover up the lapse or to withdraw from social situations. Covering up did not prevent one's self-concept from being diminished, but at least it reduced the social damage. This woman was unable to remember the plays in her regular card game:

I lose track, yes, so I quit the game . . . I had to give up a lot of jobs . . . because I can't handle it. . . . I gave up all those things because I felt I don't qual-ify and I don't want to expose myself. (p. 456)

Some causes of memory loss are treatable. Yet, Cromwell argues that women may accept forgetfulness and withdraw from valued so-cial situations without pursuing treatment. As with osteoporosis, the threat of one's aging and mortality and the stigma of infirmity and incompetence may be greater than the will-ingness to risk humiliation in pursuing av-enues for improvement.

Urinary Incontinence

One of the most stigmatized conditions of aging is urinary incontinence. Skoner and Haylor (1993) interviewed midlife women and Dowd (1991) interviewed a group of older women. Both found that incontinence was a threat to participants' self-esteem and social function-ing. The greatest threat was having an acci-dent in public, and women's memories of such humiliation were vivid. Other threats were odors or other exposure of their problem: "And my dress . . . I was never so embarrassed in my life . . . Others could see that it was wet . . . I'm telling you, it's embarrassing" (Dowd, p. 181). In order to normalize their lives, women sought to take charge of the problem. Among the adjustments were reducing fluid and caffeine intake, wearing dark clothing, parking or sitting near a bathroom, finding out through trial and error how often to use the bathroom, trying different sanitary pads or products to find the ones that were most effective without undue discomfort or visibility, and trying to fit pelvic muscle strengthening exercises into their daily routine.

The women in this study who had had incontinence the longest had achieved the smoothest functioning with the problem, having learned over time what contingencies to prepare for. Some women sought medical advice during these periods of breakdown, but none decided to use medications or surgery. They made sense of incontinence by viewing it as a normal female condition. They were willing to go to great lengths to live with it rather than to expose themselves to embarrassment or a sense of being "over the hill" by seeking more invasive treatment.

Osteoporosis

As at earlier ages, before taking on a new health promoting behavior, older women must be convinced that they face real harm, and that action will prevent harm without causing distress or social rejection. It has long been known that the risk of osteoporosis in old age can be reduced somewhat by regular weight-bearing exercise, adequate calcium intake, reducing alcohol and caffeine intake, and medications, including estrogen therapy. However, in interviews with older European-origin women in California, Magit (1994) found that osteoporosis was linked in their minds to loss of attractiveness, infirmity, vulnerability, and going downhill toward death, and they went to great lengths to distance themselves from the possibility of osteoporosis. Several had been diagnosed with osteoporosis, and yet they were adamant that they did not have it to a serious degree.

I knew what osteoporosis was. I had this stereotypical view of it, which was hunched-up old ladies whose bone mass had lost its density and

who were now suffering from something called "soft bones." . . . I, of course, was not in that category. (p. 166)

Like women at risk of heart disease, women in Magit's study compared themselves favorably to others who clearly had worse disease, citing their sturdy ancestors who had given them good bones. Living in southern California, they were deeply influenced by a cultural context in which **ageism** prevailed. They also felt it was unseemly or inappropriate to discuss intimate concerns or ask assertive questions of physicians. They didn't want to be perceived as whining, hypochondriac older women. In this context, they made only small, personally acceptable changes that did not increase their sense of impending disability and death.

Fear of Becoming a Burden

A major worry of older individuals is becoming a burden on others. Not only does this threaten a self-image of self-sufficiency and competence but it also alters long-term relationships and living conditions. Covan (1998) found that a group of older Florida residents living in a lower-middle-class retirement community went to great lengths to hide their increasing frailty. Being busy was highly valued as a sign of vigor and popularity: "You can interview me but I go for my walk at 6:00; then I play shuffleboard and then I work out at the gym" (p. 425). Yet, as time went on, illness and infirmity could not be kept secret. "Care sharing" was a way of maximizing social support in a community in which all were aging and increasingly dependent on others. Aged adults cooperated to hide evidence of frailty.

Assistive devices and health-care services were kept out of sight, and elders kept busy as much as possible to display their well-being. When unable to be active socially, the preference was to care for oneself in private, stockpiling food, staying near the toilet, and waiting out the illness rather than asking for help. The next best approach was to seek support from one's partner or spouse, even when this support included cleaning up bodily wastes and performing intimate tasks. Neighbors or health care professionals were seen as the last resort.

In a third study of self-care in late life, Berman and Iris (1998) interviewed ethnically diverse older women and men in the Chicago area and discovered three distinct approaches to self-care that crossed all ethnic and economic groups and were rooted in personal self-perceptions and priorities. The first approach was to "do and think for yourself," believing that health-focused actions made a difference to well-being. Based on their own rationales, these individuals developed daily routines and preventive measures, some using help from health professionals and others using their own judgement. A second group felt unable to do anything about their own health and let others take care of them; they saw their functional losses as inevitable results of aging. The third group did not pay much attention to their health; they saw living life as having higher priority than focusing on the physical changes of aging. They did not feel they had significant health problems regardless of their diseases or diagnoses. In all cases, elders filtered professional advice through their personal beliefs and priorities as they considered health promoting actions.

Based on the studies described here, we can see that as individuals age they maintain a strong sense of personal dignity and desire for self-determination. Women go to great lengths to conceal bodily and cognitive failings. An identity as a vigorous and capable adult continues to be valued into old age.

Health professionals can assist older women to take advantage of preventive and protective interventions while maintaining as much dignity and personal control as possible. It is important to accept that aged individuals may have definitions of their desired quality of life that contrast with the model seen as desirable by health professionals. For example, a woman with urinary incontinence who chooses to use protective garments for years rather than undergo a brief but profoundly embarrassing surgery is making a reasonable decision. At the same time, elders must be kept informed of alternatives that may improve their well-being and must not be sidelined as too old or stubborn to learn or change. As with women at midlife, health professionals can build trust and mutuality in communications with older women by drawing on their life experiences and self-knowledge when creating care plans that support elders' desired levels of self-determination.

The studies in this chapter suggest that women's lives during their careers and reproductive years are both enriched and complicated by their unique cultural worldviews, personal experiences, and commitments to others. Health and health promotion are defined and weighed from within these webs of competing concerns, and health only becomes a priority over time through personal experience. Those with the greatest resources for help with caregiving demands see the greatest range of possibility for personal change. Others appraise their barriers and then choose pathways that facilitate the well-being of loved ones before their own.

Health professionals can use these studies as reminders that no health-related decisions are made in a vacuum. We must explore with women the pressures and demands in their lives and the possibilities they see as open to them within their cultural understandings. By providing reliable information about health, and by problem solving with women to help them weave health promoting action into the complexities of their lives, professionals can increase trust by demonstrating that they are aware of realities of everyday life and at the same time help to raise women's consciousness of possible alternatives. A therapeutic partnership should be based on mutual goal setting, rather than simply replicating the oppressive authority that dominates other arenas of many women's lives.

CONCLUSION

I challenge nurses to consider the following points, gleaned from the studies described in this chapter, about selected women's *own* perspectives of promoting their health:

- Health is experienced as an interplay of body, mind, and spirit. It requires harmony and freedom from worry as well as from unpleasant or functionally disabling symptoms.
- Family care-giving responsibility holds primacy over personal health promotion unless resources are available to support both. The value placed on health promoting self-care increases over the lifespan, as knowledge increases and other responsibilities wane.

- Socially desirable self-image holds primacy over health-related benefits when considering the adoption of behavior change or seeking help with a health problem.
- Poverty, poverty-related transience and time commitments, racism, ageism, and sexism block women's access to health promoting resources they otherwise would use.
- Cultural patterns and racism affect the support sought by women outside the family and their expectations of relationships with health professionals.

Qualitative research to date suggests that despite women's strengths and resourcefulness, the complexities of their lives require them to build motivation in relation to behavior changes that promote and sustain health. This sense of possibility is found when daily crises become manageable and women's self-concepts include a sense of capability. These two areas can be targets of health professionals' interventions. When providing accurate information about steps women can take to promote health, nurses' respectful, attentive interactions can foster women's self-esteem. Concrete strategizing for dealing with daily obstacles to health promotion within an individual woman's life context can bring the seemingly impossible within reach. Nonetheless, small steps are the best starting point for change. Visible, tangible results that have value within an individual's experience and culture are needed if her health promoting action is to be sustained.

Lewis and Bernstein (1996) commented that in access to health care, "The greatest barrier of all is the lack of respect for minority women's value systems and ways of expressing themselves" (p. 55). The studies described in this chapter suggest that this statement holds true for all women, not only those in ethnic or cultural minority groups. Women's value systems and cultural norms for health are complex and diverse regardless of age group and socioeconomic category. It would be a great wrong if the largest obstacle to women's achievement of high-level wellness within a biomedical health care system was others' unwillingness to meet them where they are: to assist them to achieve health promotion that is consistent with their lives.

Health professionals must value women's opinions and choices before they can be successful in facilitating health promotion in women's multidimensional lives. This is not to say that the narrow options visible to a woman raised in poverty and disadvantage should be the only goals for health promoting professionals. Using our own qualitative knowledge of how structural inequality affects our clients' health, professionals can speak out in political and social arenas to help bring opportunities and resources within reach of all. Then women will be able to move to higher definitions of health: beyond survival in their parent and worker roles, to relief of stress and symptoms, and then toward greater energy, wholeness, and satisfaction—and health.

REFERENCES

Anderson, F. (1992). *A grounded theory study of women's perceptions of cardiovascular risk.* Unpublished dissertation, University of Washington, Seattle.

Berman, R., & Iris, M. (1998). Approaches to self-care in late life. *Qualitative Health Research, 8,* 224–236.

Blumer, H. (1969). *Symbolic interactionism: Perspective and method.* Berkeley, CA: University of California Press.

Buck, M., & Gottlieb, L. (1991). The meaning of time: Mohawk women at mid-life. *Health Care for Women International, 12,* 41–50.

Choudry, U. (1998). Health promotion among immigrant women from India living in Canada. *Image: Journal of Nursing Scholarship, 30,* 269–274.

Covan, E. K. (1998). Caresharing: Hiding frailty in a Florida retirement community. *Health Care for Women International, 19,* 423–439.

Cromwell, S. (1994). The subjective experience of forgetfulness among elders. *Qualitative Health Research, 4,* 444–462.

Davis, R. (1998). Coming to a place of understanding: The meaning of health and illness for African American women. *The Journal of Multicultural Nursing and Health, 4*(1), 32–40.

Dickson, G. (1994). Fifty-something: A phenomenological study of the experience of menopause. In P. Munhall (Ed.), *In women's experience* (Vol. 1., pp. 117–157). New York: National League for Nursing Press.

Dowd, T. (1991). Discovering older women's experience of urinary incontinence. *Research in Nursing and Health, 14,* 179–186.

Esacove, A. (1998). A diminishing of self: Women's experiences of unwanted sexual attention. *Health Care for Women International, 19,* 181–192.

Glaser, B., & Strauss, A. (1967). *The discovery of grounded theory: Strategies for qualitative research.* New York: Aldine de Gruyter.

Hautman, M. (1996). Changing womanhood: Perimenopause among Filipina-Americans. *Journal of Obstetric, Gynecologic, and Women's Health Nursing, 25,* 667–672.

Hautman, M., & Harrison, J. (1982). Health beliefs and practices in a middle-income Anglo-American neighborhood. *Advances in Nursing Science, 4*(3), 49–63.

Juarbe, T. (1998). Cardiovascular disease-related diet and exercise experiences of immigrant Mexican women. *Western Journal of Nursing Research, 20,* 765–782.

Kearney, M., Murphy, S., & Rosenbaum, M. (1994). Learning by losing: Sex and fertility on crack. *Qualitative Health Research, 4,* 142–162.

Keller, C. (1993). Developing and sustaining valued health behaviors in young African-American women. *Health Values, 17*(3), 49–56.

Lewis, J., & Bernstein, J. (1996). *Women's health: A relational perspective across the life cycle.* Boston: Jones & Bartlett.

Magit, J. (1994). *Discrete distancing: A substantive theory of postmenopausal women and osteoporosis.* Unpublished doctoral dissertation, University of California, San Francisco.

Matteson, P. (1995). *Advocating for self: Women's decisions regarding contraception.* Binghamton, NY: Haworth Press.

Purkis, M. (1997). The "social determinants" of practice? A critical analysis of the discourse of health promotion. *Canadian Journal of Nursing Research, 29*(1), 47–62.

Quinn, A. (1991). A theoretical model of the perimenopausal process. *Journal of Nurse-Midwifery, 36,* 25–29.

Redfern-Vance, N, & Hutchinson, S. (1995). The process of developing personal sovereignty in women who repeatedly acquire sexually transmitted diseases. *Qualitative Health Research, 5,* 222–236.

Rodriguez, R. (1993). *Female migrant farmworkers: The meaning of health within the culture of transience.* Unpublished dissertation, Texas Woman's University, Houston, TX.

Silko, B. (1993). *Midlife women's balanced health and ability to function through the process of self-care.* Unpublished doctoral dissertation, University of Washington, Seattle.

Skoner, M., & Haylor, M. (1993). Managing incontinence: Women's normalizing strategies. *Health Care for Women International, 14,* 549–560.

Thompson, E. (1995). *A descriptive study of women who have successfully quit smoking.* Unpublished doctoral dissertation, College of Education, Georgia State University, Atlanta.

Watson, J., Cunningham-Burley, S., Watson, N., & Milburn, K. (1996). Lay theorizing about "the body" and implications for health promotion. *Health Education Research, 11,* 161–172.

Woods, N., Laffrey, S., Duffy, M., Lentz, M., Mitchell, E., Taylor, D., & Cowan, K. (1988). Being healthy: Women's images. *Advances in Nursing Science, 11*(1), 36–46.

Wuest, J. (1997). Fraying connections of caring women: An exemplar of including difference in the development of explanatory frameworks. *Canadian Journal of Nursing Research, 29*(2), 99–116.

Wuest, J. (1998). Setting boundaries: A strategy for precarious ordering of women's caring demands. *Research in Nursing & Health, 21,* 39–49.

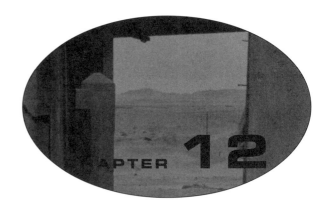

Mental Health Promotion

CATHERINE WILLINSKY
BONNIE PAPE

This chapter is based on a process that began in 1997. At that time, the co-authors began to explore the concept and applications of mental **health promotion.** The context was our workplace, the Canadian Mental Health Association (CMHA); our work was funded by the relatively vnew Mental Health Promotion Unit of Health Canada. But our motivation extended beyond professional to personal. For many years we had participated in vigorous debate about the subject of mental health promotion, and we were delighted to have the opportunity to explore it and perhaps move toward consensus.

The two sides of the debate could be summarized as follows. Those who favored a more general approach to mental health argued that it is a component of everyone's lives, and therefore it is most important to address the issues that everyone shares. These include managing stress, dealing with life transitions, and coping with work and family issues. Others made the case for the plight of the mentally ill, and the need for focusing on the specific issues related to their mental illness. These include marginalization, homelessness, and powerlessness. Perhaps, as you are reading this, you are already feeling more comfortable with one of these sides than the other. You may have participated in similar discussions. We hope this chapter will help you, as the process helped us, to understand that this dichotomy is in many ways a false one.

In recent years we have been hearing more and more about "Mental Health Promotion" from academic and health care settings, policy circles, and community programs. Although many people claim to be putting the concept into action, there are different notions about what the term means and what its applications might be (Canadian Public Health Association, 1998). Some people believe mental health promotion is a "soft" concept that applies to anything that makes people feel good. Others see it as public education efforts to raise awareness for managing life situations.

Most people think mental health promotion applies to everyone, but there are those who feel it should focus only on the "well" population. Sometimes mental health promotion can seem to mean so many things that it does not mean anything at all (Secker, 1998).

In fact, research from a number of sources shows that mental health promotion is a useful concept that has significant potential for contributing to the mental **health** of individuals and communities (Joubert & Raeburn, 1997). Its purpose, captured in its name, is to foster, protect, and improve mental health. This seems simple enough, but just what is mental health? How is it achieved? The search for answers to these questions is the continuing goal of mental health promotion efforts and the purpose of this chapter.

A Brief History of Mental Health Promotion

Although many of the concepts embedded in mental health promotion are not new, as an area of study, knowledge development, and practice, it has a relatively short history. Because mental health promotion emerged from the fields of health promotion and mental health, definitions of these concepts are a useful place to begin.

Health promotion was defined in 1986 as "the process of enabling individuals and communities to increase control over the determinants of health and thereby improve their health" (World Health Organization, Ottawa Charter for Health Promotion, 1986). A useful definition of mental health can be found in a 1988 Canadian federal government document, *Mental Health for Canadians: Striking a Balance* (Health and Welfare Canada, 1988). This discussion document introduced a definition of mental health as "the capacity of the individual, the group and the environment to interact with one another in ways that promote subjective well-being, the optimal use and development of mental abilities (cognitive, affective, and relational), and the achievement of individual and collective goals consistent with justice and the attainment and preservation of conditions of fundamental equality" (p. 7).

These definitions of health promotion and mental health contain significant points that have informed subsequent discussions of mental health promotion. Specifically, ideas about encouraging people to take charge of the circumstances that affect their mental health, promoting well-being, building capacity, and enhancing social justice or equity continue to be germane to developing notions of the mental health promotion concept (Health Canada, 1996).

A 1996 Health Canada international workshop on mental health promotion, organized by the University of Toronto's Centre for Health Promotion, achieved consensus around the following definition:

Mental health promotion is the process of enhancing the capacity of individuals and communities to take control over their lives and improve their mental health. Mental health promotion uses strategies that foster supportive environments and individual resilience, while showing respect for equity, social justice, interconnections and personal dignity. (Centre for Health Promotion, 1997)

Concurrent with this meeting, the Canadian Mental Health Association (CMHA) was also engaging in a process to understand mental health promotion as it related to the associa-

tion's mission—to promote the mental health of all people. Accordingly, we reviewed the available literature, which consisted mainly of government publications and conference proceedings rather than peer-reviewed papers (Secker, 1998) and identified and interviewed a number of key informants—academics, consumers, and practitioners—in order to develop a snapshot of how mental health promotion is understood. Happily, the CMHA process and the Centre for Health Promotion meeting had consistent results. CMHA's literature review and interviews yielded a number of components in common with the above definition.

> **Mental health promotion aims to enhance control and resiliency.**

Distilling information from the various sources, we can suggest some key elements of mental health promotion. A sense of control over one's health, and resiliency (or the ability to bounce back from life's difficulties) are two fundamental goals. Steps toward these goals tend to involve environments that foster social justice, social support, and participation in decisions about one's life and health. Mental health promotion can focus on the individual, the family, or the community level, and applies to all people, including those with mental disorders (Hodgson, Abbasi, & Clark, 1996).

> **Mental health promotion addresses issues that affect everyone.**

Mental health promotion is a complex concept that requires an expanded analysis in order to be fully understood. The following model, which anchors this chapter, is proposed as a framework to enable further analysis of the concepts. This model explores the various routes to good mental health, which include enhancing individual and community capacity as well as improving the physical and social environment. It requires us to consider the critical points in the life cycles of individuals and communities, when interventions or particular coping skills may be needed: events in the lives of individuals such as bereavement, birth of a child, divorce, illness, and events affecting whole communities, such as the closure of a local industry. Thus individual and collective strengths, the external environment, and the journey through life are all fundamental pieces of the picture that leads toward optimal mental health.

To develop a complete picture of mental health promotion, one must consider not only where and how to intervene to improve mental health, but also what outcomes to look for, and how to know when we have been successful in achieving those outcomes. Additionally, efforts to promote mental health must address the fundamental issues of health promotion, and hence must be situated within the context of the broader determinants of health such as socioeconomic status, housing, social support, equity, racism, violence, and so on. Figure 12–1 is our proposed conceptual model of mental health promotion that builds on all these approaches.

To help make the broad concept of mental health promotion more manageable, we explore it in terms of the concepts in Figure 12–1.

Issues and Settings: The Focus for Mental Health Promotion

When and where should one carry out mental health promotion activities? Some strategies, like general public education campaigns to raise awareness about mental health, may happen any place, any time. However, for most activities, it is necessary to identify particular situations or settings to ensure that mental health promotion efforts are focused on and relevant to the people they are designed to serve. It is then possible to develop the most appropriate strategies to strengthen the ability of individuals and communities to deal with each situation. Some specific examples of issues and settings follow.

Life Transitions

The journey through life takes us through a number of stages or transitions. We can all identify such times in our own lives: beginning school, adolescence, facing questions of sexual identity, leaving home, marriage, the birth of a child. Most of us also encounter unexpected situations or events that are out of our own control, such as unemployment, job relocation, family breakdown, health care restructuring, closure of a key industry, pressures of population expansion, and transition resulting from urbanization and immigration. Because stresses on individuals, families, and communities tend to increase during any such times of transition, mental health promotion activities should be considered for these transition periods.

Crisis Events/ Chronic Situations

Situations such as accidents, chronic illness, abuse, addictions, poverty, racism, and long-term unemployment also place a great deal of stress on individuals, families, and communities, and increase the potential for mental health problems to develop. These risk factors must be considered in order to design interventions likely to promote long-term mental health for different populations, at various times in the life cycle, and for groups with specific needs.

Settings

Particular physical and social environments, such as schools, workplaces, recreation facilities, and residential and health care settings, are the focus of many effective mental health promotion efforts. The aim is to develop healthy and supportive environments within the identified settings.

Disability/Disorder

Mental health promotion activities can contribute to the richness and quality of life for people with any disease or disability. What makes the mental health promotion approach different from more clinical approaches? The key difference is mental health promotion's focus on individual strengths and community capacity rather than on disability, disorder, or dysfunc-

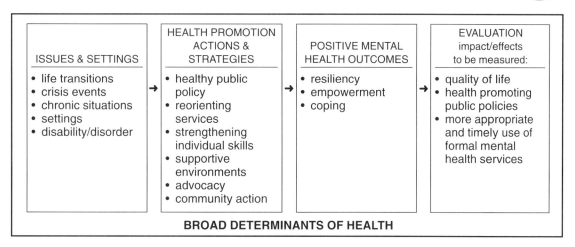

ISSUES & SETTINGS	HEALTH PROMOTION ACTIONS & STRATEGIES	POSITIVE MENTAL HEALTH OUTCOMES	EVALUATION impact/effects to be measured:
• life transitions • crisis events • chronic situations • settings • disability/disorder	• healthy public policy • reorienting services • strengthening individual skills • supportive environments • advocacy • community action	• resiliency • empowerment • coping	• quality of life • health promoting public policies • more appropriate and timely use of formal mental health services

BROAD DETERMINANTS OF HEALTH

FIG. 12–1. Conceptual Model of Mental Health Promotion.

tion. Community capacity refers to the ability of community members to use the assets of its residents, associations, and institutions to improve quality of life.

There is sometimes confusion about what part, if any, mental health promotion can play to combat mental illness. Mental health promotion efforts are not intended to cure, treat, or prevent major mental illnesses. What mental health promotion *can* do, however, is provide strategies that build on the strength and power of people with mental disabilities, thereby maximizing their mental health. Mental health promotion efforts can also build community capacity by fostering acceptance and awareness to combat the discrimination that people with mental illness face (Tudor, 1996).

> Mental health promotion aims to enhance the well-being and quality of life of the population at large as well as specific groups within the population.

Actions and Strategies: How to Promote Mental Health

What do mental health promotion strategies look like? The following actions and strategies outlined in the Ottawa Charter (World Health Organization, 1986) are means to promote individual and collective health. We will look at each one in relation to mental health promotion.

Developing Healthy Public Policy

Mental health promotion goes beyond clinical care, and even beyond programs. It places mental health on the agenda of policy-makers in all sectors and at all levels, directing them to be aware of the mental health consequences of their decisions and to accept their responsibilities for mental health. Because so many of the factors affecting mental health are beyond the control of the individual, simple programs alone are too limited. In addition to programming, there is also the need to change organizational and government infrastructures in order to carry out health promotion in the broad sense, and this can be achieved by developing public policies that promote mental health. Healthy public policy combines diverse but complementary approaches including legislation, fiscal measures, taxation, and organizational change. It requires coordinated action in order to identify the obstacles and move forward with more equitable health and social policies.

Reorienting Mental Health Services

The mental health sector needs to move increasingly in the direction of health promotion, beyond the provision of only clinical and curative services. When mental health services embrace an expanded mandate, which includes all the social, political, environmental, and economic determinants of health and which is sensitive to cultural needs, then they are taking more of a mental health promotion approach (Tudor, 1996).

The responsibility for mental health promotion in health services is shared among individuals, community groups, health professionals, health service institutions, and governments. Working together to provide services that promote mental health coordinates action so barriers to change can be addressed. Reorienting mental health services also requires more focused attention on mental health research and changes in professional education and training. This should lead to a change in attitude and organization of health services that refocuses on the total needs of the individual.

Strengthening Individual Skills

Many of the activities that promote mental health such as participating in decision making, managing life's challenges, and advocating for change require certain skills such as community organizing. Supporting people to acquire the necessary skills and abilities is an important strategy for mental health promotion.

Creating Supportive Environments

This mental health promotion strategy focuses on bringing about community and organizational change to create supportive and healthy environments. Mental health promotion is far more likely to be sustained where environments are flexible and accommodating (Health and Welfare Canada, 1990). An organizational change approach to mental health promotion brings together people from many backgrounds and disciplines. For example, expertise in industrial development and organizational dynamics can be combined with mental health knowledge to develop workplace mental health promotion programs that focus on a healthy work culture (Galbally, 1994).

Effective mental health promotion includes the development of healthy organizations such as healthy families, healthy local communities, and healthy schools and workplaces so the mental health of individuals within those settings can be supported and sustained by the organizations in which they live, go to school, work, and play, at every stage of life.

Advocacy

Advocacy refers to the actions of stakeholders to influence the decisions and actions of communities and governments that have some control over the resources that influence health. A number of mechanisms for action fall into the category of advocacy. Advocates can provide mental health information to decision-makers, and promote public involvement in decisions about mental-health-related issues. They can also direct attempts to influence appropriate levels of government to take actions that will improve the mental health of specific individuals and the broader community. For example, mental health promotion advocates would be likely to press for more funding for actions that empower the community rather than the funding of more medical interventions.

Strengthening Community Action

Mental health promotion works by encouraging effective community participation in setting priorities, making decisions, planning strategies, and implementing them to achieve better mental health. At the heart of this process is the empowerment of communities, and their ownership and control of their own endeavors and destinies. Community action refers to the process of involving members of a community in the identification and reinforcement of those aspects of everyday life, culture, and political activity that are conducive to mental health. This might include supporting political action to modify the environment, reinforcing social networks within a community, and developing the material resources available to a community.

Positive Mental Health Outcomes

What are the outcomes that mental health promotion aims to achieve? Table 12–1 identifies resiliency, empowerment, and coping as positive mental health outcomes. A brief exploration of these will help to clarify the elusive concept of mental health.

Resiliency

A recurring theme in discussions of a mental health promotion approach is resiliency. In this context, resiliency is commonly understood to mean the quality that allows an individual or group to function well despite negative odds: "Life is a constant up and down, and we can never get rid of problems, crises, sorrow and pain. Being able to bounce back in the face of these inevitabilities is an important aspect of mental health" (Joubert & Raeburn, 1997).

> **Mental health promotion attempts to increase people's ability to deal with life's challenges.**

Two fundamental concepts are associated with resiliency: risk factors and protective factors (Health Canada, 1995). *Risk* involves experiencing a number of stressful life events (e.g., moving, transitions) or a single traumatic event (e.g., divorce, bereavement). *Protective factors* are defined as the skills, personality factors, and environmental supports that contribute to resiliency. They provide a buffer as well as a reservoir of resources to deal effectively with stress. Understanding the ways individuals respond to adverse life circumstances lies in identifying protective factors rather than identifying factors that counter risk (Dyer & McGuinness, 1996).

Empowerment

A feeling of control over one's life, empowerment, can enhance the ability to bounce back from life's challenges. Empowerment is the bedrock upon which mental health promotion efforts are built. Empowerment means having a sense of control over one's life, and is crucial for us all, whoever we are and wherever they live. Having a sense of control over one's life is strongly related to feelings of well-being, both for individuals and groups. Whether in the workplace, at home, or in the community, whether young or old, whether or not a person has a diagnosed mental illness, the mental health of all people

is enhanced when they are empowered and have a sense of control over their own lives (Health and Welfare Canada, 1988). This fundamental principle can be applied whenever and wherever mental health promotion activities take place.

Coping

Coping refers to the cognitive and physical skills and resources available to and used by individuals, families, and communities to help them deal with the problems, stresses and strains of daily living, or life events causing stress (Health and Welfare Canada, 1988). Everyone experiences stressful events in their lifetime, but there are strategies that can make the events more manageable. For example, reframing a community issue to view it in a more positive way, or practicing relaxation techniques to deal with stress can help people to cope with difficult circumstances and thus enhance mental health. As one person put it, mental health promotion can help to normalize daily experiences by validating people's feelings and acknowledging stress, and by focusing on coping rather than diagnosing.

Evaluation: How To Know We Have Been Successful at Mental Health Promotion

It is difficult to determine the effectiveness of mental health promotion activities, because there are many variables at play at any given time. This does not mean that programs are not effective, just that further work must be done so we will be able to gauge the impact they are having.

In order to evaluate mental health promotion efforts effectively, the desired outcomes must be identified (e.g., capacity building of individuals and groups) and a variety of indicators developed that measure change. The most effective interventions are those that are directly relevant to the individuals and groups they are designed to serve.

Effective programs have generally been developed and implemented with a clear understanding of the relationship between the goals of the program and the social environment in which the individual or group lives

(Jonah, 1996). Examples of some possible success indicators are improved quality of life, more equitable, participatory and empowering public policies, and more appropriate and timely use of the formal mental health service system. Further attempts to promote mental health should focus on the importance of evaluation so effective interventions can be applied in different settings.

Contrasting Mental Health Promotion with Similar Ideas

Mental health promotion is often confused with the similar concepts of prevention and health promotion in general (Secker, 1988). This is understandable because there are many common elements and few clear parameters. Nevertheless, there are certain distinguishing characteristics we can identify that set mental health promotion apart from similar ideas.

Prevention

The term prevention is commonly used interchangeably with mental health promotion, and there are indeed areas of overlap. In particular, the concept of *primary* prevention, which targets the whole population, is virtually indistinguishable from mental health promotion.

> **Mental health promotion serves the population at large and seeks to enhance mental health, not to prevent a specific mental illness.**

Whenever we undertake mental health promotion activities to foster empowerment, resiliency, or coping, we may well be helping to prevent or minimize possible mental health problems. But the two concepts are still different in their aims and in their scope. Prevention efforts in mental health tend to be directed toward populations at risk of developing mental disorders. They seek to eliminate those factors that cause or contribute to the incidence of mental illness. Mental health promotion is a much broader concept. It serves the population at large, and seeks to enhance

mental health, not to prevent a specific mental illness. Mental health promotion initiatives have been described as "primarily educational rather than clinical in conception, their ultimate goal being to increase people's capacities for dealing with health crises and for taking steps to improve their own lives" (Goldston, 1977, p. 20).

Health Promotion

Health promotion and mental health promotion have many points in common. Both:

- focus on the enhancement of well-being rather than on illness
- address the population as a whole, including persons experiencing risk conditions, in the context of everyday life
- are oriented toward taking action on the determinants of health, such as income and housing, rather than focusing on risk factors and conditions
- include a wide range of strategies such as communication, education, organizational change, community development, and local activities
- acknowledge and reinforce the competencies of the population
- encompass the health and social fields as well as medical services (Health Canada, 1996)

The health promotion approach as outlined in the Ottawa Charter (World Health Organization, 1986) has considerable relevance for mental health promotion (Secker, 1998). A health promotion approach calls for a strong commitment to reducing inequities and helping people to cope with their circumstances. It includes fostering public participation, strengthening community health services, and coordinating healthy public policy. It also discusses creating environments conducive to health in which people are better able to take care of themselves, and to offer each other support in solving and managing collective health problems.

Because these are clearly examples of mental health promotion as well as health promotion, we must ask ourselves if there are any particular distinguishing characteristics of mental health promotion that set it apart? If health promotion is interpreted in terms of the broad, socially critical, and empowering ideals of the Ottawa Charter, then mental health promotion and generic health promotion are very similar indeed. The main distinguishing characteristic of mental health promotion is an emphasis on mental health goals and outcomes, such as resilience, empowerment and quality of life, and the inextricable link between mental and physical health.

Practical Applications

Mental health promotion is not a "program" but an approach to dealing with everyday realities (Health Canada, 1996). The broad strategies discussed earlier show that it can be implemented in a number of different ways. This section offers some concrete examples to illustrate mental health promotion in action.

Following each example, we pose several questions to provoke reflection, discussion, and debate. The questions challenge the reader to think about how health professionals can use their roles creatively to effect change at the individual, interpersonal, and collective levels. We encourage you to draw on your own practice and experience in formulating your ideas.

Mass Communications

Mass communication is a way to bring a message about health to the public. It can be through radio and television messages, magazine ads, or even billboards. The education and information can be targeted to the general public or to particular groups who are at an increased risk of developing mental health problems. Examples of the kinds of messages that have been used to raise awareness include the general importance of mental health ("Making Mental Health Matter"), and specific mental health issues such as how to deal constructively with family tensions.

Mass communications can also be used to change attitudes. In the 1980s in California there was a large-scale multimedia campaign to create more positive attitudes toward personal relationships. Using the slogan "Friends Can Be Good Medicine," it was based on the evidence linking social support and good physical and mental health (Taylor, Lam, Roppel, and Barter, 1984). The Ontario Division of the CMHA also used a multimedia campaign to challenge the stigma associated with mental illness. In a series of television advertisements and billboards, one young man says, "I'm glad my dad got sick last year." He explains that his father's illness helped him to learn a great deal about people's attitudes toward mental illness. Those who were open-minded and provided support helped his father to recover and get back to work and family life. The campaign was effective in challenging the persistent stigma that surrounds mental health problems. By causing the public to reflect on their own attitudes, it had impacts at several levels: the general public (increasing their tolerance toward those with mental illness), the family (whose issues around dealing with an ill relative to become better understood), and people with mental illness themselves (enhancing their acceptance in the community).

✳ Reflective Questions

The following questions will help health professionals to identify some ways of using mass communications to promote mental health.

1. How can mass communications be used to emphasize the importance of maintaining positive mental health?
2. Can media campaigns use mental health promotion principles of empowerment, participation, and control?
3. What strategies can be used to bridge the gap from seeing or hearing the message, to understanding, believing, and taking action?

Workplace Programs and Policies

Many initiatives that fit the description of mental health promotion have already become quite common in a variety of working environments. These include stress reduction workshops, flexible working hours, family leave (to allow workers to care for sick family members), job sharing, and employee assistance programs, which offer counseling and alternative health care. One of the most important ways to promote mental health in the workplace is to develop workplace procedures and policies that maximize employees' control over the design and organization of their work.

✳ **Reflective Questions**

The following questions will help health professionals to identify some issues regarding the
promotion of mental health in the workplace.

1. How can mental health issues be incorporated into the health agendas of workplaces?
2. What are some ways of highlighting mental
   health promotion on the agendas of occupational health and safety committees?
3. How can health professionals work to shift
   the emphasis of mental health in the workplace from responding to individual distress
   (e.g., stress management, employee assistance programs, etc.) to more of a proactive
   approach (e.g., changing the climate of the
   workplace to one that is more participatory,
   empowering, etc.)?

✳ **Reflective Questions**

The following questions will help health professionals to identify some issues regarding the
promotion of self-help/mutual aid.

1. How can health professionals encourage
   the development of a self-help group while
   supporting the autonomy of the group?
2. What are the roles professionals can play
   vis-a-vis self-help groups? What is the
   point at which the professional should step
   aside and let the group take over for itself?
3. Does providing professional assistance to
   self-help groups interfere with the purity of
   the nonprofessional self-help model? How
   can financial resources be provided for
   self-help efforts without compromising their
   autonomy?
4. Mental health promotion rests on the fundamental principles of empowerment and
   self-determination. How can funding programs balance supporting these principles,
   while allowing for flexibility and maintaining
   accountability?

Self-Help/Mutual Aid Groups

Self-help groups are voluntary, small-group
structures for mutual aid. Members typically
share a common problem or situation, and
meet for the purpose of achieving a common
goal. Many people who join such groups find
that all their needs cannot be met by the formal service system, but that self-help fills those
gaps with its round-the-clock, personal support
from equals whose understanding of the problem come from actually living with it. Self-help
also offers the opportunity for people to use
their own strengths and abilities as role models,
helpers, and advocates. Some groups (such as
Mothers Against Drunk Driving) begin as traditional mutual support groups providing help
to and by individuals, but shift to a collective
advocacy focus, catalyzing social change about
their common concern. By increasing people's
self-determination, helping them to cope with
difficult situations, and offering an avenue for
social change, these groups provide clear illus-
trations of mental health promotion.

Self-help is a popular and rapidly growing
phenomenon. As just one example of how
it can be implemented, targeted efforts have
taken place in British Columbia and Ontario
to develop self-help groups and other similar
resources (such as telephone peer support) for
seniors who are caregivers. These networks
help address many issues of senior caregivers,
including isolation, stress, and depression.

Community Development Projects

Involving a community in the identification
and reinforcement of those aspects of everyday life, culture, and political activity that are
conducive to health is known as community
development. CMHA's Framework for Support project is a good example of a community development approach to mental health
promotion. In this model, self-help groups or
other organizations run by people with mental health problems, family and friends, and
generic community groups such as religious
organizations and service clubs join together
with the formal mental health service system
to provide a complete array of potential supports and connections to community.

In a number of communities, groups have
used this community development model to
enhance employment opportunities for those
with mental health problems, to improve access to recreation and cultural settings, and to
create housing options. By enhancing the capacity of the community to accept and include
people with mental health problems, these
strategies are promoting autonomy, quality of

life, and integration—all elements that contribute to peoples' mental health.

✳ Reflective Questions

The following questions will help health professionals to identify some ways to promote community development approaches.

1. How can professionals act as a resource for
the group throughout the process of identifying issues and ways to address them?
2. What is the best way to engage communities around a particular issue?
3. How can health professionals develop relationships with communities?

Skills-Building Projects

Developing skills to strengthen our own mental health or that of others is another form
of mental health promotion. Besides the organized structures of self-help groups and organizations, naturally occurring social support is
a critical component of mental health promotion. Because informal kinds of support are
just as important to positive mental health as
organized efforts, we need to find ways to legitimize and promote them (Collins & Pancoast, 1976).

The natural processes that people carry out
in communities, such as providing social support and organizing to solve collective problems, are key components of mental health
promotion. Attempts to enhance individual
skills should recognize the importance of these
natural processes and build on them.

An example of this approach is a CMHA project called "Helping Skills," which was implemented to respond to the stress caused by the
failure of the fishery in Newfoundland. Lay-
people across the province were trained by
counsellors in the basic human skills of helping
and in clarifying areas where professional intervention is needed. The non-service-oriented
nature of the project drew on the strengths and
capacities of local people to support each other
through hard times. In the process of counseling their peers, these helpers were also increasing the community's participation in its own
health issues and deepening the community's
capacity to deal with its mental health needs.

✳ Reflective Questions

The following questions will help health professionals to identify some approaches to build
on people's capacities and skills.

1. How do you ensure that skills-building efforts do not result in programs that dupli-
cate existing professional structures or
approaches?
2. How can one participate in developing skills
without compromising others' confidence in
their own natural abilities?

Enhancing Participation

Because an important key to mental health
promotion is having a sense of control and
participation in decision making about issues
that affect one's life, programs or policies that
encourage participation are good examples
of mental health promotion activities. Policies
that support the development of consumer-
run organizations, such as the U.S. National
Self-Help Clearinghouse or the Council of
Canadians with Disabilities, promote mental
health by fostering people's participation in
decision-making processes. Those organizations and groups that are not fully run by the
constituents can still operate with a mental
health promotion approach by supporting the
active and real participation of their constituents on boards and committees, as service
providers and evaluators.

✳ Reflective Questions

The following questions will help health professionals to identify some ways to promote
meaningful participation in mental health
promotion policies.

1. What are the decision-making processes
in which meaningful participation of constituents is important?
2. What are the barriers to participation? How
can these be overcome?
3. What practical measures can be taken to
overcome barriers and encourage individuals and groups to become part of the
decision-making process? (e.g., timing of
meetings, subsidies, language, etc.).

Intersectoral Action

Different organizations, ministries, departments and levels of government are more effective when working collaboratively to address issues that impact mental health, such as economic development, housing, health care, education, and transportation. Collaborative approaches to mental health promotion draw on a broad umbrella of expertise and experience, and focus on a particular mental health issue.

The Canadian Mental Health Association's national projects on youth participation exemplify intersectoral collaboration with a mental health promotion agenda. Health Canada has supported CMHA to bring together youth and the agencies that serve them at local, provincial, and national levels to explore how young people can have a greater say in the policies and programs that affect their lives. These collective efforts raised awareness about the importance of young people's participation, and resulted in concrete policy changes to foster involvement.

✳ Reflective Questions

The following questions will help health professionals to highlight ways to promote intersectoral collaboration.

1. What is the professional's role in working with community groups to address issues collaboratively? What steps need to be taken?
2. How do you deal with competing agendas when working together?

Reflections on the Essence of Mental Health Promotion

Although mental health promotion is a complex notion, a number of key elements are evident. In discussions of mental health pro-

motion, the themes of control over one's life and the related concepts of empowerment and participation, social justice, and equity consistently emerge. Although certain at-risk groups may be targeted, mental health promotion addresses issues that affect everybody, and can be applied to individuals, families, and communities. There are particular times and settings in people's lives when mental health promotion efforts may be especially relevant, but there are also strategies that are appropriate for the general population at any time.

> Mental health promotion initiatives must inevitably relate to social and structural issues.

Interventions to promote mental health do not belong to health care systems alone. Influences from many aspects of people's lives contribute to their mental health. If mental health promotion efforts are to be successful, they must address the fundamental issues of health promotion, including the broad determinants of health such as income, housing, employment, and education (Lurie, 1995). Mental health promotion initiatives can help people fulfill their human potential by enabling them to develop their capacities and make use of available resources. The challenge that we now face is to identify clearly the elements of positive mental health, find effective strategies for achieving them, and then apply them not only to individuals, but to groups and the wider community as well.

Acknowledgements

This chapter is based on a "Social Action Series" produced by the Canadian Mental Health Association. The authors are grateful to the Mental Health Promotion Unit of Health Canada for funding support for the production of that document.

REFERENCES

Canadian Public Health Association. (1998). *Mental health promotion resource directory.* Ottawa: Authors.

Center for Health Promotion. (1997, June). *Proceedings from the International Workshop on Mental Health Promotion.* University of Toronto, Toronto, Ontario.

Collins, A., & Pancoast, D. (1976). *Natural helping networks.* Washington, DC: National Association of Social Workers.

Dyer, J. G., & McGuinness, T. M. (1996). Resilience: Analysis of the concept. *Archives of Psychiatric Nursing, 10*(5), 276–282.

Galbally, R. (1994). *Towards a health promotion strategy.* Sydney, Australia: Victorian Health Promotion Foundation.

Goldston, S. (1977). Defining primary prevention. In G. W. Albee & J. M. Joffe (Eds.), *Primary prevention of psychopathology* (pp. 18–23). Hanover, NH: University Press of New England.

Health and Welfare Canada. (1988). *Mental health for Canadians: Striking a balance.* Ottawa: Ministry of Supply and Services Canada.

Health and Welfare Canada. (1990). *Mental health services in Canada.* Ottawa: Ministry of Supply and Services Canada.

Health Canada. (1995). *Resiliency: Relevance to health promotion: Discussion paper.* Ottawa: Minister of Supply and Services Canada.

Health Canada. (1996). *Mental health promotion: The time is now.* Ottawa: Mental Health Promotion Unit.

Hodgson, R., Abbasi, T., & Clarkson, J. (1996). Effective mental health promotion: A literature review. *Health Education Quarterly, 55,* 55–74.

Jonah, N. (1996). *A guide to the literature on the effectiveness of prevention of mental health problems for those at risk.* Unpublished manuscript, Health Care and Issues Division, Health Canada, Ottawa.

Joubert, N., & Raeburn, J. (1997, Sept.). *Mental health promotion: What is it? What can it become?* Paper presented at Ayrshire International Conference on Mental Health Promotion, Ayrshire, Scotland.

Lurie, S. (1995). The need to strike a balance. *Canada's Mental Health, 43*(2), 34.

Secker, J. (1998). Current conceptualizations of mental health and mental health promotion. *Health Education Research, 13,* 57–66.

Taylor, R., Lam, D., Roppel, C., and Barter, J. (1984). Friends can be good medicine: An excursion into mental health promotion. *Community Mental Health Journal, 20,* 294–303.

Tudor, K. (1996). *Mental health promotion: Paradigms and practice.* London: Routledge.

World Health Organization. (1986). *Ottawa Charter for Health Promotion.* Geneva.

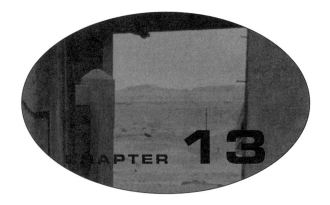

Nursing Support with Family Members of the Critically Ill: A Framework to Guide Practice

VIRGINIA A. VANDALL-WALKER

John, a 15-year-old aboriginal youth involved in a motorcycle accident, is admitted to the Intensive Care Unit around suppertime suffering from multiple fractures, lacerations and abrasions, and a closed head injury. He is unconscious but responding to deep pain. Surgery to stabilize a fractured femur and to debride wounds is scheduled for later that evening. Staff report that family members and friends are "taking over" the waiting room, requesting visitation. The nurse speaks by phone from the unit to John's mother who is in the waiting room, informing her that she will be called in to visit once admission procedures are completed.

An hour later, John's mother calls, expressing anger, impatience, and fear to the ward clerk, who then informs the nurse. The nurse admits to the ward clerk that she forgot about the family and advises the ward clerk to notify the family that they can now visit. Five individuals arrive at the nursing desk from the waiting room. The ward clerk explains to them that only two members of the immediate family can visit at a time. The three individuals who must leave the unit are obviously angry as they glance about, trying to locate John's cubicle. The nurse approaches John's mother and aunt, leads them to the bedside, and briefly explains the equipment, John's condition, and the visiting rules. She then excuses herself, noting that it is her coffee break. John's mother and aunt are left standing at John's bedside, each feeling confused, uncertain, worried, and overwhelmed.

Nursing, Support, and Families in Critical Care: An Overview

Throughout the history of nursing, the expectation has been that providing support to patients constitutes an essential component of practice. Is providing support to family members an expectation as well? If so, what is the nature of the support provided to family members by nurses and how is this nursing support implemented? A review of the literature reveals that nursing support in general has received minimal attention from nurse theorists and nurse researchers. In the literature, the term, concept, and activities of "support" are used as commonly, imprecisely, and contradictorily as they are in practice. As a result, the nature of nursing support for family members is obscured by confusion in implicit and explicit definitions of nursing support.

Extensive research has been conducted over the past two decades to examine the importance of the family to patient recovery (e.g., Heater, 1985), the many needs perceived by family members of critically ill patients (e.g., Leske, 1992a), and the importance of the nurse in assisting family members of critically ill patients to meet their needs (e.g., Leske, 1992a). This knowledge has not, however, been readily translated into practice. Why does this research-practice gap persist? I suggest that the lack of both a meaningful and clear explanatory model about what constitutes nursing support with family members, and of an organizing framework for nursing support interventions with family members, has hampered the application of the research.

In an attempt to address this knowledge imbalance, I have developed the Nursing Support with Families (NSWF) Framework, to guide nursing actions that promote the health of family members of the critically ill adult so they can, in turn, help their critically ill relatives. This framework evolved over the past decade from my reflections on clinical practice, an extensive review of the literature (Richardson, 1998), and a concept analysis of nursing support for families in critical care (Richardson, 1994). I break down the complex, abstract, and heretofore ill-defined concept of nursing support with family members of the critically ill adult into more identifiable and manageable components. This way, interventions may be more frequent, thoughtful, intentional, and integrated into the delivery of care to the patient, not an "add-on if I have time."

In presenting the NSWF Framework, I explore the links between support and nursing in general, among the various types of support, and among nursing support, critical care family member needs, and critical care family member health.

To illustrate the NSWF Framework, I include actual case studies of family members experiencing a critical illness. These clinical exemplars are specific to the critical care situation, the main focus of my nursing practice. I encourage readers to consider cases from their own populations of interest to determine the relevance of the NSWF framework to their practice. I welcome readers' comments concerning the applicability of this framework to their practice, to assist with its continued development.

Definitions

Nursing support with family members of a critically ill adult is defined broadly as: the dynamic interactive assistance provided by the professional nurse, comprised of health promoting activities that are situation-specific and finite and aimed at minimizing the negative impact of the critical care experience for both individual family members and the family unit (Richardson, 1994). Health is defined as the physical, mental, spiritual, and social integrity of both the family unit and individual family members. The health of the family unit and of individual family members influences their ability to be resilient and to adapt in the face of adversity.

To facilitate ease of communication, the terms "family" and "families" are used throughout this chapter to specifically denote family members of critically ill adults. If the family system/unit is being referred to, it will be explicitly stated. The family is defined as consisting of whomever the person identifies. "This definition helps remove the nurse's value judgements from the realm of practice" (Leahey & Wright, 1987, p. 4).

Nursing and Support Linkages: Exploring the Ambiguity

In this section, I briefly explore the linkages among nursing, support, nursing support, and other types of support to reveal the problematic ambiguity that prevents a clear understanding of the concept of nursing support. A more comprehensive discussion in the concept analysis of nursing support (Richardson, 1994) is available on request from the author.

Nursing and Support

As noted, there has historically been the explicit and implicit assumption that nurses should and do to provide support to patients. Florence Nightingale (1860) implied that psychological, informational, and social support were important aspects of nursing. She exhorted nurses to give pleasure to the sick and to advocate on behalf of the patient when it came to limiting visitors.

More recently, influenced by Maslow's (1968) theory about the hierarchy of needs, Henderson (1997) suggested the following definition of nursing:

The unique function of the nurse is to assist the individual, sick or well, in the performance of those activities contributing to health or to its recovery (or to a peaceful death) that the person would perform unaided given the necessary strength, will, or knowledge. (p. 22)

The current focus on providing nursing care that is holistic and contextual includes the family as well as the ill individual as necessary recipients of care. This shift in focus influenced Henderson (1997) to expand her definition to include health promotion activities with the family as a component in the provision of care to the sick. Henderson's definition, which formed the cornerstone of modern philosophical and theoretical understanding about professional nursing, speaks to the significance of the nurse's role in becoming involved only when there is a need and/or request, and only to the extent that the patients (and/or family) require. Implied in Henderson's definition is a respect for the individual's strengths and capabilities. The nurse is not to "take over" or control, but to assist until such time as the individual can again resume self-care, or care of his/her family member, that is, to be a "substitute" to provide what is lacking. This explanation of the role of the nurse correlates well with the health promotion focus of the NSWF Framework presented in this chapter, which suggests the "how to" of the provision of nursing support for families in critical care. Henderson's explanation of the role of nursing informed the concept analysis of nursing support and the resultant definition of nursing support (Richardson, 1994).

Defining Support and Nursing Support

Support is one of those concepts that is in such common use, both within and external to the nursing discipline, that an explicit definition pertinent to nursing practice has been largely overlooked. Many nurse-theorists imply support in their models and theories and some use the term specifically, but to my knowledge none have *defined* it explicitly. Additionally, the literature is rife with inconsistencies, so that at times, two or three compound terms are used interchangeably (e.g., social support and professional support). Definitions are frequently circular. Following the various definitions of support and nursing support, I explore such concepts as social support, and professional, surrogate, or objective social support. These terms are presented to highlight the ambiguity that exists both in the literature and in practice, and to advocate for a more rigorous usage of the term "support."

Dictionary Definition of Support

According to *Webster's New World Dictionary* (Neufeldt & Guralnik, 1991), the term support is derived from the Latin "sub" meaning *under* and "portare," *to carry,* that is, to carry or bear from underneath, bearing up, or upholding. All the definitions cited are closely related: to keep from falling or sinking; to give courage, faith, or confidence to; to help or comfort; to give approval to or be in favor of; to maintain or provide for with money; to maintain, sustain; to hold up or serve as a foundation or prop for; to promote the interest or cause of; to advocate; to help prove; and to corroborate or vindicate.

It is interesting to note that synonyms such as "assist" and "aid" imply different hierarchical roles. The provider of "aid" is in a primary or superior role. The provider of "assistance" is in a secondary or subordinate role (Neufeldt & Guralnik, 1991). All definitions imply one-way help, rather than the reciprocal help that is inherent in the social support definitions discussed in the section, Defining Other Types of Support.

Nursing Support with Families

Nursing support with families of the critically ill adult is health promoting. An acceptance of the inherent value of the family unit and of each family member, and a belief in their abilities to be resilient and adapt in response to crisis, are fundamental presuppositions. Nursing support promotes family and individual integrity by sustaining, augmenting, or restoring these abilities. There are four dimensions of nursing support: emotional, instrumental, informational, and spiritual. These dimensions result from activities associated with connecting, empowering, being instrumental, and discovering meaning (Richardson, 1994; see Fig. 13–1).

The term "assistance" corresponds most closely with the somewhat subordinate role of the nurse in reinforcing the autonomy and strength of the family members. The nurse's cues come from the family. Support is provided where and when it is needed and/or requested. The intent in providing support does not include an expectation of reciprocity (an exchange of benefits); however, reciprocity is frequently an outcome.

In the following section I briefly present the theoretical and research literature about a range of types of support that I considered in developing my definition of nursing support with families.

Defining Other Types of Support

The following is a synopsis of the definitions of social support and professional support (sometimes referred to as objective support or as surrogate social support). Many authors have subsumed all types of support, no matter who the provider is, under the primary label of social support. However, the definitions provided for social support often include dimensions that do not apply to the support that nurses provide. This discussion is presented to illustrate the ambiguity and imprecision that exists in the literature about support, and attests to the value of seeking clarity about a concept and activity considered by many to be fundamental to the practice of nursing.

Social Support

Norbeck (1981) defined social support as mutual assistance that is exchanged among persons who have a social connection, such as family, friends, neighbors, colleagues, and self-help groups, and is not restricted by time and situation. Gottlieb (1983) defined social support as "verbal and/or non-verbal information or advice, tangible aid, or action that is proffered by social intimates or inferred by their

presence and has beneficial emotional and behavioral effects on the recipient" (pp. 28–29). Shumaker and Brownell's (1984) definition includes reciprocity as an integral component of social support. Resources are exchanged between participants to enhance the well-being of the recipient of social support. All three of these definitions exclude consideration of nurses providing social support: Norbeck's because mutual assistance and social connection are not foundational to the nurse-patient relationship; Gottlieb's because he states that the support is provided by social intimates, which nurses are not; and Shumaker and Brownell's because of the expectation of reciprocity, not an expectation of nurses, though it frequently and ideally results.

Stewart (1989) cited Rook and Dooley's cautionary comment, that "social support achieved through interventions should not be assumed to be equivalent in its form or effects to social support normally available from one's family and friends" (cited in Stewart, p. 102). Several years later, Stewart and colleagues (1997) defined social support as "interactions with family members, friends, peers, and health professionals that communicate information, esteem, aid, or emotional help" (p. 95). I question why the form of support provided by professionals would be termed social support if the forms and effects are different as suggested by Rook and Dooley (as cited in Stewart, 1989). The Stewart and colleagues' (1997) broad definition of social support does allow for the consideration of nursing support as one expression of social support, because reciprocity, exchange of resources, and social intimacy are not included. The question I raise is whether this umbrella definition muddles the understanding of both social support and nursing support, or whether it provides a basis from which nursing support could be investigated as *unique* and therefore be better understood.

Laireiter and Baumann's (1993) comprehensive analysis of the field of empirical studies on social support highlighted the following significant points: Individuals do not find every supportive action helpful; in times of crisis, individuals who have knowledge of the situation become more significant providers of social support; in everyday community life, professionals are considered less significant providers of social support than in the clinical settings; at times of crisis, the core support system is less effective; and patients found nurses the most important supporters for psychological and instrumental needs. These results raise the question of whether it is social support that is being provided in times of crisis or whether the nature of the support changes from "social" to "professional." Earlier, Gardner and Wheeler (1987) had discussed the vague and inconsistent definitions of social support, arguing that support provided by nurses should be studied separately from social support even though there are some conceptual similarities.

Langford, Bowsher, Maloney, and Lillis (1997) presented a concept analysis of social support based on their review of the literature. In this analysis, they identified emotional support, instrumental support, informational support, and appraisal support as defining attributes of social support. Reciprocity must be present for social support to continue. These defining attributes occur in the presence of antecedents (social network, social embeddedness, and social climate), and the results are positive: health and well-being. Certainly, these antecedents are not required for the provision of nursing support, indicating a significant difference between actions deemed to be evidence of social support, and those that provide evidence of nursing support. Hupcey (1998) also completed an extensive review of the literature on social support in order to clarify the concept. She proposed the following definition of social support: "a well-intentioned action that is given willingly to a person with whom there is a personal relationship and that produces an immediate or delayed positive response in the recipient" (p. 313). This definition clearly removes the professional from the sphere of providers of social support.

Professional, Objective, and Surrogate Support

Norbeck (1988) noted that professional support (sometimes referred to as direct support, objective support, or surrogate social support) exists within the context of professional relationships involved in a health care situation, and ends when the professional service is no longer required. It is not reciprocal. This support is primarily solicited during a crisis when the usual social supports prove inadequate to sustain the family. The professional support required is of high intensity and relatively short duration, and consists primarily of emotional or psychological, instrumental, and informa-

tional support. A number of other authors such as Warren (1999) cite Norbeck in their discussion of professional or objective support. Kupferschmid, Briones, and Dawson (1991) discuss critical care nurses' support for families and patients as objective social support, frequently necessary as a result of hospitalization. This objective social support includes emotional, informational, instrumental, spiritual, and appraisal assistance. Reciprocity is not addressed, nor is objective social support operationally defined in their study. Most recently, Hinds and Moyer (1997) defined professional support narrowly, primarily as informational support.

In her writings on social support, Stewart (1989, 1993) and Stewart and colleagues (1997) follow the lead of Norbeck (1988) in labeling as surrogate support the support provided by nurses during periods of crisis or transition. Stewart and colleagues discuss the roles the nurse plays in enhancing and mobilizing social support indirectly and directly. Surrogate support is provided when nurses play a more direct role in enhancing the patient's social support. Stewart (1989) also speaks of nurses providing instrumental support.

Gardner and Wheeler (1987) discuss the vague and inconsistent definitions of support and social support, arguing that they should be studied separately even though there are some conceptual similarities. More recently, Hupcey and Morse (1997) pose the critical question I have been asking for some time: "Can a professional relationship be considered social support?" They argue that "significant differences exist between social support and professional support [many due] to the nature of the relationship between the provider and recipient of support" (p. 275). Hupcey and Morse's ideas resonate for me. They challenge traditional thinking about social support and extend our understanding of the complex phenomena of social support and nursing support.

Practitioners with other populations and from other disciplines need to explore the concept of support to further refine it in light of their experiences. I am confident that such inquiry will reveal that there is overlap among practice disciplines and client populations in their understandings and actions of support. It is premature at this time, however, to propose a broad "professional support" definition that would encompass the practice and populations of other professionals, such as teachers, social workers, and physicians.

The Family, Critical Illness, and Nursing Support

During times of stress, most families are able to support, comfort, and give their members a sense of belonging. When the nature of the crisis involves a threat to one family member's life however, and requires urgent or emergency admission to hospital and especially to a critical care unit, the family must yield responsibility for their ill relative to professionals (Heater, 1985; McClowry, 1992). Critical care nurses are primed to provide all measures of support for their patients. In contrast, family members of critically ill patients have difficulty securing support from nurses to augment their indigenous supports (Halm, 1990). In critical care areas, support for the family is frequently hit and miss, dependent on such factors as time, personality, experience, and inclination. In fact, critical care nurse-family interactions have been described by family members as limited, stressful, and less than satisfying (Chesla, & Stannard, 1997; Rodgers, 1983). Often families are viewed as sources of stress by nurses (Gardner & Stewart, 1978). Rodgers (1983) suggested that a nurse's interaction with families in critical care is also limited by a perceived lack of knowledge in dealing with the family, and by the primary focus being on the care of the patient.

Family members may experience feelings of helplessness and hopelessness, states that are associated with an inability to provide emotional support to their ill relatives (Krantz, 1980), and suppression of their own immune systems (Stewart, 1993). As well, multiple nursing studies have demonstrated that the negative effects of the critical care experience on family members may last long past the acute stage (e.g., Titler, Cohen, & Craft, 1991).

The scenario presented at the beginning of the chapter about John and his family illustrates these points graphically. The nurse provided a degree of "informational support," only one dimension of nursing support for families as it is defined in this chapter. In some situations with family members, informational support is adequate in and of itself. In the case of John's family, it is clearly not enough to help family members cope with the shock of the crisis they are experiencing. The nurse's actions did not go far in promoting the health of John's family. Time appeared to be an issue. John's mother and aunt were left standing alone at the bedside, feeling confused, bewildered, afraid, and angry. I am convinced that these emotions, common to family members experiencing a critical care event, can be mitigated by the provision of nursing support. The result of receiving comprehensive nursing support is that family members would feel reassured about the care being provided, empowered by the information learned about treatments and the active role they could play in care, and valued and respected as important members of the health team. Some of the stress due to uncertainty and feelings of powerlessness inherent in critical care situations is avoided. The critical care nurse who provides nursing support to family members is promoting family and individual health by assisting family members in their adjustment to the new reality.

Interventions with family members in critical care must be focused on their perceived needs, assessed from systems and individual perspectives that recognize that these needs are dynamic. If interventions are based on the nurse's perspective, it is not clear whose needs are being met. Molter (1979) conducted a landmark study of a variety of family members' perceptions of their needs, using a 45-item questionnaire she developed—the Critical Care Family Needs Inventory (CCFNI). The results suggest that the need for hope, information, and support were very important for family members in critical care. During the 1980s there was a proliferation of quantitative research using Molter's (1979) and subsequently Molter and Leske's (1983) CCFNI. Leske (1992c) conducted a meta-analysis of the results of 21 studies of critical care family needs that used the CCFNI for data collection. Combined, these studies included responses from a total of 905 family members. Leske identifies five need categories: assurance, proximity, information, comfort, and support. The variety of resources, support systems, and supportive structures that family members need after a critical illness to achieve emotional, spiritual, financial, and personal stability are described as "support needs."

Open visitation (e.g., Krapohl, 1995), family presence during resuscitation (Hanson & Strawser, 1992), counseling interventions (Bunn & Clarke, 1979), family conferences (Atkinson, Stewart, & Gardner, 1980), and support groups (e.g., Halm & Alpen, 1994; Hildingh, Fridlund & Segesten, 1995) are family interventions that have been investigated. Leske and Jiricka (1998) suggest that interventions to mobilize family strengths may help promote family adaptation following a critical care event. Results from all of these studies demonstrate the value of these different interventions to family members in critical care settings.

There has been very limited research about nursing behaviors perceived as supportive by family members, beyond the frequently investigated provision of information (e.g., Leske, 1992b, 1992c; McGaughey & Harrisson, 1994). Irwin and Meier (1973) conclude that families of terminally ill patients identified the following as supportive behaviors: being honest, giving clear explanations and information about the patient's condition, making the families and patients comfortable, and showing interest by answering questions.

This very brief overview of the literature about family members in critical care identifies the need for a theoretical framework to help nurses identify and use interventions that meet the reported needs of family members. Improved and focussed interventions can better promote the health and well-being of individual family members and consequently of the family unit as a whole. The NSWF Framework is presented next: its assumptions, core concepts, informing theories, and practice theory.

The Nursing Support with Families (NSWF) Framework

The NSWF Framework is proposed to help nurses implement the nursing process with family members in critical care. This framework was derived from ethics research that identified providing nursing support as the focus for nursing actions that are based in a context of valuing (Davies & Oberle, 1990). I labeled as "nursing support" those nursing interventions that focus on promoting family member and system adjustment and adapta-

tion, with the objective of optimizing family integrity in the critical care situation. I completed a concept analysis of nursing support (Richardson, 1994) and a meta-review of the critical care literature about families (Richardson, 1998) that were pivotal to the development of the NSWF Framework.

The Framework is composed of three theoretical components: the core concepts, informing theories, and the practice theory. The schematic representation of this model is depicted in Figure 13–1. Assumptions deemed critical to understanding the context within which the NSWF Framework is situated are:

1. Nursing as a profession exists in response to a societal mandate.
2. The family is important to patient recovery.
3. Each family member is of value and deserving of being treated with dignity.
4. All individual members and the family as a whole have inherent strengths and resources.
5. The nurse-family relationship is dynamic and situation-delimited.
6. Reciprocity is not a property of nursing support, although it is frequently an outcome.
7. The goal of nursing is patient and family integrity.
8. The family and nurse should agree on nursing interventions with family members.

Core Concepts

Roach's (1984) basic tenet that "to care is human; to be human is to care" (p. 1) is a core principle underlying the NSWF Framework. Supporting is one of the ways in which caring is conveyed or demonstrated. Anyone who cares has the potential to be supportive. The metaphor for critical care nursing support for families is portrayed in Figure 13–1 as a clover leaf germinated from the "Human Caring Seed."

Other leaves (not depicted in the diagram) could represent social support and support received from other health care professionals (such as physicians, social workers, etc.), indicating that in caring for the critical care patient and family, a collaborative support approach is required to ensure patient and family integrity. Together the "support" leaves and stems would constitute a collaborative

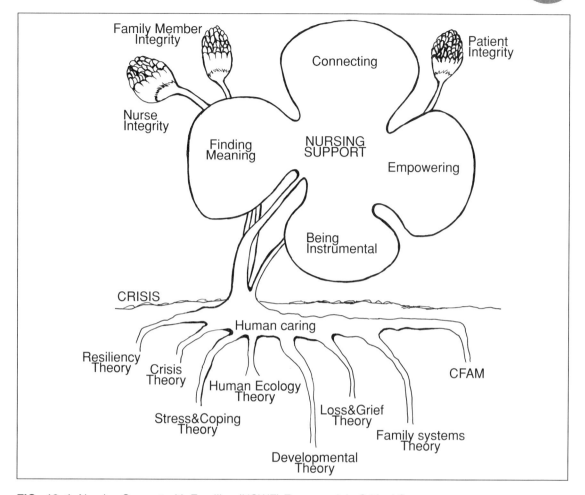

FIG. 13–1. Nursing Support with Families (NSWF) Framework in Critical Care.

support network that potentially exists around a family in response to the critical care situation. The outcome of *nursing* support, then, is the co-constitution of family-and-nurse integrity, always within the context of other sources of support.

Watson's (1988) theory of nursing focuses on humanistic and altruistic values, and provides guidance to the application of the "informing" theories outlined in the following section. According to Watson, caring includes a spiritual and metaphysical dimension and is concerned with preserving, protecting, and enhancing human dignity in a fragmented, technology-dominated environment. The Canadian Nurses Association (1997) has formalized this valuing process by declaring those values held collectively by nurses: choice; dignity; health and well-

being; confidentiality; fairness; and safe, competent, and ethical practice. The stalk of the four-leaf clover depicts this valuing, necessary for nursing support to occur.

Henderson's (1997) goal of nursing (cited previously) informs nursing support as depicted by the four-leaf clover metaphor. In promoting independence (or peaceful death), the nurse respects the individual's strengths and capabilities, and strives to assist as needed and as requested, until the individual can assume self-care or resume care for the family member. The nurse serves as a "substitute for what the [individual] lacks" (p. 23). Nursing actions, then, are focussed on health promotion activities with patients and family members.

Levine's (1991) Conservation Model offers support of the ethic that one duty of nursing is to cause no harm (nonmaleficence), either physically or emotionally. Levine views the ability to maintain balance through methods of conservation as something that affects adaptation to illness. Energy, structural integrity, personal integrity, and social integrity all require conservation. Adaptation is defined as the process of change whereby individuals retain integrity within the realities of their environments. Although Levine uses the terminology "patient," the model fits for the family just as well. In the diagram, the outcome of maintaining or promoting integrity is depicted by the flowers that develop from the clover plant.

Theories Informing the Provision of Nursing Support

Various theories were chosen to inform and direct the provision of nursing support. As such, they are depicted in the schematic portrayal of the NSWF Framework as the nutrients in the soil that the roots of the clover plant draw upon; these theories inform the nurse in the process of enacting support. Not all of these theories are referred to at the same time or all the time, and in fact, many of them overlap. In different situations, different theories not shown in the diagram may also inform the nurse. Theories are drawn upon based on the individual family system and family member situation. This eclectic approach is useful because no one theory encompasses every element of the critical care experience of families (Wright & Leahey, 1991).

I have chosen eight theories/models to present here, because these are particularly useful to me in the assessment and intervention domains of caring for families experiencing a critical illness. These theories, models, or frameworks help to explain family responses to the critical care event and help me to direct the choice and/or development of intervention strategies to meet families' needs. The necessarily brief explanation provided for each does not include discussion of the limitations of the theory nor identified researchers and those authors who have subsequently refined it. I encourage readers to examine additional original and later sources to gain more in-depth understanding of these theories and models, and also to consider other theories that may be useful for inform-

ing the provision of nursing support for their own client populations.

Developmental Theory (Carter & McGoldrick, 1989)

As in the case of each individual, the family has a life cycle that includes pivotal events or periods such as marriage, childbirth, adolescence, and death. Developmental theory can help nurses to assess individual family member roles, tasks, and functions over time.

Human Ecology Theory (Bubolz & Sontag, 1993; Bronfenbrenner, 1989)

The ecological perspective views each family member's development within the family system environment, and the family unit's development within the community environment. The environmental context of the family unit and of the community must be taken into consideration during all phases of the application of the nursing process with family members.

Family Systems Theory (Broderick & Smith, 1979)

This theory, rooted in General Systems Theory, views the family as a system composed of members who are interdependent; when one member becomes ill, all family members are somehow affected (Williams, 1974). The family's response affects the patient as well (Doherty, 1985). Family members are complex subsystems within the family system, separate from, yet open to, the environment.

The health care system is also an open system, and nurses, as subsystems of the health care system, constitute key figures with whom critical care families interact. Critical care family members' perceptions of their needs affect their interactions with nurses, as do nurses' perceptions of critical care family needs. Nursing interventions affect the family, and family actions have an impact on the nurse (Doherty, 1985). One of the advantages of applying a family systems framework to the critical care family situation is that it helps to explain the responses of individual members from within the context of the family as a whole.

Loss and Grief Theories (Carlson & Blackwell, 1978; Rolland, 1990)

Grief is considered to be a process through which a person attempts to recognize, resolve, or adjust to loss. Carlson and Blackwell (1978) define loss as any changes in the individual's situation that reduce the probability of achieving implicit or explicit goals. Anticipatory loss is a syndrome experienced by those who begin the grieving process prior to the actual loss and may serve as a valuable coping mechanism enabling the family to rehearse different scenarios of loss (Rolland, 1990).

Stress, Coping, and Crisis Theories (Lazarus, 1966)

Many scholars have proposed frameworks to explain stress and coping, which generally merge systems theory and the developmental approach. One such theory, Lazarus's theory of stress, appraisal, and coping (1966), has as an underlying premise the importance of determining the factors appraised as stressful in order to develop strategies to improve family member coping.

A crisis is a limited period in which an individual or group is exposed to threats and demands that are at or near the limits of their ability to cope (Lazarus, 1966). During this period (usually lasting less than six weeks), a window of opportunity exists during which people are more trusting, open, and amenable to suggestions and interventions. The goal of crisis intervention is to facilitate the family's return to at least pre-morbid functioning.

Resiliency Theory (McCubbin & McCubbin, 1996)

Resiliency theory helps the nurse to assess the appraisal of the event and the family system strengths and resources, all of which influence adaptation to a crisis. This theory provides a framework for identifying interventions to promote a family resiliency.

Calgary Family Assessment Model (CFAM) (Wright & Leahey, 1991)

The CFAM, though not a theory, is included here because it is a useful framework for helping the nurse organize and interpret observations with family members. The CFAM yields family system structural, developmental, and functional information, through the use of tools such as the family genogram and ecomap. All family systems have strengths that can enhance family life. Identifying individual family strengths as well as problems, as they pertain to the family system as a whole

and the various subsystems, are essential for determining appropriate interventions.

Nursing Support with Families Practice Theory

The final component of the NSWF Framework, the practice theory is derived directly from the concept analysis of nursing support (Richardson, 1994). All the categories chosen from the literature about the needs of families in critical care were determined to fit under the umbrella label of nursing support. This is in contrast to Leske (1992a), who identified support as only one of the five categories of needs. The dimensions of nursing support are identified as informational, instrumental, spiritual, and emotional. These four dimensions capture all the activities performed by the nurse that together entail nursing support with families (see Table 13–1).

I use the CFAM as an assessment tool to help identify family member needs, strengths, roles, and interrelationships. Based on the assessment, the nurse chooses from the array of nursing support referents as perceived by family members, a sample of which are presented in Table 13–1. These referents are divided into subjective (i.e., the family member perceives it, e.g., he/she perceives the nurse to be empathetic), and objective (i.e., the nurse can be seen to "perform" these actions, e.g., appropriate gestures and responses). In clinical practice, the subjective referents provide cues to direct specific interventions that can be more objectively measured—the objective referents—and therefore ultimately evaluated. More research attention needs to be focused on the referents of nursing support for families so that reliable and valid methods of measuring the occurrence of nursing support can be developed.

Dimensions of Nursing Support

In selecting the dimensions of nursing support during the development of the NSWF Framework, all uses of the term support were considered, including those that were compound terms, such as professional support, direct support, emotional support, and so on. Three of the dimensions of social support proposed by Langford, Bowsher, Maloney, and Lillis (1997) were chosen (informational, instrumental, and emotional), and the additional dimension of

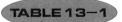

TABLE 13–1

DIMENSIONS, ACTION CATEGORIES, AND REFERENTS OF NURSING
SUPPORT WITH FAMILIES (NSWF)

Dimension	Action Category	Subjective Referents	Objective Referents
Emotional Nursing Support	Connecting	**Demonstrate:** Empathy	**Provide:** Presencing Listening
		Respect	Information
		Concern	Presencing Touch (as appropriate)
		Trustworthiness	Honest reassurance Explain role Explain procedures
		Caring	Social chitchat Touch (as appropriate)
		Valuing	Sharing of info/common bond Requesting a photograph of the patient Asking about patient's life before
Instrumental Nursing Support	Being Instrumental	**Promote:** Comfort	**Provide:** Telephone, blankets, food, sleep, & bathing facilities nearby Comfortable chairs at bedside
		Proximity	Open visitation Waiting room nearby Encourage family to engage in care Phone calls about changes
		Understanding	Advice Clarification Atmosphere that invites questions
		Patient and family interests	Advocacy
		Financial security	Referral to a social worker
Informational Nursing Support	Promoting Empowerment	**Promote:** Understanding	**Provide:** Answers to who, what, where, why, how? Suggest a contact person
		Learning	Technology and treatment info How to provide patient care
		Control	Descriptions of staff functions Nurse-family-physician meetings Opportunities to give care
		Questioning	Nurse-family-physician meetings
		Trust	Honest information Information about credentials
		Validation	Honest praise Referral to support group
		Self-confidence	Encourage questions and suggestions for care Praise for care provided Nonthreatening environment
Spiritual Nursing Support	Discovering Meaning	**Promote:** Hope	**Provide:** Listening for sources of hope (faith, organ donation, etc.) Hopeful and honest demeanor Realistic appraisal of patient condition
		Prayer	Referrals to clergy Time and quiet place for prayer
		Understanding of why?	Listening
		Understanding	Discussion of possibility of disability, death

spiritual support was included based on my experience and a review of the literature specific to this dimension. Critical care nurses and families are confronted with life-and-death decisions at every turn. Family members' needs to maintain hope and to answer the question "why?" pervades the experience. Spiritual support is much broader than, but inclusive of, religious faith.

The four dimensions of nursing support result from the actions of connecting, being instrumental, promoting empowerment, and discovering meaning. These action categories are inextricably interrelated and dependent on the existence of a context in which families as well as patients are valued. The four-leaf clover in Figure 13–1 depicts this graphically, with valuing being the stem supporting the leaf whose leaflets represent the action categories. In fact, one can think of these action categories as developing from: (1) the core concepts that address human caring, valuing of all persons/families, and promoting integrity; and (2) the theories that help to inform the choice of interventions.

The four sections, or the leaflets that form each leaf, are joined in the center, sharing common "space." This aids in visualizing that the four action categories are not mutually exclusive and that certain referents of support are shared by two or more categories. In Table 13–1, I have outlined the links among the dimensions of nursing support, along with the action category that relates to each dimension, and the actions (referents), both subjective and objective, that the nurse adopts in providing nursing support.

Action Categories

The four action categories related to each of the dimensions are explained below. Specific nursing activities for each category are noted in Table 13–1. As a result of these actions, family members in critical care perceive that the nurse supports them.

1. *Connecting* is defined as a dialogic experience involving speaking, hearing, looking, and touching (Pierson, 1999) that leads to a sense of connection, engagement, attachment, or bonding between a nurse and the family member(s) (Clayton, Murray, Horner, & Greene, 1991). There are three components: making the connection, sustaining the connection, and breaking the connection (Davies & Oberle, 1990).

2. *Being instrumental* involves being an instrument of, doing for or with, taking action, or facilitating family members in some tangible way. This includes promoting comfort, proximity, and understanding as well as acting as an advocate on behalf of the family.

3. *Discovering meaning* refers to assisting the family members in their search for understanding about the situation and for hope, in both the spiritual and temporal domains, through activities such as listening, praying, referring family members to clergy, or encouraging other spiritual rituals or practices.

4. *Promoting empowerment* involves actions to promote a degree of family control over their experiences in critical care through such actions as demonstrating respect, allowing open visitation, encouraging family members to be involved in direct care, and providing honest information.

Patient and family integrity are depicted by the flowers that develop as a result of the positive interrelationship of all the support activities provided during the critical care experience by all professional personnel and family members involved. Nurse integrity frequently results as well, depicted by an additional clover flower.

Now let us review a case from my practice in which nursing support for family members was totally absent (of all dimensions of nursing support). As you read, try to identify the missing dimensions and activity categories.

✳ **Reflective Questions**

1. Would you agree that the defining dimensions of support (informational, emotional, spiritual, and instrumental) are completely absent from this example, replaced by distancing or rejection?
2. Why was nursing support not provided to these parents?
3. Should the nurses have provided some measure of support to the parents?

Clinical Example: Case Study

A CONTRARY CASE

A 10-month-old infant who sustained a massive closed head injury is transferred from a rural hospital on total life support to an urban medical center. Parental abuse is suspected. Shortly after admission to the trauma room in the emergency department, staff members are informed that the parents have arrived. No one present verbally or physically responds to this information. An hour later the social worker is observed ushering the parents to the baby's bedside and leaving. No staff members acknowledge their presence in any way. The room is silent. The parents are tearful and visibly upset. All staff members continue to ignore them; there is no touching, no talking, no eye contact.

Now contrast this scenario with another scenario from my clinical practice—one that manifests all the dimensions of nursing support.

The Call for Nursing Support

Professional nurses working in critical care environments are in a prime position to initiate interventions to promote the health of family members while providing the necessary care to the patient. Time need not be a factor if family members are incorporated into the delivery of patient care, either by being encouraged to be present during nursing care activities, or by being encouraged to provide direct care under supervision of the nurse. In this chapter, these interventions and the context for them were grouped under the label of the NSWF Framework, which is based on a definition of nursing support that is similar to, yet different from, social support. Whether nurses respond to the challenge to include family members in their domains of care depends in large measure on the theoretical framework that is applied in practice. The NSWF Framework proposed in

this chapter is one framework that can be adopted to guide nursing practice with families in critical care. The long-term outcome of comprehensively supporting families as they experience the trajectory of a family member's critical illness is improved coping, adjustment, and adaptation for the family. The integrity of the individual and family systems of all involved are promoted. In turn, satisfied, supported family members are better able to work in collaboration with staff and effectively provide social support to the patient in either the recovering process or the dying process.

✳ Reflective Questions

Now that you have completed reading this chapter, recall your responses to the questions presented at the beginning of the chapter. Have your responses changed? How?

1. What nursing actions, if any, would you suggest with the family presented in the opening scenario? Why?
2. In your view, who comprises the "family"?
3. What do you think about open visitation in critical care units? Is this a health promoting practice? If yes, for whom?
4. Can and should you respect and value all your patients and their families? Why or why not?
5. Should the "bedside" nurse work at building a relationship with family members? Why or why not? If yes, how?
6. Who should be responsible for health promotion interventions with family members in critical care? In general units? In acute care? In the community? Why (in each case)?

BOX 13−1

CASE STUDY

Mr. Gee, a 46-year-old divorced, childless, and recently unemployed computer technician, was admitted to the ICU following an unwitnessed beating in which he sustained a Lafort III skull fracture. He had been at a family reunion, where he was attacked by a relative. On admission, Mr. Gee was unconscious, though intermittently very restless, requiring restraints to prevent him from pulling out his endotracheal tube inserted for airway protection. His blood-alcohol level was elevated. The ICU staff nurse admitting Mr. Gee asked the unit clerk to determine if any family members were in the hospital.

BOX 13–1 (cont.)

About fifteen minutes after admission, the family members were called and advised that Mr. Gee's nurse would meet them in the waiting room. On arrival in the waiting room, his nurse introduced herself, explained her role, reassured the family members that Mr. Gee's condition was stable, and asked their relationship to him and what they knew of his injuries. She very briefly described what they would see and hear, including people, alarms, and equipment, as well as Mr. Gee's appearance and his level of consciousness. She encouraged them to feel free to ask her questions at any time. She then took them into the unit, standing nearby as they oriented themselves to Mr. Gee and the environment, noting their apprehension about getting close to the bedside. The nurse asked his mother if she would like to hold Mr. Gee's hand. She responded tearfully in the affirmative, observing cautiously, "I don't want to hurt him." The nurse reassured Mrs. Gee that holding her son's hand would cause no harm and might bring him comfort. The nurse was about to take the mother's hand when she noticed Mr. Gee's sister approaching closer. The nurse watched as the daughter supported her mother in touching her son.

Chairs were provided for the family members, who were encouraged to stay as long as they wished. Questions about equipment, alarms, and care were asked and answered. When the nurse performed a procedure, she explained her actions to both Mr. Gee and his family and talked with the family about him. The picture of a gentle, caring, and very reserved individual was lovingly painted, his passion for mountain climbing and solitude evident in all they said. The horror of this trauma, sustained as he tried to prevent his inebriated nephew from driving, resulted in the family grasping to make some sense of this situation: "He wouldn't hurt a flea."

The family was asked if they had a photograph of Mr. Gee that they could leave at the bedside to help staff better identify with him because he could not communicate. Mrs. Gee remarked that that was a wonderful idea. The nurse waited respectfully while the family prayed for the recovery of Mr. Gee, and afterward, hung his mother's rosary above his bed, at her request. Based on the information that his condition, though serious, was stable, the family decided that Last Rites would not be requested yet, but the nurse would call the Roman Catholic chaplain.

Shortly thereafter Mr. Gee's family decided to leave. His mother took the nurse's hand saying, "I can get a little sleep now. I know you'll be here with Donny. Thank you so much." The nurse reassured his family that she would be called if there was any significant change. His sister was identified by the family as the contact person. The mother left while the sister remained behind. She approached the nurse and asked if the family should get a lawyer for Donny or whether they should take pictures as she felt that someone should know how bad Donny's injuries were. The nurse suggested contacting the police investigator in charge of the case who would be in the best position to advise them. His sister agreed, and after commenting on the excellent care, departed, saying she would call in the morning.

The resident arrived to assess Mr. Gee, and after glancing at the lab results and report of the CAT scan, commented, "Saturday night and another drunk. Look at this alcohol level. And there's brain atrophy indicative of alcoholism. He's probably going to go through withdrawal." The nurse gave her verbal physical assessment of Mr. Gee, concluding with details of the precipitating events, and information about Mr. Gee having climbed Mount Kilimanjaro. The resident replied, "Who would ever have guessed?"

This scenario includes all of the critical dimensions of support: informational, instrumental, emotional, and spiritual. The nurse played the supporting role by:
1. connecting with the family, by talking about the wedding and Mr. Gee;
2. promoting empowerment by deferring to the daughter in terms of support at the bedside for the mother, asking for Mr. Gee's photograph, providing information, and encouraging family presence to help allay uncertainty and fear; and
3. being instrumental by acting as Mr. Gee's advocate with the resident on behalf of the family, and by providing chairs for comfort, and beginning the process of discovering meaning with the family through listening, respecting their praying, and referral to the clergy.

And *very important:* This support was provided at the bedside to the family members during the course of administering to the physical and comfort needs of the patient and in no way detracted from the care provided to the patient.

REFERENCES

Atkinson, J. H., Stewart, N., & Gardner, D. (1980). The family meeting in critical care setting. *Journal of Trauma, 20,* 43–46.

Broderick, C., & Smith, J. (1979). The general systems approach to the family. In W. Burr, R. Hill, I. Nye, & I. Reiss (Eds.), *Contemporary theories about the family* (Vol. 2, pp. 112–129). New York: Free Press.

Bronfenbrenner, U. (1989). Ecological systems theory. In R. Vasta (Ed.), *Annals of Child Development.* Greenwich, CT: JAI Press.

Bubolz, M. M., & Sontag, M. (1993). Human ecology theory. In P. G. Boss, W. J. Doherty, R. LaRossa, W. R. Schumm, & S. K. Steinmetz (Eds.), *Sourcebook of family theories and methods: A contextual approach* (pp. 419–448). New York: Plenum Press.

Bunn, T., & Clarke, A. (1979). Crisis intervention: An experimental study of the effects of a brief period of counseling on the anxiety of relatives of seriously injured or ill hospital patients. *British Journal of Medical Psychology, 52,* 191–195.

Canadian Nurses Association. (1997). *Code of ethics for registered nurses.* Ottawa: Author.

Carlson, C., & Blackwell, B. (1978). *Behavioral concepts and nursing intervention.* Philadelphia: Lippincott.

Carter, B., & McGoldrick, M. (1989). Overview: The changing family life cycle. In B. Carter & M. McGoldrick (Eds.), *The changing family life cycle: A framework for family therapy* (pp. 3–28). Needham Heights, MA: Allyn & Bacon.

Chesla, C. A., & Stannard, D. (1997). Breakdowns in the nursing care of families in the ICU. *American Journal of Critical Care, 6,* 64–71.

Clayton, G. M., Murray, J. P., Horner, S. D., & Greene, P. E. (1991). Connecting: A catalyst for caring. In P. L. Chinn (Ed.), *Anthology on caring* (pp. 155–165). New York: National League for Nursing Press.

Davies, B., & Oberle, K. (1990). Dimensions of the supportive role of the nurse in palliative care. *Oncology Nursing Forum, 17,* 87–93.

Doherty, W. J. (1985). Family interventions in health care. *Family Relations, 34,* 129–137.

Gardner, D., & Stewart, N. (1978). Staff involvement with families of patients in critical care units. *Heart & Lung, 7,* 105–110.

Gardner, K. G., & Wheeler, E. C. (1987). Patients' perceptions of support. *Western Journal of Nursing Research, 9*(1), 115–131.

Gottlieb, B. H. (1983). Social support strategies: Guidelines for mental health practice. Beverly Hills, CA: Sage.

Halm, M. A. (1990). Effects of support groups on anxiety of family members during critical illness. *Heart & Lung, 19,* 62–71.

Halm, M. A., & Alpen, M. A. (1994). Support groups: An annotated bibliography for critical care nurses. *Critical Care Nurse 14*(3), 118–128.

Hanson, C., & Strawser, D. (1992). Family presence during cardiopulmonary resuscitation: Foote Hospital emergency department's nine-year perspective. *Journal of Emergency Nursing, 18,* 104–106.

Heater, B. (1985). Nursing responsibilities in changing visiting restrictions in the intensive care unit. *Heart & Lung, 14,* 181–186.

Henderson, V. (1997). *Basic principles of nursing care.* (3rd ed.). Washington, DC: International Council of Nurses.

Hildingh, C., Fridlund, B., & Segesten, K. (1995). Cardiac nurses' preparedness to use self-help groups as a support strategy. *Journal of Advanced Nursing, 22,* 921–928.

Hinds, C., & Moyer, A. (1997). Support as experienced by patients with cancer during radiotherapy treatments. *Journal of Advanced Nursing, 26,* 371–379.

Hupcey, J. E., (1998). Social Support: Assessing conceptual coherence. *Qualitative Health Research, 8,* 304–318.

Hupcey, J. E., & Morse, J. M. (1997). Can a professional relationship be considered social support? *Nursing Outlook, 45,* 270–276.

Irwin, B. L., & Meier, J. R. (1973). Supportive measures for relatives of the fatally ill. *Community Nursing Research, 6,* 119–128.

Krantz, D. S. (1980). Cognitive processes and recovery from heart attack: A review and theoretical analysis. *Journal of Human Stress, 6*(3), 27–38.

Krapohl, G. L. (1995). Visiting hours in the adult intensive care unit: Using research to develop a system that works. *Dimensions of Critical Care Nursing, 14,* 245–258.

Kupferschmid, B. J., Briones, T. L., & Dawson, C. (1991). Families: A link of a liability? *AACN Clinical Issues, 2,* 252–257.

Laireiter, A., & Baumann, U. (1993). Network structures and support functions. In H. Veiel & U. Baumann (Eds.), *The meaning and measurement of social support* (pp. 33–55). New York: Hemisphere.

Langford, C. P. H., Bowsher, J., Maloney, J. P., & Lillis, P. P. (1997). Social support: A conceptual analysis. *Journal of Advanced Nursing, 25,* 95–100.

Lazarus, R. (1966). *Psychological stress and the coping process.* New York: McGraw-Hill.

Leahey, M., & Wright, L. M. (Eds.). (1987). *Families and life-threatening illness.* Springhouse, PA: Springhouse.

Leske, J. S. (1992a). Needs of adult family members after critical illness. *Critical Care Nursing Clinics of North America, 4,* 587–595.

Leske, J. S. (1992b). The impact of critical injury as described by a spouse: A retrospective case study. *Clinical Nursing Research, 1,* 385–401.

Leske, J. S. (1992c). Effects of intraoperative progress reports on anxiety of elective surgical patients' family members. *Clinical Nursing Research, 1,* 266–277.

Leske, J. S., & Jiricka, M. K. (1998). Impact of family demands and family strengths and capabilities on family well-being and adaptation after critical injury. *American Journal of Critical Care, 7,* 383–392.

Levine, M. (1991). Introduction to patient-centered nursing care. In K. Schaefer & J. Pond (Eds.), *Levine's conservation model: A framework for nursing practice.* Philadelphia, PA: F. A. Davis.

Maslow, A. (1968). *Toward a psychology of being.* (2nd ed.). Princeton, NJ: Van Norstram.

McClowry, S. G. (1992). Family functioning during a critical illness. *Critical Care Nursing Clinics of North America, 4,* 559–564.

McCubbin, M., & McCubbin, H. (1996). Resiliency model of family stress, adjustment and adaptation. In H. McCubbin, A. Thompson, & M. McCubbin (Eds.), *Family assessment: Resiliency, coping and adaptation* (pp. 1–64). Madison, WI: University of Wisconsin Press.

McGaughey, J., & Harrison, S. (1994). Understanding the pre-operative information needs of patients and relatives in intensive care units. *Intensive & Critical Care Nursing, 10,* 186–194.

Molter, N. (1979). Needs of relatives of critically ill patients: A descriptive study. *Heart & Lung, 8,* 332–339.

Molter, N. C., & Leske, J. S. (1983). *Critical Care Family Needs Inventory (CCFNI).* Copyright 1983. Available from authors: University of Wisconsin at Milwaukee.

Neufeldt, V., & Guralnik, D. (Eds.). (1991). *Webster's new world dictionary.* (3rd college ed.). New York: Webster's New World.

Nightingale, F. (1860). *Notes on nursing.* New York: Dover Publications.

Norbeck, J. (1981). Social support: A model for clinical research and application. *Advances in Nursing Science, 3*(4), 43–59.

Norbeck, J. (1988). Social support. *Annual Review of Nursing Research, 6,* 85–109.

Pierson, W. (1999). Considering the nature of intersubjectivity within professional nursing. *Journal of Advanced Nursing, 30,* 294–302.

Richardson, V. A. (Vandall-Walker, V. A.) (1994). *Concept analysis of nursing support.* Unpublished manuscript. Athabasca University, AB.

Richardson, V. A. (Vandall-Walker, V. A.) (1998). *Adult critical care family research: Three decades reviewed.* Unpublished manuscript. Athabasca University, AB.

Roach, S. M. S. (1984). *Caring: The human mode of being: Implications for nursing.* Toronto: University of Toronto Press.

Rodgers, C. D. (1983). Needs of relatives of cardiac surgery patients during the critical care phase. *Focus on Critical Care, 10*(5), 50–55.

Rolland, J. (1990). Anticipatory loss: A family systems developmental framework. *Family Process, 29,* 229–243.

Shumaker, S., & Brownell, A. (1984). Toward a theory of social support: Closing conceptual gaps. *Journal of Social Issues, 40*(4), 11–36

Stewart, M. J. (1989). Social support intervention studies: A review and prospectus of nursing contributions. *International Journal of Nursing Studies, 26,* 93–114.

Stewart, M. J. (1993). *Integrating social support in nursing.* Newbury Park, CA: Sage.

Stewart, M. J., Ellerton, M. L., Hart, G., Hirth, A., Mann, K., Meagher-Stewart, D., Ritchie, J., & Tomblin-Murphy, G. (1997). Insights from a nursing research program on social support. *Canadian Journal of Nursing Research, 29*(3), 93–110.

Titler, M. G., Cohen, M., & Craft, M. (1991). Impact of adult critical care hospitalization: Perceptions of patients, spouses, children, and nurses. *Heart & Lung, 20,* 174–182.

Warren, C. M. (1999). Professional nursing support for culturally diverse family members of critically ill adults. *Research in Nursing and Health, 22,* 107–117.

Watson, J. (1988). Nursing as human science. In *Nursing: Human science and human care, a theory of nursing* (pp. 11–26). New York: National League for Nursing.

Williams, F. (1974). The crisis of hospitalization. *Nursing Clinics of North America, 9*(1), 37–45.

Wright, L., & Leahey, M. (1991). *Nurses and families.* Philadelphia: F. A. Davis.

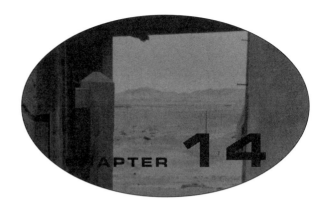

Governing the Health of Populations: Conversations in the Clinic

MARY ELLEN PURKIS

Engaging in the practice of **health promotion** places nurses in a paradoxical position. On the one hand, the sciences informing the knowledge base of health promotion draws in large part on epidemiological studies. This knowledge can be used to help people make healthy choices about the food they eat, the kind of exercise they engage in, strategies for building and developing strong social networks, and so on. On the other hand, nurses' predominant mode of practice is with individuals or with small family groups. Although we might want to engage in health promotion in our practice, many nurses find it difficult to translate available health promotion knowledge into their everyday work with individuals and families.

When you talk with nurses, they tell you why they are interested in engaging in health promotion—they believe health is good. Perhaps they even assume that most individuals they encounter want to be healthier—but whose definition of health is being drawn on when we say this? Think about encountering a young patient in hospital who has been admitted with cellulitis because of repeated IV injections of heroin? Can we assume this patient wants to be healthier? If so, what might health mean to her? How will we work toward a goal of promoting health under these circumstances?

What this example brings to light is that there are different interests at play in this business of defining and promoting health. In this chapter I want to challenge you to think about health promotion as a form of government—both literally

and metaphorically. Local and federal governments are interested in increasing the numbers of healthy citizens because it costs them less money to govern healthy people than those who are sick and in need of care. Governments have always required large numbers of healthy citizens to form armies to fend off foreign dangers. Healthy, contented citizens are less likely to rise up and challenge a government's legitimacy to govern.

But health promotion professionals have a different set of reasons for motivating citizens to take up healthier lifestyles. Often health professionals talk about helping people maximize their potential—to be everything they can be for themselves, not for their government. Nurses and other health professionals also talk about health promotion as a more advanced form of practice than traditional forms of practice—an advancement in their own careers. But for nurses to be able to do the work of health promotion, the people they work with also need to be brought along to think about promoting health. This is perhaps the most difficult work.

In the study reported later in this chapter, mothers marvel at the uniqueness of each one of their children. But they do not think about each one developing at a different pace—a pace that health promoters are interested in for reasons of maximizing the potential of the baby. But when these mothers attend a community health clinic, where the baby's development becomes the focus of conversation with the nurse, the mothers do become interested in the babies' differing rates of development. Even though individual parents, nurses, and state officials seek the same outcome of a healthy citizen, the sketches presented illustrate that each wants this outcome for different reasons.

In their everyday work with people in hospitals and communities, nurses must negotiate the difficult terrain between a knowledge base that provides a particular direction for practice, but does not account for the diverse interests of all those concerned with producing healthy citizens. Nurses must figure out what Foucault (1991) has called "the problem of government." This "problem of government" means that some very particular questions must be asked and answered within the context of practice. For instance, how to govern oneself (how to be a good member of the profession of nursing); how to be governed (how to develop a productive relationship with coworkers and managers); and how to govern others (how to work with parents in such a way that my knowledge and expertise as a health professional is heard and taken up) are questions that give unique form to health promotion practices of nurses.

Does it seem too extreme to equate the work of nurses with the work of governing? Read on and see if the equation bears itself out.

The Problem of Theory for Nursing and Health Promotion

It is not enough to seek structures in language, thought or the human beings who speak, think or know. In all these cases one can connect characteristics of the structure of language, thought or knowledge with the functions they have in and for the life of human beings in groups.(Elias, 1989, p. 68)

Academic nursing has long struggled to narrow the proposed gap between "theory" and "practice." This work is somewhat surprising because our historical memory suggests that the theory of practice came late in our development, with the move of nursing into the academic realm. At that time, a shift in our collective understanding of the relationship between theory and practice took place. Having entered the scene rather late, theory was now to be taken up by practitioners as coming *ahead of their practice*: that is, that theory should *inform* practice.

There are clear advantages for a profession like nursing in such a formulation of the "theory-practice" divide. Where theory can be said to guide practice, then predictions about good practice can be made. Predictions can also be made about the outcomes of good practice. In an age of accountability such as that of modern health service delivery, such abilities to predict cannot be ignored. But, as Elias (1989) warns, "*it is not enough* to seek structures in language, thought or the human beings who speak, think or know" (p. 68, emphasis added). The relationship between theory and practice widely accepted as accurately representing the current state of affairs in fact institutes the divide between theory and practice. Theory is taken as the "structure" of practice. If we take up Elias's formulation and seek to "connect characteristics of the structure of language, thought or knowledge with the functions they have" (p. 68) in everyday life, the divide vanishes. Practice *is* theoretical!

In this chapter, the location of theory in relation to practice will be examined. This examination will reflect Elias's (1989) concerns to connect structures found in language, thought, and knowledge with the functions, or as I will refer to them here, the effects those structures have in everyday nursing practice. My interests in recasting the relationship between theory and practice in this way are two. First, I wish to challenge the claim that nurses require specific training and the adoption of particular theories to guide their practices of health promotion (Canadian Nurses Association, 1988; Labonte, 1997; Meleis, 1990; Pender, 1996). This call for training arises from an assumption that theory comes before practice and the associated, though rarely articulated, assumption that practice is not, itself, already theoretical. This is my second and related interest: to demonstrate, through detailed description, that practice is *already* theoretical and as such, has effects that have largely been ignored in writings about nursing practice. I do not mean that those who write about nursing practice know about the effects and have simply ignored them. Rather, in adopting a stance regarding a particular relation between theory and practice, their descriptions of practice slice away evidence of these effects (Purkis, 1994). In an era when the demand to demonstrate effective outcomes has become so prevalent, it is important to explore all avenues that might help us provide such demonstrations.

Practitioners have become familiar with the demands, building over the last decade of the twentieth century, to demonstrate effectiveness in practice. Such demonstrations are problematic within the context of health promotion. Even though it is relatively easy to account for the successful completion of 30 coronary artery by-pass surgeries, it is much more difficult to account for having prevented 1,500 such surgeries through advocating the uptake of nutritional and exercise programs designed to reduce arteriosclerosis.

Nursing has an additional problem in this realm of health promoting practice. How do we account for our practice as *nursing* practice when the theory of health promotion tells us that the patient is to be understood as controlling how and when to make changes in his or her own lifestyle? Theories of health promotion, with their assumptions that speech, thought, and knowledge are separate things, regularly fail to appreciate how the very act of a nurse speaking with a patient involves an intricate *process* of discipline. This is not to say that speech constrains. Speech (thought, knowledge) also enables meanings to be produced. So we cannot avoid the discipline of our speech, knowledge, and thought. We can, however, describe it and explain how, as an integral part of our practice, it is effective in particular sorts of ways.

If we are going to open up other possibilities to examine how theory and practice relate beyond one totalizing view that theory comes before practice, we need to examine practice from a different location. The dominant understanding of the relationship between theory and practice suggests that we need to locate ourselves in theory, say theory of health promotion and, from there, evaluate how well practitioners are doing against the dictates of the theory. Instead of this, I will locate myself in practice and, from there, describe the effects of nursing practice.

To remain consistent with my own philosophical position in this chapter, I acknowledge that, of course, these descriptions that I offer are not arising in any sort of "pure" way from the data collected during my ethnographic research study of nursing practices of health promotion (Purkis, 1993). Indeed, my descriptions reflect disciplined readings that are informed by the work of social theorists (Elias, 1989; Fernandez, 1986; Latour, 1987; Munro, 1998a, 1998b; Rose, 1996), sociologists (Armstrong, 1983; May, 1992a, 1992b; O'Brien, 1994, Petersen & Lupton, 1996) and nurses (Allen, 1995; Bjornsdottir, 1996; Heslop, 1998; Latimer, 1997, 1998; Mueller, 1995; Nelson, 1997, 1999; Parker, 1997; Purkis, 1994, 1997, 1999; Rudge, 1998). In different ways, each of these authors seeks to disrupt taken-for-granted ideas about theory and practice. Their insights in this regard are helpful in broadening the debate on "effectiveness" in nursing practice and how we can use alternative means to describe the effects of nursing practice. From here, we can begin to discuss whether these are the effects our clients and we believe we should be achieving.

Nursing and Governmentality

The chapter began with a challenge to think about nursing as a form of government. I want now to push that challenge a little further. To begin, I would ask you to think about nurses being *positioned* within a wider health care system. As knowledgeable members of a system that is organized around medical practice, nurses are positioned to translate technical information about health and illness in ways that are meaningful for people seeking assistance. In the community, nurses are also positioned to translate knowledge about health and illness as it is understood within families and give that knowledge a "professional" turn. Nurses are disciplined members of a professional group who take their responsibilities to care for the sick and improve the health of the wider population seriously. It is from this place of serious engagement in the work of nursing that client populations come to be treated (by nurses and by society as a whole) as appropriate populations for nursing care. We know who we are and what we are about. In order to go about our work, we require patients or clients. We transform people into patients or clients so we can achieve our professional aims. It is in this transformation of people into populations and with the effects of such transformational practices that this chapter will explore. As such, nursing will be studied as a particular instance of what Foucault (1991) describes as "governmentality." Only a very brief introduction to this concept will be provided here. Descriptions of practice within a community health clinic will be presented in the following sections to illustrate the ways in which this notion of governmentality is a significant one for those interested in critically examining the effects of contemporary nursing practice.

Studies of governmentality must necessarily be concerned with studies of conduct. For Foucault (1991), the notion of conduct refers to something much broader than "activities" or "behavior." Conduct refers to an association of, on one side, specific apparatuses or techniques, and on the other, a complex of knowledges organizing everyday life. So, Foucault's concern is not with a particular outcome but with complex processes. For instance, consider the word *conduct* in relation to the nursing practice in a public health clinic: the term "conduct" is used here to refer to the way in which techniques used by nurses to determine a child's "development" are *produced by* knowledge (statistically derived predictions about "normal" biological and psychological development) but are also *productive of* knowledge (effectiveness of parenting skills). These knowledges are taken up both by parents and nurses and are used by them to make meanings about any number of things like the relative health of a particular child in contrast to his brothers and sisters or about the ability of a woman to successfully fulfill the role of mother. It is important to note that these meanings do not reflect an objective form of truth but rather are shot through with beliefs held by people occupying particular positions. The techniques are designed by nurses to signal to parents how to adjust their practices in the home in order to keep their child's development within "norms." So, conduct refers not just to the surface *actions* of nurses or parents. Conduct also refers to the ways in which all actions constitute knowledge about parenting; knowledge that, beyond the walls of the clinic, *incorporates* systems of order taken by nurses as crucial for the ongoing progress of society.

In his writings on governmentality, Foucault (1991) was interested in demonstrating how the practices of everyday life, practices like those involved in taking one's child to the community health clinic, constitute processes of ordering. The aim of these ordering processes is, according to Foucault, to facilitate the practices of government. Through such processes, governing is no longer just the responsibility of one, single authority but, in addition (indeed, by multiplication), is accomplished everywhere through disciplined practices of managing populations. The example of the baby clinic is exemplary in this regard: Nurses monitor children's physical development and provide instructions for parents about how to improve on these developmental activities in the home. Thus, the aims of society for a healthy population are being affected through the everyday work of nurses in the clinic and, from there, by parents in the home. How these processes are enacted will now be examined.

Getting a Measure on Health

In the community health clinic, measurement is influential. Measurements of each child are taken prior to counseling sessions with the nurse. Measurements are not merely functional. That is, they not only provide the nurse with information to show parents, they are also drawn on in the constitution of hierarchical or asymmetrical relations between parents and nurses. For instance, measurements are obtained in such a way that nurses occupy the position of expert; only the nurse reads the weight, she[1] conveys this information to the parent, usually after converting the measurement from the metric system into the imperial system. The nurse then makes another translation when she turns the number into an "X" on a graph—a graph that bears no resemblance at all to the physical appearance of the child. Parents occupy the position of helper; they hold the baby still while the nurse places the tape measure in a very precise and presumably knowledgeable way against the baby's body. Parents wait to be told about how their babies measure up.

The taking of measurements serves to apply a frame to the child's body. Because, as I have noted, the measurements bear no resemblance to the physical appearance of the child, the frame is drawn on as a resource by the nurse to accomplish her position of expertise in relation to the parent. Having been measured, the child is no longer unique and therefore "unknown" to the nurse. The nurse

---

[1]Female gender in reference to nurses is used throughout the chapter because this reflects the makeup of nurses observed during the research.

now, through the device of measurements, "knows" about the child. She can approach the child knowledgeably through the transformations she accomplishes. For a while at least, the parent turns over expertise to the nurse. In so doing, parents also turn over the forms through which their child will be represented during the encounter. That is, although parents might represent their child as "quieter than her older brother" or, "the apple of his mother's eye," once in the clinic, the nurse's approach to the child takes place through a deferral of these other forms of representation (Latour, 1987). Measurements *facilitate* an approach to the child for the nurse. However, they facilitate it by slicing away other forms of representation that might arise from experiences parents may have of their child. To the extent that nurses are successful in deferring the parent's rendering of the child, the nurse controls her own "size" within the clinic. Latour argues that the accomplishment of "size," and particularly asymmetrical size, is an effect of power and, as such, has an important influence on the production of meaning. Concerns with relative "size," therefore, are significant, as the following example demonstrates.

In the following scenario, Helen, the clinic nurse, begins a counseling session with Anne, mother of Tom and Dan. It is Tom who has been brought to the clinic for immunization on this particular occasion. He is four months old. His brother Dan is three years old. Anne holds Tom on her lap while she and Helen talk. Dan plays on the floor with toys brought to the clinic by his mother. Tom has been weighed and measured by Helen, and they settle in the more private clinic office where Helen shows Anne the results of the measurements.

HELEN: OK. This young man . . . is a big boy.
ANNE: Uh hmm.
HELEN: Here's his, now I've put it in just that shade over the four months /[2]
ANNE: / yeah /
HELEN: / and he's *ju-u-st* below the ninetieth percentile for length /
ANNE: / uh huh /
HELEN: / so he's mo-o-oved up tremendously 'cause he was just above average /

---

[2]Diagonal marks (/) indicate an overlap of conversation. Three dots (. . .) indicate a brief pause or that conversation trails off.

ANNE: / Yeah /
HELEN: / And his weight is just a bit below seventy-fifth so actually you can see that calorie growth has gone length-wise and he needs to fatten up a little. Eat a little bit more. Slow down his activity, whatever.
(Anne laughs.)
HELEN: Yeah, sometimes that length will parallel off while the other . . .
ANNE: Dan was always tall, he was always up in the ninety . . .
HELEN: Yeah, well, he's certainly not underweight. *(Helen glances over to where Dan is playing beside Anne's chair.)*
ANNE: No, he's not suffering at all.

Helen begins the encounter with the measurements in hand. She has translated the measurements from raw numbers into "X's" on a graph. She joins the "X's" from Tom's previous visit to the clinic at two months of age. In so doing, Helen positions herself to offer a particular interpretation of Tom's growth. Slicing away Anne's understanding of Tom by focussing on the graph, Helen gains size in relation to Anne.

The transcript suggests, through conversational tactics such as "yeah" and "uh-huh," that Anne is "following" Helen through the interpretation of the "X's." She gives Helen the floor and, for a while, allows Helen's representation of Tom to stand. Then, Helen goes too far. She overextends her interpretation. Helen is serious in her instruction to Anne that action should be taken in order to bring Tom's weight and height measurements into alignment. But Anne's laughter at Helen's instruction signals that, rather than taking the instruction seriously, Anne has read Helen's suggestion as an attempt at humor.

Helen's position in the clinic as someone who has legitimacy to instruct new mothers is in jeopardy. Realizing suddenly that Helen is "serious," Anne's next comment that Tom is growing in a similar pattern as his older brother "saves" both Helen and the graph. Helen has been unsuccessful in slicing away all of Anne's experience. In order to save the graph and herself (for further instruction), she must agree with Anne's representation of the two children as growing in similar ways. She must also align with Anne to agree that Dan, the older child, gives every appearance of normal growth and development: "He's certainly not underweight."

This reading, or interpretation, of clinic practice draws on the work of Bruno Latour (1987). Latour's work offers an analytic perspective permitting a serious regard for all practices constituting nursing care in the clinic. It also enables an analysis that treats practice as *in process*. This example illustrates how Helen, a highly experienced clinic nurse, launches into what she would describe as a "typical" encounter with a mother in the clinic. But no matter how mundane an interaction might appear at the outset, there are always surprises in practice. One moment Helen is completely at ease in her role as clinic nurse. The next moment her very credibility as someone with legitimate authority to instruct new moms is in question. Practice is always *in process*.

This is not to say that *anything* is possible. Practice is structured in ways that privilege some people and materials over others. Nurses offer *advertisements for order*[3] in their conversations that, when picked up by parents, mean that health gets promoted in particular ways. For instance, even though Helen and her graph are influential in organizing what gets talked about in terms of the baby's development, Anne's laugh disrupts the flow of conversation. Helen's ability to treat the graph as the sole definer of Tom's development is not fixed. There are other readings that could be made. Anne's preferred reading would be to treat her child's *appearance* as more significant in terms of "evidence" of healthy development than the translation of her child's body into *measurements* depicted on the graph. So the

graph, typically not challenged by parents attending the clinic, remains viable as a clinic artifact. But it no longer has the strength and size it was observed to have in other nurse-parent encounters.

A nurse's ability to apply standards drawn from measurements onto the child's body positions her to interpret what the measurements mean and how they will be used during the interaction. However, as this first example demonstrates, nurses cannot take their interpretations for granted. Challenge is possible, though rarely observed in the clinic. Most often, measurements of the child's body puts the nurse in a strong position not only to influence how the measurements are to be read, but the extent to which those readings are considered valid. The taking of measurements plays a significant part in confirming asymmetrical relationships.

Audit: A Site for Health Promotion

Interpretations of each child's measurements serve an important part in accomplishing asymmetry of relations between parents and nurses. However, because it is not an entirely secure means to achieve asymmetry, it is supplemented by other features of practice. Once measurements are interpreted and the interpretations conveyed to the parent, nurses engage in a process of seeking accounts from parents about their child's development. The "audit" of parental accounts is the primary "site" of work in the clinic and is the innovative feature adopted by nurses to accomplish an economic form of health promotion.

Parental accounts are organized within a context of mutual obligations to account and to attend to the accounts given during clinic visits. As part of the audit, "parental concerns" are constituted as "needs." An example will demonstrate how these features operate. Diane, the nurse, engages mother, Sylvia, in conversation about baby, Liz.

DIANE: So, she's been OK the last little while? No health concerns or . . .?
SYLVIA: No, no. She did have a little bit of a rash for a while and I think we've figured that one out now . . . so . . .
DIANE: Oh, where did she have her rash?
SYLVIA: Everywhere.
DIANE: Oh, really? What do you think it was?

---

[3] "Advertisements for order" is a phrase employed to describe patterned phrases used by nurses in the clinic. Strategic use of these phrases by nurses was observed to provide parents with categories around and through which they could organize their accounts about their children. As such, the organization of accounts of childhood development is framed by nurses while filled out by parents. That parents were easily able to "fill out" the categories suggests that these categories are not unfamiliar to parents. That is, parents have been primed to fill in the categories through their own access to knowledge about childhood development from reading that they have done at home, or through conversations with parents with children of a similar age to their own. As will become clear later in the chapter, parents' willingness and ability to engage in such framed conversations around topics such as childhood development means that the nurse's influence can extend well beyond the geographic boundaries of the clinic.

SYLVIA: I think it was baby lotion. I think she was allergic to baby lotion. She had it *all* over her body 'cause when we /

DIANE: / Really? Was it a perfumed one?

SYLVIA: . . . It was the baby . . . [name] baby lotion.

DIANE: Oh, really? And as soon as you quit using it, it seemed to go away?

SYLVIA: And actually it was coincidental that we did it 'cause we started her on formula about the same time so uhm, we thought it was formula. So we changed to soy, uh soy at one point and she reacted to that, she just threw up everything. So uhm, we couldn't figure out what it was and then the doctor told us to try a [cream] with uhm, cortisone. As soon as I started that it went away like, right now. So we, and then she hasn't had it since and we put her back on the formula so we figured it must be the baby lotion.
(Liz makes talking noises.)

DIANE: Some of those baby lotions are really scented and, I mean babies don't need all those perfumes and /

SYLVIA: / No /

DIANE: / it's more really for the adults!

SYLVIA: That's right! So we don't use it at all any more and she's fine now.

DIANE: OK, so she's on formula now?

This exchange between mother and nurse is, like the one in the preceding example, typical of conduct during a clinic visit. Diane begins with a vague question about Liz's health: "So, she's been OK the last little while? No health concerns or . . . ?" Enacting an *advertisement for order* in the clinic, Diane underlines her invitation to talk with the cue of "health concerns." This is an example of nurses building in redundancy to their talk, "ordering" Sylvia to frame her response narrowly against the breadth of possibilities available within an account of how the baby is "OK."

Sylvia's response to Diane's question is significant. It is important to note that Sylvia has a choice at the outset of this conversation. She can choose to offer an account of a health concern or she could simply indicate everything is fine. Having raised a concern about a rash, Sylvia immediately indicates that Liz only had the rash for "a while" and that it is now resolved. But the "concern" has been launched and it is available for nurse Diane to follow up on. Indeed, several other interesting possibilities arise: Liz is now on formula; the

rash was read by Sylvia as a reaction to the formula, so a decision was made to start Liz on a soy milk product; there was a more significant reaction to that; Liz and Sylvia have been to see the doctor; lotions have been prescribed; and so on. Sylvia's account offers a minefield of possibilities for a nurse interested in promoting health!

Sylvia may feel she has offered too much information. The "concern" about the rash closes with a statement from Sylvia that they have learned from this episode: They do not "use [the baby lotion] at all any more," and, perhaps more firmly that the baby is "fine now." There are no other concerns.

But Sylvia has not achieved sufficient size to control this conversation. There is material available for nurse Diane to proceed with. She picks up on the mention of formula and the conversation proceeds through an account of the details of feeding regimes.

The topics for discussion are not likely surprising to any one with experience in early childhood development. What is interesting to note, however, is the manner in which these topics come up for discussion. In only one instance during the observations of nurse-parent encounters were nurses unsuccessful in stimulating a parent to offer an account such as that provided by Sylvia. This regularity, this *conduct,* is significant in relation to one of the "problems" of this form of nursing practice called health promotion. Specifically, I refer to the "problem" of accounting for effective nursing practice when it is patients who carry out the work of promoting their own health. The work of getting parents to produce accounts of their child's development can help us examine how nurses are successful governors of parents so that parents routinely offer accounts of their parenting activities in response to quite vague prompts on the part of the nurse.

Nurses in the clinic work with assessment forms that demand particular kinds of information be obtained during each clinic visit. Typically, however, rather than relying on that form to direct their practice, nurses elect to employ this other, more *conversational* model to activate their interactions with parents. Conversations of the sort seen between Sylvia and Diane can be said to be successful on two counts. First, they are productive of talk that permits nurses to complete the assessment form (and therefore to be seen by clinic managers as governing themselves well as nurses).

But conversation is also successful in that the identification of concerns can be read (by parents certainly, but also, to some extent, by nurses) as *having arisen from parents directly* and *not* through the use of the clinic's assessment form. It is to the conversational model used in the clinic that I will turn next to explore its use as a preferred and local model for guiding health promoting practice in the clinic.

Conversation and Friendliness in the Clinic

The preceding examples are designed to illustrate that "conversation," as it is used in the clinic, is neither incidental nor natural. Instead, "conversation" represents a skilled and strategic mode of practice employed by nurses as necessary in their accomplishment of health promotion. This may be read by some as too calculating an account of health promoting work. However, in the sections that follow, I demonstrate that these practices are representative of nurses' serious attempts to successfully govern themselves and the people they work with.

To deny the significance of conversation as a disciplined approach to practice is to do one of two things. First, it is to treat nurses as lacking agency in their workplace, that they have no choices in some matters. This undermines opportunities for exploring the systematic ways in which asymmetries in practice settings are enacted *through* nurses' agency (and therefore removes possibilities for considering new ways for conducting practice). Second, it is to treat the context of practice as exerting force over human actors, which again removes agency and suggests a more rationalized frame for practice than the examples presented thus far support. Therefore, my analysis proceeds on the understanding that actions engaged in by both nurses and parents are knowledgeable and reflective of organized and organizing understandings of social situations. This is not to say, however, that nurses and parents come to the encounter equally capable of organizing.

The notion of the life-world gains importance here. The life-worlds of the clinic and of the home serve as structural reference points contributing to organized and organizing conduct. The aim in the following examples is to illustrate the extent to which conduct in the clinic has an effect on parental conduct in the home. I want to explain and illustrate the ways in which practices enacted in the clinic cut across life-worlds, influencing the nurses' life-world and the parent-child life-world in particular, and different, ways. As the concept "life-world" suggests, the concern here is to show how spaces are defined and differentiated from one another. In the following pages, I describe a pattern that was observable in the clinic encounters. The pattern involved nurses treating the clinic, and specifically the office where counseling sessions were conducted, as a principal work site. Within this site, problems in need of instruction were raised to the surface. The problems were of a particular sort. That is, where a variety of problems were available to the nurse, she would select one or two for which she already had a solution readily available. These problems were then removed from the entanglements of their site of origin, the home, and discussed in a much more abstract way in the "cleaner," more standard (to the nurses) context of the clinic. Parents were then left with the work of re-contextualizing instructions into their particular home circumstances. This work involved parents having to make accommodations within the life-world of the home. That is, in order to follow the instructions given by the nurse in the clinic, the home underwent adjustment to accommodate the nurse's instructions.

The example of mother Marcia and her four-month-old baby, Kim, provides an opportunity to examine some features of how the life-world of the clinic operates in relation to the life-world of the home. Nurses from the clinic had seen Marcia and Kim on two previous occasions. The first contact was during a home visit shortly after Kim's birth. The second contact took place at the clinic when Kim was two months old. Marcia has returned with Kim, now four months old, for the next immunization in the series. Kim's weight at this visit was found to have decreased as represented on a graph. Nurses had told me that they used the graph to "alert" them to situations where a child may not be gaining weight sufficiently. If a child's weight was "seen" to be dropping over time, staff members would take this as an "alert" that they "should be watching . . . seeing what's happening." This particular case offered just such an "alert." Yet, no follow-up was suggested nor instituted.

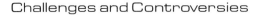
I do not want to treat this as an example of practice "gone wrong," but rather to treat the case as an instance of how prevailing images of work are brought to bear on such "problems" in order to *enact "watching" from the clinic itself.* As a negative case of clinic policy, the example can be used to further demonstrate the extent to which audit stands as the central "site" of practice.

Constructing a "Need"

The sequence of the visit was no different than any other observed at the clinic. Measurements were taken out in the waiting room and then Marcia was invited by nurse Helen to enter the private office. Through the entire interaction with Marcia, Helen gives no verbal indication that she is anything but supportive of Marcia's maternal conduct. After Marcia leaves, Helen recounts to me quite another understanding of Marcia: Helen believes Marcia is "insecure" and "doesn't pick up on things right away." In an interview with me immediately following the encounter between Helen and Marcia, Helen suggested that the measurements were important in her understanding of the "problem":

HELEN: See, it started above the fiftieth, leveled to just above the twenty-fifth, now it's just above the tenth.

In the interview with me later, Helen compares Marcia with another mother whom she had also "counseled" on this particular day:

HELEN: This last one [Marcia] is more insecure as to how things are going. Obviously doesn't pick up on things right away.

Helen's interpretation of the encounter suggests just how deeply influenced she is not only by the measurements, but the measurements within the context of her "reading" of this mother's conduct in the clinic.

Returning now to the encounter between Helen and Marcia, Helen starts by relaying the measurements to Marcia. Helen was visibly somber as she began to interpret the results of the measurements to Marcia:

HELEN: OK, let me show you where she's at here. She's . . . moved down a *little* off the seventy-fifth to just above the fiftieth for *length* . . .

MARCIA: Um hmm . . .
HELEN: She's slowed up a bit. She didn't *gain* a tremendous amount here. She's moved . . . on the tenth percentile /
MARCIA: / Oh! /
HELEN: / and she was on the twenty-fifth so . . . Has she been ill or not feeding as good or just, really, activity changed that she's just really more and more active?
MARCIA: Yeah, I find that she's really more and more active.
HELEN: Yeah, she's *burning* those calories.
MARCIA: Yeah, she used to sleep a *lot.* She used to sleep, you know, eight to . . . well, no, actually from about nine o'clock to about seven and then /
HELEN: / ten hours . . .
MARCIA: . . . yeah from about eight to twelve. From one to four and *now* she's starting to, you know /
HELEN: / Not sleep as much /
MARCIA: / Yeah /
HELEN: / and so she's burning more of the . . .
MARCIA: Yeah, the nights more is, is the same but the morning is just two hours and then in the afternoon maybe an hour and a half /
HELEN: / Ah *ha!* /

Using the graph to "show" Marcia the changes, Helen makes a series of moves beginning with the height and then the weight measurements: showing by saying what she sees (Foucault, 1973). Marcia expresses surprise at this information. Helen offers a number of labels for "problems," which serve as advertisements for ordering a work space for the visit: She suggests that Kim might have been "ill" or "not feeding as good" or that her "activity" level might have increased. Helen "secures" a cause ("more and more active") for the problem by offering Marcia a menu of options.

Helen's "view" of development is tightly coupled with the growth chart. As a device for structuring the clinic visit, the chart's most narrow use is employed to quickly set up boundaries around a "problem." The problem of "insufficient weight gain" rests entirely on the technological device of the graph to provide visible "evidence" of the status of the problem. Drawing on Marcia's "account," Helen identifies the cause for this problem—increased activity. Helen then supplements Marcia's account with a technical account of the problematic weight gain ("she's *burning* those calories").

Once "activity level" is settled between them as a device for ordering the conversation, Marcia supports the construction of the problem by providing further accounts of Kim's behavior in the home. Sleep is raised as a prime indicator of activity levels. Marcia supplies "guesses" regarding Kim's activity level.

Instruct-able Problems

Helen's work involves "pulling a problem through" by attending to cues appropriated from the parental account. We saw this previously when Diane pulled feeding practices through Sylvia's account in the preceding example. Input from the parental account gives the "problem" local significance. "Local," however, must be understood as local to the clinic. It is important to recognize that the construction of a workable problem has *not* taken account of the home context. Instead, the problem of "increased activity" arises out of advertisements for ordering work *in the clinic.* Because feeding advice is one aspect of work in the clinic, a problem is structured around the notion of a child who is burning excessive calories. Helen has successfully established space for work. Helen's "instruction" to Marcia is to begin feeding Kim solids immediately:

HELEN: OK. Now I'll tell you what they said last time and you tell me what's new. OK, they've put down that she was breast on demand. What do you notice that she's leveled out too? How frequent are her feeds now?
MARCIA: Uhm, . . . yeah they're, . . . let's see, . . . uh . . . twice in the morning and . . . uh . . . three . . . three or four in the afternoon.
HELEN: OK, so there's about . . . six feeds and then does she feed at nighttime?
MARCIA: No, she goes right through at night.
HELEN: Ah-h-h, . . . OK. And [Helen sighs] were you going to consider some solids in the next little while?
MARCIA: Yeah, I was thinking at . . . maybe at five and a half or six months.
HELEN: OK. See how she does with her nursing. If she still keeps pipped up there as far as not settling down, just because her weight is, is, is dropped that *bit* so that it's well *below* what her height is I might say, even though she hasn't made that six month mark, now's an ideal time to get some extra calories in her /

MARCIA: / Oh! OK /
HELEN: / Yeah. *Not* so that it affects her nursing.

Helen's questions in this segment position Marcia in particular ways. First, Marcia is positioned so that she must provide a "schedule" of feeds. Second, she is positioned to "consider" changing the form of food given to Kim.

Note the ways in which the "problem" is located within the interaction. Rather than leaving it open for Marcia to define signs of weight-loss that she has noticed (other than the one of increased activity, which the problem was initially constructed around), Helen defines and locates the problem with direct reference back to the measurements. The instruction to feed Kim solids is legitimated by Helen "because her weight is, is, is dropped that *bit* so that it's well *below* what her height is." The weight "loss" is made visible by Helen through reference to another measurement—that of height. The "problem" is defined and sustained through reference to the measurements. Helen speaks as an "expert" member of the life-world of the clinic. There is no indication that Helen takes advantage of, or "appropriates," any aspect of Marcia's life-world to construct the "problem." As the following illustrates, this has implications for how the problem is addressed once Marcia returns home.

"Abstracting" Problems in the Clinic

The effect of the process in the previous example is to "abstract" aspects of conduct away from the life-world in which they arise. Abstracting involves a construction of a problem that draws entirely on structures informing practice at the clinic. Abstract must be understood not in its adjectival sense—as a description of a cognitive process engaged in by the nurse. Rather, "abstract" is used here as a verb. The action denoted by the verb is the formulation of an instruct-able problem. Helen *abstracts* Marcia's faltering account of how frequently she feeds Kim into the cleaner, more precise language of the clinic ("OK, so there's about six feeds").

This clarification is important. I do not wish to suggest the description of a cognitive process but rather an inter*action*al one—a material one. The effects of power in the clinic are observable in these terms. In this way, the "abstracting" of accounts represents "typical" conduct in the clinic. The effect is that problems are "wrapped up" in clinic devices: devices for "seeing" them as problems and devices for "solving" the now visible problems. Abstracting, as a disciplining action engaged in by nurses, represents a central aspect of the nurses' expertise in the clinic. The nurses' ability to abstract problems from the audit of "concerns" facilitates her ability to instruct during the encounter.

Abstracting also represents a solution to one of the problems posed by the work of health promotion. In the introduction I raised the problem of enacting a practice visibly different from the "old ways" of so-called traditional, problem-oriented nursing practice. Exploitation of the parents' obligation to account for their child's development enables nurses to instruct parents toward forms of health that can be said by the nurse to have arisen out of the parent's own account—as though the account appeared spontaneously. As illustrated previously, however, this formulation of the appearance of parental accounts renders invisible the significant ordering work sustaining the rich spaces within which health promoting work proceeds. The powerful effects of the conversation observed between Helen and Marcia are only evident when we challenge the taken-for-granted notion that theory drives practice.

Re-contextualizing Abstract Instructions

At an interview in Marcia's home two weeks after her encounter with Helen in the clinic, Marcia gave some indication of how she had "worked out," or re-contextualized, the instructions given to her:

MARCIA: Yeah, I did take her advice in feeding her rice pablum. I started that and she seems to be taking it really good so I must have been doing that for the past, it must be going on two weeks.

ME: And have you noticed any change in Kim?

MARCIA: Not really, not in weight wise like I don't think her legs are chubbier or anything but she's a little bit more active so maybe it is giving her a little bit more energy and helping her to grow.

What Marcia "notices" as a difference is not in weight, but that Kim is "a little bit more active." Marcia concludes that this may be attributable to the rice pablum, understood by her as giving Kim "more energy."

The discrepancy between the "cause" constructed by Helen in the clinic about why Kim was not gaining sufficient weight and Marcia's measurement of "success" of the remedy must be taken seriously. In response to Helen's menu of reasons why Kim's weight had not increased as expected, Marcia stated that she had noticed Kim had become much more active lately. However, back in Marcia's life-world, that is, in her own home two weeks later, Marcia tells me that since she has been giving Kim the pablum, Kim is "a little bit more active."

Earlier in this interview in Marcia's home, she had pointed to some of the "stresses" defining her life-world as a wife and mother of two small children:

MARCIA: It has been a little stressful, you know, mentally because my husband doesn't have a job so it's you know, we're thinking of ways of trying to get rent together and you know things and yet kind of really maintain a character, just hold ourselves together and of course having the little one [Andrew] being so demanding. Kim is quiet, she just occupies herself and does a little bit but he [Andrew] is really demanding and he likes a lot of attention and I find a lot of, I guess maybe rebellion in a way that he doesn't feel like he's getting enough attention.

It should be noted that this account was stimulated by the first question asked at this research interview. An "opening" question was asked regarding how Marcia presently viewed her state of health. It took very little prompting to surface the account. I would argue that it was, therefore, an account that was also available to Helen, the nurse.

There are a number of important points to be made here. First, this account should not be treated as more "valid" than the one obtained by Helen in the clinic. Rather it reflects an account of the life-world stimulated by different institutional constraints (Lyotard, 1984) than that of the account arising in the clinic. The structures enabling, but also constraining, this account of "stress," are *different* from those structures informing the account given to Helen in the clinic regarding how Kim had been feeding.

This insight needs to be pressed further. In light of the "stresses" defining her perceptions of the home environment, it seems reasonable to suggest that, in response to Helen's question about the feeding pattern Kim had "leveled out to," Marcia may not have noticed any pattern at all until she was positioned by Helen's question to provide an account. As the transcript illustrates, when Marcia was asked by Helen in the clinic what Kim's "feeds" had "leveled out to," Marcia was left struggling to provide an account.

In contrast to her account of Kim's feeding regime in the clinic (framed by the life-world of the clinic), the account provided during the interview in her own home suggests that Marcia and her husband are struggling to "get rent together" and "just hold ourselves together," struggling to "maintain a character." Marcia describes her two-year-old boy, Andrew, as "so demanding." Kim, on the other hand, is described as "quiet, she just occupies herself." Given this description of their home situation, it seems plausible that in the turmoil of the day-to-day struggle of keeping the family's collective head above water, Marcia has simply not noticed Kim's growth patterns at all. Kim is a quiet baby amidst the stress and demands of Marcia's life-world. Being a quiet baby, Kim is gaining weight at a very slow rate because her "requirements" are not being noticed above the other demands Marcia is bombarded with on a day-to-day basis.

The discrepancy in Marcia's account can be commented on further. As an effect introduced by the research design itself, this "account" is stimulated by the connection between myself, as the researcher, and the clinic visit where Marcia and I first met. Under ordinary circumstances, an account of the clinic visit would not be sought, although a comment from a neighbor or friend may stimulate a similar sort of account. I recognize that my close connection with the clinic may have an additional influence on the client's attempts to remember the visit, to recall it: to re-visit the visit. Thus, the discrepancy is not as significant for its relative "inaccuracy" as it is for its sense of "accommodation." The problem constructed within the life-world of the clinic has been re-contextualized in Marcia's account two weeks later into the life-

world of the home. As a result, difficulties in "fit" arise, compromises are made to definitions applied in the clinic, and a "new," accommodated account of the child's status is available to the parent for use when someone calls on them to account again.

Making Accommodations in the Life-World

The analysis of Marcia's visit to the clinic and my subsequent visit with her in her home illustrates that parents engage in a significant amount of work around the visit to the clinic. They position themselves to offer accounts to the nurse and then afterwards, to make some form of accommodation for the definition made of their life-world during the clinic visit. As we saw in the example of Marcia and daughter Kim, the account provided in the clinic may contrast radically with understandings of the day-to-day life-world. In the clinic Marcia tells Helen that Kim has been much more active (and this is why her weight has reduced) whereas when I visit in the home, Marcia tells me that the food is making Kim more active—suggesting she had noted Kim's lethargic behavior prior to instituting the new feeding routine.

We can think about these positions that parents assume in relation to nurses and to the visit to the clinic as "preparation," and it is this preparation by the parent that in part sustains "obligations" on the part of parents to give accounts, and on the part of nurses to attend to those accounts. However, as my examples indicate, I am suggesting a preparation that is well prior to the visit itself. This state of preparedness from which parents approach the clinic influences the readings parents make of "regions" in the clinic and how they appropriate meanings made in those regions to accommodate the life-world of their own home.

The effect of making "accommodation" is important to understand practice in the clinic as an example of governmentality. In the next section, I examine accommodations as powerful effects of wider disciplinary processes implicated in the constitution of members' relative size in relation to one another. I propose one explanation of how conduct between nurses and clients in the clinic can be understood in a way that foregrounds practice as a *mutual* accomplishment.

The Convenience of "Fracturing" the Life-World

The predominant location for encounters between nurses and clients was observed to be the clinic. Even where nurses did venture out into the community, the manner in which clients' living areas were rearranged and the conduct of the visits suggested only that a transfer of the life-world of the clinic to a different location was occurring, not an accommodation for different life-worlds. During immunization clinics, *parents bring children to the nurse*. The significance of this move should not be lost in the detail of the visits themselves. The atmosphere of the clinic, friendly but efficient, offers sharp contrasts with the atmosphere of the home. Shifting the "site" of practice away from observation (associated perhaps with more traditional forms of practice such as hospital nursing) to the audit of client accounts represents a radical turn *away from surveillance* of the "visible" *toward a cross-checking of reportable conduct*. This radical turn marks a significant relocation for nursing "action." It is important to note that relocating action from observation to the auditing of accounts takes advantage of a significant feature of the life-world of community nursing practice. In fracturing the life-world of clients coming to the clinic, nurses need to find different ways of constituting knowledge for their practice. Because they rarely observe everyday parenting, they turn instead to *accounts* of parenting. Nurses rely on parents making some aspect of their life-world of the home present for the nurse in the clinic. Giddens (1984) describes such a reliance on accounts as practice that takes account of conditions of "presence availability." Giddens takes these conditions to be pervasive in our society—largely arising out of our increased reliance on computers and other mediated forms of knowledge. Within this study of nursing practice, nurses' reliance on conditions of presence availability has particular effects that can be explored.

For example, Helen's assessment of Marcia's abilities as a mother ("she doesn't pick up on things") stands in contrast to her relatively supportive stance within the encounter. Helen's support of Marcia can be read as exemplifying a "cynical" stance taken by nurses in relation to their practice in the clinic. Nurses in this study treated it as widely known that parents would literally and figuratively dress their children up to bring them into the clinic. The cynicism inherent in such knowledge surely underpins the radical turn away from surveillance—the nurse cannot treat the appearance of the child and the parent as trustworthy. So instead, nurses shift their practice toward a more "visible" cross-checking of reportable conduct. A vague but disciplined question about "concerns" enables subsequent questions about feeding regimes and then about sleeping patterns. The account offered by the parent must maintain a certain level of internal consistency—the parent works hard to ensure this. But where inconsistencies are heard by the nurse, such inconsistencies can be picked up as opportunities to instruct.

The conditions supporting these shifts from observation to auditing accounts find sympathy in Foucault's (1991) distinction between sovereign states and the "art of government":

"The common good" refers to a state of affairs where all the subjects without exception obey the laws . . . the good is obedience to the law, hence the good for sovereignty is that people should obey it . . . Now, with the new definition given by La Perrière, with his attempt at a definition of government, I believe we can see emerging a new kind of finality. Government is defined as a right manner of disposing things so as to lead not to the form of the common good . . . but to *an end which is "convenient" for each of the things that are to be governed*. (p. 95, emphasis added)

The possibility that parents may refuse an instruction (such as was the case where mother Anne took nurse Helen's instruction as humorous) suggests that arguments designed to regulate health through the development of "laws" are largely anachronistic in a modern society. More importantly, given that parents *can* refuse instruction, where instructions *are* followed, we can expect to find, not a docile obedience to a "common good," but rather an intricate series of relations that lead members to follow the instruction presented as a "convenience."

Marcia's account to me two weeks after the clinic visit that, having followed Helen's instruction to feed Kim, she now observes Kim to be "a little more active," might, at first glance, appear to contradict the move to convenience. Surely, given Marcia's stressful and hectic world, it is more convenient to have a quiet baby. But, against Helen's interpretation of Marcia, I would argue Marcia *was* "picking up on things." She is a "good" mother—albeit a highly stressed one. She desires a healthy child. She sees the feeding as "helping (Kim) to grow." *She had an interest* in taking up the instructions offered at the clinic.

This is the economical and convenient model of practice that nurses have worked out. It is hardly necessary any longer to move away from the clinic: The clinic does so much of the work of preparing parents for the visit that nurses can, with just one or two small instructions, effect quite remarkable changes in far distant locales out in the community.

By tapping into such parental interests, a "procedure of power" emerges in which, drawing on particular "tactics" (Foucault, 1991, p. 95), such as conversational techniques, the generation of parental accounts of development by nurses in the community health clinic can be understood as a form of governmentality. Tracing a child's development represents a location where both nurses and parents have an "interest": nurses in recording such development and parents in having development confirmed. Here are the grounds for translations (Callon, 1986; Latour, 1987) of those interests to occur. As "experts in normality" (Foucault, 1979, p. 228), nurses situate themselves as the purveyors of practical knowledge for parenting. Parents come to the clinic in a "stripped-down" version of their day-to-day life-world of child rearing, ready to produce accounts of parental conduct. Rather than employing visual surveillance, linked to the existence of "laws" for the common good (Foucault, 1991, p. 95), nurses at the clinic "cross-check" reportable conduct as a means of effecting governmentality at the "site" of the audit. The "convenience" of having development confirmed by clinic workers means that clients fracture their own life-world, as a form of translation, through their very approach to the clinic. Parents position themselves in relation to the nurse as if they wish to fulfill their own interests.

Governing the Health of Children

For Foucault (1991), governmentality involves an intricate operation of power. This power operates by setting its sights on particular groups of people (such as "parents" and "children") and, by establishing relationships of risk management, domination can be mobilized in ways that ensure economic running of the state through the work of individual members of society. The clinic represents a very specific institutional locale where procedures such as measurements of children's bodies are used to make calculations about parenting abilities. An analysis of the calculations is offered to parents early in the visit through very particular tactics of "friendly conversation." By exploring these friendly conversations as part of the methodology of governing, we can see that the friendliness serves a purpose: that of enrolling parents for the disciplinary purposes of state welfare.

As we have seen, the interpretation of measurements can be taken quite seriously by parents, as in Marcia's case, or they can be "laughed off," as in Anne's. But laughing off the interpretation does not mean rejection of the encounter in its entirety. Anne accommodates her own "error" in thinking that Helen had made a joke. The graph and Helen's position as an influential actor in the clinic may be altered but ultimately, both Helen and Anne have an *interest* in maintaining a relationship, albeit that their interests may be quite different. This is, indeed, a "complex form of power," dynamic in its moment-to-moment expressions and shifts. But it has a target: the family—and perhaps more precisely, the health of children within families.

The analysis I have made of these interactions between nurses and mothers is that these exercises of power represent an economic and convenient form of practice. And here I must underline again the significance of the nurses turning away from the more widely accepted understanding of practice where nurses make observations of bodies and, on the basis of that visual surveillance, enact disciplining practices of health care. Discourses of health promotion have penetrated the practices of nurses to such an extent that nurses in the clinic have shifted the site of knowledge generation away from the body into the auditing of parental accounts of their children's "growth and development." Granted, there is still an opportunity, it might be argued, to observe the body during the taking of measurements at the desk. But a policy change in the clinic serves to illustrate again my point about the turn toward the audit. Just prior to the conclusion of my fieldwork, nurses in the clinic had made a decision that, in order to "save time" for their interviews with parents, they would no longer completely undress children prior to weighing and measuring. Heavy outer clothing would be removed but other items of clothing would remain. This suggests that it is the measurement and not the body that the nurse is interested in. Given the important place that measurements consistently played for each nurse in launching the "conversation" in the interview room, this choice may not be surprising, but it must be treated seriously as arising out of a form of knowledge that organizes conduct in the clinic.

Conduct in the clinic then is:

(f)ormed by the institutions, procedures, analyses and reflections, the calculations and tactics that allow the exercise of this very specific albeit complex form of power, which has as its target population, as its principal form of knowledge political economy, and as its essential technical means apparatuses of security. (Foucault, 1991, p. 102)

And it is through the "apparatuses of security," the ways in which nurses' instructions tap into the interests of parents to ensure them that they are doing everything they can to foster the healthy development of their child, that governmentality has its most profound effect. Even though the "problem" with Kim's development was constructed in the clinic through conveniences that seemed to be nonsensical to an observer, they had an effect. And in this particular case, a "good" effect. The instruction to begin feeding Kim earlier than clinic policy dictated meant that a child whose presence was hardly noted by her mother, a child who seemed at some risk of simply fading away, became a bit brighter and therefore perhaps more noticeable again amidst the troubles of Marcia's everyday life.

Gordon (1991) has commented on a certain form of optimism in Foucault's later works. That optimism is apparent here. And, it speaks to *the limits of health promotion.* Although the effects nurses have from the clinic are far-reaching and, at times, based on only constructions of convenience, *the only effects that they can have are those that are understood as credible by those being governed*: parents and, perhaps in a different way, children. As Gordon (1991) reads this,

---

Foucault seems to think that the very possibility of an activity or way of governing can be conditional on the availability of a certain notion of its rationality, which may in turn need, in order to be operable, to be credible to the governed as well as the governing: here, the notion of rationality seems clearly to exceed the merely utilitarian bounds of a technique or know-how . . . [and] that ideas which go without saying, which make possible existing practices and our existing conceptions of ourselves, may be more contingent, recent and modifiable than we think. (p. 48)

This is optimistic for parents. As Anne discovered, a mere laugh demonstrates the contingency of the nurse's position as expert. And perhaps it is optimistic for nurses too. Within the home, it is more difficult for nurses to issue instructions: In the home, parents are operating more acutely within their own life-world. The nurse must work much harder to bring the life-world of the clinic to bear upon parents there. Although the nurse cannot know for certain that a parent will take up her instructions, the analysis demonstrates that nurses are far more effective than they give themselves—and the parents they work with—credit for. Parents prepare themselves for the visit to the clinic. They dress their children up, and in so doing, assume a stance toward the nurse. It is surely one in which a mother's position as ultimately responsible for her child cannot be questioned—even when there is "evidence" that her abilities might be questioned. But in drawing on parental interests as a convenience, instructions issued in the clinic are re-contextualized within the life-world of the home. In the home, instructions have very clear and specific effects. But significantly, *these are not effects that the nurse can predict.*

Theories operating in practice are those concerned with carefully managing the relationship between parent and nurse. Nurses cannot push parents too far. Parents cannot take advice from nurses too lightly, not if the relationship is going to be sustained. What a prescriptive theory (that is, one that seeks to position itself ahead of practice, to *predict* practice) misses is that parents will make translations of instructions issued in the clinic once they return home. Only by treating actions observed in the clinic as already theo- retical can we expose the powerful effects embedded in nurses' decision to adopt a conversational technique within which to undertake their work. And then, by following parents back into their homes, to be able to expose the multiple ways in which friendly conversations from the clinic come to govern parenting practices in the home.

✸ Reflective Questions

1. When you reflect on your own practice setting, can you describe routine patterns of conduct engaged in by nurses? By patients or clients?

2. In what ways do these patterns of conduct predispose things so as to lead to an end that is "convenient" for members of the professional care team and the clients or patients toward whom that care is said to be directed?

3. When the relationship between theory and practice is challenged such that we treat practice as theoretical we can no longer predict the outcomes of practice. Thinking about practice as theoretical shows up the dynamic and contingent character of nursing practice. Using what you know about Marcia's life-world, how might you engage in a relationship with Marcia if you were the community health nurse?

4. Is it paradoxical to say that nurses can promote the health of their clients?

REFERENCES

Allen, D. (1995). Hermeneutics: Philosophical traditions and nursing practice research. *Nursing Science Quarterly, 8*(4), 174–182.

Armstrong, D. (1983). The fabrication of nurse-patient relationships. *Social Science & Medicine, 17,* 457–460.

Bjornsdottir, K. (1996). The construction of a profession: A study of the history of nursing in Iceland. *Nursing Inquiry, 3,* 13–22.

Callon, M. (1986). Some elements of a sociology of translation: Domestication of the scallops and the fishermen of St. Brieuc Bay. In J. Law (Ed.), *Power, action, belief: A new sociology of action?* (pp. 196–233). London: Routledge & Kegan Paul.

Canadian Nurses Association. (1988). *Health for all Canadians: A call for health-care reform.* Ottawa: Author.

Elias, N. (1989). *The symbol theory.* London: Sage.

Fernandez, J. W. (1986). *Persuasions and performances: The play of tropes in culture.* Bloomington, IN: Indiana University Press.

Foucault, M. (1973). *The birth of the clinic: An archæology of medical perception* (A. Sheridan, Trans.). London: Routledge.

Foucault, M. (1979). *Discipline and punish: The birth of the prison* (A.M. Sheridan-Smith, Trans.). Harmondsworth: Penguin.

Foucault, M. (1991). Governmentality. In G. Burchell, C. Gordon, & P. Miller (Eds.), *The Foucault effect: Studies in governmental rationality* (pp. 87–104). Hemel Hempstead: Harvester Wheatsheaf.

Giddens, A. (1984). *The constitution of society.* Cambridge: Polity Press.

Gordon, C. (1991). Governmental rationality: An introduction. In G. Burchell, C. Gordon, & P. Miller (Eds.), *The Foucault effect: Studies in governmentality* (pp. 1–51). London: Harvester Wheatsheaf.

Heslop, L. (1998). A discursive exploration of nursing work in the hospital emergency setting. *Nursing Inquiry, 5,* 87–95.

Labonte, R. (1997). Community and public health: An international perspective. *Health Visitor, 70*(2), 64–67.

Latimer, J. (1997). Giving patients a future: the constituting of classes in an acute medical unit. *Sociology of Health & Illness, 19,* 160–185.

Latimer, J. (1998). Organizing context: Nurses' assessments of older people in an acute medical unit. *Nursing Inquiry, 5,* 43–57.

Latour, B. (1987). *Science in action: How to follow scientists and engineers through society.* Cambridge, MA: Harvard University Press.

Lyotard, J.-F. (1984). *The postmodern condition: A report on knowledge* (G. Bennington & B. Massumi, Trans.). Manchester: Manchester University Press.

May, C. R. (1992a). Individual care? Power and subjectivity in therapeutic relationships. *Sociology, 26,* 589–602.

May, C. R. (1992b). Nursing work, nurses' knowledge and the subjectification of the patient. *Sociology of Health & Illness, 14,* 472–487.

Meleis, A. I. (1990). Being and becoming healthy: the core of nursing knowledge. *Nursing Science Quarterly, 3*(3), 107–114.

Mueller, M. (1995). *Organizing participation: An ethnography of "community" in hospital.* Unpublished Doctoral Thesis, University of Edinburgh.

Munro, R. (1998a). Disposal of the gap: The production and consumption of accounting research and practical accounting systems. *Advances in Public Interest Accounting, 7,* 139–159.

Munro, R. (1998b). On the rim of reason. In R. Chia (Ed.), *In the realm of organization* (pp. 142–162). London: Routledge.

Nelson, S. (1997). Reading nursing history. *Nursing Inquiry, 4,* 229–236.

Nelson, S. (1999). Entering the professional domain: The making of the modern nurse in 17th century France. *Nursing History Review, 7,* 171–187.

O'Brien, M. (1994). The managed heart revisited: Health and social control. *Sociological Review, 42,* 393–413.

Parker, J. (1997). The body as text and the body as living flesh: Metaphors of the body and nursing in postmodernity. In J. Lawler (Ed.), *The body in nursing* (pp. 11–29). Melbourne: Churchill Livingstone.

Pender, N. (1996). *Health promotion in nursing practice.* (3rd ed.). Stamford, CT: Appleton & Lange.

Petersen, A., & Lupton, D. (1996). *The new public health: Health and self in the age of risk.* St. Leonards, NSW: Allen & Unwin.

Purkis, M. E. (1993). *Bringing "practice" to the clinic: An excavation of the effects of health promotion discourse in a community health clinic.* Unpublished Ph.D. Thesis, University of Edinburgh.

Purkis, M. E. (1994). Entering the field: Intrusions of the social and its exclusion from studies of nursing practice. *International Journal of Nursing Studies, 31,* 315–336.

Purkis, M. E. (1997). The "social determinants" of practice? A critical analysis of health promoting discourse. *Canadian Journal of Nursing Research, 29*(1), 47–62.

Purkis, M. E. (1999). Embracing technology: An exploration of the effects of writing nursing. *Nursing Inquiry, 6,* 147–156.

Rose, N. (1996). Psychiatry as a political science: Advanced liberalism and the administration of risk. *History of the Human Sciences, 9*(2), 1–24.

Rudge, T. (1998). Skin as cover: The discursive effects of "covering" metaphors on wound care practices. *Nursing Inquiry, 5,* 228–237.

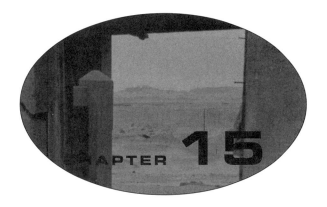

Human Genome Project: Implications for Nursing Practice*

CINDY L. MUNRO

Mary, age 45, is recovering from breast cancer surgery. Her two daughters, Anne, age 25, and Jennifer, age 23, are visiting. Mary is very concerned that she may have "given a bad gene" to her daughters. Anne is interested in whether or not genetic testing could tell her more about her risks of getting breast cancer like her mother, but Jennifer would prefer not to know. In fact, Jennifer says, "I really don't want my sister to seek testing— we're pretty close, and if her test results are bad, I know she won't be able to keep it from me. I just don't want to know! What difference would it make to my life anyway?"

Health care is undergoing a dramatic shift in views about health and disease that is fueled by an explosion in genetic information. The potential impact of this shift can be appreciated by reflecting upon the influence of a previous paradigm shift—the acceptance of germ theory in health care. Although widely accepted today by both health care providers and consumers, the concept that microorganisms can cause specific diseases was a radical notion when Semmelweis attempted to institute hand-washing in obstetrical practice in 1850. Subsequent acceptance of the role of microorganisms in human health and disease yielded a very different approach to understanding disease, dramatically altered health care practices, and reduced morbidity and mor-

tality in certain infectious diseases such as puerperal fever.

Today we are on the threshold of changes in health care that will be more far-reaching than those brought about by the influence of germ theory. Information gained through the Human Genome Project will substantially revise our understanding of disease susceptibility and causation, and will lead to sweeping changes in health care practices. Although it is possible to speculate about potential effects of the Human Genome Project on health care and nursing practice, the project is likely to generate effects that are as yet unimagined. This chapter reviews the establishment of the Human Genome Project, reports on current progress of the project, and identifies some implications of the project for health care generally and nursing specifically.

The Human Genome Project

The Human Genome Project is a worldwide research initiative that was initiated by the United States Department of Energy (DOE) and the National Institutes of Health (NIH) in 1987, a multidisciplinary collaboration to understand the basis of heredity. The Human Genome Project is expected to discover all of the human genes and make them accessible for in-depth biological study (Department of Energy, 2000). The DOE, as a descendant of the Atomic Energy Commission, became in-

*An earlier version of this paper was published in *Neonatal Network, 18* (3), 7–12, 1999 as "Implications for Nursing of the Human Genome Project."

terested in the concept of sequencing the human genome because of a long-standing need to improve methods used to monitor changes in genetic material caused by radiation (Patrinos & Drell, 1997). Serious consideration of the feasibility of an attempt to ascertain the complete human genetic sequence was initiated at a DOE-sponsored international conference in 1986. NIH interest in the project arose from a recognition of the importance of genetic information in human disease (Fink & Collins, 1997). In 1988, following a National Research Council report that recommended federal support for a human genome sequencing project, the DOE and NIH signed a memorandum of understanding outlining development of the project. The project officially began on October 1, 1990; completion was projected for 2005. Costs were estimated at $200 million per year, for a total estimated cost of $3 billion. In addition to American involvement, human genome centers were established in other countries including Canada, England, France, and Japan (Munn, 2000). In addition to the federally funded Human Genome Project, Celera Genomics Corporation (led by Dr. J. Craig Venter) are contributing to sequencing efforts (White House, 2000).

The Human Genome Project articulated several goals for what was anticipated to be a 15-year project period. First and foremost, the project seeks to develop maps of the 24 human chromosomes (22 autosomes, X and Y). In addition, a goal was established to map and begin to sequence model organisms, including yeast, the nematode, and the fruit fly (Munn, 2000). Because it was clear at the initiation of the project that laboratory methods for sequencing would need to be improved if the project were to meet its stated timelines within the budget projections, goals were included that addressed enhanced DNA sequencing technology and technology to support it (such as what was required to analyze and store data), and research training. Additional goals were set to guide technology transfer and the handling of data, data collection, management, and distribution. Importantly, the project goals not only focused on science and technology but also ethical, legal, and social issues arising, and related policy options.

In addition to overall goals, interim goals for the first five years of the project were devel-oped; these goals dealt primarily with the process of the research. The project has stayed remarkably on target, and original estimates of time and cost have so far been accurate. In the third year of the project (1993), the 5-year goals were revised to direct additional efforts for the 1993–1998 period (Collins & Galas, 1993; Revised 5-year research goals, 1993). The original first 5-year goals were met (Genome Project, 1995), and the 1998 interim goals were accomplished on schedule.

Mapping and Sequencing of the Human Genome

The primary goal of the Human Genome Project is to map all human genes and complete the sequencing of human DNA. A gene is a section of DNA that serves as the blueprint for making a cellular product (Munro & Pickler, 1996). At the project outset, the number of human genes was estimated to be more than 50,000; more recent estimates suggest that the human genome includes 70,000 to 100,000 genes (Rowen, Mahairas, & Hood, 1997). The fundamental building blocks of DNA are the nucleotides, or bases; the human genome is comprised of approximately 3 billion nucleotide base pairs (Rowen, Mahairas, & Hood, 1997).

Genetic mapping is a process that identifies the locations of specific DNA segments relative to each other. These specific DNA segments can be genes or can be stretches of DNA that do not serve as a blueprint for making proteins. Genetic mapping can be compared to having a road map of an interstate highway with exits for cities sequentially numbered. From such a map, the location of cities relative to each other is apparent, but the physical distance between them may not be precisely determined. In sequencing, the exact order of the nucleotides is determined. In the highway analogy, sequencing would provide mile markers that would give information about the exact physical location of cities and other roadway features.

In the spring of 2000, researchers announced that they had completed a rough draft of the map of the Human Genome (White House, 2000), with the location of more than 9,272 genes established (Count of genes, 2000). In addition, many specific DNA sequences known as "expressed sequence tags" have been isolated; expressed sequence tags are fragments of genes. These expressed sequence tags probably represent about 40,000 to 50,000 genes, and work is continuing on mapping these sequences (Rowen, Mahairas, & Hood, 1997). The mapping goal of the Human Genome Project is to establish a marker every 100,000 bases across each chromosome (Department of Energy, 2000). A marker is a group of nucleotides on a chromosome that can be used to identify a segment of that chromosome. At present, about 95 percent of the genome has marker sequences spaced about 200,000 bases apart. Large-scale sequencing of the human genome was begun in 1996 (Department of Energy, 2000). About 2 percent of the 3 billion base pairs of human DNA have been sequenced.

Mapping and Sequencing Model Organisms

In addition to Homo sapiens, the Human Genome Project established a goal of mapping and sequencing the DNA from several other selected organisms. The mouse (Mus musculus), a roundworm (Caenorhabditis elegans), the fruit fly (Drosophila melanogaster), baker's yeast (Sacchromyces cerevisiae), and a bacterium (Escherichia coli) were selected for study. These organisms were selected because they are commonly used as model systems of human conditions. Many people are familiar with the contributions of mice, fruit flies, and E. coli bacteria to biological inquiry. The roundworm and yeast are frequently used in studying cellular development.

Progress on sequencing model organisms is related to genome size. Sequencing of the Escherichia coli genome is complete, as is sequencing of Baker's yeast, the roundworm, and the fruit fly. The mouse (who has the largest genome of the model organisms selected for sequencing) is approximately 0.2 percent complete.

Investigators have completely sequenced 11 other bacterial genomes to date: Hemophilus influenzae (an important pathogen in bacterial meningitis in infants), Helicobacter pylori (involved in peptic ulcer disease), and Mycoplasma genitalium (found in non-gonoccocal urethritis) have been sequenced by The Institute for Genome Research (TIGR) (Fleishman, et al., 1995; Fraser, et al., 1995; Tomb, et al., 1997). Sequencing of microorganisms may yield valuable insights about their ability to cause disease.

Ethical, Legal and Social Implications

At the initiation of the Human Genome Project, a commitment was made to devote 5 percent of the project budget to consideration of ethical issues related to the project. The Committee on Ethical, Legal, and Social Implications (ELSI) was formed to address related project goals. ELSI was to become instrumental in informing both policy development and service delivery.

Initially, ELSI focused on issues related to privacy of genetic information, use of genetic information in the clinical setting, fairness in use of genetic information, and professional and public education (Department of Energy, 2000). When interim goals for the Human Genome Project were developed in 1993, the following ELSI goals were articulated (Collins & Galas, 1993):

1. Continue to identify and define issues and develop policy options to address them.
2. Develop and disseminate policy options regarding genetic testing services with potential widespread use.
3. Foster greater acceptance of human genetic variation.
4. Enhance and expand public and professional education that is sensitive to sociocultural and psychological issues.

ELSI formed a Task Force on Genetic Information and Insurance, which published recommendations in 1993. Central to the work was the recommendation that genetic information (as well as other information about past, present, or future health status) should not be used to deny health care coverage or service—an issue of particular relevance in the United States in which health insurance is offered through for-profit companies (Hudson, Rothenberg, Andrews, Kahn, & Collins, 1995). The Task Force further recommended that genetic services should be offered comparably to nongenetic services and should encompass appropriate genetic counseling, testing, and treatment within a program of primary, preventive, and specialty health care services for individuals and families with genetic disorders and those at risk of genetic disease (Insurance Task Force, 1993). At the time that the Task Force worked, a national health care plan was vigorously debated in Congress. Although a national plan for health care was not subsequently approved by Congress, the recommendations have impacted federal legislation. The U.S. Equal Employment Opportunity Commission has ruled that genetic discrimination in employment decisions is illegal, and the Federal Health Care Portability and Accountability Act of 1996 does prohibit use of genetic information in decisions related to health insurance eligibility (Department of Energy, 2000). In the past, information about potential for genetic disease that was identified through in-utero genetic testing was used to deny or limit health care coverage to neonates. Through addressing such issues as this and a host of other complex and contentious issues, ELSI creates an environment in which discriminatory practices may not prevail.

The activities of ELSI were evident in a recent initiative affecting neonatal health care, an initiative of particular interest to nurses who care for neonatal clients and their families. ELSI established a Task Force on Genetic Testing that specifically addressed issues related to genetic testing in neonates, a contentious area especially in regards to screening practices. In its final report published in 1997, this ELSI Task Force recommended that neonate screening tests occur in accordance with their general recommendation that clinical validity and utility of a test (its ability to point to safe and effective interventions) should be established prior to its widespread use for screening in clinical practice, and that the test should provide benefit to the person being tested. They recommended that, prior to testing information, parents are engaged in a discussion about screening, including why it should be done with full disclosure of potential risks and benefits of doing so. The Task Force recommendations were written to discourage the use of neonatal testing to identify couples at risk of birthing a future child with a genetic disorder unless such testing benefits the infant to whom the test is administered; if tests are to be administered solely to identify future risks for parents, the parents should be apprised of this prior to screening, and written consent must be obtained. If the tests are used in development of new tests and include any information identifying the infant, the Task Force recommends that parental consent be obtained.

Implications for Health Care

New understandings related to genetic information are likely to affect even greater changes in understanding of disease susceptibility and causation, and to be accompanied by substantive changes in health care practices and therapeutics. The "age of genetic health care" may emphasize identifying susceptibilities to disease prior to the onset of detectable pathology, understanding pathophysiology of human responses at a molecular level, designing rational interventions based on enhanced understanding of molecular pathophysiology, and new ways of collaborating with consumers regarding their care.

The genetic health care approach might lead to different treatment approaches for patients with the same disease, based on the individual patient's genetic profile. For example, several genes are being investigated in relationship to breast cancer. Both the BRCA1 and BRCA2 genes are tumor suppressor genes; a mutation in either gene has been identified in some women with familial breast cancer. Changes in the BRCA1 gene have been implicated in increased risk for both breast cancer and ovarian cancer. However, changes in the BRCA2 gene do not appear to increase risk of ovarian cancer. At present, knowledge about the particular mutation carried by a woman with breast cancer is not helpful in directing prevention efforts, therapy, or follow-up. However, one might speculate that in the future follow-up for breast cancer might be tailored to an individual's genetic risk profile. Indeed, it is conceivable that as knowledge expands related to how these genes increase susceptibility for breast cancer, therapeutic interventions offered to a patient might be customized to her genetic profile.

An interest in genetics as a contributor to health and illness is beginning to permeate the United States public. For example, genetic information can be found as the subject of cartoon strips. In one cartoon, a character states, "This article says a melancholy personality may be inherited," to which another replies, "Yes, if you have blue genes!" (Thaves, 1993). Genetic influences are invoked for both physiologic and psychologic factors.

Recent polls indicate that many consumers are open to including genetic information as part of the health record and genetic diagnoses. A Harris poll conducted in the United States in April 1995 reported that 56 percent of respondents said that DNA databases containing "genetic fingerprints" of all newborns would be very or somewhat acceptable. In the same sample, 68 percent said they would be likely to ask physicians for genetic tests if the tests were available at a reasonable price.

However, consumers' interest in testing depends on which tests are available and individual perception of benefits from test results (Brownlee, Cook, & Hardigg, 1994). Comparing the case of adenomatous polyps with Huntington's disease is illustrative of this. Persons identified by family history to be at risk for familial adenomatous polyposis may be followed aggressively to detect the development of polyps. In these individuals, colectomy is frequently recommended if polyps are found because of the high risk for colon cancer. For individuals with a family history risk of familial adenomatous polyposis, DNA testing for the mutation related to the disease holds high potential benefit. A DNA test that indicates an individual does not carry the genetic mutation associated with familial adenomatous polyposis can obviate the necessity for frequent screening for polyps and for prophylactic colectomy. In contrast, many of those who are at risk for Huntington's disease because of family history decline DNA testing. In the case of Huntington's disease, which has no effective prophylactic or therapeutic options, benefit in knowing one's genetic profile is not as easily demonstrated.

As additional genetic information becomes available, increased interest has been focused on multigene effects, environmental effects on phenotype (Kaiser, 1997), prognosis, interventions, and prevention strategies. At issue is whether providers and consumers will view genetic information as fortune telling or weather forecasting. If genetic information is viewed as "fortune telling" as simplistic genetic determinism or predestination, patients may either be immobilized by fear of their future health or unwilling to participate in prevention or treatment strategies. If, however, the "weather forecasting" view of genetic information as a predictor of potential risk is dominant, individuals might be motivated to participate more fully in health promotion or early detection activities.

Gene therapy provides a novel new treatment modality that is likely to be an important part of therapeutic intervention in the future (Pickler & Munro, 1995). Gene therapy is currently in the experimental phase. The first gene therapy trial was begun by Blaese in 1990, with 186 clinical trials in gene therapy currently operating in the United States. An additional 32 projects involving introduction of genes in human subjects are in progress, but do not have a therapeutic purpose (The Office of Recombinant DNA Activities, 1997). Of the therapeutic clinical gene therapy trials, 31 investigate single gene mendelian diseases; 13 diseases are represented in these 31 trials, and 16 of these trials are focused on cystic fibrosis. The largest number of projects (130) are concentrated in the area of cancer, and 21 trials are directed to treatment of human immunodeficiency virus infection. Four other non-mendelian diseases are represented in clinical trials as well. The science of gene therapy is still young; dramatic clinical results have not yet been demonstrated, but exciting potential exists.

The public's expectations of the health care system may be altered by the increase in genetic information, availability of genetic tests, and gene therapy trials. Identification of involvement of a particular gene in disease generally precedes understanding of the mechanism of that genetic alteration and may precede the ability to intervene therapeutically. At least 29 DNA-based genetic tests are currently available in clinical practice (Casey, 1997), although in many cases therapeutic intervention is not possible. Costs generally range from $150 to $1,500, although individual tests may be higher (for example, $2,400 for BRCA1 or BRCA2). However, there may be unrealistic public pressures to incorporate genetic information into clinical practice prematurely. In addition, the public's definition of what is healthy, normal, or desirable are likely to be altered by enhanced information related to genetics (Munro, 1995).

Implications for Nursing Practice

Nurses play an important role in assisting clients and their family members to realize the benefits of the Human Genome Project and the new paradigm of genetic health care. The Human Genome Project has recognized nurses as vital participants in the field of genetic information. The ELSI Task Force on Genetic Testing stated, "Nurses have much to offer people before, during, and after the genetic testing process. Because of their vast numbers and the wide range of health care activities they can perform, nurses can play an important role in providing care for those undergoing genetic testing. Nurses should be provided with additional education and training that can increase their effectiveness in providing education for people undergoing genetic testing" (Holtzman & Watson, 1997).

As additional genetic tests and gene-based therapies become available, parents will have many questions. They are likely to request information and support from the nurse caring for their child, and to expect the nurse to have the ability to correctly interpret genetic information, and the skill to translate the information into a form that they can use in decision making. Continued expansion of the nurse's knowledge base is essential as new information becomes available.

Information from the Human Genome Project will continue to expand the knowledge base about risks of susceptibility to disease. Although understanding single gene mendelian diseases, such as phenylketonuria and cystic fibrosis, will remain important in providing competent care, future knowledge about the importance of multigene interactions and the influence of environment on disease occurrence or severity will require nurses to consider genetic information in planning and implementing care for all patients/clients.

Nurses have an excellent opportunity to contribute to the body of nursing knowledge regarding genetic information and its effects on patients. For example, nurses might investigate strategies for risk factor identification or risk factor modification in genetically susceptible populations. Nurse researchers could study responses to genetic information, including how people deal with uncertainty and guilt. Designing and testing the effectiveness of coping strategies would enhance nurses' ability to assist parents and improve care. In addition, nurses might become involved in social justice issues related to the Human Genome Project, including access to and cost of testing and therapies, public education, and the development of culturally and linguistically appropriate patient education materials. The new paradigm of genetic health care will focus on the family rather than the individual, will be concerned with interactive lifestyle counseling for risk reduction, and will need to be responsive to the complexities of genetic screening, genetic diagnoses, and genetic interventions or therapies. Nurses already possess strengths in family-centered care and anticipatory guidance, and nurses are demonstrated leaders in health care ethics. The strengths of nursing will serve the public well as society moves into the post-Human Genome Project era of health care.

✳ Reflective Questions

1. How is knowledge of disease susceptibility obtained through genetic testing different from knowledge of disease susceptibility gained through family history?

2. How would you respond to a family situation like the one presented in the chapter opening?

3. How do you respond to Mary's concerns? Can Jane's request to know her genetic status be balanced with Jennifer's desire not to know?

4. What health promotion activities would you recommend to Jane and Jennifer based on Mary's diagnosis, or based on results of genetic testing? Would your recommendations differ from those for women without a family history or genetic testing for breast cancer?

5. Genetic susceptibility to disease has been likened to a weather report (but is NOT a crystal ball!). How does this view of genetic susceptibility to disease influence your health promotion activities?

REFERENCES

Brownlee, S., Cook, G. G., & Hardigg, V. (1994, August 22). Tinkering with destiny. *U.S. News and World Report*, 59–67.

Casey, D. 1997. What can the new gene tests tell us? *The Judge's Journal, 36*(3), 14–19. Also available: *http://www.ornl.gov/TechResources/Human_Genome/publicat/judges/judge.html.*

Collins, F., & Galas, D. (1993). A new five-year plan for the U.S. Human Genome Project. *Science, 262,* 43–46.

Count of genes by chromosome. (2000). [Online]. Available: *http://gdbwww.gdb.org/gdbreports/CountGeneBy-Chromosome.html.*

Department of Energy. (2000). Human Genome Project Information. [Online]. Available: *http://www.ornl.gov/TechResources/Human_Genome/home.html.*

Fink, L., & Collins, F. S. (1997). The Human Genome Project: View from the National Institutes of Health. *Journal of the American Medical Women's Association, 52,* 4–7,15.

Fleischmann, R. D., Adams, M. D., White, O., Clayton, R. A., Kirkness, E. F., Kerlavage, A. R., Bult, C. J., Tomb, J.-F., Dougherty, B. A., Merrick, J. M., McKenney, K., Sutton, G., FitzHugh, W., Fields, C., Gocayne, J. D., Scott, J., Shirley, R., Liu, L.-I., Glodek, A., Kelley, J. M., Weidman, J. F., Phillips, C. A., Spriggs, T., Hedblom, E., Cotton, M. D., Utterback, T. R., Hanna, M. C., Nguyen, D. T., Saudek, D. M., Brandon, R. C., Fine, L. D., Fritchman, J. L., Fuhrmann, J. L., Geoghagen, N. S. M., Gnehm, C. L., McDonald, L. A., Small, K. V., Fraser, C. M., Smith, H. O., & Venter, J. C. (1995). Whole-genome random sequencing and assembly of Haemophilus influenzae. *Science, 269,* 496–512.

Fraser, C. M., Gocayne, J. D., White, O., Adams, M. D., Clayton, R. A., Fleischmann, R. D., Bult, C. J., Kerlavage, A. R., Sutton, G., Kelley, J. M., Fritchman, J. L., Weidman, J. F., Small, K. V., Sandusky, M., Fuhrmann, J., Nguyen, D., Utterback, T. R., Saudek, D. M., Phillips, C. A., Merrick, J. M., Tomb, J.-F., Dougherty, B. A., Bott, K. F., Hu, P. C., Lucier, T. S., Peterson, S. N., Smith, H. O., Hutchison,C. A. III, & Venter, J. C. (1995). The minimal gene complement of Mycoplasma genitalium. *Science, 270,* 397–408.

Genome Project finishes fifth year ahead of schedule. (1995). *Human Genome News, 7*(3–4), 1.

Holtzman, N. A., & Watson, M. S. (1997). Promoting safe and effective genetic testing in the United States: Final report of the Task Force on Genetic Testing. [Online]. Available: *http://www.nhgri.nih.gov/ELSI/TFGT_final/.*

Hudson, K. L., Rothenberg, K. H., Andrews, L. B., Kahn, M. J. E., & Collins, F. (1995). Genetic discrimination and health insurance: An urgent need for reform. *Science, 270,* 391–393.

Insurance Task Force makes recommendations. (1993). *Human Genome News, 5*(2), 1.

Kaiser, J. (1997). Environment Institute lays plans for gene hunt. *Science, 278,* 569–570.

Munn, M. (2000). What is the Human Genome Project? [Online]. Available: *http://www.genome.washington.edu/UWGC/tutorial/default.htm.*

Munro, C. L. (1995). Genetic technology and scientific integrity. In F. L. Macrina (Ed.), *Scientific integrity: An introductory text with cases* (pp. 309–330). Washington, DC: American Society for Microbiology.

Munro, C. L., & Pickler, R. H. (1996). The basis of heredity: A genetic primer. *Neonatal Network, 15*(7), 7–10.

The Office of Recombinant DNA Activities. 1997. Human gene therapy protocols (as of 10–14–97). [Online]. Available: *http://www.nih.gov/od/orda/protocol.htm.*

Patrinos, A., & Drell, D. W. (1997). The Human Genome Project: View from the Department of Energy. *Journal of the American Medical Womens Association, 52,* 8–10.

Pickler, R. H., & Munro, C. L. (1995). Gene therapy for inherited disorders. *Journal of Pediatric Nursing, 10,* 40–47.

Revised 5-year research goals of the U.S. Human Genome Project October 1, 1993, to September 30, 1998 (FY 1994–1998). (1993). *Human Genome News, 5*(4), 2.

Rowen, L., Mahairas, G., & Hood, L. (1997). Sequencing the human genome. *Science, 278,* 605–607.

Thaves, B. (1993, June 3). Frank and Ernest. *Richmond Times Dispatch*, n. p.

Tomb, J. F., White, O., Kerlavage, A. R., Clayton, R. A., Sutton, G. G., Fleischmann, R. D., Ketchum, K., Klenk, H. P., Gill, S. R., Dougherty, B. A., Nelson, K., Quackenbush, J., Zhou, L., Kirkness, E. F., Peterson, S., Loftus, B., Richardson, D., Dodson, R., Khalak, H. G., Glodek, A., McKenney, K., Fitzegerald, L. M., Lee, N., Adams, M. D., Hickey, E. K., Berg, D. E., Gocayne, J. D., Utterback, T. R., Peterson, J. D., Kelly, J. M., Cotton, M. D., Weidman, J. M., Fujii, C., Bowman, C., Watthey, L., Wallin, E., Borodovsky, M., Hayes, W. S., Karp, P., Smith, H. O., Fraser, C. M., & Venter, J. C. (1997). The complete genome sequence of the gastric pathogen Helicobacter pylori. *Nature, 388,* 539–547.

The White House. (2000). President Clinton announces the completion of the first survey of the entire human genome: Hails public and private efforts leading to this historic achievement. [Online]. Available: *http://www.ornl.gov/hgmis/project/clinton1.html.*

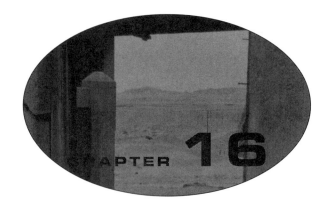

CHAPTER 16

What Is Quality Care? A Hospital Health Promotion Perspective

ALEX BERLAND
LYNNE E. YOUNG

One guy came to us with a diagnosis of leukemia. He had a history of abusing his wife. She was then four months pregnant and their lifestyle must have been just abominable. She came with him to the hospital. The thing we had to deal with was how he behaved. Everybody was scared to death of him on the first day that he was there because he was so abusive and threatening. We decided that we had to come up with some way of letting this guy express his anger that would be acceptable to us and still develop some kind of relationship with him. So we got him doing relaxation tapes, which was a real hard sell, but eventually he did get on with those. Now whether that made any impact on him when he left, I don't know. For his wife, we also had to do a lot of nutritional teaching with her because she had no idea how to look after herself being pregnant. They never showed up for follow-up appointments so I don't really know what happened.

This story, told by a medical nurse working in a teaching hospital, illustrates what is key in the practice of **health promotion** in hospital settings: the capacity to see beyond the patient's diagnosis and to care for the whole person, a caring process that takes into account the individual's social context, including family life. A diagnosis of leukemia in a family member is but one aspect of life for this family, who, because of multiple stressors, seem to be in a high-risk state. Indeed, the leukemia treatment may be the most predictable aspect of patient and family care facing the nursing staff, certainly the most

familiar. Protocols for chemotherapy are clearly and thoroughly delineated for nurses; however, what guides health promotion practice for these same nurses beyond nutrition education is much less certain. In contrast, research about conditions like heart disease and diabetes have led to standardized health promotion strategies for patients with these conditions and in some cases their family members.

As research on health promotion strategies accumulates, evidence provides the basis for health promotion practice. Knowledge about what strategies are effective in promoting health accrues as a result of well-designed evaluation studies. Evaluation research generates knowledge about what patients and their families perceive, learn, and do as a result of health promotion efforts by nurses, and illuminates contextual factors influencing their capacity to engage in health promoting practice. Evaluation research measures patient outcomes in relation to providers' knowledge about what constitutes effective treatment, sometimes without equitable consideration for the health-related expectations of patients and their families. How can we ensure that evaluation consistently captures data about patients' perceptions of what contributes to their **health**?

This chapter delineates key questions to guide the evaluation of quality care in hospital nursing, and proposes what needs to be considered when planning a study designed to evaluate quality care, care that is effective and health promoting.

As a hospital manager concerned about the quality of care[1] offered in my (Berland) institution, posing the previous question uncovers focused areas for action in my everyday work. For the purposes of illustration, I recount a typical incident that prompted me to reflect on the question, what is quality care? Several months ago, family members complained that their relative was told nothing about his surgery and "aftercare." They reported that when they confronted the surgeon he replied, "Well I did explain the surgery and follow-up to him (referring to the patient) in the office. But, you know, he's old and confused and I think he did *not* get it." Reflecting on this situation, it occurred to me that this was an example, not of quality care characterized by a health promotion approach, but rather the care provided to this vulnerable man could be characterized as "health demotion." Thus, as a manager responsible for the delivery of care that is health promoting, scenarios like this one prompt me to explore how such situations can be addressed at the system level, the level at which my actions as manager can stimulate change. (See Chap. 10 for a full discussion of definitions of health.)

Health promotion in hospitals is a paradox. Although current definitions of health promotion emphasize empowerment (World Health Organization, 1984, 1986), hospitals take away individual control from patients by imposing schedules, treatments, diet, and clothing (Lupton, 1994). Even in the opening story, although nurses engage in what is held to be a health promoting activity, it is they who define and control the health promotion agenda for the man and his wife. What is not apparent in the story are the contextual factors impacting the nurses' health promotion practice. In a study exploring hospital nurses' perceptions of their role in health promotion (Berland, Whyte, & Maxwell, 1995), we found that nurses' time constraints, workload, and morale affect all their activities, but especially how they promote health. As well, we found that lack of knowledge about health promotion, cultural factors, and discomfort with the health promoting role affect nurses' ability to care for patients in a manner that is health promoting.

[1]Quality of care is conceptualized for the purposes of this chapter as care comprised of the delivery of effective treatment during which the expectations of the patient and their family are met, and the health of the patient and family is promoted.

Since this study was conducted in the early 1990s, restraints in health care delivery have escalated and nursing positions have been cut back. This has exacerbated the pressures on nurses to fit ever more tasks into their work lives, leaving less time for what is perceived by nurses as quality patient care (Shindul-Rothchild & Gordon, 1998). We suggest that nurses' capacity to enact their role in health promotion is increasingly compromised during this time of restraint. How can we keep quality care on the health care agenda for patients and their families in this time of restraint? And, how can we improve the health promotion dimension of quality care?

Compared to community-based studies, research on hospital health promotion is sparse, providing nurses with minimal empirical evidence upon which to base their health promotion practice. Contributing to this, in our experience, is the lack of acceptance by the biomedical research community of the relative importance of exploring the effectiveness of hospital-based health promotion nursing strategies when compared to the importance attached to researching drugs and biomedical technologies. Health promotion research is often not well accepted as rigorous science by the scientific establishment in the hospital setting where clinical trials are designed within limited views of health (as the absence of disease). Health promotion research in the hospital setting and the methods used to establish the effectiveness and efficacy of health promotion are considered pioneering. In spite of these differences, everyone agrees that the goal of hospital care is to deliver high-quality care, care that improves health. Hospital-based health promotion in our view is central to this mission.

Now we have another question: How do we evaluate quality care? This is a complex and messy topic. There is considerable uncertainty and disagreement about what to measure, how to measure quality of care, and whether measurement is the only and best evaluation strategy to employ in such research.

Because patients' definitions of health often differ from providers' definitions, and nurses' perceptions of quality care that is health promoting may differ from what is acceptable by the institution, a key starting point is to be clear about "Who is asking the question?" and "To what end?" Providers and health care system leaders generally define health as the absence of disease, whereas patients and often nurses define health more broadly, as a resource for living, a feeling of energy, or balance (WHO, 1984, 1986).

In the section entitled "What factors do patients and providers agree constitute quality care?" we discuss some commonly shared viewpoints among providers and patients. Then we ask, "How do providers view quality care?" In this section of the chapter, we describe the findings of a study in which hospital nurses speak about their efforts to include health promotion in their practice. In the section, "How do patients define quality, health promoting care?" we describe findings from a major study in which hospital patients expressed their issues of concern. In the two concluding sections, we introduce a framework for thinking about what we do not know and how we may proceed to improve the quality of health promotion in a hospital setting.

Who Is Asking the Question?

Evans (1984) sheds light on this question by pointing out that information shared between health care providers and their patients is asymmetrical, that is, one party knows more than the other. To use an analogy to explain this notion, think about common commercial transactions: Consumers may not know how a product is made and they likely have no knowledge about the technical components or operating principles, knowledge held by those producing the item. (Think about your microwave oven—or your computer!) What consumers do know, however, is what the product will do for them and how to make it work. They know better than the producer what value, or potential value, the product has for them in their everyday lives. In health care, however, asymmetry of knowledge goes beyond the technology and its components to bodily sensations and to patients and their family members' perceptions of the quality of their lives. Patients are generally not interested in the intricate details of health care technology. Most patients know their own body's symptoms, sensations, and what affects the quality of their lives. They do not know how a particular treatment will affect them, mostly because they frequently have no other experience to use as a guide: A gallbladder can only be removed once. Rather, patients want health; they seek health care expecting that it will improve their health (Evans, 1984).

Providers, primarily in response to the demands of the health care system, define health and treatment outcomes that count for them. Providers practice according to the knowledge that they have about what affects the health of a particular patient, knowledge gained through repetitive contacts under specific conditions: that is, "so many gall bladders, only so much variation." (One notable exception may be in mental health.) Predictability reduces uncertainty. For the consumer, acute episodes of illness and early stages of chronic disease are novel events. The consumer lacks the provider's experience at classifying and categorizing symptoms into meaningful diagnoses, thus the asymmetry of information between patients and providers. This asymmetry results in a "gap" in perceptions of quality. What counts as quality differs for providers and their patients. Health care received does not always result in health perceived. As Evans (1984) notes with customary pithiness, "If health could be purchased directly, no difficulty would arise" (p. 73). Instead, patients seek or undergo health care, expecting it to provide restored or improved health. When results are less than expected, patients may feel betrayed, or at least underserved. From the provider perspective, however, the results perceived to be inadequate or lacking from the consumers' perspective, may be perfectly adequate and expected. How might we close this gap? How can we ensure that providers understand patients' perceptions and expectations when quality holds different meanings for each of them, and there is a power differential in the caring arena between the provider and the consumer?

Previously, quality in health care was evaluated according to structures or processes (Donabedian, 1988). The structural dimension is assessed by examining the credentials of health professionals charged with particular health care responsibilities in an institution. An example of a pertinent evaluative question might be, "Is that diabetic teaching nurse appropriately credentialed for his job description?" A related evaluative process question would be, "Are glucometer readings recorded regularly?" More recently, health-related patient outcomes have been recognized as an appropriate focus for evaluation, for instance, "Can a diabetic patient independently maintain acceptable serum glucose

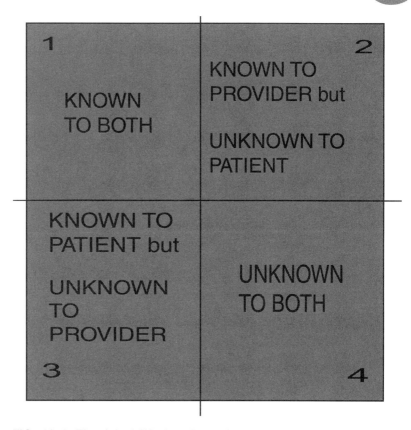

FIG. 16–1. The Johari Window. It can be used to illustrate domains of awareness (Luft & Ingham, 1955).

levels?" This shift to patient outcomes is one step toward using a patient-centered approach to evaluating quality. However, even with this commendable shift of focus, gaps in perceptions persist. In grappling with how to understand and address these gaps, one tool that we have found useful for thinking through what contributes to this perceptual gap is the Johari Window. This model evolved from the field of cognitive psychology, where it was used to illustrate domains of awareness (Luft & Ingham, 1955). The model comprises a two-by-two table of four domains: (1) subject matter that is known to both; (2) what is known only to one party; (3) what is known only to the other; and (4) what is unknown to both (Fig. 16–1). Using this model, we can begin to articulate what is known and not known to various stakeholders.

This idea is not a model for health promotion, nor for evaluating quality. Rather it is a conceptual tool for thinking about how different parties view the same experience. We use it here to illuminate patients' and providers' shared and different perceptions of high quality, health promoting care. Although patients' and providers' perceptions, facts, and experiences that affect their definitions of what comprises the desired quality of care may be different, they may also be shared. For instance, both view the diagnostic triad—rubor, rigor, calor (redness, swelling, fever)—as meaningful symptoms that point to infection, and both can directly observe whether these symptoms improve with care. These shared definitions comprise the first quadrant of the model.

In the second quadrant, the provider's perception may be termed "quality of examination." We sometimes refer to this domain as "clinical quality" or "quality of fact." It arises from measurable, usually quantifiable, com-

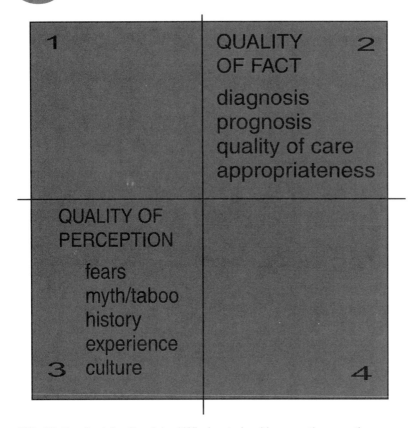

FIG. 16–2. Applying the Johari Window to health promotion practice: gaps in perceptions of patients and providers.

ponents such as signs, symptoms, and test results that may have no significance to the patient.

The patients' "quality of experience" occupies the third quadrant. This is usually based on qualitative sensations, such as pain and fatigue, or feelings of competence or humiliation. This is sometimes referred to as "service quality" or "quality of perception" and refers only to what is known to the patient.

Neither patient nor provider knows the content of the fourth quadrant, by definition. The contents are as yet unmeasured and unfelt components of quality. Once known, these quality indicators would move to one of the other three quadrants.

To illustrate the model, we apply it to understanding the situation of a patient with dermatitis, a common skin affliction. Both patient and care provider probably agree on the nature of the problem because both can directly observe certain aspects: areas affected; the size, color, and profile of the le-

sions or rash; whether treatment is reducing the symptoms; and so on. The patient is unlikely to know the diagnostic pathway in the provider's thought processes, considerations such as whether this is a topical manifestation of a systemic disease, or aspects of the provider's thinking such as prognosis and treatments (although the introduction of web technology is changing patients' level of interest in, and knowledge about, diagnostic issues). These all belong in the second quadrant, that is, what is known only to the provider (Fig. 16–2). The provider, similarly, cannot independently assess the degree of itching, the sleep disruption, or the effect on body image experienced by the patient. These belong in the third quadrant, along with other considerations such as fears about the proposed treatment, cultural taboos such as exposing one's body to someone of the opposite gender, financial worries about prescription costs, and concerns about others' reactions.

This is our concern: How do we improve quality from the patient's perspective, particularly in the hospital setting? The following sections are organized around the four domains of the Johari Window model.

What Factors Do Patients and Providers Agree Constitute Quality Care?

In the first domain of the model, then, are those things that both providers and patients know. These are elements that all would agree indicate quality care. In the hospital setting, for instance, the impact of conventional health promotion activities, like teaching about diabetes, can be measured by pre- and post-tests. We can assess, for instance, what patients know about the interaction of diet, exercise, and medication.

There is, however, another problem in reaching mutual agreement about how quality care should be evaluated. Do we measure only quality indicators that are well recognized like those mentioned earlier, or do we collaborate with patients and their families to determine what is meaningful to them, gen-

---

TABLE 16—1

EXCERPT FROM A CHARTER OF PATIENT'S RIGHTS IN A PSYCHIATRIC HOSPITAL

Part II -- Charter of Patient Rights Guidebook
Quality of Care/Therapeutic Rights

Right # 5:

"The right to a second medical opinion and to have hospital staff facilitate the obtaining of this second opinion."

Clarifying Statements:

■ Patients have the right to obtain a second opinion from a licensed physician on both medical and psychiatric treatment issues. The attending physician does not have the right to deny someone's request for a second opinion.

■ Hospital staff will assist the patient in obtaining a second opinion.

■ Patients can ask for a second opinion verbally.

■ Patients can put requests for a second medical opinion in writing and will have their request signed by the staff and returned to the patient. The staff will document the request on the patient's chart.

Policies Referred to:
PAT-100 (Second Medical Opinion)

Second medical opinions may be requested from physicians external to Riverview Hospital as well as internally. Hospital staff are to assist the patient in obtaining access to external resources who can help the patient locate a physician the patient feels is suitable.

Example: Prabha feels that the doctor is changing her medications too often, or recommending a course of treatment that she is unsure about. She requests a second opinion. At her doctor's request a doctor from another ward reviews her chart and meets with Prabha to discuss her treatment.

erating new items for evaluation, such as how patients adapt their insulin regulation to special occasions or unexpected events?

For the last decade, most hospitals have prioritized quality-of-care measurement. Clinical Quality Indicators (CQIs) or Key Performance Indicators (KPIs) are now established as the "Holy Grail" for quality measurement. These indicators are usually quantitative performance measures, such as readmission to hospital, waiting times, and adverse incidents. Unfortunately, there is truth to the folk saying, "Not everything that counts can be counted." Certainly many hospitals attempt to include patients' perceptions in designing CQIs and KPIs (Wolf, 1995). However, patients' perceptions of quality care may be largely related to process factors, factors that are challenging, if not impossible, to capture quantitatively. The ideal is to design CQI and KPI measurement tools with input from patients. This is further discussed below.

In some jurisdictions, patients' charters have been developed as a way to begin closing the gap between providers' and patients' perceptions of quality care. Such charters are printed and made widely available to providers and patients to begin the process of ensuring a shared understanding of expected standards. These charters attempt to create a "Bill of Rights" or guarantee of service standards for patients, and go some way to ensuring that practice standards are transparent to consumers. At one long-stay psychiatric hospital (Riverview Hospital, 1998), a patients' charter was developed with extensive patient, family, and advocate involvement (For an excerpt see Table 16–1). This became a way of jointly establishing expectations about quality of service.

Unfortunately, even when providers know what patients want, they do not always address their needs. Shared decision making is not a cultural norm in North American health care systems. Rather, the valuing of expert knowledge over lay knowledge predominates in hospital settings, creating a power differential between health care providers and consumers that influences how quality care is understood and therefore evaluated. For instance, for many decades Jehovah's Witnesses wished to avoid blood transfusions, a request that was treated as unreasonable in many hospitals until scientific evidence pointed to the increased number and seriousness of blood-borne diseases such as AIDS.

How Do Providers View Quality Care?

The quality of care provided in hospitals is an ongoing social concern. All hospitals in Canada participate in a regular accreditation process to identify strengths and areas for focused development. The accreditation process is an opportunity for hospital personnel to analyze the quality of care when they are providing accrediting bodies with information about the effectiveness of care, teaching programs, and overall hospital performance. In this section, we discuss how providers define quality as it relates to formal program evaluation and overall hospital effectiveness. As well, we provide an overview of new practice trends.

Formal Program Evaluation

In a landmark work in this field, Donabedian (1988) developed a widely used evaluative framework based on structure, process, and outcomes, a framework that remains current today. It is complementary to the idea of the Johari Window because Donabedian posits that providers and patients may have different perceptions of the three components of quality care: structure, process, and outcome. For instance, providers may value the training of staff and assessing competence as key indicators of the structure of quality care. Here, standards are applied in the evaluation of a professional's performance. Yet, in my role as manager, I (Berland) have observed situations in which patients do not understand health professionals' qualifications, let alone the capabilities of their caregivers. In my interactions with patients, when I posed the question "Who is the most caring person you have encountered in the hospital?" I was surprised to learn that some patients felt that the housekeeper was the most caring person they encountered during their hospital stay.

Another example of the differences in perception between providers and patients about quality care is evident in situations in which there is a perceptual gap about the value of a procedure, such as surgery. Providers may value healthy wound healing and timely discharge as indicators of a successful outcome. For a patient who expects improved functioning and undisrupted body image, surgery that results in negligible functional improvement and altered body image may be considered unsuccessful. This suggests that providers should explain in detail, from their position as expert, what patients might expect from a procedure with a view to preventing gaps in perceptions of what counts as a successful outcome.

Evaluating quantitative dimensions of health promoting interventions is possible, as is evident in the diabetic teaching example. We can count the total number of diabetic teaching sessions, the credentials of the educators, the percentage of newly diagnosed patients with diabetes who are contacted before discharge. But what is the impact of all this activity? Do we also measure the proportion of diabetic program graduates who have achieved effective blood glucose control six months later? Long-term outcomes are what matter to patients, although these are rarely measured due to methodological difficulties and practical challenges.

Overall Evaluation of Hospital Effectiveness

As mentioned earlier, the typical hospital is evaluated in multiple ways by external agencies. These include inspections that examine radiology and lab facilities, for example, or processes for credentialing health professionals such as dieticians or pharmacists by their professional associations. Teaching hospitals are more rigorously scrutinized than others. Such assessments have clearly defined expectations, typically focusing on structure and process. Patient satisfaction surveys, the impact of treatment, and quality of life measures are included in some hospital-wide assessments. Nonetheless, corporate provocateurs ask, "How much time is spent talking about the most important things with the most important people—the patients and their families?" Sadly, as expected, and not as much as may be optimal or ideal.

The Canadian Council for Health Facilities Accreditation (CCHFA) plays a very significant role in accrediting or rating agencies. In late 1997, the CCHFA created a national

steering committee to develop a framework for quality indicators (Heidemann, 1997). With a view to addressing apparent weakness and gaps in the quality evaluation process, these indicators go beyond what was once evaluated and include measures of continuity, effectiveness, appropriateness, and accessibility. Following a pilot project in 20 hospitals and a national education program, these indicators have been incorporated into an accreditation process.

Many major teaching hospitals have independently developed Quality Indicators (Barnsley, Lemieux-Charles, & Baker, 1996). Primarily corporate indicators that focus on a variety of quality measures, they are useful for comparing performance over time, or for comparing one agency's performance against that of others. Such initiatives provide a retrospective analysis of quality performance. Quality improvement, a forward-looking process, requires such comparisons as a basis for developing and evaluating new initiatives. Typically though, these indicators are a first step in assessing quality performance and refer only indirectly to patients' perceptions of quality care. This is not a criticism. From the perspective of a hospital manager, it is essential to assessing the quality of care by focusing first on high-yield issues, such as those targeted in Quality Indicator evaluations. Hospital nurses, as stakeholders with a primary interest in health promotion, play a key role in ensuring that health promotion principles are incorporated into the ever-evolving lists of quality indicators. Presently, the Quality Indicators movement, in its early stage of development, is just a baby-step in the right direction.

Exploring New Practice Trends

In 1991 and 1993, two exploratory studies examined health promotion practice by acute care nurses (Berland & Whyte, 1993; Berland, Whyte, & Maxwell, 1995). The data were gathered during focus group discussions and a survey targeting nurses working in a variety of acute care hospitals. Although these studies focused only on process, they revealed important findings about the way nurses define quality in their health promoting practice. The nurses noted that a major component of their health promotion role involves personalizing the institutional environment, a health promotion challenge and truly a paradox. One nurse observed:

In this big institution—patients walk in and check all their rights and all their privacy and all their personality at the door . . . [the nurse] can make people feel more comfortable where they are, and let them know where the boundaries are.

In personalizing the hospital environment, the nurse strives to give the patient some measure of control by creating a comfortable climate and providing an orientation to the hospital environment.

Nurses in the focus group study were committed to maximizing the control patients have while hospitalized, and view this as both enabling of and fundamental to their patients' health. The following exchange among study participants illustrates this point:

NURSE 1: So many patients come into the hospital, and even if they have been fairly well in the community, assume a sick role. With a lot of elderly people it is assumed that the nurse will be there and [the patient may say] "Oh, I can't bathe myself" where yesterday morning at home she gave herself a good wash.

NURSE 2: You give them the right to take control of themselves.

NURSE 3: Ask whether they want to do this or don't want to do this.

NURSE 1: Or even just to say "No, you can still take care of yourself, despite the fact that you are in the hospital. It doesn't mean that all of a sudden you have to lay flat on your back."

NURSE 3: We are going to help you to do this— but you can still do that.

NURSE 1: Yes, if we didn't take away all the control, it would be easier for people to stay healthier.

Working collaboratively with those in their care is one strategy nurses can use for restoring patients' control over their own health. One tactic mentioned is to "translate the language for them and put it in a context they are familiar with. [Then] they might not assume a sick role so readily and feel loss of external control." One nurse described this tactic of translating the language:

*Maybe if we can encourage people to think of themselves as consumers of health care . . . patients automatically will think, "My money, so therefore I have a right to demand certain things." Translated that way you help em-*power them to say, "I have a right to proper medical care, and a right to ask for this, and a right to do what I can do in the situation. And a right to refuse service if I disagree."

Patient contact is at the heart of the nurse's role in health promotion, according to the study participants. However, this patient contact can also involve more than just traditional one-to-one interactions. Some nurses mentioned that they preferred to facilitate small-group sessions for some topics rather than undertaking individual patient teaching sessions, not a typical hospital nursing function. One participant explained: "For some topics, there are things that are pertinent to all patients . . . they get so much support from each other and so much information from each other." Facilitating group sessions was viewed by focus group participants as relevant and preferable for addressing topics such as medication management and preparation for hospital discharge. Fostering mutual aid did not always occur in a formal group setting. As one focus group participant observed:

Sometimes if you see that one patient has a need you think another patient could help (maybe they have had the same sort of procedure or they are going through the same thing), you can go and talk to one of the patients and say, "Mr. Such-and-Such down the hall is going through a similar thing and you've had this a little bit longer, would you like to go and talk to him?" And you can facilitate it.

In spite of nurses' best intentions and creative approaches, nurses in these studies reported substantial barriers to their health promotion practice, citing time constraints, workload, and attitudes on the unit as key influences. As well, the survey results indicated that lack of knowledge about health promotion, cultural factors, and discomfort with the health promoting role affect nurses' ability to care for patients in a manner that is health promoting. In a recent analysis of hospital nurses' health promotion practice, Robinson and Hill (1999) reported similar factors to those found in our studies and recommended that hospital managers should organize health promotion education sessions for nurses, create supportive work environments, and foster interdisciplinary collaboration. Gebbie (1998) observes that lack of funds is a barrier to establishing hospital-based health promotion programs such as comprehensive cancer prevention and screening programs. To overcome this barrier, Gebbie suggests that clinicians should become part of community-based initiatives such as local health boards or cancer societies to ensure that hospital health promotion programs are on community-based funding agendas.

Despite occasional studies examining hospital health promotion (Baskerville & Le-Touze, 1990; Hendryx, 1993; McBride & Moorwood, 1994), there is a paucity of research that addresses hospital health promotion practice. A major deficiency exists in research about the complexities of nurses' hospital health promotion practice. For example, hospital care plans, practice guidelines, or care maps have evolved to include various health promotion activities, yet little is known about their effectiveness in promoting health. Such tools (care maps in particular) have potential to be useful frameworks for evaluating the effectiveness of what is deemed to be quality care as implemented in everyday practice. Did we actually do what we said we would do? Variance from care maps and compliance with practice guidelines would permit a patient-focused analysis. If care maps and practice guidelines were also to include health promotion activities, focused health promotion research could occur using these tools as evaluation frameworks. Knowledge to guide hospital health promotion practice could then be generated about the complexities and effectiveness of nurses' health promotion work and patients' and families' responses to it.

How Do Patients View Quality Care?

Quality from the patient's perspective comprises many facets, some of which can be measured: waiting time for appointments, predictability of scheduled surgery, and turnaround times for the reporting of results. Although access to health care services and information as measured by these indicators may not have a primary effect on treatment outcomes, they can significantly impact a patient's personal anxiety and disrupt family life and relationships. There are numerous factors that affect patients' perceptions of quality care that, because of their complexity, are difficult to conceptualize and therefore to measure. Researchers at a Canadian teaching hospital surveyed patients and staff to assess the quality of care as seen "through the patient's eyes" (Charles et al., 1994; Bradley, 1986). These surveys revealed many disturbing things. Although patients rated overall quality of care high, over one-third stated that communication, physical care, pain, and discharge planning were not well managed. Survey analysis pointed to groups less well served than others: younger patients, female, single, admitted through the emergency department, and generally sicker.

Using the findings of such surveys to educate staff is a strategy that can catalyze change at the unit or ward level; for instance, informing nurses on a surgical unit that 25 percent of their own patients reported that no one talked to them about risks of surgery in ways they could understand, 21 percent did not understand the results of their surgery, 28 percent said that their fears and anxieties about the operation were not discussed, and 26 percent said they had more pain than they expected, raises nurses' awareness of areas of practice that require planning, collaboration, and new approaches to care. Informing nurses that patients stated emphatically that they did want to be involved in decisions about their care; that over 90 percent said that even if their medical news was bad, they wanted to know; that patients said they want to know about options for their treatment, and that they want their family to be fully informed about diagnosis and treatment, provides nurses with direction for how to approach interactions with patients and their family members. Thus, feedback such as that reported in this survey focuses areas for performance improvements. Surveys such as these may be powerful incentives to change practice toward that which is more health promoting, particularly when supported by staff education, formal policies, and ongoing evaluation.

There is only one way to understand how patients define quality. We must ask them. We health care providers need to define our success in terms of the well-being of our patients from their perspectives. Then, patients will assist us in defining success. We need multiple visions, rather than just one corporate vision. Yet, there is much to discover about quality care. What do we know about what we do not know? The fourth domain of the Johari Window is certainly the hardest to think about: This is the area that is unknown to both providers and patients. Knowing that we do not know is an important first step. But then what?

Probing What Is Unknown to Either Patient or Provider

In preparing for a major fundraising campaign, staff at one Canadian teaching hospital engaged a marketing firm to develop a marketing strategy (Vancouver Hospital, 1993). Marketers felt that it was crucial to understand patients' perceptions and ideals about the hospital and its place in the overall health care system. Using a commercially oriented agency with novel approaches brought new insights to hospital managers. The marketing agency exposed about 50 patients in six focus groups to various projective techniques, for example, bubble drawings, epitaphs, and collage-building, as a way to learn about the patients "mind set" about the hospital. Their findings indicated that patients subconsciously fear hospitals because they symbolize illness. Illness and hospitals have identical meanings in patients' experiences: lack of control, a state of dependence, restriction, and loss of freedom. The patients also feared "The System" with its "high tech" focus, a focus that in their view eclipsed a value for "people skills" they described as:

"They communicate at every level."

"They listen and allow me to ask questions."

"They educate me before I come in and before I leave."

So far these comments seem predictable and obvious to me (Berland) from the perspective of a health care manager. But when asked about the ideal relationship between a patient and a hospital, the patients' answers surprised me. For many of the focus group participants, the relationship, was captured in the phrase, "*an atmosphere of drunken intimacy.*" In such an environment it was felt that patients could ask for anything based on a healthy exchange of information. Some referred to a teacher-student relationship where the ultimate goal is to guide the student to independence.

These patients described a respectful partnership as the ideal. They recognized their reliance on providers' expertise, hence, in their view, it would not be an equal partnership.

But they also recognized that trust could be abused if there was no effort at collaboration and sharing of expertise. Therefore, they saw communication as the biggest indicator of respect and one that would in turn lead to their trust.

Choosing pictures to illustrate this ideal relationship, they selected a friendly senior professor coaching a student; a pair of ballet dancers, one balancing the other in a graceful pas de deux pose; two rowers in a light scull, straining for an unseen goal; and a team of baseball players swarming around their captain, spontaneously celebrating a victory—no white coats; no machines that go "ping!"

Education and Research: The Key to Improving Communication Between Patients and Providers

Not only do providers need to know more about what patients know, but patients need to know more of the things that providers know. Transferring knowledge from pro-

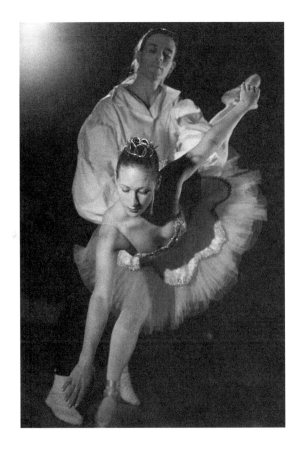

viders to patients is the traditional health education model. With new electronic technologies, this can now be simultaneously individualized and impersonal. Patients come to their doctors' offices carrying sheaves of pages printed from the Internet. "*I think I have this condition,*" they may say "*and this is what I want you to do about it.*" They have taken our indiscriminate health education model and turned it back on us.

Our challenge as health promoters will be to transform the mass production model of patient education to which our patients are exposed via the Internet into a mass customization model. We must provide individualized service from a wide range of possible options, including the Internet, patient education materials produced by hospital patient education departments, government, and voluntary organizations such as the American Heart Association and the Arthritis Society. This will require developing programs that account for broadly conceived individual differences, for example, age, culture, gender, and educational level, and tailored for delivery in a particular moment to a particular person and his or her family members. Many people, for instance, will manage quite well in a diabetes education program based on classroom or small-group instruction, but people who speak little English will require a supplementary program.

Professional development programs must focus on the individual in the context of his or her family and community. Patients often manage their own health supported by a network of others; they may let us help. For instance, women with breast cancer may need nurses' assistance to decide what information is appropriate to share with family members. A nurse can provide these women with opportunities to practice information-sharing interactions with family members using strategies such as role-playing. Such strategies can help women to anticipate the variety of responses from their children, spouses, or work colleagues. Role-playing—seeing ourselves from outside—can help women develop empathy for what family members are feeling. Strategies such as this have potential to contribute to the improved health of our patients and their family members. Evaluating strategies such as this will contribute to knowledge development to support the health promotion practice of hospital nurses.

Involvement in the process of their own care seems well established in the first domain of the Johari Window, what is understood by both providers and patients. What is not so clear is how much patients want to be involved at the health care system level. More involvement by patients is an article of faith for many in the health promotion field. However, neither providers nor patients are very clear about how the general public can best be involved in health care system improvement. This is a critical area for research, so that evidence leads to improvements in practice. (See Chap. 5 of this volume.)

A formal strategy to involve patients in planning and service development has been built into the health care reforms in many jurisdictions. Community members now have more representation either informally as individuals or as part of interest groups or formally as system governors, for example, as members of community health center boards. What can they achieve in these roles? Complex administrative matters requiring financial, legal, and human resources expertise are beyond the scope of most lay health board members. On the other hand, they are experts in community values, priorities in service needs, and patient perceptions of quality care. Effective orientation and training of community board members is critical for their success in directing a complex system (Office of the Auditor General, 1998). Beyond this, there must also be skillful elicitation of the lay board members' expertise and knowledge of the lived experience of health in setting goals and priorities.

Finally, one strategy to uncover patients' perceptions of quality care is to identify the rainmakers—those who bridge the cultural gap between patient and provider. Perhaps these are providers who have become patients. Sometimes an exceptional patient finds the reachable moment in a practitioner. Sometimes, it is research that brings forward the perspective of the patient to providers. (See Chap. 4 of this volume.)

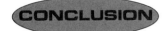

I have a patient now who is terminal. He cannot be cared for at home due to his medication. He is also a heavy smoker. At this point in his life, I don't think we could stop him smoking. So we allow him to live as normally as possible. We ask the family to take him for car rides outside; they take him to a restaurant; they take him to smoke in the roof-top garden. He is dressed in his normal clothes; he socializes; he participates in activities like aerobic exercises; he goes for outings with the other patients.

Here is a nurse who provides quality care in consultation with the patient and his family. What counts as healthful is defined by the patient and his family from their perspectives. The final outcome isn't going to improve the patient's health when defined as the absence of disease, the health professional's perspective. Nonetheless, by working from the patient's perspective on health, his or her satisfaction with the care he or she receives in hospital will improve beyond what is possible when applying standardized institutional prescriptions for care. What is quality care? It's all a matter of perspective.

REFERENCES

Barnsley, J., Lemieux-Charles, L., & Baker, G. R. (1996). Selecting clinical outcome indicators for monitoring quality of care. *Health Care Management Forum, 9,* 5–10.

Baskerville, B., & LeTouze, D. (1990). Facilitating the involvement of Canadian health care facilities in health promotion. *Patient Education and Counseling, 15,* 113–125.

Berland, A., & Whyte, N. (1993). *Hospital nurses and health promotion.* Vancouver, BC: Registered Nurses' Association of British Columbia.

Berland, A., Whyte, N., & Maxwell, L. (Young, L. E.) (1995). Hospital nurses and health promotion. *Canadian Journal of Nursing Research, 27*(4), 13–31.

Bradley, C. F. (1996). *In pursuit of quality.* Vancouver, BC: Vancouver Hospital.

Charles, C., Gauld, M., Chambers, L., O'Brien, B., Haynes, R. B., and Labelle, R. (1994). How was your hospital stay? Patients reports about their care in Canadian hospitals. *Canadian Medical Association Journal, 150,* 1813–1822.

Donabedian, A. (1988). The quality of care: How can it be managed? *Journal of the American Medical Association (JAMA), 266,* 1817–1821.

Evans, R. (1984) *Strained mercy: The economics of Canadian health care.* Toronto: Butterworth.

Gebbie, K. M. (1998). Payment for cancer prevention: community and government perspectives. *Cancer Practice: A Multidisciplinary Journal of Cancer Care, 6,* 47–50.

Heidemann, E. (1997). *Current and future challenges for quality management.* Toronto: Insight Press.

Hendryx, M. S. (1993). Rural hospital health promotion: Programs, methods, resource limitations. *Journal of Community Health, 18,* 241–250.

Luft, J., & Ingham, H. (1955) The Johari Window: A graphic model of interpersonal awareness. *Proceedings of Western Training Laboratory in Group Development.* Los Angeles: UCLA Extension Office.

Lupton, D. (1994). *Medicine as culture: Illness, disease and the body in Western societies.* Thousand Oaks, CA: Sage.

McBride, A., & Moorwood, Z. (1994). The hospital health promotion facilitator: an evaluation. *Journal of Clinical Nursing, 3,* 355–359.

Office of the Auditor General. (1998). *A review of governance and accountability in the regionalization of health services.* Victoria, BC: Province of British Columbia.

Riverview Hospital. (1998). *Patients' charter of rights.* Coquitlam, BC: Author.

Robinson, S. E., & Hill, Y. (1999). Our healthier hospital? The challenge for nurses. *Journal of Nursing Management, 7,* 13–17.

Shindul-Rothchild, J., & Gordon, S. (1998). Market driven health care and its impact on nurses. *Revolution-Journal of Nurse Empowerment, 4,* 92–97.

Vancouver Hospital. (1993). *Foundation marketing study.* Vancouver, BC: Author.

World Health Organization. (1984). *Health promotion: A discussion document on the concepts and principles.* Copenhagen: WHO Regional Office for Europe.

World Health Organization. (1986). *Ottawa Charter for health promotion.* Ottawa: Canadian Public Health Association & Health and Welfare Canada.

Wolf, G. (1995). Creating an environment for reengineering. In S. Blancett & D. Flarey (Eds.), *Reengineering nursing and health care* (pp. 100–117). Gathersburg, MD: Aspen.

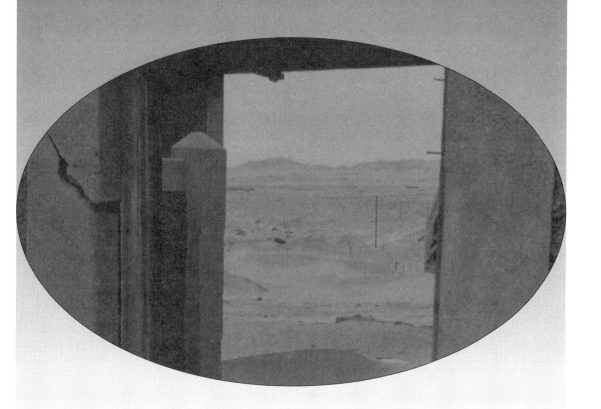

SECTION FOUR

Health
Promotion
Research

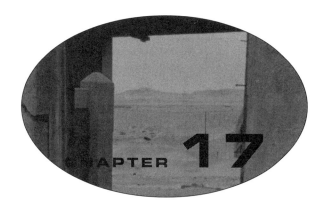

CHAPTER 17

Perspectives on Learning and Practicing Health Promotion in Hospitals: Nursing Students' Stories

MARCIA D. HILLS

A student completing the first-year nursing program writes:

I cannot believe that I am in the last three weeks of my first year of nursing. Where has the time gone? When I look back over the year, there were many times when everything seemed to have its own place. It was frustrating not doing a lot of hands-on work in the beginning and instead doing a lot of talking. But when it comes down to it, the "hands-on" skills have been the easier of the two to learn. You can "train" almost anyone to go through the motions. Becoming part of the patient's health team, to talk and listen to their needs, to understand and believe that the patient[1] has rights and beliefs about his/her own health; that has been the challenge of the first year . . .

I feel that I have gained the confidence and education to successfully achieve what is asked of me as a first year nurse. I have achieved everything from doing bed baths, to repositioning and turning, to vital signs, and medications, enemas, commodes, assisting with feeding, understanding the use of oxygen, charting . . . and the list could go on. Yet, the most important thing that I have learned is that the hands-on skills are not the only things that make a nurse. It has been exciting to see the pieces fall into place. As I look back to September, everything seemed to be in its own place:

[1]In this chapter, the terms patient and client are used interchangeably.

biology, health, professional growth, psychology. Now at the end of my first year as I look back, I realize that it all has become one—nursing; and I am becoming a nurse.

✳ Reflective Question

This student's reflections capture the essence of a first-year student's experience of learning to practice nursing from a health promotion perspective. How does it relate to your experience of practicing nursing?

The architects of an innovative nursing program in Canada envisioned health promotion as a viable and exciting curriculum framework for educating nurses for the 21st century. The curriculum that they designed is based in its entirety on the philosophy and principles of health promotion. Students are steeped in the rhetoric and discourse of health promotion, and the students' clinical experiences are chosen deliberately to provide for a wide range of health promotion experiences in both institutional and community settings. This health promotion curriculum and the process used for developing it are described elsewhere (Hills & Lindsey, 1994; Hills, Lindsey, Chisamore, Bassett-Smith, Abbott, & Fournier-Chalmers, 1994).

In an earlier study, experiences of students educated in this nursing program were examined for evidence of health promotion practice in hospitals (Hills, 1998). This chapter builds on that earlier research by analyzing the links between students' learning and their practice. This chapter reveals that students who are educated from a health promotion perspective do indeed practice in a way that reflects the central tenets of health promotion upon which their program was based. This chapter describes the tenets and related assumptions, introduces the study that was used to gather students' accounts of their hospital clinical experiences, includes illustrative narrative accounts of students' clinical experiences, and provides a critical analysis of the relationship between the students' clinical practice and the central tenets of health promotion.

Health Promotion: What's in a Definition?

The term **health promotion** is often used indiscriminately to capture many health initiatives. Within the context of this chapter, health promotion has the specific meaning described as follows and is perceived as being distinct from lifestyle change, illness prevention, or health education. Health promotion, for the purposes of this nursing program and this chapter, is defined as "a process of enabling people to increase control over and to improve their **health**" (World Health Organization, 1986). The endorsement of this definition by the nursing program architects impacted upon their development of the curriculum and of the processes that were to be used to educate future nurses.

Three pillars of health promotion are embedded in this definition. So defined, health promotion is first and foremost *about people* and only subsequently about health. Because health promotion is concerned with people, the nature of health professionals' relationships with people is of utmost importance. *Empowerment* is a second concept embedded in this definition. Issues of power and control lie at the heart of all nursing health promotion practice. The definition implies a third and related concept. If people are to increase control over and improve their health, they need not only the power to do so but also the requisite knowledge and skills. Health promotion practice is also about *enabling*. Al-

though described in differing terms, these three tenets—the primacy of people, empowerment, and enabling—are generally considered the pillars of health promotion (Labonte, 1993; Raeburn, 1992; Raeburn & Rootman, 1999; Wallerstein & Bernstein, 1994).

✳ Reflective Questions

1. How do you conceptualize health promotion?

2. What do you think are the central tenets of health promotion?

The Three Pillars and Related Assumptions

The Primacy of People

People are at the heart of nursing health promotion practice. Acceptance of this adage means acceptance of certain assumptions that underlie it. Students educated in this nursing program are taught to value and care for the person, not to focus upon the disease. Further, they are taught that it is the person and the relationship with that person, not the skill or task being done for the person, that is the core of health promotion nursing practice. They are taught to value the uniqueness and diversity of individuals. Respect for differences, whether of race, culture, sexual orientation, or ways of thinking about the world, is inherent in a health promotion perspective. Students are taught that people experience the world as whole human beings and make meaning of the world that they experience. Therefore, students are encouraged to view people as whole beings who cannot be separated into component parts.

Although it is common in nursing to describe people as bio-psycho-social beings, this language still suggests that you can know parts of a person; therefore, within the health promotion curriculum, this type of language is avoided. Because the health promotion curriculum is informed by a phenomenological theoretical orientation, students are taught that people are always situated in time and place, and cannot be understood outside of that context. This assumption is particularly significant in hospital-based nursing. In very simple terms, it is the realization that people do not live in hospitals but rather in homes and communities and that, consequently, nurses need to deal directly with people's social, political, and historical contexts, recognizing the impact of this context in relation to health choices. The overall intention of this nursing program is that students will learn to value people and their experiences as central to nursing rather than thinking that diseases or skills are the primary focus of nursing. This focus on people and their health and healing experiences is consistent throughout the curriculum.

✳ Reflective Questions

1. How does your health promotion practice recognize the primacy of people and their experiences?
2. What strategies do you use to keep people at the center of your care?

Empowerment

Empowerment is a pivotal concept throughout health promotion (Freire, 1972; Labonte, 1993; Raeburn, 1992; Raeburn & Rootman, 1999; Rappaport, 1981; Wallerstein & Bernstein, 1994). This nursing program includes hospital clinical experiences; therefore, it is important to understand health promotion nursing practice in the context of a hospital setting as well as in community settings. Furthermore, the majority of students will graduate to work in hospitals. This chapter deals only with a restricted view of the concept of empowerment: empowerment in its relationship to the nurses' roles with individuals and families in hospitals. Individual and family empowerment, implications for the nurse's roles, and the resulting client-nurse relationship, all within the hospital context, are germane to this chapter.

As Labonte (1993, p. 49) explains, "the empowering act exists only as a relational act of power taken and given in the same instance." In hospital settings nurses do have more power than clients so they need to learn to develop relationships with clients in which power is negotiated. Nurses have power in their knowledge, not only of the medical con-

dition and how to assist the client to heal, but also of the system and the rules by which it functions.

Nurses always have a choice of using their power to create "power over" or "power with" relationships with their clients. "Power over" relationships value nurses' knowledge over the clients' knowledge and nurses with "power over" relationships attempt to educate clients to hospital routine and the hospital's way of doing things. The nurse is in charge and knows what is best for the client. Clients who resist the good intentions of the nurse are often labeled "noncompliant." In contrast, "power with" relationships are characterized by valuing the clients' experiences, conveying respect for patients and their points of view, and co-creating a shared understanding of the situation that the clients are experiencing. In the BC Program, students are taught how to negotiate power and how to create "power with" relationships.

The valuing of egalitarian relationships is based on the belief that there is a reciprocity between power and control and that, in order for there to be more equitable relationships, those in power must be willing to give up control so that others may share their power. This is critical in the relationship between nurses and clients. Shared power does not negate health professionals' responsibilities, skills, or knowledge. It is the coupling of the nurses' knowledge with the patients' understanding and experience that creates the basis of care planning and decision making.

Hegemony is a critical concept that is related to empowerment. Hegemony refers to the ability of a dominant group to control the actions or behaviors of others. . . . Hegemonic power is that form of power-over that is invisible, internalized, structured within the very nature of our day to day living so that we come to take it for granted. (Labonte, 1993, p. 50)

Students are taught to recognize the prevailing hegemony within the health care system and to create a counter hegemony by understanding the systemic nature of some issues and the impact of this institutional ethos on people who work in the system. In addition, they are encouraged to attempt to overcome the hegemony by establishing egalitarian relationships.

Students learn health promotion strategies that seek to empower and emancipate. "Empowerment . . . thus embodies an interactive process of change, where institutions and communities become transformed as people who participate in changing them become transformed" (Wallerstein & Bernstein, 1994, p. 142). Empowerment comes from the act of finding one's voice and that can only occur in conditions of justice and equity.

✸ Reflective Questions

1. Think of a time when you were engaged in an empowering experience with a client(s). What were the key elements in the situation that made it empowering?

2. Think of a time when you were engaged in a situation with a client and you used your power "over" the client. What might you do differently if you were confronted by a similar situation in the future?

Enabling

Enabling is closely related to empowerment but it deserves separate attention. To increase control over and to improve one's health, one must be not only *empowered* to do so but also *able* to do so. To be able, one must possess the requisite skills, resources, and knowledge. The fundamental assumption underlying the notion of enabling is that people have capacity—to identify their own needs, to solve their own problems, and to generally know what is best for them in a given situation. If you believe that people have capacity, you can act in ways that develop ability and that are empowering. If, on the other hand, you do not hold this belief, it will be difficult to do either.

To enable clients, nurses need to develop collaborative relationships with them and begin "where the client is." Historically, nursing has not done so. Although some theorists (Newman, 1986; Parse, 1990; Quinn, 1989; Watson, 1988) have advocated for a more humanistic enabling approach, a problem-oriented approach that is built upon a deficit model of care continues to dominate nursing practice. This problem orientation is clearly reflected in the use of nursing process and nursing diagnosis. "The nursing process of assessment and intervention is inherently a medical model approach requiring the nurse to label a person and intervene with universal advice, often without acknowledging the uniqueness of the person or the meaning of the experience" (Morgan & Marsh, 1998).

Furthermore, nursing has been reluctant to trust people to act in their own best interests. "On the whole, professionals do not trust ordinary people, seeing them as lacking knowledge, living inappropriate lifestyles, absconding with resources, and generally not doing what they should to keep themselves healthy" (Raeburn & Rootman, 1999, p. 19). By contrast, from a health promotion orientation, people are viewed as experts about their bodies and their experiences. Nurses focus on clients' strengths and see people as their own best resource who often need only support or understanding to better appreciate their health issues or problems. They include the clients as partners in the care planning process.

From a health promotion perspective, health and illness are understood to co-exist and are not points on a continuum. People who are experiencing health issues often view themselves as healthy because health is individually defined and best understood by the person experiencing it. People experience similar health issues differently so nurses must rely on clients to share their experiences of a given health issue. Nurses educated with a health promotion perspective learn to initiate their care by eliciting the client's story. They are taught to place great faith in the client's experience and to use the client's story as a starting point to plan care. Then, based on the client's experience and the nurse's knowledge, a plan of care is developed collaboratively. Clients are trusted and seen as a valuable resource in care planning.

Health promotion can be thought of as a paradigmatic approach to health and health care. It is an acceptance of certain beliefs, values, assumptions, and central tenets that results in a particular "way of being." And so, in this nursing program, nursing content that historically would be presented by discussing diseases is instead organized within the themes of people's experiences with health and healing. Clients are viewed as facing challenges and nurses act as facilitators to assist clients to deal with these challenges. It is hoped that this approach will result in a health care practice that reflects a particular worldview.

✳ Reflective Questions

1. How does your practice reflect this enabling stance?

2. What strategies do you use to develop collaborative relationships with your clients?

3. How do you incorporate the client's story into your plan of care?

The Research with Students

This section briefly describes the data collection methods used to gather nursing students' accounts of practice experiences in hospital settings and the subsequent analysis of the data that was performed to examine whether the central tenets of health promotion were present in the students' descriptions of their practice.

Data Collection

Twenty-four students enrolled in either the second or third semester of the nursing program volunteered to participate and their signed informed consents were obtained. Their clinical experiences consisted of approximately six hours each day for two days a week over a 14-week semester. All collected information was coded to ensure anonymity and confidentiality.

Qualitative research methods were used to collect the data. One of the methods, the Iterative Dialogue Review Process, had been developed specifically to encourage students to critically reflect on their clinical experiences; it is described in detail elsewhere (Hills, 1998; Hills, Tanner, Calnan, Greene, & Belliveau, 2000). This process consists of several stages: (a) students write stories (narratives) from their clinical experiences in their "reflective journals"; (b) these stories are analysed by the students using a framework developed for this purpose; (c) these stories and analyses are submitted to the appropriate faculty members for review; (d) the faculty respond

to the students' critiques by raising questions that will assist the students to reflect further on the experiences that have been described; (e) these notes, questions, and comments are returned to the students; and (f) the students respond to the faculty members' comments. The compilation of the narratives, reflections, and student-faculty dialogue comprise the data for the study.

Each semester, students submitted five or six stories that were generated from their clinical experiences. They were asked to give as much detail as needed for someone else to understand their intentions, feelings, and thoughts as the situation unfolded. To assist students in choosing appropriate stories from their practice, students were given guidelines that had been developed for similar research (Benner & Tanner, 1987; Hills et al., 2000). The students were asked to choose an incident in which they felt their intervention really made a difference in patient outcome, either directly or indirectly (by helping other staff members); an incident that went particularly well; an incident in which there was a breakdown (things did not go as planned); an incident that was ordinary or typical; an incident that captured the quintessence of what nursing is all about; an incident that was particularly demanding; or an incident that stood out for some reason.

After writing their narratives, students were asked to critically reflect on their experience using an analytical framework developed for this purpose (Hills, Chisamore, & Hughes, 2000). New insights were developed as students engaged in a reflective process, which assisted them to re-evaluate their experiences and, therefore, to link new ideas with existing knowledge and feelings, and to translate thoughts and ideas into action (Boud, Keogh, & Walker, 1985). Faculty reviewed students' journals, posed strategic questions to encourage further reflection, and then returned the journals to the students for their comment. In this way, an iterative dialogical process was created between the teacher and the students.

Data Analysis

For the purpose of this chapter, a thematic analysis of the students' journals containing the narratives, reflections, and student-teacher dialogue was conducted using van Manen's recommendations (1990). This analysis focused on revealing links between students' descriptions and interpretations of their experiences and the central tenets of health promotion that were identified as forming the basis of the curriculum. The journals were read several times in their entirety to grasp a sense of the whole experience that each student described. The narratives and journals were read again to search for meanings in order to identify stories that reflected the central tenets of health promotion. This process is "more accurately a process of insightful invention, discovery, and disclosure . . . grasping and formulating a thematic understanding is not a rule bound process but a free act of 'seeing' meaning" (van Manen, 1990, p. 79).

Student Examples

The analysis revealed evidence of the three central tenets of health promotion that are intrinsic to this nursing program and are clearly reflected in students' narrative accounts of their clinical experiences. The following excerpts from students' journals are illustrative.

The Primacy of People

Students consistently described the importance of placing the person at the center of his or her care. As one student explained, "a patient is a person first and a patient second." Another stated, "The man who was my patient who passed away was also someone's husband, someone's father and someone's friend."

This repeated focus on the person reflected students' ability to incorporate their learning about nursing as being primarily concerned with people and their experiences of health and healing rather than being concerned with disease. The following narrative eloquently highlights this point. The student wrote:

A friend of mine died the other day. I didn't know her very well but in the short time that I knew her I learned a lot about myself. She was in hospital because of a bacterial infection, possibly tuberculosis, and I as a nursing student was asked if I wanted to be assigned to care for her. Usually I am quite eager to get a chance to increase my knowledge about different disease processes and to help others understand their situation, I found myself

hesitating to take her as a patient. You see, she was HIV positive. I tried to sort out the different feelings I was experiencing, the biggest one being fear.

Fear immobilized me. I found that I couldn't think clearly but I really was hoping that I wouldn't have to be her nurse. At that point I can honestly say that I cared more about myself than I did about her. I worried about somehow getting infected; I thought of what I might be bringing home to my children. I approached her bed with hesitant steps and introduced myself. She was very pleasant and very willing to have a student care for her. She told me that she was also a nurse and could remember what it was like being a student. Then very efficiently, she explained to me about the equipment around her and what the doctor was attempting to do for her while she was in hospital. That day and the next, we spent some time getting to know one another.

Over the next few weeks I chose her as my patient assignment. As my fear dissipated and my knowledge of her illness grew, I began to understand some of what she was going through. I also began to see how other nurses were caught up in their fear. When she would press her call bell, a nurse would answer over the intercom and avoid entering her room. When staff did enter her room, they would put gloves on, even if they were not doing an invasive procedure. No one touched her other than to do something with her equipment, and even then they did not linger long at her bedside. I felt myself bristling at the injustice and unfairness, although I am ashamed to say that I didn't speak up for her when others would make assumptions about her. The world of a student is a double-edged sword. I was only there two days a week and I felt powerless to help her.

As her illness progressed, she experienced behavioral changes and would occasionally lash out at me. Although she was sometimes quite demanding about the way things were done, I was able to look beyond the behavior and appreciate her frustration. Because others had not taken the opportunity to get to know the person, they saw only the disease and labeled her accordingly.

This woman taught me that fear is natural but we can get beyond it if we take the first step. When we learn about our fears we are able to look beyond them. I call her my friend because she did everything that friends do for one another, and I tried to do the same for her. Sadly though, she died alone in a hospital filled with people too afraid of the illness to care for the person. She had hopes and dreams just as you and I do. Despite the struggle near the end of her life, no one stayed with her to face the inevitable, to calm her fears, to tell her that she would be missed. I wish I had thanked her for helping me to make the journey from ignorance to knowledge. I will miss her, but she will always be with me as will others who have taught me so much about caring.

The student demonstrated respect and caring for this woman as she described how she learned from her and was able to look beyond her behavior, even when she "lashed out at her." Her description and criticism of others that seemed to work from a perspective that focused more on the disease than the person demonstrates the value the student placed on a person-centered approach to care.

There exists an ongoing debate among faculty members who teach in this nursing program about the emphasis during the first year on the development of this person-centered orientation. Faculty members often wonder if there should be more focus on developing nursing "technical" skills. The journal excerpt that opens this chapter captures what many students describe as the frustrations and rewards of learning to place people at the center of their care. This student has learned to place the "skills" within the context of caring for people. She embraces this health promotion philosophy and recognizes its value as a way of being with clients. Looking at the earlier quotation from her reflective journal, we see her initial frustrations of attending to biology, psychology, and nursing courses, and not getting to the "hands-on work" in clinical practice. Instead, it seemed to her that nursing was "doing a lot of talking." On reflection, however, she discovered that for her, the technical skills were easier to learn to do than the relating to people, her patients. Being a health promoting nurse is more than "training" in psychomotor development. "Real" nursing has fallen into place: "Becoming part of a patient's health team, to talk and listen to their needs, to understand and believe that the patient has rights and beliefs about his/her own health has been the challenge of this first year."

In another example, a student described how she overcame her nervousness about performing a skill by understanding the impact that her decision might have on her client. She wrote:

I think my narrative regarding changing the catheter is a good illustration of the health and healing domain. I overcame my own uneasiness regarding the situation because it was important for me to preserve Mr. P's personhood. If I backed out of his care because of my own insecurities, it might convey the message that I'm more concerned about me rather than him. It would be terribly degrading for him. I feel I am also developing an open, caring approach to my practice. At times, as a student, this becomes difficult when I become more concerned with the task at hand than the person for whom I am performing the task. I would hope that as time progresses, an open, caring manner will become second nature in my practice.

The student shows that she values having the person as being central to her care even to the displacement of technical skills. People, not skills or tasks, are the primary focus of nursing. Interestingly, the student concludes not with the hope that she will become more skillful but with the hope that she will become caring!

✳ Reflective Questions

1. What stands out in these stories as significant to your own practice?

2. What story from your practice comes to mind as you read these students' stories?

Empowerment

Students' stories about empowerment provide strong evidence for health promotion practice. The students consistently spoke of the need for clients to be in control of decisions about their health care and often reported planning their care based on the clients' expressed desires. Client participation in planning and decision making is evident repeatedly. Students not only showed a willingness to alter hospital routines to suit their clients' needs, but they also questioned why this was not done by others. They consistently reflected a desire to develop "power with" relationships and they often criticized other nurses who seemed to create "power over" relationships with their clients.

One student who had admitted a woman who was to have open heart surgery had the opportunity to accompany this client to the operating room and recovery room. She described her experience in the recovery room as she attempted to establish a "power with" relationship with her client. She wrote:

Although the patient, an 80-year-old woman, had appeared pleasant and calm pre-operatively, in the recovery room the patient quickly became labeled "very confused, agitated and combative." I observed one RN pass this judgement to another RN and when the patient became more vocal she was told to "shut up." I was stunned and pretended not to hear. The patient did calm down but when I sat with her I apologized for having an RN speak to her that way. I explained that they were pressed for time and had a heavy work load. . . . I made sure that I was there for the patient and I tried to explain what the nurses were doing and what their rationales were. What I observed was nurses explaining something briefly but never really clarifying if the client understood or had any questions. . . . She ended up being a "noncompliant patient" because she didn't understand what was happening. I spoke softly in her ear and she seemed to respond. She wanted me to look after her and she didn't want to deal with the RN. I explained my role as a student but this was followed by the RN saying to the patient, "You're stuck with me for 10 more hours Grace, you can take it or leave it. I feel like you are wasting my time when you know we are here to help you." Are we really there to help by this kind of statement? Do we allow her to express her own control? Do we help her powerlessness?

At the end of the day I was so mad at myself for not saying something to the RN. I felt shocked, frustrated and a mere observer. I felt I would be in the wrong to critique the RN. Showing the other side of a "role model" seemed to be the most appropriate thing to do. I showed the RN how I would communicate with the client. The client responded to my questions, she asked more questions until everything was clarified and she became more co-operative and less agitated. I demonstrated empathy towards her family and told them that this type of agitation was common after surgery. The RN was busy adjusting her work schedule when she could have spent a little time easing the family's suffering. The family was relieved once I spent some time explaining things to them.

This student chose to facilitate a "power with" relationship with the client. She was empathic and respectful of the client and her family's experiences. "The process of empowerment is to a large extent controlled by the nurse. Empowerment is as much a process as it is an outcome. It is not just something that happens, but a process that is facilitated" (Caraher, 1998, p. 55). In contrast to the RN, the student gave up control and negotiated power with the client. She shared her knowledge and discussed issues with the client and family. Hegemony is also present in this story as the student, "knowing" not to criticize the RN, tries to create a counter-hegemony by being with the client in a way that she knows is different than the norm.

In another story, the student questions whose needs are being met and why hospital routines are not altered more to fit the patient's needs. The student described:

My patient was going for an X-ray and had his last pain medication at 0730hrs. The porter came for him at 1010hrs. I knew I could not give him his morphine as the order read q3h. I should have either told the porter to come back in a half an hour or given the patient some Tylenol. I would not have done this without asking the RN first, but it was ordered PRN. I feel that the patient's

needs were not being met. The X-ray departments . . . expected that the patient would fit into their schedule. I should have been an advocate for the patient. So what if their schedule was upset? That patient was in a lot of pain and was one day post-op. I did say to the RN, "Can't they bring up a portable X-ray machine?" She said that they are in short supply. That is when I should have spoken up.

Another example of hegemony was last week while I was at coffee. Physiotherapy came and took my patient to the physio room. I was planning the morning so that I could give my patient's meds at 1000hrs. Physio usually came at 1030.They must know by now the patients' medication times. I went to the physio room and suggested that I give them there. . . . They did not seem too happy because it took 15–20 minutes but I thought, "the patient is the priority here." Maybe next time they will inform us if they need to come early. I have noticed with physio they seem to come when they decide to. I can sure see how important it is to critically question the hegemony of current nursing practice.

This student challenged the dominant institutional norms, taken-for-granted assumptions and procedures. By questioning traditional practices the student exemplified her willingness to change the system to better meet her client's needs.

One student described a situation in which she tried to individualize nursing care to accommodate the client's desires. However, the client was not sure about how to respond to the idea that he could have some say in his care. The student explained:

I spent a great deal of time talking to him and giving him choices in the care I was going to provide for him. For example, when would he like to be washed up or when would he like to go for a walk. He would say to me "You're the one running the show, it doesn't matter what I want." I would reply, "Yes it does, you have a say in the care you receive."

Here, even the patient had accepted the hegemony!

One student described the tension between enabling and empowering clients, on the one hand, and professional responsibility on the other. She wrote:

I must admit I squirmed somewhat when the speaker today advocated giving clients control over their care because they know what's best for them. I agree that they know what's best for them but I guess I have questions regarding responsibility. Our system doesn't allow for us to sign over our responsibilities to the client so that if we allow the client to have the control over their care (which, in a perfect world, they should have) and something goes sideways we are ultimately liable. Is there some system wherein we can sign our responsibilities over to them and therefore they get their control and we can freely give them that control without fear of liabilities? Maybe really listening to our clients and trusting that they know best is the answer—it is certainly more of a challenge. I can see the need for change in our system when dealing with clients who want to have more control over their care. I'm having trouble perceiving its implementation but it all begins by questioning the hegemony of our system today and then perhaps we can work towards the change tomorrow.

Clearly, there are aspects of the current hegemony that are troubling for this student. She seemed to appreciate the importance of people having control over factors affecting their health but questioned how this can actually happen. She has not yet learned how to share power without negating the nurse's responsibility, skills, or knowledge.

In another situation, the nursing staff was concerned about a patient who was taking vitamins for her multiple sclerosis. The staff was concerned that the client was being taken advantage of by the vitamin salesperson and that she was not accepting her condition. The student has a different interpretation of this situation. She explained:

The client said that the vitamins have really improved how she feels. She says that she knows she is supposed to accept the MS and she says that she does. She takes the vitamins to deal with the fatigue. She really believes that they work and says that she's not nearly so tired as she used to be. . . . She says that they are all natural things and won't harm her. The vitamins are obviously giving her some hope. She realizes it's not going to cure her. She just wants to have some control and the highest quality of life that's possible.

Perhaps the differing points of view, student versus nurse, derive simply from different starting points of accepting and not accepting that the client has the capacity to know what is best for herself.

✳ Reflective Questions

1. What is your reaction to the way the nurses behaved in these stories?
2. How might you have responded in these situations?
3. What are you left wondering about?

Enabling

Students' stories demonstrated their desire to work with clients in a way that was enabling.

This often involved developing a partnership with clients so that the students and clients could work together sharing knowledge, ascertaining what the clients already knew and what other understanding or knowledge was required.

One student described how, by developing a collaborative relationship and eliciting the client's story, she encouraged the client to identify her own needs and assisted her in getting the resources that she needed.

I have discovered that almost all the time even the most intractable of patients will blossom and unfold if you just give them a few minutes of undivided attention. There have been at least a half a dozen times in the last two weeks that I have been able to use warmth, humor, and presencing with nearly miraculous results when dealing with patients who have had a wide variety of diagnoses. One lady whose husband was on the telemetry side was waiting for surgery the next morning on the gyne side and was feeling very scared and unsure about a lot of things; like who would care for them when they left the hospital, they had no resources to access. She was worried about pain and how long she would be in the hospital, she even considered canceling the surgery that she had waited months to get. Just listening to her and letting her speak was calming for her and afterwards I was able to reassure her that should the need arise we could set up some home care for her or whatever they might need to get over this bump in their lives. I gave her a small hug and she clung to me for quite some time and tearfully said thank you. Later, when she was on the gyne end I would sit with her for a bit and she said that I was the only one that ever came in and said good morning to her. I cannot say that this is true or not but I know that she was glad of me.

This student saw potential in her client. She understood the importance of simply being with the client rather than trying to fix the problem. She saw the client as a person who was facing challenges and discussed with the client ways of dealing with these issues in the context of her life.

Another student described how she used information gained from the patient to plan appropriately for the insertion of a nasal gastric tube. As she explained:

*Reflecting on the insertion of the NG tube, I believe this experience falls well into the parameters of the health and healing domain [a term used to describe an aspect of nursing **praxis**]. By involving and encouraging the patient in the procedure, I was able to maximize the patient's participation and control. For example, I discussed his previous experience with an NG tube in place. He was able to tell me of his sore nostril and the discomfort associated with the positioning of the tape se-*

*curing the tube in place. I believe there was good commu-
nication between the patient and myself allowing me to
provide optimal emotional support and attend to his
comfort needs.*

Another story tells how the student
learned that simply giving information may
not be enabling and that nurses need to know
what the clients understand about the information they receive. The student wrote:

*The first day I was on the ward I accompanied a nurse as
she talked to a patient who was being discharged that
day. As the nurse talked to the patient, she interjected
questions to test the patient's knowledge of her condition
as well as what activities would be appropriate while recovering from her open heart surgery. One interesting
discrepancy arose in that the patient was not aware that
she couldn't drive for up to six weeks after the surgery, if
not longer, depending how the sternum heals. The patient was not aware of this thinking that she could put a
pillow under her seat belt and drive off.*

*This interchange between the nurse and the patient
reinforced for me the fact that you can explain procedures
and guidelines to a patient; however, sometimes I think it
is too much information to assimilate at one time and it is
best to continue to communicate with the patient about
their understanding and knowledge of the surgery and
recovery process. Fortunately for this patient, the nurse
realized that the patient had not understood that she
could not drive a car for another couple of months and
reinforced this with the patient and explained to her the
reasons for this.*

The important point for the student is
knowing where the client is coming from,
knowing what the client understands about
the information that has been shared. Too
often, nurses assume that if patients are told
something, they understand it and they can
then care for themselves. As is demonstrated
in this story, through the process of critical dialogue, nurses can know what clients already
know and what else they need in order to
care for themselves.

The final story, an account of a student's
experiences and her reflections upon them,
demonstrates how she saw her client as being
the expert about her healing experience. It
also clearly contains many other references to
the assumptions that underlie all three of the
central tenets of health promotion practice:

*During my first day of clinical practice for this semester, I
was involved in an incident in which my intervention
really did make a difference in patient outcome. My
client, Mrs. J., 74 years old, was two days post-op for a
Rt. hemiarthroplasty. Mrs. J. was using a PCA for pain*

*control and was to undergo her first session with physio-
therapy.*

*Upon the initial assessment of my client, I inquired as
to whether or not she was experiencing any pain. On a
scale of 1–10 she gave a figure 3 to indicate her pain
level. She stated that she pushes the morphine release
button frequently in order to ensure the pain doesn't become any greater. She also told me that the PCA had
"gone on the blink" during the night and was not providing her with adequate pain relief. She said she had
pushed her button several times, yet the morphine was
not being released. This problem had been confirmed in
morning report. I later learned that the [pump] had not
been recording the number of "pushes" through the
night. As a result, Mrs. J. received a new PCA early in
the morning.*

The Issue
*While I was in with Mrs. J., the anesthetist came in to see
her. She told Mrs. J. that she felt the PCA was no longer
required and that an oral pain medication would be prescribed instead. Mrs. J. became visibly upset and told the
anesthetist that she was not yet ready to come off the
PCA. The anesthetist insisted that she was "obviously"
ready to come off it as she had not pushed the button all
night. Mrs. J. further explained that the PCA had not
been working properly and that she indeed had pushed
the button several times through the night. The anesthetist replied, "That's fine but I believe you're ready for
oral pain relief now anyway." The anesthetist left the
room to go write the d/c orders for the PCA. I stayed with
Mrs. J., knowing that she would likely want to discuss
this further. Mrs. J. was very upset and in tears. She was
concerned that she wouldn't be able to take the pain. She
also stated, "I will not even attempt to move my leg if I'm
in any kind of pain."*

My Thoughts and Feelings
*"Pain is what the person experiencing it says it is!" Mrs.
J. is still experiencing a lot of pain and doesn't feel she is
ready to be off the PCA. She would feel better if she could
have it for one more day. She has also stated that she will
not attempt to ambulate if she experiences any pain.
Therefore, by discontinuing the PCA she will experience
increased anxiety possibly leading to increased pain possibly leading to decreased mobility leading to potential
respiratory problems and compromised tissue integrity.*

*At this same time, I was also concerned with some is-
sues surrounding my clinical practice. . . . Would the
staff think I was being critical of the way things were
done here? Would they think I was overzealous and
overreacting to Mrs. J.'s needs? Would this diminish my
chances of having any future credibility on this unit? All
these thoughts and questions came to mind as I reflected
on Mrs. J.'s dilemma.*

My Actions
*Mrs. J.'s needs were much more of a priority than my
concerns over what the staff may be thinking of me. I am
a very strong patient advocate and am not able to down-
play or ignore my patient's needs at any expense. I approached the RN and anesthetist and asked about the*

PCA. "Is it standard practice to d/c it two days post-op?" They informed me that 2–3 days was about the norm, but that Mrs. J. wasn't really needing it any more. I told them that she did need to have the PCA one more day and that she was still pushing the button frequently. The anesthetist said that she wasn't pushing it very much as it showed no record of this through the night. She also said that oral pain relief would be sufficient. I explained that my client was very anxious about potential pain and would not attempt to ambulate if any pain were present. I further informed them that Mrs. J. stated that she would at least try to ambulate with physiotherapy today providing she has use of the PCA. This machine seemed to provide her with a feeling of confidence and control over her situation. The RN did then reaffirm that this was a new PCA and that the faulty one had not been recording the frequency of pushes throughout the night. The anesthetist replied that she was unaware that my client had pushed the button during the night (although Mrs. J. had told her this earlier). As a result of my intervention, the anesthetist and RN agreed to leave the PCA in place for another day.

I was pleased with the outcome of my intervention. My client was now less anxious and would at least make an effort with physiotherapy today. My need for credibility seemed unimportant now!

The student acted as a patient advocate out of a deep sense of trust in the patient's experience. She saw the patient as being in the best position to name the experience and she rec-ognized that she couldn't assume that what works for one client will work for another. "Pain is what the person experiencing it says it is!" She enhanced the client's capacity for health by advocating for the client's voice to be heard. This student's approach to care is reminiscent of MacLeod-Clark's (1993) description of health nursing:

A health model of nursing encompasses the fact that each individual's need for care is different and that whenever possible, patients and clients should be involved in decisions about and be able to participate in their care. Health nursing focuses on maximising the potential for health and independence. It builds on people's existing knowledge and experience, helps them become more autonomous and empowers them to take responsibility for their own health. (p. 258)

> ✳ **Reflective Questions**
>
> **1.** In what ways does your practice reflect this description of health nursing?
> **2.** In what ways do the students' stories resonate with your own experiences?

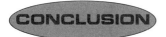

CONCLUSION

The evidence of the three tenets in students' narrative accounts suggests that students who are educated with a health promotion perspective do value and attempt to practice in that way. Students' assessments reveal that they believe that this approach makes a difference to clients and that, in fact, clients are getting better quality care. The students' stories leave no doubt that they believe that practicing in a way that attends to the primacy of people and that is empowering and enabling is a worthwhile way to practice nursing.

It remains troubling that too often the professionals with whom the students worked did not hold the same values and seemed unaware of the impact of their practice on client care. Students' caring health promotion perspective often stood out in stark contrast to the "less caring" manner of the institution's staff! This seems to indicate that the current hegemony militates against the kind of practice that these students embrace. More research is needed to better understand the hegemony of current nurses' practices.

Acknowledgements

The authors wishes to acknowledge the contribution of the faculty and students at Camosun College, Victoria, BC, for their participation in the study from which this chapter was drawn.

REFERENCES

Benner, P., & Tanner, C. (1987). Clinical judgement: How expert nurses use intuition. *American Journal of Nursing, 87*, 23–31.

Boud, D., Keogh, R., & Walker D. (Eds.) (1985). *Reflection: Turning experience into learning.* London: Kogan Page.

Caraher, M. (1988). Patient education and health promotion: Clinical health promotion—the conceptual link. *Patient Education and Counselling, 33*, 49–58.

Freire, P. (1972). *Pedagogy of the oppressed.* London: Penguin Books.

Hills, M. (1998). Student experiences of nursing health promotion practice in hospital settings. *Nursing Inquiry, 5*, 164–173.

Hills, M., Chisamore, M., & Hughes, M. (2000). *Clinical evaluation in a caring curriculum: Development of an appraisal framework.* Unpublished manuscript, University of Victoria, Victoria, BC. (in review)

Hills, M., & Lindsey, L. (1994). Health promotion: A viable curriculum framework for nursing education. *Nursing Outlook, 42*, 158–162.

Hills, M., Lindsey, L., Chisamore, M., Bassett-Smith, J., Abbott, K., & Fournier-Chalmers, J. (1994). University-college collaboration: Rethinking curriculum development in nursing education. *Journal of Nursing Education, 33*, 220–225.

Hills, M., Tanner, C., Calnan, R., Greene, E., & Belliveau, D. (2000). *Clinical evaluation in a caring curriculum: Encouraging reflective practice through an iterative dialogue review process.* Unpublished manuscript, University of Victoria, Victoria, BC.

Labonte, R. (1993). *Health promotion and empowerment: Practice frameworks.* Toronto: Centre for Health Promotion & ParticipACTION, University of Toronto.

MacLeod Clark, J. (1993). From sick nursing to health nursing: Evolution or revolution? In J. Wilson-Barnett & J. MacLeod Clark (Eds.), *Research in health promotion research and nursing* (pp. 249–255). London: Macmillan.

Morgan, I., & Marsh, G. (1998). Historic and future health promotion contexts for nursing. *Image: Journal of Nursing Scholarship, 30*, 379–383.

Newman, M. (1986). *Health as expanding consciousness.* St. Louis, MO: Mosby.

Parse, R. (1990). Health: A personal commitment. *Nursing Science Quarterly, 3*, 136–140.

Quinn, J. (1989). On healing, wholeness, and the haelen effect. *Nursing and Health Care, 10*, 553–556.

Raeburn, J. (1992). Health promotion research with heart: Keeping a people perspective. *Canadian Journal of Public Health, 83*(1), 20–24.

Raeburn, J., & Rootman, I. (1999). *People-centered health promotion.* Chichester: John Wiley.

Rappaport, J. (1981). In praise of paradox: A social policy of empowerment over prevention. *American Journal of American Psychology, 9*, 1–25.

van Manen, M. (1990). *Researching lived experience.* London, Ontario: Althouse Press.

Wallerstein, N., & Bernstein, E. (1994). Introduction to community empowerment, participatory education and health. *Health Education Quarterly, 21*, 141–148.

Watson, J. (1988). *Nursing: Human science and human care. A theory of nursing.* New York: National League of Nursing

World Health Organization. (1986). *Ottawa charter for health promotion.* Copenhagen: Author.

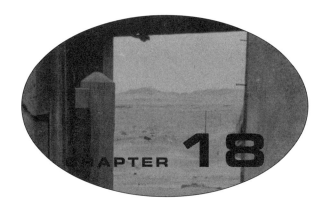

APTER **18**

Meditation-Based Stress Reduction: Holistic Practice in Nursing Education

ANNE BRUCE
LYNNE E. YOUNG
LINDA TURNER
RENA VAN DER WAL
WOLFGANG LINDEN

Meditation takes time; it's time I sometimes don't have. . . . I just wish it could be incorporated into the nursing curriculum. I think it would be really beneficial because our stresses carry over to the patients that we take care of, right? And with the knowledge we have to manage our stresses, we could use meditation as a teaching tool.

Third year baccalaureate nursing student

Alternative approaches, such as meditation, are being used increasingly in health care practices to support health and healing. Like many mind-body interventions, meditation is being explored scientifically within more liberalized interdisciplinary research settings (Murphy & Donovan, 1999). As a self-care practice, meditation shows promise in addressing health issues of stress that afflict so many of us in contemporary society. In this chapter we explore how meditation has been used as a stress reduction intervention with nursing students. In addition, we address how attending to stress reduction and students' experiences of stress within the curriculum helps to embody the principles of health promotion as presented throughout this book.

As in society at large, the experience of stress among nursing students is a critical issue. Empirical evidence indicates that student nurses experience high levels of stress and higher levels of physiological and psychological symptoms when compared with students in other health-related disciplines (Beck, Hackett, Srivastava, McKim, & Rockwell, 1997; Haack, 1988). If ignored, stress will impact negatively on the health of student nurses and, in turn, the future of health care. The issue of student nurse stress came to the attention of faculty in a baccalaureate nursing program in Western Canada during a course in which students had an opportunity to discuss the stressors in their lives and its effects on their health and school performance. Consequently, students and faculty engaged in a community development initiative focused on addressing students' stress. Through collaborative efforts among students, nursing and psychology faculty, and community-based clinical nurse specialists, a mindfulness-based stress reduction program was offered to one cohort of university nursing students. To assist us in determining the effectiveness of this program, a pilot evaluation was conducted to examine program outcomes on the health and well-being of participating nursing students. Students included both third-year baccalaureate and post-RN nursing students.

In this chapter, we explore the mind-body practice of meditation with particular emphasis on its conceptual basis as a stress-reduction intervention. Links between stress management and meditation are presented in the description and discussion of the findings of this evaluation. The relevance of offering student nurses an opportunity to practice mindfulness meditation as part of their course work is underscored in reviewing relevant research in this domain.

Holistic Practice in Nursing Education

Holistic education can be broadly described as a collection of attitudes rather than a defined system of pedagogy (Miller, 1988). As a worldview, holism honors the unity of all life, going beyond a modern dualistic view of subject and object, material and immaterial, reason and intuition, and body and mind (Dacher, 1997; Dewey, 1939). Through holistic nursing curricula, students gain a broader vision of health and healing that embraces both the mechanistic workings of the body and mind and a more expansive view integrating body/mind/spirit/environment.

Meditation is a practice embedded in this expansive view of the human condition. Interest in meditation and Eastern techniques of consciousness transformation is increasing in North America. Although mystical awakening in some form is found in most cultures (Taylor, 1999), Asian traditions of meditation are the primary source for most health care practices integrating mind-body approaches. In trying to define meditation, it is important to consider meditative techniques within the cultural and spiritual traditions in which they are embedded. As meditation practices are adapted into Western cultures, their foundations in Eastern systems of thought must be understood if a trustworthy interpretation is to be made (Taylor). Towards this end, we explore meditation generally as a family of practices and follow this with specific attention to mindfulness meditation and its origins in Buddhist traditions.

Meditation: A Holistic Practice

Meditation is a generic term referring to disciplines that cultivate particular ways of paying attention in one's life. The disciplines range from the act of inward contemplation, to placing attention on an object of meditation, to the experience of complete absorption in the object of attention (Murphy & Donovan, 1999; Walsh, 1982). There are also misleading understandings of meditation commonly held in North America. For example, meditation is often understood to be: (1) a state of relaxation that is psychologically and physically beneficial; (2) a dissociated state in which one experiences a trance-like condition; and (3) a mystical state in which higher realities or religious objects are experienced (Varela, Thompson, & Rosch, 1991). Although these perceptions are accurate, they are misleading. The implication is that meditation is something applied in order to get away from the mundane, perhaps stressful, state of reality. Verala and colleagues (1991) explain that meditation is intended to be quite the opposite. Rather than moving away from, meditation assists in moving closer to whatever one is experiencing. Meditation is described as seeing our psychological situation very precisely and directly. The practice of meditation develops one's capacity to:

Abide wakefully within whatever experience is arising. When there is no identification either with the observer or the observed, awareness remains undisturbed by any divisions, and a new freedom, freshness, clarity, and compassion become available. (Welwood, 1996, p. 109)

Therefore, meditation can be viewed as the intentional self-regulation of attention from moment to moment (Goleman, 1991).

Mindfulness Meditation

Mindfulness meditation is primarily derived from Buddhist traditions and has been extensively researched by Jon Kabat-Zinn since the 1980s (Kabat-Zinn, Lipworth, Burney, & Sellers, 1987; Kabat-Zinn et al., 1992; Kabat-Zinn, 1996). In understanding mindfulness, it may be helpful to begin with defining its opposite, *mindlessness.* Langer (1992) associates habitual and automatic behavior that occurs with little or no conscious awareness with the state of mindlessness. We can no doubt all recall times when we suddenly realize we have consumed an entire meal without really being aware of the experience. Not only being "lost in thought," as this example implies, but an overreliance on already determined conceptual categories is an aspect of mindlessness. Relying too heavily on predetermined concepts such as "anxiety," "stress," or "patient" may interfere with one's capacity to see what is actually going on in a situation. For example, nurses who too quickly identify a patient with the concept of "noncompliant" may overlook other aspects of what is going on during interactions with that person. The state of mindlessness leaves one oblivious to novel or alternative aspects of a given situation. Ellen Langer (Langer & Imber, 1979; Langer & Rodin 1987; Langer, Perlmuter, Chanowitz, & Rubin, 1988), a psychologist, has done extensive research demonstrating the negative implications of mindlessness for learning, behavioral competence, memory, and health.

In contrast, *mindfulness* is a state of conscious awareness. Varela, Thompson, and Rosch (1991) define mindfulness as a process wherein,

---

The mind is present in embodied everyday experience; mindfulness techniques are designed to lead the mind back from its theories and preoccupations, back from the abstract attitude, to the situation of one's experience itself. (p. 22)

Attending to whatever arises in the mind, the meditator notes sense perceptions, thoughts, and emotions without judgement. Mindfulness meditation encourages an exploratory and experiential perspective toward whatever object presents itself in the mind at any given moment. Mindfulness meditation practice gradually develops the ability to be present with one's mind and body both in formal meditation practice and in everyday living (Varela, Thompson, & Rosch, 1991).

The initial stages of this form of meditation usually involve practice in concentration meditation to develop a degree of stability of attention. Once grounded in moment-to-moment awareness of the primary object, the meditator then engages in a process of free attention, placing his/her attention on whatever mind-object is most prominent. The meditator is encouraged to investigate this mind-object from a stance of calmness and neu-

trality, free of judgment, self-involvement, and conclusions. (Miller, 1993, p. 179)

As the meditator's mindfulness deepens, she or he is able to embrace the present moment as it is, free of reactive and habitual thoughts and behaviors. In relation to stress management, Kabat-Zinn (1990) claims that increasingly direct contact with the present moment provides a person with the capacity to respond with greater awareness in discerning the nature of an encounter. That is, one can respond rather than react in deciding whether an encounter is benign, threatening, or stressful. Moreover, continued mindful practice leads to deepening understanding of our habitual reactive responses, and the nature of mind itself (Delmonte, 1987; Miller, 1993; Trungpa, 1973; West, 1987).

Integrating East and West: Stress, Coping, and Adaptation Theory

Mindfulness meditation has been successfully adapted by Kabat-Zinn (1990) into a mindfulness-based stress reduction (MBSR) program. Within this program, theories of stress and coping are drawn from the work of Lazarus and Folkman (1984). Lazarus and Folkman define stress as a response to a person-environment event that is perceived by the person to tax or possibly exceed his or her resources for managing it, and also as a threat to well-being. Appraisal, according to this theory, is the process through which a person perceives, then assesses, and evaluates the stress-related nature of a situation or demand. The degree of emotional distress that an individual experiences will depend on what is at stake in the transaction, and the degree of perceived threat, loss, or harm. Consequently, one's ability to cope with stressful demands depends on several factors, including one's appraisal of the situation, the resources available, and the nature of the situation.

Within Lazarus and Folkman's model, coping is concerned with what the person actually thinks or does in a given context, along with changes in these thoughts and actions across encounters. However, appraisal processes are not necessarily conscious and may be shaped by agendas below the person's immediate awareness. This view of appraisal and coping is highly congruent with mindfulness meditation that looks at moment-to-moment awareness of thoughts and actions and provides space in the appraisal process for attentive response rather than habitual reaction.

Mindfulness-Based Stress Reduction

The theory and practice of mindfulness are not mysterious or mystical. The aims are simply to come to know one's own mental processes as thoroughly as possible in order to understand and have some control or nonreactive relationship with them. A further aspiration is to gain freedom from a habitual mind and its unknown and seemingly uncontrollable states (Deatherage, 1979). To this end, Kabat-Zinn's (1990) mindfulness-based stress reduction model has contributed enormously in introducing Eastern meditative practices and perspectives into Western society. The MBSR program is a client-focused approach that uses training in meditation for coping with stress, illness, and pain (Kaplan, Goldenberg, & Galvin-Nadeau, 1993; Kabat-Zinn, Lipworth, & Burney, 1985; Kabat-Zinn et al., 1987; Kabat-Zinn & Chapman-Waldrop, 1988; Kabat-Zinn et al., 1992).

The MBSR program originated with the Stress Reduction Clinic at the University of Massachusetts Medical Center in 1979. Since its inception, more than 10,000 medical patients have been through the basic program. MBSR has a high rate of program completion and adherence, as well as clinical effectiveness documented in a series of outcome studies examining patients with chronic pain, anxiety, and panic disorder (Kabat-Zinn, 1982; Kabat-Zinn & Chapman-Waldrop, 1988; Kabat-Zinn et al., 1985; Miller, Fletcher, & Kabat-Zinn, 1995). The underlying assumption of the MBSR is that every individual has inner resources that can be mobilized through mindfulness meditation to assist in health and healing. As a resource-oriented rather than problem-oriented approach, the MBSR is a commitment to the belief that there is more right with an individual than there is wrong, no matter what is going on for that person.

The core of the MBSR program is an eight-week course during which participants undergo training in the daily practice of mindfulness meditation and its application in everyday life. The program requires an openness to self-exploration through commitment to a 45-minute-per-day meditative practice including several exercises that help participants explore inner and outer realities. Examples include enhancing awareness through asking participants to describe in detail their physical and mental reactions to both a pleasant event and a stressful experience. After the fifth week of the program, a one-day silent retreat is held.

The program introduces participants to a variety of meditation techniques, including body scan, breathing meditation, and Hatha Yoga. Awareness of body sensations is fostered through bringing one's attention to different parts of the body using a mental body scan. The foundation practice of sitting meditation uses both concentration and mindfulness and attends to awareness of breathing. Instruction in Hatha yogic postures are done slowly and consciously to enhance awareness of body sensations, movement, and breathing. Attitudinal factors that constitute the major pillars of mindfulness practice are integrated throughout. These include cultivation of nonjudging, patience, trust, nonstriving, acceptance, and letting-go. Meditation is introduced as practicing the simple act of carefully paying attention and experiencing one's life in the present moment.

Mindfulness Meditation and Health: The Evidence

During the past 25 years, scientific investigation into meditation as a self-care technique has grown. Murphy and Donovon (1999) conducted an extensive review of research into the physical and psychological effects of meditation from 1931 to 1996. Most of the 1,300 studies examine concentration techniques such as transcendental meditation, with mindfulness-awareness techniques only beginning to be studied in the late 1970s. Kabat-Zinn and colleagues (1992) have scientifically documented the clinical effects of mindfulness meditation training on psychological symptoms. They reported that providing a MBSR program within a group setting effectively reduces symptoms of anxiety and panic. These reductions can be maintained in patients with medically diagnosed general-ized anxiety disorder, with a majority of these patients still demonstrating positive changes at a three-year follow-up.

Research with patients suffering from chronic pain has demonstrated that mindful-ness training can be effective in pain man-agement (Kabat-Zinn, 1982; Kabat-Zinn et al., 1985; Kabat-Zinn & Chapman-Waldrop, 1988). This research suggests that the MBSR program may be beneficial for reducing stress-related psychological symptomatology and enhancing coping with chronic pain.

A few studies have recently been conducted where the MBSR program has been offered to students within the university setting. One study examined the effects of mindfulness-based stress reduction on medical and premed-ical students (Shapiro, Schwartz, & Bonner, 1998). Findings indicated a significant reduc-tion in state and trait anxiety, psychological distress, and depression, with increases in overall empathy levels and scores on a mea-sure of spiritual experiences. This growing body of research suggests that mindfulness meditation as a treatment approach is show-ing promising results in reducing stress and stress-related disease in student populations. Thus, we concluded that the MBSR program would be an appropriate program to offer stu-dent nurses and that evaluating its use would be a valuable contribution to the growing body of empirical literature in this domain.

Evaluation of the Mindfulness-Based Stress Reduction Program

Because there was no evidence that the MBSR was an effective intervention for re-ducing stress and improving the health of stu-dent nurses, we launched a pilot evaluation to begin addressing this gap in knowledge. The evaluation addressed process, impact, and outcome objectives (Green & Lewis, 1986). We addressed process objectives dur-ing focus group sessions by asking partici-pants to describe their experiences of the MBSR program specifically related to per-ceptions of and satisfaction with the physical environment, teaching instruction, and the stress reduction strategies introduced during the program. Impact and outcome objectives were also examined during focus group ses-

sions by asking students to speak to the im-pact of the program on their lives in general, and specifically as it affected their stress, health, and school performance. Impact and outcome objectives were further evaluated by gathering data about health status indicators, stress, and school performance using question-naires and visual analogue scales with partici-pants in experimental and control groups. Undergraduate nursing students were involved as research assistants in all aspects of the study. After an orientation, two nursing stu-dents conducted the focus group interviews, administered and collected questionnaires and physiological measures, and assisted in the analysis of qualitative data. The pilot pro-ject received ethics approval from the appro-priate university review committee.

In this before/after, randomized, quasi-experimental design, 15 students participated in each of the treatment and control groups (N = 30). Psychological symptoms of stress were measured using three questionnaires: the Health Status Profile (SF-36V2), Symptom Checklist-90-Revised, and Antonovsky's (1987) Orientation to Life Questionnaire (OLQ). The Health Status Profile (SF-36V2) was adminis-tered to measure the overall health status of participants (Ware, 1993). The instrument uses 36 questions to assess major health con-cepts including physical functioning, body pain, general health, vitality, social function-ing, and emotional and mental health. The Symptom Checklist-90-Revised (SCL-90R) was used to measure physical and psycholog-ical symptoms of stress. This instrument was developed and later revised by Derogatis, Rick-els, and Rock (1976) and Derogatis (1983), respectively. The questionnaire contains 90 items measuring physical and psychological symptoms and has been used extensively by Kabat-Zinn and colleagues in research studies to identify outcomes related to the MBSR program. The third instrument was Antonov-sky's (1987) Orientation to Life Question-naire (OLQ). This instrument measures Sense of Coherence, a dispositional orientation that reflects an individual's capacity to respond to stressor situations. The OLQ is a 29-item, seven point Likert-type scale. All three of these measures have good reported reliability and validity.

Visual analog scales (VAS) were used as subjective measures of perceived stress, over-all school performance, capacity to meet deadlines, and attendance at class. Physiological measures included blood pressure (sitting), pulse, and salivary cortisol as indicators of the stress response. Thus, we used qualitative and quantitative methods. All students who expressed interest also provided written consent and were randomly assigned to the treatment or the wait-list control group for the matched control group design. Quantitative data were gathered before and after the MBSR program, whereas qualitative data were collected three times: during focus group sessions held prior to the first MBSR session, mid-way through the 8 week program, and after the final MBSR session.

MBSR: Determining Its Impact

Process, impact, and outcome data were gathered qualitatively during focus group sessions, and are presented here before our report of the quantitative findings. The textual data were analyzed for themes and relationships drawing from methods described by: Guba and Lincoln (1989); Strauss and Corbin (1998); and Thorne, Reimer Kirkham, and MacDonald-Emes (1997). Throughout the focus group sessions, discussion turned frequently to how being in a university nursing program impacted on respondents' health and capacity for scholastic performance. Seeking to find balance and juggling multiple life events within the constraints of time were pervasive challenges for these students. The process of seeking to find a balance was perceived as stressful, but failure to achieve balance added to this stress, because students experienced lack of balance as significantly affecting their physical, emotional, mental, and social well-being.

Seeking to Find Balance

Students spoke of the challenge of maintaining their health while in the nursing program. When asked how they view health, students described it as a balance between the spiritual, mental, physical, social, and psychological aspects of their lives. Health meant being physically active, eating well, thinking clearly, being emotionally stable, and having time for family or significant others. For them, one did not have to be disease-free to be healthy. They claimed that health was an important factor in preventing illness and a pre-

cursor for being able to take care of others, a capacity they considered essential in their roles as nursing students. Their studies were identified as a significant factor impacting the balance in their lives, and therefore their health. The following quotations are verbatim from focus group transcripts with baccalaureate and post-RN nursing students.

Last year I just had a great balance but then school started and it was really hard to try to hold that balance. So, I'm not as healthy . . . I still exercise and try to eat right.

Losing their sense of balance was related to increased stress levels that resulted in physical and psychological symptoms. Physical symptoms included nausea, difficulty breathing, anxiety attacks, pounding heart, crying, gastrointestinal distress, and fatigue. Psychological symptoms included anger, frustration, irritability, depression, lack of motivation, fear, and feeling emotionally labile. Regarding the mental dimension of health, students spoke about how stress interfered with their ability to focus and concentrate. Further, students described the social costs of being in school: lack of time for friends and emotional outbursts that disrupted intimate relationships. They described the consequences of losing their balance in terms of: missing classes, spending increased amounts of time in bed, spending increased amounts of time watching TV, experiencing decreased productivity, having an increased sense of distraction, increased nibbling of food with subsequent weight gain, increased likelihood of getting ill, decreased ability to make thoughtful decisions, feelings of social isolation, and decreased amounts of exercise. From these descriptions, a picture emerges of young adults with a clear idea about how health operates for them, an awareness that going to university impacts the balance in their lives, but at the same time, a reduced capacity to avert the negative effects of stress in their everyday lives.

Juggling to Achieve Balance

Student nurses describe an experience of juggling many different facets of their lives. These include demands from the work they did for remuneration; managing finances; school (deadlines, classes, difficult readings, papers, exams, marks, practica); relationships with family, friends, and/or significant others; and the expectations of others. Juggling multiple demands led students to feel that they had lost their balance in life. They described struggling to regain that balance, although they sometimes paid a price in terms of their health. One student commented about this phenomenon:

It's a lot to juggle but I seem to do it, somehow. I guess when the stress gets a lot for me, I get sick. . . . That's what I am right now. . . . Lots to juggle.

When students had multiple life events to manage, the limiting factor appeared to be "time." Students had too many obligations to fulfill within a predetermined period of time. Caring for themselves was the first demand to go:

For my health right now, I have bronchitis related to doing too many things at once and getting a little run down with so many obligations to fulfill: work, school, family, friends. It's just been way too busy. I haven't been taking good care of myself.

Impact of Taking the MBSR Program

Student nurse participants described aspects of the program that were enabling, as well as the challenges posed by the MBSR program. They told of gaining insight into how they manage multiple demands, a beginning step toward learning new ways to manage their lives. The MBSR was effective in providing participants with an opportunity not only to learn new skills, but also to learn new ways of thinking about the multiple demands of their lives. They told of how they learned to "let go" of stress. Letting go of stress freed a space for evaluating the various stresses they faced. Central to the "letting go" process was learning to attend to their body's cues of stress. As one student put it,

It makes you more in tune with your health, when you aren't healthy, and when your body is not feeling healthy. I learned how to deal with it, to recognize that I was not balanced.

Thus, they began to pay attention to their bodily reactions to various situations. They subsequently developed awareness of their overall responses to stress.

Students were taught different techniques that required practice and training (meditation, body scan, yoga, being mindful, and breathing). They told us that these techniques were not integrated into their lives immediately, but required continual practice

and reminders. Many experienced frustration and impatience as they realized how restless their minds were and how difficult it was to apply the techniques.

At least I'm trying to do it; sometimes it only lasts for five minutes 'cause I just can't do it. I'm not good enough yet for meditation, I'm still so overwhelmed with so much in my head that I find it really hard to just meditate.

As they practiced the techniques, many students remarked on their enhanced capacity to be "aware of what's going on" and "being able to focus." As the program progressed over the eight weeks, participants began to trust more in themselves and their own experiences.

We sit there and we meditate, and it's like we're dealing with our own stuff. It's not someone telling us what it is. Rather than someone saying what's right or wrong, [you begin to] believe what you feel.

Time seemed to be a major consideration in determining which techniques they chose to practice. Students varied in the amount of time they devoted to practice. Although some committed to minimal practice, or attempted to complete all the practice assignments, others tried to integrate the awareness practices into their daily activities. Sitting meditation, being "mindfully present," and mindfully breathing were skills that required little time and could be practiced almost anywhere. Those skills that took less time and could be practiced in multiple locations were more likely to be used, whereas skills that took more time (body scan and yoga), and had to be practiced in specific locations were used by participants with specific needs such as back pain.

Students also varied in how new skills were integrated into their lives and which skills they used. For example, one student described how she breathed deeply many times throughout the day as a reminder to be present. Other students use their daily walk to class or the corner store to practice being mindful. An outcome of practice for some was alterations in ways of thinking, perception of time, and perceptions of life events. Taking time between the stressor and the re-action to the stressor was a strategy that allowed some students to begin to manage stress rather than getting lost in it.

However, despite the challenges of learning these new skills, all reported that they saw

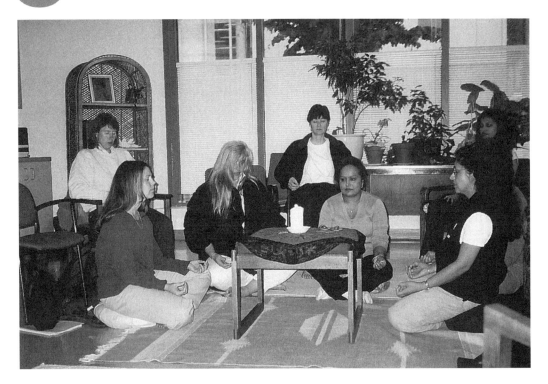

value in the techniques that were taught and plan to continue to try to integrate the skills into their lives.

Before the course, I wouldn't have made time for myself because of guilt. . . . I don't have time for this, I don't have time to enjoy or go for a walk. But now because we have to do that for this course and then seeing the benefits from that, that's why we incorporate it in our lives. We have permission but now we know that it works and it's a good life skill to incorporate [into our lives].

Another student reflected that she learned more than skills, she acquired a new philosophy:

You don't need to do all of the techniques to realize you're not present. You don't need all that stuff to tell yourself that there are more important things in life than what you're stressing out about—usually it's minor inconveniences. The whole philosophy of the MBSR class has taught me that it's usually never that important. So the philosophy, I think, can be enough without the skills.

Thus, students were able to increase control over their lives through enhanced awareness of their reactions to stressful experiences, such as writing papers and preparing for an exam with a broader perspective about what is important. They felt empowered to achieve and maintain a balance in their lives because

they did not let university stresses rule. They told how they began to take time from their studies to be with friends and family members, and to go for walks, runs, or workouts. They told us that they had experienced a change in perception of how time flows, a change that resulted in a reduction of fluctuations between extreme ups and downs of "panic" level stress and bottomed-out "no stress." One student reflected:

It's taught me to step back and not take things so personally, just accept what I have to do and find creative ways to solve problems. It's a fact of life. You have to jump through the hoops, but it's the way you jump through the hoop that can be the difference.

Some students reported that they were teaching these skills to others, family members, significant others, or patients. In addition, post-RN students who worked as nurses found the skill of being present with their patients enhanced care:

[I use the skills] at work, too, with patients. As nurses, we have so many tasks to do and we're pressed for time, it makes such a difference when you can zoom in on one patient and you're totally there. They feel it right away. They tell you more, they touch you and they want you to stay with them. There's power in the moment when you're really centered. . . . I feel it.

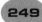

These experiences were powerful rein-forcements of the value of MBSR techniques for these students.

MBSR Evaluation: Measuring Outcomes

Quantitative analyses of health indicators, stress, and school performance reinforce the findings of the qualitative component of this study. We adopted a matched control design comparing mindfulness meditation outcomes with a no-treatment control group. This de-sign has the advantage of permitting the cal-culation of statistical effect sizes that are useful indicators of treatment benefit, espe-cially when there is a lack of statistical power because of the small sample sizes that pre-clude meaningful significance testing.[1]

Effect sizes (in this case Cohen's d) (Cohen, 1977) integrate information about mean changes and the variability of these mean changes across different people. It is widely accepted to label scores as follows: $d = .2$ (or thereabout) are considered small, $d = .5$ is a moderate effect size, and $d = .8$ is con-sidered a large effect. Scores of available meta-analytic reviews in therapy outcome literature consistently conclude that the ef-fects of psychological therapy tend to fall be-tween $d = .5$ and $d = 1.0$, with the larger values generally seen if only pre- and post-tests are compared in the absence of any con-trol treatments.

The results from this analysis clearly sup-port the qualitative statements made by the study's participants. The quantitative results are described by clustering the available out-come variables into subgroups that are simi-lar in nature, that is, related domains of functioning. For example, one such grouping is "Psychological Symptoms" (feeling rushed, confused, disoriented, etc.); another is the av-erage scores from the SF-36V2 Health Status Profile scale, which assesses health-related quality of life. Health-related quality of life is different from "Psychological Symptoms" be-cause people often provide seemingly incon-gruous reports; that is, they may be happy although in pain or depressed in the absence of physical health concerns. In addition, it

is worth looking at "Sense of Coherence," which provides some indication of the partic-ipants' sense of direction and meaning in life, or a degree of spiritual anchoring. Also of in-terest are physical symptoms, which are often indicative of perceived stress (feeling aches and pains). Even though symptoms of stress are obvious targets for a stress reduction in-tervention, one may also want to test whether stress reduction produces more ancillary ben-efits than could arise if stress is effectively re-duced. Such a test of the generalization of benefits was made by studying academic out-comes, that is, grade point average, ability to meet deadlines, and perceived ability to regu-larly attend classes. In total, this provided five classes of variables pertinent to study.

For simplicity, the results (expressed as ef-fect sizes d) are displayed in Figure 18–1, or-ganized by categories of meaning.

As Figure 18–1 indicates, there are a num-ber of differences between the treated and the control participants, and the figure offers a clear pattern of results. The MBSR interven-tion produced small-to-moderate effect sizes for health-related quality of life, for sense of coherence, and for medical symptoms. It had essentially no effect for academic performance and showed that psychological symptoms had by far the greatest decrease. Despite the small sample and inherent lack of statistical power, the psychological symptom changes are suffi-ciently large to also reveal a statistically signif-icant difference between MBSR intervention and the control group.

In sum, these results show that the benefit is most apparent for psychological symptoms and that only a moderately sized sample is needed to show the benefits of meditation for nursing student stress. Students in this pilot study who learned mindfulness meditation reported enhanced awareness of their physi-cal, emotional, and mental responses to stress. Students reported experiencing the difference between mind*less*ly reacting to situations and mind*full*y being present to what was happen-ing. Some reported a heightened awareness of the effects of stress that resulted in "letting go" of their habitual stress reactions. These reports are considered in light of the finding of reduced psychological symptoms including decreased feelings of being rushed, confused, and disoriented. The capacity of mind-body approaches to elicit a sense of letting go is re-ported elsewhere (Kern & Baker, 1997). In-

---

[1]For further discussion of significance testing see Munro (1997).

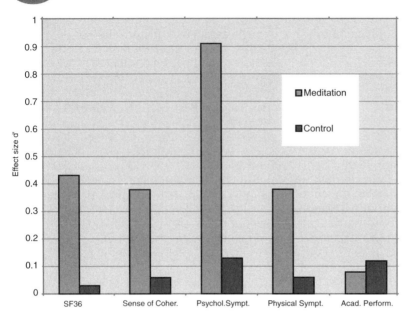

FIG. 18–1. Effects of Mindfulness Meditation.

terestingly, the pilot study corresponds with other studies reporting positive psychological outcomes in managing stress after a relatively short (8 weeks) training period (Astin, 1997; Shapiro, Schwartz, & Bonner, 1998). Even though decline in academic performance was not significant, we questioned our current measures and whether academic performance can be appropriately measured over such a short time.

In addition to the benefit of letting go of habitual reactions to stress, students in this MBSR evaluation noted that they developed an enhanced awareness of their mind and body that empowered them to manage their stress, and that participating in the MBSR created a sense of community. Roth (1997) observes something similar in an evaluation of the MBSR with inner-city patients suffering with pain:

Among patients who participate fully in the program . . . initial relief of suffering occurs within the first few weeks of the program. . . . As their practice continues and deepens, patients realize that more is happening than symptom relief. Patients begin to experience subtle and profound shifts within themselves, which yield new ways of interacting with their world. (p. 54)

Students report learning to shape their responses to stressful situations by cueing into their physical, emotional, and mental responses, then activating new-found stress management techniques such as mindful breathing. Over the eight-week program, they began to see the "bigger picture," which allowed them to step back and not take things so personally. Thus, students began to look beyond their self-fixated orientation. The MBSR was a vehicle that allowed students to learn to connect more intimately with themselves and with others. There are many advantages of short courses like the MBSR and the implications for other populations including faculty, caregivers, family members, and adolescents that warrant further investigation.

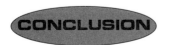

Often nursing curricula are designed to teach health promotion concepts that are essential in preparing future nurses for the complex health environments they will face.

However, without adequate care and attention to how these concepts are enacted and modeled in the educational environment, students receive mixed messages, and often learn only the rhetoric of health promotion. Being able to "walk the talk" between what is taught about self-care practices and what is supported by educational institutions is an ongoing challenge. Pedagogical integrity is at risk if the curricular content links only to the clients nurses care for while overlooking the health needs of the students themselves. Educational institutions need to reorient nursing curricula making healthy nursing students a priority, because it is the healthy nurse that has the inner resources to care and the energy to provide competent and compassionate nursing care.

Addressing stress as a mind-body interaction affecting health and school performance has afforded us an opportunity to explore meditation as a congruent holistic health promoting intervention. As a self-care practice, mindfulness meditation was reported to be beneficial to individuals and to the collective. Equally important was the perceived congruence of educational content with how students learned to care for themselves as they strive to incorporate notions of health promotion into their professional and personal lives. In closing, one student aptly sums up these notions in recommending that self-care strategies such as the MBSR be incorporated into the learning experiences and curriculum.

I think these strategies and methods of coping with your stress are something that all of our peers should have. Since health promotion is the area we're learning about, it would be beneficial [to be actively practicing it]. Experience helps you understand it from theory to practice.

Acknowledgements

The authors would like to acknowledge the contributions of Suzanna (Suzie) Janosek and Lian McKenzie, University of Victoria School of Nursing students, who contributed enormously to the Student Nurse Stress Project 1997–1999.

REFERENCES

Antonovsky, A. (1987). *Unravelling the mystery of health.* San Francisco: Jossey-Bass.

Astin, J. (1997). Stress reduction through mindfulness meditation: Effects on psychological symptomatology, sense of control and spiritual experiences. *Psychotherapy and Psychosomatics, 66,* 97–106.

Beck, D., Hackett, M. B., Srivastava, R., McKim, E., & Rockwell, B. (1997). Perceived level and sources of stress in baccalaureate nursing students. *Journal of Nursing Education, 36,* 180–186.

Cohen, J. (1977). *Statistical power for the behavioral sciences* (Rev. ed.). New York: Academic Press.

Dacher, E. S. (1997). Towards a post-modern medicine. *Complementary Therapies in Nursing & Midwifery, 3,* 66–71.

Deatherage, G. (1979). The clinical use of "mindfulness" meditation techniques in short-term psychotherapy. In J. Welwood (Ed.), *The meeting of the ways: Explorations in East/West psychology* (pp. 208–216). New York: Schocken Books.

Delmonte, M. (1987). Meditation: Contemporary theoretical approaches. In M. A. West (Ed.), *The psychology of meditation* (pp. 39–53). Oxford: Oxford Science Publications.

Derogatis, L. R. (1983). *SCL-90-R: Administering, scoring & procedures manual—II.* Towson, MD: Clinical Psychometric Research.

Derogatis, L. R., Rickels, K., & Rock, A. F. (1976). The SCL-90 and the MMPI: A step in the validation of a new self-report scale. *British Journal of Psychiatry, 128,* 280–289.

Dewey, J. (1939). The unity of the human being. In J. Ratner (Ed.), *Intelligence in the modern world* (pp. 819–835). New York: Random House.

Goleman, D. (1991). A Western perspective. In D. Goleman & R. Thurman (Eds.), *MindScience: An East-West dialogue* (pp. 3–6). Somerville, MA: Wisdom.

Green, L. W., & Lewis, F. M. (1986). *Measurement and evaluation in health education and health promotion.* Palo Alto, CA: Mayfield.

Guba, E. G., & Lincoln, Y. S. (1989). *Fourth generation evaluation.* Newbury Park, CA: Sage.

Haack, M. (1988). Stress and impairment among nursing students. *Research in Nursing & Health, 11,* 125–134.

Kabat-Zinn, J. (1982). An outpatient program in behavioral medicine for chronic pain patients based on the practice of mindfulness meditation: Theoretical considerations and preliminary results. *General Hospital Psychiatry*, *4*, 33–47.

Kabat-Zinn, J. (1990). *Full catastrophe living: Using the wisdom of your body and mind to face stress, pain, and illness.* New York: Delacorte.

Kabat-Zinn, J. (1996). Mindfulness meditation: What it is, what it isn't, and its role in health care and medicine. In Y. Haruki, Y. Ishii, & M. Suzuki (Eds.), *Comparative and psychological study on meditation.* Eburon: Netherlands

Kabat-Zinn, J., & Chapman-Waldrop, A. (1988). Compliance with an outpatient stress reduction program: Rates and predictors of program completion. *Journal of Behavioral Medicine, 11,* 333–352.

Kabat-Zinn, J., Lipworth, L., & Burney, R. (1985). The clinical use of mindfulness meditation for the self-regulation of chronic pain. *Journal of Behavioral Medicine, 8,* 163–190.

Kabat-Zinn, J., Lipworth, L., Burney, R., & Sellers, W. (1987). Four-year follow-up of a meditation-based program for the self-regulation of chronic pain: Treatment outcomes and compliance. *The Clinical Journal of Pain, 2,* 159–173.

Kabat-Zinn, J., Massion, A. O., Kristeller, J., Peterson, L., Fletcher, K., Pbert, L., Lenderking, W., & Santorelli, S. (1992). Effectiveness of a meditation-based stress reduction program in the treatment of anxiety disorders. *American Journal of Psychiatry, 149,* 936–943.

Kaplan, K., Goldenberg, D. L., & Galvin-Nadeau, M. (1993). The impact of a meditation-based stress reduction program on fibromyalgia. *General Hospital Psychiatry, 15,* 284–289.

Kern, D., & Baker, J. (1997). A comparison of a mind/body approach versus a conventional approach to aerobic dance. *Women's Health Issues, 7,* 30–37.

Langer, E. (1992). Matters of mind: Mindfulness/Mindlessness in perspective. *Consciousness and cognition, 1,* 289–305.

Langer, E., & Imber, L. (1979). When practice makes imperfect: The debilitating effects of overlearning. *Journal of Personality and Social Psychology, 37,* 2014–2025.

Langer, E., & Rodin, P. (1987). The prevention of mindlessness. *Journal of Personality & Social Psychology, 53,* 280–287.

Langer, E., Perlmuter, L., Chanowitz, B., & Rubin, R. (1988). Two new applications of mindlessness theory: Aging and alcoholism. *Journal of Aging Studies, 2,* 289–299.

Lazarus, R. S., & Folkman, S. (1984). *Stress, appraisal and coping.* New York: Springer.

Miller, J. (1988). *The holistic curriculum.* Toronto: OISE Press.

Miller, J. (1993). The unveiling of traumatic memories and emotions through mindfulness and concentration meditation: Clinical implications and three case studies. *Journal of Transpersonal Psychology, 25,* 169–180.

Miller, J., Fletcher, K., & Kabat-Zinn, J. (1995). Three-year follow-up and clinical implications of a mindfulness meditation-based stress reduction intervention in the treatment of anxiety disorders. *General Hospital Psychiatry, 17,* 192–200.

Munro, B. (1997). *Statistical methods for health care research* (3rd ed.). Philadelphia: Lippincott.

Murphy, M., & Donovan, S. (1999). *The physical and psychological effects of meditation* (2nd ed.). Sausalito, CA: Institute of Noetic Sciences.

Roth, B. (1997). Mindfulness-based stress reduction in the inner city. *Advances: The Journal of Mind-Body Health, 13,* 50–58.

Shapiro, S., Schwartz, G. & Bonner, G. (1998). Effects of mindfulness-based stress reduction on medical and premedical students. *Journal of Behavioural Medicine, 21,* pp. 581–599.

Strauss, A., & Corbin, J. (1998). *Basics of qualitative research: Techniques and procedures for developing grounded theory.* Thousand Oaks, CA: Sage.

Taylor, E. (1999). Introduction. In E. Taylor (Ed.), *The physical and psychological effects of meditation* (pp. 1–30). Sausalito, CA: Institute of Noetic Sciences.

Thorne, S., Reimer Kirkham, S., MacDonald-Emes, J. (1997). Interpretive description: A non-categorical qualitative alternative for developing nursing knowledge. *Research in Nursing & Health, 2,* 169–177.

Trungpa, C. (1973). *Cutting through spiritual materialism.* Berkeley, CA: Shambhala.

Varela, T., Thompson, E., & Rosch, E. (1991). *The embodied mind: Cognitive science and human experience.* Cambridge, MA: MIT Press.

Walsh, R. (1982). A model for viewing meditation research. *The Journal of Transpersonal Psychology, 14,* 69–84.

Ware, J.E. (1993). *SF-36 Health Survey (SF-36).* Boston: Medical Outcomes Trust.

Welwood, J. (1996). Reflection and presence: The dialectic of self-knowledge. *The Journal of Transpersonal Psychology, 28,* 107–128.

West, M. (1987). Traditional and psychological perspectives on meditation. In M. A. West (Ed.), *Meditation: Contemporary theoretical approaches* (pp. 5–22). Oxford: Oxford Science Publications.

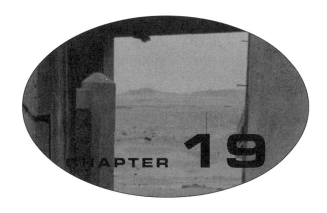

CHAPTER 19

Midlife Women's Empowerment Process within a Group

ELIZABETH BANISTER

Local women have the opportunity to engage in dialogue about their changing bodies within the context of a menopause group that meets weekly at a local health clinic. The 12 women in the group call themselves the *50-Over Group.* The group is facilitated by a nurse and is designed as a self-help group. As a guest speaker for one of the group's meetings, I had the honor of witnessing a lively group discussion about issues pertaining to **midlife** women. I vividly recall Judith's (a group member) comments: "People need to pay attention to women's midlife changes and take them more seriously." Judith elaborated: "When I joined the group three months ago I had many questions about feeling so emotionally and physically vulnerable. It was the first time in my life I felt that I did not have a handle on things." The answers had not been easy to come by for Judith. Prior to coming to the group, weeks had gone by, then months, with increasing feelings of vulnerability. She explained that her doctor had suggested using hormone replacement therapy. But for Judith, "the hormones didn't work for me. . . . my periods were weird and it started worrying me. I didn't know what I was doing to myself. So I got off that."

At that point in the meeting, a lively discussion ensued. Judith's comments provoked Ann to share an experience that was similar. A few months earlier, Ann found herself having to pull herself "out of the depths" and of "not knowing what was going on." At that time, her doctor had suggested Prozac, an antidepressant, which "is

the favorite that everyone tries." But for Ann, as with other group members, the monthly prescription cost was beyond her means.

The group continued sharing and discussing personal experiences and information related to midlife changes. At the meeting's close, the members' collective focus had shifted to telling each other about "alternate things" they had used for their symptoms of menopause. As Sandra put it, "I've tried all sorts of other things. What I've tried isn't anything that the medical profession has told me. And I think this stuff is working for most of us because we are taking charge of our lives and it's working." Clearly, group participation had benefits for these women, as myths and misconceptions about women at midlife were balanced by personal accounts of their changing bodies—and where, as experts of their own experience, a wealth of knowledge and information emerged. For this group, sharing their experiences and knowledge enabled the women to demystify some assumptions about menopause and to connect with collective power to promote and improve health.

It can be hard to be a woman at midlife these days. Many women may experience the midlife transition as disempowering, despite the current climate in which midlife events such as menopause are more openly acknowledged and discussed than in the past. This disempowerment may stem from many factors, some of which relate to ageist[1] and sexist[2] assumptions about aging women in our society, others of which spring from lack of consistent and reliable information available about midlife issues such as menopause and sexuality. Because of these factors and the increasing proportion of women who are experiencing midlife in Western society (Foot, 1996), it is important that we acknowledge some of the barriers facing such women and facilitate ways in which they can take control of their own health. One such venue is to provide opportunities for women to collectively share their midlife knowledge and expertise, where, as feminist historian Heilbrun (1988) noted, the truth of female experience emerges. The intent of this chapter is to describe, from a health promotion perspective, some of the ways in which my research project with women at midlife provided such a venue for sharing, and to discuss the ways in which they used the group to empower themselves to participate actively in their own health care. I begin by providing some background to the study and briefly outlining the methodology that was used. I then attempt to provide the reader with a sense of the research setting. I conclude with a discussion of broader implications for health care.

Background of the Study

Midlife is described as a time of biological, cultural, and social transition in the course of a woman's development, but very little is known about how midlife women themselves experience this stage in their lives (Baruch & Brooks-Gunn, 1984; Gergen, 1990). Apart from studies of menopause, many of which have been drawn from populations representing health care providers' clientele, little attention has been given to women's midlife issues. Because the samples chosen for these studies were not representative, the perspectives of women's midlife experiences that emerged from such work were often incorrect (Baruch & Brooks-Gunn, 1984; Gergen, 1990), portraying women's midlife transition as a time of crisis, emotional distress, and turmoil (Gergen, 1990; Quinn, 1991). Furthermore, the majority of research relates to a different cohort than that of the **"baby-boomers"** who are now entering the middle years (Woods & Mitchell, 1997). More recently, some women-centered researchers have made attempts to provide a greater understanding of midlife events, such as menopause, by listening to the voices of women themselves (Bond & Bywaters, 1998; Daly, 1995; Engebretson & Wardell, 1997; Hunter & O'Dea, 1997; Jarrett & Lethbridge, 1994; Jones, 1994; Quinn, 1991). However, descriptions of midlife women's own concerns, such as physiological changes that have an impact on sexual functioning and numerous losses (including loss of youthful appearance), have been scarce in the literature.

In an attempt to explore the sources and implications of this gap in our knowledge (Gergen, 1990; Hunter & Sundel, 1994; Lippert, 1997; Mansfield, Theisen, & Boyer, 1992), and to contribute to rectifying this shortcoming, I undertook a study to discover the meaning of midlife experience for women who themselves were experiencing this developmental transition (Banister, 1999b). My research question was: What are midlife women's perceptions of their changing bodies? I chose an ethnographic method (Spradley, 1979), because this would enable me to study the influence of the social and historical context upon the women's experiences. This method is rooted in anthropology, wherein the researcher attempts to capture individuals' perceptions of meanings and events within specific contexts (Agar, 1986; Spradley, 1979). This research approach is primarily an inductive method grounded in empirical data (Glaser & Strauss, 1967) provided by participants' thick descriptions (Geertz, 1973), descriptions that represent the central elements of individuals' meanings of their experiences (Denzin, 1989). New questions and theories are developed from these data.

I collected data through individual (Kvale, 1996) and group interviews (Morgan, 1988) and participant observation (Spradley, 1980) with 11 women ages 40–55. Because the voices of women from marginal groups are underrepresented in developmental and health-related research, I purposely selected the participants with variation in cultural background, employment status, marital status,

[1]In their book entitled, *Women and gender: A feminist psychology,* Unger and Crawford (1992) refer to ageism as negative attitudes toward the aged. Ageism encompasses discriminatory practices based on such attitudes.

[2]Sexism refers to the belief that women are valued in terms of their physical attractiveness and use to men (Unger & Crawford, 1992).

ableness, and sexual orientation. Nine of the women identified themselves as white, one as Aboriginal, and one as Asian. Four women were employed full time, two part-time, and two unemployed; three women were out of the workforce due to early retirement, disability, or serious illness. Regarding marital status, five of the women were married, one had never married, and five were divorced or separated. Two members of the participant group were lesbian. I conducted a total of 23 one-hour individual interviews (two consecutive interviews took place with each participant; one woman was interviewed three times).

Following completion of the individual interviews and analysis of the transcripts, I conducted three consecutive group interviews (Morgan, 1988) to verify the domains that had emerged, to add to theory development, and to allow the participants to collectively share their experiences of the research and insights into the midlife transition. All 11 individual participants attended at least one group meeting, with an average of eight per group. Together, all individual and group interviews spanned an entire year.

Analysis focused on discovering meaning of midlife women's experiences of their changing bodies and was based on the premise that participants organize their knowledge about their world into categories (Spradley, 1979). Through immersion in the data, categories and subsequent themes emerged, representing common threads of meaning among the women's narrative accounts (Fetterman, 1989; Spradley, 1979). A recursive process among data collection, analysis, and further questioning and observation continued until theoretical saturation had been reached, or when new instances of the phenomenon no longer led to new categories (Lincoln & Guba, 1985). Prior to and during each interview, I encouraged discussion of the emerging analysis among the women for verification and additional information (Lincoln & Guba, 1985).

Rich data emerged from both the individual and group interviews. For many of the women, both interview approaches offered a rare opportunity to share their midlife experiences of issues such as menopause, sexuality, and their changing physical attractiveness. The women spoke candidly and openly, expressing a full range of thoughts and emotions related to their midlife experience.

Within the group interview context, however, group interaction produced insights *beyond* those obtained in the individual interviews, facilitating an empowerment process that provided groundwork for social and political action. It is to this process that I devote the remainder of this chapter.

What Is Empowerment?

First, it is important that we understand the use of the word "empowerment" as it relates to this chapter. In the health promotion field, the term "empowerment" has two primary meanings: (a) the individual's development of autonomy and self-control, and (b) the "development of collective influence on the social conditions of one's life" (Young, 1994, p. 48). Both meanings are relevant to my study and to the interpretations presented here. Although it is assumed in practice that clients are able to empower themselves, and that empowerment cannot be given to clients (Gibson, 1991), certain conditions can facilitate processes of empowerment. To demonstrate the ways in which the conditions of my study facilitated a movement toward empowerment for the participants, I present glimpses into the three group interviews, which, as mentioned earlier, were held near the end of my study. I begin with the first group meeting, held approximately three weeks after completing the entire set of individual interviews. Verbatim slices of conversation illustrate the ways in which an empowerment process unfolded as the women collectively shared their experiences of their changing bodies.

Setting the Stage for Group Interaction

Each woman came to the initial group meeting with a degree of comfort with having participated in at least two consecutive individual conversations with me. The individual interviews had, in themselves, provided an opportunity for the women to gain more awareness of their struggles, confusion, and isolation related to their experiences of their changing bodies. The rapport already established during these conversations seemed to create an interest for each participant to find out what other participants were saying about the midlife experience, and to provide a bridge for the women to step into the unknown territory of sharing with others their perceptions of their changing bodies. In this transition from individual to group conversations, many also expressed a desire to continue their involvement beyond that of participating in the individual conversations in the hopes that they would be able to share stories collectively with other women who held in common the fact that they had participated in the research. They believed that doing so might "help break some of the silence surrounding the experience" of midlife for women.

I chose a convenient central location for the first group meeting, accessible for those requiring bus transportation. Even so, I was overwhelmed by the women's support for this second stage of data collection when nine of the original 11 participants appeared one by one at the door. My part in creating a relaxed atmosphere was providing cheese, slices of fruit, a variety of juices, and some homemade muffins, and arranging the seating at a round table, with ample room for a wheelchair. The "finger food" was strategically placed so that the women could easily help themselves throughout the meeting.

The First Group Meeting: A Shift in Agenda

For all my planning, serendipity played a part in the first meeting prior to the tape recorder being turned on. Despite the fact that I had deliberately included a person with a disability in the sample, I neglected to check whether washrooms were accessible to wheelchair users. Unfortunate as this incident was, it provided an unexpected lesson in disempowerment, and perhaps contributed to setting the stage for the important work that occurred during the session. It also gave me a very clear indication of the tone that the group would likely take, of values held by the members (including myself) and of the ways in which the participants would respond to each other's unsettling midlife narratives shared within the group.

This same participant spoke of her experience of living with a physical disability and her perception of the ways in which people

respond to her when she is in her wheelchair. This event helped raise the group's consciousness of the difficulties with using a wheelchair, and stimulated a lively discussion and genuine interest in hearing more from the woman who brought the topic to the forefront.

I was pleased to note that the wheelchair-using participant was comfortable enough to voice her concerns within a group, which consisted of strangers and myself, who, in my position as the researcher, may have been viewed as being in a position of power (Chinn, 1995). Also auspicious was the fact that the others in the group were immediately supportive and sympathetic, willing to discuss a sensitive topic, giving, taking, and inquiring of one another. And, for myself, I was able in this situation to meet the participants as peers, rather than as "subjects" in my study. I was aware that in also being a woman at midlife, I could enhance the research process by sharing my own experience and by engaging in continual reflection of my midlife transitions (Banister, 1999a).

I believe that the inaccessible bathroom incident served two functions: it established an incipient focus of interest in empowerment, and it helped to build initial rapport among this small community of women. It seemed to affirm for everyone involved that the group would be a comfortable place in which the participants could each be safely vulnerable enough to collectively share some of the intimate details of their midlife experience, assured that their audience would be interested and caring.

Once the participants were comfortably seated around the table, I switched on the tape recorder placed in the middle of the table and began the group interview. I started out by reminding the women of the importance of maintaining confidentiality within the group. After our introductions, I stated the purpose of the meeting, reviewed the tentative agenda that I had created beforehand, and asked for additions or deletions. I reminded the women that the purpose of the meeting was to bring them together to continue discussing their concerns about their changing bodies but this time with one another. I also explained that I hoped to present them with the tentative analysis of the individual interview data to see whether it fit with their understanding of their experiences of midlife. I then invited the women to take turns and share a few words of their experiences of participating in the study up to that point.

The women were animated, almost all speaking at once:

JUDITH[3]: I enjoyed the process of the interview thing. It was very strange for me to take that time to reflect on myself. I guess it's really strange for me to have the chance to talk about my experience and what it's like to be me.

CORINNE: I was just starting to really think about things and then I thought about a whole lot of things afterwards, when the interview was through. That was quite an experience!

SANDRA: It's been a delightful process for me, I've really, really enjoyed it! I was really looking forward to being here and meeting the other women that are in the project.

BETH: It's been very interesting. It definitely makes you reflect on your problems and the things going on for you.

LILLIAN: A few years ago when I really saw the major physical changes mostly in my face—I had quite a lot of difficulty with that. I think more recently that I feel a lot better about accepting the changes as they happen. I don't know if that had to do with the study but it was sort of happening around the same time. I'm a lesbian and in my community there is a lot more acceptance of aging.

Unlike the women above, Suzanne shared an unanticipated result of her participation in the research process, one that left her feeling uncertain about what to expect during that evening's meeting:

SUZANNE: For me, one of the things that I was hoping for was to begin to see some clarity and to get rid of all the confusion. What in fact happened was the more I thought I was answering questions the more questions that came up. I'm trying to get comfortable with that sense of ambiguity and that there is no real answer—to begin to accept that.

The women did not spare themselves from responding to Suzanne's questioning, particularly related to the vast amount of information about menopause on booksellers' shelves and the confusing messages conveyed in some of them. Indeed, after completing my final analysis of the entire set of data, this theme, initially voiced by Suzanne, emerged as one of the major themes in the midlife experience of women; that is, "having more questions" about what to expect as their bodies aged (Banister, 1999b).

The women's comments on their experience of participating in the project were enlightening in a number of ways. Within the general sense of excitement and engagement, a number of insights emerged. It was acknowledged that our society provides little opportunity for self-reflection, particularly as supported by a nonjudgemental listener. The process of the individual interviews was understood as somehow providing an impetus for further thought, inquiry, and self-exploration, a process that led to insights regarding the events of one's life and the discovery of a new focus. For some participants, even those who struggled with issues of self-esteem, a movement toward self-acceptance had been precipitated. Suzanne's remark went further, implying that uncertainty and ambiguity are underlying components of transition and growth and the related need to embrace rather than avoid these initially uncomfortable feelings.

Besides being simply informative for me and adding to the analytic content, this exercise furthered the process that was occurring in the group in an unexpected way. Clearly, each of the participant's responses quoted earlier reveals an attitude or view that can be a precursor to the development of empowerment. Indeed, as the meeting continued and the participants spoke of themselves and listened to one another, the level of empowerment rose, as exemplified by the fact that they turned the meeting to their own needs.

As mentioned earlier, my plan had been to begin the meeting by asking the women to verify eight hypothetical domains or categories I had developed up to that point through the analysis of the individual interviews. These domains had been previously written on a flip chart with room to add the women's comments about each as the group conversation progressed. The women, however, had more pressing issues to discuss and I quickly abandoned my influence over the direction of the interview. I was aware that a

---

[3]To maintain confidentiality, I have changed all information that might identify the women.

shift in power often takes place in group interviews due in part to the mere number of participants having control over the interaction (Wilkinson, 1998, 1999). With humility, I put my planned agenda aside for later, realizing that by "letting go of control" (Chinn, 1995), space could be created for further spontaneous sharing and support.

Suzanne's acknowledgement of her confusion and uncertainty about her changing body prompted most of the women to explore their experiences more deeply and meaningfully than they would have if they had just been recounting events. For example, right after she spoke, others quickly jumped in, anxious to share stories of confusion and discomfort about their midlife experiences of their changing bodies. The women expressed confusion about the use of hormone replacement therapy, drugs prescribed by physicians for treating "symptoms" of menopause. Uncertainty and skepticism prevailed about the benefits versus risk factors involved with use of these drugs. The question of who ultimately benefits from the prescription of these drugs was also discussed. This moved into a discussion of the women's disillusionment with the medical profession's approach to some of their concerns. I observed the women carefully, noting the lively and emotionally laden discussion that took place around this disillusionment:

LILLIAN: Elizabeth interviewed me before Christmas and then somebody gave me Germaine Greer's book, *The Change*. I have some difficulties with Germaine Greer's attitude. She was extremely negative about many things and very arrogant. But there was enough really solid evidence in that book to really make me want to burn a path to the doctor's office and raise hell because she had so much evidence about how the medical profession treats us, especially around menopause.

Lillian's remarks kindled a collective voice of frustration: at times, physicians' explanations of women's midlife changes were incongruent with their own experiences, and distorted their expectations of bodily changes. The women wanted more information to answer their questions with a view to filling noticeable gaps in their knowledge. I realized, however, that they were not particularly interested in the "expert advice" from health care professionals. Instead, these women found value in the knowledge and wisdom that emerged from sharing their own experiences *with one another.*

The women told one story after another, and I watched, fascinated by the interactions that seemed like the women had known each other for a very long time. They listened carefully to one another's stories validating each other's concerns. Some women, who were at first reticent, became outspoken, encouraged by the openness of others. Sandra, for example, shared a narrative of her confusion:

SANDRA: I have gone to a number of doctors about my health. I don't know what is going on! I may have a hormone imbalance or something, but the feedback I'm getting is that I'm perfectly healthy. I get the feeling that it's all in my head. I find if I question the doctors, they take it as being confrontational.

When Sandra said this, a tone of collective empathy seemed to permeate the room. Exchanging looks, Mary tried to put Sandra at ease:

MARY: I don't think there's anything wrong with questioning. It's good. I think it's very important.

One after another, the women spoke of difficulties they had experienced with obtaining useful information about their midlife changes. Sharing their stories of physical change reassured some that they were not "losing their minds," that they had a right to question that their bodies were "feeling different." As it turned out, the willingness to question their situation was an important part of taking control of their own health.

The building of relationships that was taking place among this small community of midlife women fostered an environment of openness and trust in which personal and shared exploration of midlife experiences could take place. As the women shared their stories, I reflected on how much the conversation was taking on an air of empowerment. Unfolding as a collective network of support, the group became a place in which each member's contribution was valued and treated in a nonjudgemental way. The conversation continued. I listened, stepping in at times only to keep the flow of ideas generating:

JUDITH: Male physicians don't seem to care enough to find out what is wrong emotionally because it isn't in their realm of consciousness.

LOUISE: Women's experiences weren't taken seriously and men never had those problems.

JUDITH: They didn't have much sympathy or understanding because they hadn't gone through those things, they didn't know what it was like to have hot flashes or PMS.

SAMANTHA: It was easy for them to say, "Oh well, female problems are all in their minds."

Louise's voice shook as she confided her disappointment with her female physician:

LOUISE: I was really unhappy with the female physician that I'd switched to because I went thinking it would be wonderful. But then I noticed that when I got into the issues, I asked my physician about some sexuality questions and some menopausal questions, and she laughed! I was really distressed about that!

A chorus of gasps echoed in the room. Attention stayed focused on Louise:

BETH: She laughed, because?

LOUISE: I'm not sure. I think it was more, she was uncomfortable with the subject matter.

CORINNE: Well, women—they're all trained in the same medical schools.

MARY: That's true. Yeah!

SAMANTHA: Usually by male physicians.

The women nodded vigorously; they understood exactly.

I was fascinated with this milieu of consciousness-raising in which participants discussed the broader context of their concerns. In their own way, the women articulated some of the basic social factors such as **ageism** and **sexism** influencing their experience. The subject of alternative medicine came up as they questioned their situation.

BETH: I don't know, maybe someday something like midwifery will develop where we will have women's health experts to turn to.

The women seemed to welcome the shift in subject, reflecting more liberating attitudes that enable women to make proactive choices about their health. The power of the group was charged with a collective energy even more political than before:

JUDITH: It's taking the lack of trust and doing something about it. I feel I'm being more proactive in my health care. I'm not assuming that the medical profession knows everything.

LOUISE: Our generation is questioning whether you listen to the advice of a regular doctor, whether you seek alternatives, or whether you try and do all these other things to improve your health.

CORINNE: I think women are just becoming more aware and educated and assertive.

As the women sought out alternatives to the perceived inadequate forms of health assistance provided by the "mainstream," they moved toward assuming responsibility for their own well-being, not only physically, but also mentally and spiritually. Some women described how medicine was just not as efficacious as some alternative means. Predictably, the idea of seeking alternatives for their complaints was at times discouraged by their physicians:

SAMANTHA: I started going for massage therapy, which was outright laughed about. My doctor thought the idea was ridiculous. "If you think it will help go ahead, but it really won't help you" type of attitude.

SANDRA: You know, if you talk to the medical profession about a variety of alternative things they really don't want to talk about it, so I've just been focusing on them anyway.

BETH: I think doctors should consider alternative methods too. They shouldn't say, "Well, if you don't want to take hormones, if you don't want to take antidepressants, there is nothing I can offer you." That's nonsense!

LOUISE: The medical profession should get into the 21st century and look not at just conventional medicine but alternate measures, sort of holistic treatment.

JUDITH: I stopped taking antidepressants and hormones and started on something else, alternate things, herbals and so forth. And then, I started feeling better, physically. I had a little more energy, and was not quite as depressed. That got me reading more and finding out more. I started to get a little angry too because I didn't get any help with ordinary conventional medicine. So that was kind of a spur, just getting a little angry, just finding my own answers.

The opportunity to collectively voice frustration and anger within a mutually empathic and supportive group environment helped to mobilize the women's energies and resistance to the seeming invisibility of their concerns. The discussion of the lack of consistent information about their physical changes prompted the women to question and challenge traditional cultural constructions of their experiences, indicating their resistance to negative attitudes about aging women. And in fact, this resistance to the cultural discourse was justified. As described next, personal experience helped many participants in this study to challenge some of the myths of midlife women's sexuality. Within the group interview context, what started out as a discussion of their experiences of their changing bodies ended with a request to meet again, to focus on the nitty-gritty of the topic of women's sexuality.

It was five minutes before the first group was to end when Corinne spoke up. Not able to contain herself any longer, she looked around and addressed the group. With the women's initial awkwardness having disappeared, Corinne posed a question that brought the group to the main intersection between the first and second group meeting:

CORINNE: I know what we haven't talked about . . . we haven't talked about sex!

SANDRA: Are you allowed to have two groups before you're finished?

JUDITH: Two hours isn't that much time; it's totally fun!

LOUISE: I think sex is another big topic. *(laughter)*

MARY: It is for me!

LILLIAN: I'd like to come back as a group together and discuss sexuality issues and a number of other things.

SAMANTHA: I'd love to come back!

BETH: I'd like to have another group meeting.

ELIZABETH: *(Interviewer without hesitation)* Of course!

Satisfied that a second meeting was possible, we collectively chose a tentative date and time that would work and agreed to meet in the location as before. There was unanimous agreement, however, that the time and date may have to change to accommodate the two members who had been absent for this discussion.

Second Group Meeting: Talk about Sex

Three weeks later the second group meeting took place. It was attended by eight participants from the first group and one additional woman from the original sample, attending the group for the first time. After my experience of having had my agenda for the first group meeting co-opted by the group, I made sure to establish the agenda for the second group meeting through consensus with the group members. The main agenda item to emerge was "discuss sexuality." By the time the women had settled in, it didn't take long for the conversation to begin. As it turned out, this meeting was even more candid than the first. The advent of the group was exhilarating and this tone continued until the two hours was up. I was touched by the women's energy, and from a health promotion perspective, came to appreciate even more the power of engaging in mutual dialogue of individuals' health-related concerns.

No one knew exactly how this second meeting would unfold, but what became apparent was the way in which the participants were collectively challenging assumptions of sexual decline in aging women. Because the topic of women's midlife sexuality mattered to the group, they responded to each other's narratives with a level of openness and intimacy, which I had never observed in a research context before. Most of the women confessed to discovery of a new sense of sexual desire and fulfillment, despite the societal belief that women deny their sexuality as they age:

JUDITH: I think sex is a great thing for menopausal women! It's a great cure-all!

(General agreement)

CORINNE: Sex is very powerful!

MARY: It's communication between people.

LOUISE: You feel freer, more relaxed

The women smiled knowingly. Their sharing helped some to collectively contradict some midlife misconceptions and provided a microcosm of support for the numerous transitions taking place at this stage of life. The women's honesty continued to intrigue me and the appreciation I had been feeling shifted to a deep sense of reverence. I came to realize the power of the group for validating the concerns of individual members.

Like the first meeting, the second one was characterized by a shift. The first meeting had embodied a shift from a gathering of discrete individuals into a community, the members of which became comfortable with and supportive of one another. The second group built on this familiarity and support, providing an environment in which an important issue could be explored productively. A collective process of empowerment among the women seemed to be taking hold.

Aspects of this process, observable during this second group meeting, included the decision and commitment to work on a meaningful topic that was potentially uncomfortable, if only because it is not a subject of everyday conversation. The choice of this topic revealed the level of trust and intimacy already attained in the group. Furthermore, because of its importance, this topic provided an impetus to increase both the level of trust and the sense of community within the group. Another characteristic of the topic of sex illustrates a further aspect of the empowerment process: because midlife women's sexuality is restricted as a topic for everyday conversation, the very act of discussing it is a challenge to mainstream culture (see Banister, 1999a). However, a much more active challenge was elicited when the taboo against discussing this topic had been broken; an alternative, nonmainstream, ad hoc culture began to develop, in which group members could affirm the positive aspects of their own experiences. These positive aspects are in contradiction to mainstream society and its devaluing of midlife women's sexuality. This led to further challenging of this taboo as represented in mainstream cultural attitudes and values fostered in the media and elsewhere. From there, it was a natural step for the women to articulate the ways in which their personal lives were socially constructed, and constrained by power relations and by mainstream cultural assumptions that devalue aging women. The conversation had taken on a more political tone.

Third Group Meeting: Reaching Out

After the second session, I realized how much the women had come to interpret their situations through a socially conscious lens, working collectively to discuss ways that other women in the community could obtain a broader scope of information about emotional and physiological changes associated with their midlife physical changes. During the third group meeting the possibility of reaching out to other women filled the room with excitement:

SAMANTHA: I think it's important to be able to get together with a group, a disparate group of women, where not everybody is just like me; to be able to throw out our anxieties, put them on the table and get feedback from people. I think the isolation and the fear is quite huge.

LOUISE: It's peer information; it's not just an expert telling us. We're peers. We're all going through it. We have the same experience.

SANDRA: But there's still those other people around who are getting misinformation or not much at all from their doctors if they do talk to them. I don't!

CORINNE: I'm concerned about the women we can't reach in this way.

MARY: I think the majority of women still are having negative experiences.

BETH: And you can see why younger women might have anxiety because all they've heard from their mothers and from the medical profession is a total lack of any accuracy and information and total lack of feeling and empathy.

CORINNE: I think there's a need for a woman's health collective that would draw from a wider population of women. Like the *Boston Health Collective* that came out of the 70s.

MARY: Yeah, I think there's a need for something like that perhaps with one of the community health centers like the [name] Community Project.

JUDITH: Wouldn't it be great if we could get something like this going and then we could send out things regularly to the medical profession, flyers to the doctors' offices, saying, "If you want to talk about menopause, contact so-and-so."

The women were committed to continue demystifying (Chinn, 1995) issues that relate to midlife women's changing bodies by talking about such issues with women outside the group. They hoped that further dialogue with other women might have a "ripple effect" on other women, thereby contributing to women's ability to take charge of their own health.

As the group came to an end, there was unanimous agreement among the women about the value of sharing their perceptions of their changing bodies with each other, which provided them with invaluable information based on their own knowledge and wisdom. At that time, I asked the participants to share with other group members their experiences of having participated in the group:

MARY: My awareness of myself as I am at midlife has probably changed in that it's becoming more positive and that's the positive influence of this group.

JUDITH: I think we're all ready for this next step and we've all gone through the craziness and the confusion.

My final analysis of the data obtained from both individual and group interviews revealed that the women in the study experienced an assortment of many characteristics of empowerment. In particular, the group experience had an emancipatory benefit for most of the participants (Banks-Wallace, 1998), contributing to a process that was self-enhancing and empowering. For most of the women, a shift in perspective took place, representing a sense of agency related to their own health care choices and perceptions of their changing bodies.

Implications for Health Promotion

I have attempted to show in this chapter the ways in which a research project, intended to explore women's midlife experience of their changing bodies, was co-opted by the study participants to become a venue by which they were able to move from a state of questioning and confusion, toward political action. We, as health promotion practitioners, hope that clients attain empowerment within

enabling conditions that are co-created between our clients and ourselves. The process that occurred during this study exemplifies the co-creation of an enabling condition within which the movement toward empowerment was facilitated.

As health care professionals, we must examine our own attitudes and practices, and policies within the health care system, in light of how we currently strive to help women gain control over their own health. During this reflective process, we can explore the extent to which aspects of our professional work counteract, or contribute to, midlife women's dissatisfaction with the current state of health care. It is imperative that we seriously reflect on the broader context in which we address women's health issues.

It is important that, as practitioners, we provide opportunities for women to talk with one another about their midlife experiences. My research corroborated what feminist researchers have already documented: Group interviews help participants' co-construct meaning within a social context (Kitzinger & Barbour, 1999; Wilkinson, 1998, 1999). We can help women in a variety of contexts overcome some of the barriers to empowerment by providing opportunities for them to engage in dialogue with one another and share knowledge of their midlife experiences. Consciousness-raising conversations are dialogical (Young, 1994). Through the give and take of discussion, the participants in my study constructed an understanding of their personal lives as socially conditioned. This indicates that if health care professionals provide environments in which such dialogue may occur, the participants in such groups may come to trust their own expertise and to seek solutions congruent with their health-related values. Health care professionals can further this process by posing critical questions at strategic points during such dialogue. Consider how such actions would contribute to rebuilding women's trust in health care professionals!

This chapter recounts what I believe are the salient features of a process of empowerment that occurred serendipitously as a by-product of a research study. The group interview experience became a mechanism for enhancing the women's midlife empowerment process. The fact that this process occurred during a research project indicates to me that, given the right conditions, almost *any* group of midlife women could work together to develop a small community in which members can generate for themselves, and for one another, a movement toward empowerment.

✳ Reflective Questions

1. What key components of health promotion can you identify in the process that unfolded in the group?

2. How did the women's willingness to question their situations (e.g., the lack of consistent information about their changing bodies) contribute to their empowerment process? Why is this important?

3. What role did the women's collective anger toward the medical profession contribute to their empowerment process?

4. This chapter illustrates ways in which women collectively challenged cultural assumptions of health-related issues such as sexuality. How does this relate to the concepts of health promotion? What is the role of health practitioners for facilitating women's ability to challenge cultural assumptions related to women's health?

REFERENCES

Agar, M. H. (1986). *Speaking of ethnography.* Beverly Hills, CA: Sage.

Banister, E. M. (1999a). Evolving reflexivity: Negotiating meaning of women's mid-life experience. *Qualitative Inquiry, 5,* 3–23.

Banister, E. M. (1999b). Women's mid-life experience of their changing bodies. *Qualitative Health Research, 9,* 520–537.

Banks-Wallace, J. (1998). Emancipatory potential of storytelling in a group. *Image: Journal of Nursing Scholarship, 30,* 17–21.

Baruch, G. K., & Brooks-Gunn, J. (1984). Introduction: The study of women in mid-life. In G. Baruch & J. Brooks-Gunn (Eds.), *Women in mid-life* (pp. 1–8). New York: Plenum Press.

Bond, M., & Bywaters, P. (1998). Working it out for ourselves: Women learning about hormone replacement therapy. *Women's Studies International Forum, 21*(1), 65–76.

Chinn, P. (1995). *Peace and power: Building communities for the future* (4th ed.). New York: National League for Nursing Press.

Daly, J. (1995). Caught in the web: The social construction of menopause as disease. *Journal of Reproductive and Infant Psychology, 11,* 115–126.

Denzin, N. K. (1989). *The research act* (3rd ed.). Englewood Cliffs, NJ: Prentice Hall.

Engebretson, J., & Wardell, D. W. (1997). Perimenopausal women's alienation. *Journal of Holistic Nursing, 15,* 254–270.

Fetterman, D. M. (1989). *Ethnography.* Newbury Park, CA: Sage.

Foot, D. (1996). *Boom, bust & echo.* Toronto: Macfarlane, Walter & Ross.

Geertz, C. (1973). *The interpretation of cultures.* New York: Basic Books.

Gergen, M. (1990). Finished at 40: Women's development within the patriarchy. *Psychology of Women Quarterly, 14,* 471–493.

Gibson, C. H. (1991). A concept analysis of empowerment. *Journal of Advance Nursing, 16,* 354–361.

Glaser, B. G., & Strauss, A. L. (1967). *The discovery of grounded theory.* New York: Aldine de Gruyter.

Heilbrun, C. G. (1988). *Writing a woman's life.* New York: Ballantine Books.

Hunter, M. S., & O'Dea, I. (1997). Menopause: Bodily changes and multiple meanings. In J. M. Ussher (Ed.), *Body talk* (pp. 199–222). London: Routledge.

Hunter, S., & Sundel, M. (1994). Mid-life for women: A new perspective. *Affilia, 9,* 113–128.

Jarrett, M. E., & Lethbridge, D. J. (1994). Looking forward, looking back: Women's experience with waning fertility during mid-life. *Qualitative Health Research, 4,* 370–384.

Jones, J. (1994). Embodied meaning: Menopause and the change of life. *Social Work and Health Care, 19,* 43–65.

Kitzinger, J., & Barbour, R. S. (1999). Introduction: The challenge and promise of focus groups. In J. Kitzinger & R. S. Barbour (Eds.), *Developing focus group research: Politics, theory and practice* (pp. 1–20). Thousand Oaks, CA: Sage.

Kvale, S. (1996). *Interviews: An introduction to qualitative research interviewing.* Thousand Oaks, CA: Sage.

Lincoln, Y. S., & Guba, E. G. (1985). *Naturalistic inquiry.* Beverly Hills, CA: Sage.

Lippert, L. (1997). Women at mid-life: Implications for theories of women's adult development. *Journal of Counseling and Development, 76,* 16–22.

Mansfield, P. K., Theisen, S. C., & Boyer, B. (1992). Mid-life women and menopause: A challenge for the mental health counselor. *Journal of Mental Health Counseling, 14,* 73–83.

Morgan, D. L. (1988). *Focus groups as qualitative research.* Newbury Park, CA: Sage.

Quinn, A. A. (1991). A theoretical model of the perimenopausal process. *Journal of Nurse-Midwifery, 36,* 25–30.

Sandelowski, M. (1986). The problem of rigor in qualitative research. *Advances in Nursing Science, 8*(3), 27–37.

Spradley, J. P. (1979). *The ethnographic interview.* New York: Holt, Rinehart & Winston.

Spradley, J. P. (1980). *Participant observation.* New York: Holt, Rinehart & Winston.

Unger, R., & Crawford, M. (1992). *Women and gender: A feminist psychology.* Philadelphia: Temple University Press.

Wilkinson, S. (1998). Focus groups in feminist research: Power, interaction, and the co-construction of meaning. *Women's Studies International Forum, 21,* 111–125.

Wilkinson, S. (1999). Focus groups: A feminist method. *Psychology of Women Quarterly, 23,* 221–244.

Woods, N. F., & Mitchell, E. S. (1997). Women's images of mid-life: Observations from the Seattle mid-life women's health study. *Health Care for Women International, 18,* 439–453.

Young, I. M. (1994). Punishment, treatment, empowerment: Three approaches to policy for pregnant addicts. *Feminist Studies, 20,* 33–57.

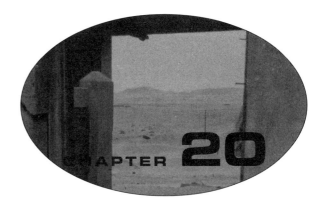

CHAPTER 20

Family Health Promotion within the Demands of Pediatric Home Care and Nursing Respite

VIRGINIA E. HAYES
PAMELA J. McELHERAN

I hope you don't mind me saying this to you, but I found the questions [on the written questionnaire] ridiculous. I filled in all the little boxes, but I think the questions are superficial. You really want to know the impact my son's illness has had? All right, then, you need to get at the way it has . . . affected each and every one of us and our plans and dreams. . . . It is the totality of its effects, its all-encompassingness that you should study. . . . OK, tell me: how do you convert this into a +3 or a −3 answer, to a decimal? How do you compare it with other [families'] reactions? I insist it is illegitimate to make comparisons. We are not things. We are not an "interpersonal problem," a "family stress."

Kleinman, 1988, p. 184

This mother of a boy with muscular dystrophy is making a plea—to be seen as a whole family, one that includes more than her son's illness and its effects on individuals, one that is more than a group of people dealing day-by-day at home with lifts, wheelchairs, medications, incontinence, a member whose mental condition is deteriorating, who cannot speak, and who has little motor control over his upper body. This is a unique *family,* whose members are trying to maintain the health of *both* the individual members *and* the family as a whole in the face of significant challenges.

To be a healthy family in the presence of a child's long-term health condition requires much

work both inside and outside the family (Hayes, 1992). This work is sometimes very demanding indeed, and frequently depends on informal and formal assistance from social networks and the community (Eiser, 1993; Hayes, 1997a; Leonard, Brust, & Nelson, 1993; Patterson, Leonard, & Titus, 1992). There is work for all members over and above the usual growth, development, and relationship building of family roles and tasks. In these "special families," any member may also add roles of health caregiver, care coordinator, or night nurse. He or she might maintain dialysis at home, suction a tracheostomy, or set up and maintain home parenteral nutrition. But as the father of a five-year-old with cerebral palsy said during a research conversation, "We just have to look at the *whole* family." The bottom line is that a family, with a child at home with a chronic condition and the extra requirements of caregiving, is also a family like any other. As the mother in this same family said, "We're trying to stay as an integrated unit in spite of the difficulties."

When the severity of the child's condition requires in-home nursing care (nursing respite services or home care provided by a qualified RN or Licensed Practical Nurse), we can be sure that demands on the family are very high. In fact, in-home nursing care for the child and his or her family introduces another set of forces or adaptations required of the members, particularly in cases when long hours and/or overnight care are provided by a professional. How does having nurses in the home affect family life? How can such families be healthy, functioning, contributing units in society in the face of their unique, difficult, and complex situations? What role do health professionals play in promoting families' health beyond attending to the special child's care requirements? How can family-level health promotion be integrated into nurses' too-brief, too-infrequent interactions with family members at home?

✳ Reflective Questions

1. Would you think that having a nurse in the home on a regular or semi-regular basis to provide respite for the family would be stress alleviating or stressful? Why?
2. What happens within families when stresses (or demands) are very high?
3. What factors affect a family's functioning in the presence of high demands?
4. When a family's resources are over-whelmed, what can the family members do? What can be done by those in the health and social professions? By policy-makers?

This chapter is about families and how they deal with having a child with a medically fragile condition at home. Although the affected children are being cared for by their families, they have health conditions that are so demanding that in-home nursing respite[1] is required to help their families remain as close as possible to

---

[1]Respite care refers to those family support services specifically aimed to provide temporary relief from the rigorous physical and emotional demands involved in caring for a family member with special needs, while simultaneously providing a positive and rewarding experience for the child with special needs (Canadian Association for Community Care, 1996, p. 5). This entails care measures or services for the child, parents, siblings, or family as a whole. Respite has been reported to reduce the burden on families raising children with chronic health concerns or disabilities at home by: relieving familial stress; improving family functioning; improving parental attitudes toward the child; and reducing social isolation. Services may be provided by volunteers or paid workers, including health care, educational, or social service professionals with a wide range of specific or general education and training.

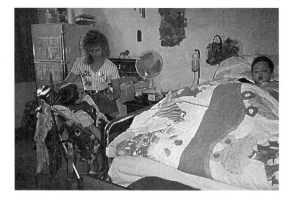

FIG. 20–1. The child's equipment can dominate a home.

being integrated, well functioning, and able to meet their members' needs. This chapter explores one theme (concept) of a grounded theory study we conducted that was designed to evaluate the effectiveness of a Nursing Respite Program (for children and their families) in British Columbia. Our thoughts are informed here as well by two subsequent projects, a national survey concerning services for children with special needs and a later **constructivist** study (Guba & Lincoln, 1994) about the best practices in children's respite care, both aimed to move families' needs onto the national health care agenda.

One of the goals of these studies was to gain and report insight about families and their experiences of living and working with children's "hi-tech" or complex care at home. In the primary study partially reported here, we collected data directly with families and individual members and their Respite Program care records. We talked with and observed family and work activities that involved parents, children, and often visited children or extended family members and adult friends, and occasionally the nurses involved with the family. In the Canadian services project (Hayes, Hollander, Tan, & Cloutier, 1997), we spoke with key informant personnel associated with home care-related agencies and from government departments that oversee programs and set policy, whereas in the best practices project (Kannon, Hayes, Radford, & Canadian Association of Community Care Children's Respite Project Group, 2000), we held focus groups and interviews with community agency personnel and groups, and with parents and other key individuals in three communities. Among our research participants were families and care providers who thought that the number of respite hours and the quality of care they were giving and receiving were adequate, and many who thought they were not. We transcribed audiotaped interviews and field notes, took notes during focus group discussions and individual telephone conversations, then coded and analyzed according to established grounded theory strategies (Glaser, 1978; Strauss, 1987; Strauss & Corbin, 1998).

This chapter highlights selected parts of these families' stories that are relevant to better understanding of the demands families face and their responses to them (a micro theory), including selected parents' own ideas about promoting individuals' and *families'* health. We conclude by looking critically at health promotion in this particular context: children's chronicity or disability[2] and nursing respite care. Our focus is on the family as the unit of care, and the unit of research. Also, the family is whatever a member considers it to be (Hanson, 2001; Stuart, 1991).

A Study of Families Living with Constant Care

Because we wish to concentrate on specific aspects of the theory generated with families that had children with significant care needs that required nursing respite, a brief orientation to our research will help to frame our interpretations and conclusions. In the overall study, our aims were to evaluate the effectiveness of a Nursing Respite Program, looking at selected child, parent, family, cost, and

program outcomes over the families' first year of receiving respite services, and to understand the impact that nursing respite has on the families receiving this form of home care (Hayes, McElheran, & Tan, 1997). Although this was a **triangulated** design, using both quantitative (theory-directed) and qualitative (theory-generating) methods and several sources of data, the theme discussed in this chapter arises from the **grounded theory** data and analyses.

In this study, a researcher would spend from two to seven hours over three visits talking with and actively observing families being families. Sometimes visits were with one caregiver or family member at home with the special child, or with more family and friends, or constituted brief or lengthy telephone conversations. Some parents kept diaries. We collected data before and twice after respite services were initiated. The over 150 hours of data from this project are varied, rich, voluminous, and were gathered and analyzed over time using the constant comparison methods characteristic of grounded theory (Glaser, 1978; Strauss & Corbin, 1998). During analyses, we worked independently and also in pairs or groups to draw out pertinent interpretations and concepts. Although space does not permit their expansion in this chapter, the analyses were also informed by pertinent literature and shaped by our practice and personal experiences and our pre-existing knowledge (Denzin, 1994; Richardson, 1994). Together, these data sources provided a myriad of examples to illustrate or "ground" our theory.

A wide range of families participated: one to six children; two-parented, lone-parented, or blended; of European, South Asian, and First Nations origin; small to substantial incomes; high school to graduate parental education; and living in rural and urban areas across our large, geographically varied province. The special children ranged in age from 13 months to 17 years (mean = 5.1 years), their siblings from 5 months to 22 years (mean = 7.7 years), and their parents' ages averaged 34.7 years (range = 21–55). Their conditions were generally complex (that is, it was the rare child who had a single medical diagnosis), and examples included chronic renal failure (one child was waiting for transplant for polycystic kidneys), liver disease, seizure disorders, brain tumors and injuries, cerebral palsy, spastic quadriplegia, post-

---

[2]Terminology is troublesome in this substantive area, due to the connotations or local usages of specific words, debates about their inclusiveness and labeling of children, and parents', children's, practitioners', and authors' preferences. In this chapter, the term chronic condition is used to denote any condition of 12 months' duration or longer that requires ongoing health monitoring and/or treatment or special health care. Its use encompasses terms such as chronic illness, disability, long-term health conditions, special needs, etc. Its use includes physical conditions, developmental delay, psychosocial problems, or states of children's health that may require highly technical interventions at home. Some examples in childhood: speech, hearing and visual disabilities; autism; diabetes; asthma; cerebral palsy; a wide range of congenital conditions such as spina bifida and complex syndromes; heart, lung, liver, kidney diseases; cystic fibrosis; and a variety of acquired conditions such as brain injury, neurological diseases, etc.

BOX 20−1

EXAMPLES OF CARE MEASURES AT HOME (NURSES AND FAMILY MEMBERS)

Assisting with activities of daily living
Care and maintenance of Total Parental Nutrition
Maintenance and monitoring of naso-gastric tube feeds
Maintenance and monitoring of gastrostomy tube feeds
Maintenance and monitoring of jejunal tube feeds
Care of ileostomy
Monitoring of bowel routine, nutrition, signs and symptoms of infection
Oral-pharyngeal suctioning
Care of tracheostomy
Maintenance and monitoring of oxygen
Maintenance and monitoring of ventilator
Respiratory assessment
Monitoring for seizures—neuro assessment
Administration of rectal valium for seizures
Administration of medications
Teaching related to medication, activity, skill, nutrition
Dressing changes
Blood sugar monitoring
Kidney dialysis

BOX 20−2

EXAMPLES OF NURSING DIAGNOSES IDENTIFIED IN CARE PLANS

Activity intolerance
Sleep pattern disturbances
Potential for infection
Self-care deficit
Knowledge deficit
Potential dehydration
Altered nutrition
Potential for constipation
Alteration in bowel elimination
Potential for injury
Potential for aspiration
Alteration in cardiac output
Alteration in respiratory function/ineffective breathing pattern
Potential for respiratory infection
Potential for parental stress
Discipline techniques
Potential for alteration in blood sugar level
Potential alteration in skin integrity
Potential altered growth and development

meningitis, hydrocephalus, developmental delays, prematurity and its associated conditions, congenital heart defects, hearing and visual disabilities, complex syndromes, esophageal reflux, and short gut syndrome. Some examples of the children's care measures and selected nursing diagnoses are illustrated in the boxed summaries. None of the children were palliative, but despite this, of the 27 families in the study, five children died during the family's one-year participation.

Trying to Have a Life

Families Living with Childhood Chronicity and Nursing Respite Care

"Trying to Have a Life" is what we call the part of the overall grounded theory that we use to describe families' experiences with a child's medically fragile or complex condition *in combination* with between 4 and 70 hours of nursing care in their homes each week (see Fig. 20–2). This phrase, "Trying to Have a Life," is used by some of the parents themselves. This is complex work, and is constant, inclusive of all family members, and tiring (Hayes, 1992). The child's chronic condition, its management, and the in-home respite care combine in multiple ways to affect the whole family. To illustrate, here are the words of a mother of three adolescent boys thinking back over years of having respite services provided at home:

When we started doing interviews for nurses . . . I told [the program consultants that] if my boys don't like [the nurses] they're not coming, because this is a family. Mark's[3] illness affects this family so Mark's care affects this family.

The implications of this mother's emphasized use of the words "illness" and "care" (that

---
[3]All names used in this chapter are fictional.

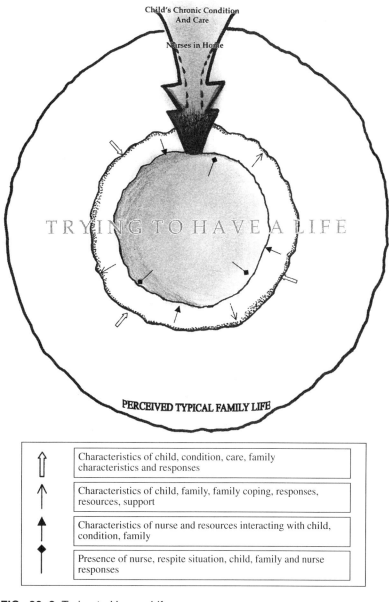

FIG. 20–2. Trying to Have a Life.

affect the whole family) are extremely significant for these families, in some cases overwhelmingly demanding.

We use the word "demands" to capture the wide range of care measures and their implications. According to the dictionary, a demand is "a strong or authoritative request," an urgent claim, a need, a requirement (Guralnik, 1970). It could be compared with the way Selye (1976) describes stress as both eu-

stress and distress—a demand on a family or individual is a force that simply "insists on being," something that requires skill or effort to ameliorate, and is not always negative. In families, demands can be on individuals or the family as a whole, and can affect development or functioning, or both. Families and their individual members respond in simple and complex ways to the interplay among the chronic condition, its management, and nurse's regular presence in the home. They share with someone from outside the family the care of children that, were it not so burdensome, parents and families would normally expect to be able to manage on their own.

Dealing with Chronicity and Respite

We introduce now the issues and demands for families that arise from our observational and conversational data and present those that pertain to the individual and family levels. We have conceptualized the family process of Trying to Have a Life in terms of two main forces impinging on what the parents in our study call Typical Family Life: those emanating from or the consequences of their children's conditions and care, compounded by those associated with having to have a nurse in the home to provide them a break from caregiving (see Fig. 20–2). Clearly, demands for families arise from the characteristics of the special child, the other children in the family, the parents, the complex or medically fragile condition(s), and the complex or highly technical care. These demands can affect the family positively or negatively (depicted in the diagram by two sets of small arrows). In addition, the characteristics of the nurses and the family members' responses to them and the respite situation (such conditions as the number of hours per week and associated resources, each introducing their own set of demands) can also affect the family positively and negatively (the other two sets of arrows in the diagram). First, we describe the nature of the individual-level and family-level demands derived from our observations and conversations with families in our study (and corroborated in our subsequent studies with different informants), and then turn to aspects of their situations that were reported to be positive and negative about each. Then we offer a rendering of what would promote family health by maximizing the "positives" and minimizing the "negatives" in families who live with both childhood chronicity and in-home respite care. We close with an interpretive account of what parents themselves see as the policy implications and solutions for their sometimes tenuous physical, mental, and social health.

> ✳ **Reflective Questions**
>
> **1.** What effects on *individual* parent(s) might you expect when a child has a chronic condition requiring in-home care? How might this change for better or worse with nursing respite care in the home?
>
> **2.** What effects on the *other children* in a family might you expect when one child has a chronic condition requiring in-home care? How might it affect their relationships with each other, with their sibling requiring care, with their parent(s), or with their friends? How might this change for better or worse with respite care?
>
> **3.** What different reactions might we see among parents in making the choice between "burnout" and having a stranger live in their house part-time? What factors might influence their reactions positively and negatively?

Demands at the Individual Level

Demands on parents who care for children requiring respite care range from minor to major, and from causing minimal to maximal disruption or accommodation. As one would expect, the demands are experienced toward the "heavier" ends of these continua, despite the provision of in-home help. Parents reported the continuous weight and responsibility of caregiving, an inability to control events in their lives the way they'd like to, the persistence of worrying, constant fatigue, and lack of time for themselves and for whole-family activities. Although rest and personal time do improve with respite care, it does not do so to the degree anticipated. In fact, parents report difficulty in giving up control, and "turning down" their vigilance. One mother explained, after saying that having respite for a second time in their lives was "excellent":

I had a lot of struggles the first time we used [respite services]. . . . I didn't have any problems with leaving her with Paulo [husband] but I had a lot of problems leaving, just period. So . . . a lot of times I didn't even go anywhere, I just stayed here and I got a lot more from just sitting here talking. . . . And I know Paulo would, he'd get annoyed. But [this time] I think . . . we were really physically and emotionally bankrupt by the time [respite started]. We were just, both of us were exhausted, and we really used the respite this time. . . . We actually got to spend some time with each other, which we hadn't done for six and a half years.

Despite their plans and dreams for how parents might use their time while their child was being cared for by a trustworthy, competent, well-trained nurse, they would not use respite time for *going out* as much as they would for *staying in,* to sleep or rest, with their "radar" turned down but not completely off. The vigilance they have become accustomed to, the responsibilities they have shouldered before respite starts are difficult to give up in many cases, whether they had been gained over a short or long time. Even with respite care, parents continue to find life stressful. Here's an interchange between a husband and wife as they explain why they are requesting additional respite hours:

Mother: *I mean [remaining as we are] is not going to benefit anybody in this family because even now I'm short tempered with Amy. I get short tempered with my husband; that's because I hold everything back not to strike out at him or anything, but I strike out at everybody else around me.*

Father: *We're all very short tempered right now.*

Mother: *The stress factor has gone down a little but not much.*

Parents in our study reported sacrificing, working hard, being restricted in their socialization outside the family, and needing to make constant adjustments. Respite services help, but not completely, and must be adequate to provide genuine relief from caregiving for *all* family members' needs.

Children are also individually affected by having a respite nurse in the home to care for their sibling with a chronic condition. During our interviews, they did not talk about these effects directly, but we made significant observations and listened to their parents describe them. For example:

I think these guys are finding it pretty frustrating. . . . Being a family then all of a sudden having to deal with—You know, somebody else in the house . . . a stranger in the house.

This mother went on to say that she expects herself "to put up with" the situation, but thinks that other members of her family are having a harder time doing so. Underscoring the intrusiveness of respite care, her com-

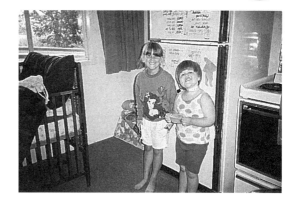

FIG. 20–3. Homes get rearranged.

ments illustrate that it is important for her that her children's relationships with each other are as much out of the "public" gaze of the respite nurse as possible.

Some parents in our study pointed to gains for their children. One mother told a story about one of her two healthy boys:

They have gone without a great deal because of Jannie [their sister], and they have never complained, and they are wonderful to her. But they've also developed. . . . Carl our youngest son, his little friend was out here on his bike—it's kind of amusing—and he fell off and I could hear him screaming out there. I went running out there and Carl's standing there looking at [his friend who] was bleeding and I said to him, "Carl what the h— are you doing? Help him up." And he looked at me and he said, "He's not blue and he's breathing so I figured he was okay." . . . Because that is the policy in our house, you never overreact because if you overreact you will panic Jannie. It has to be a sense of calm; it has to be okay.

This illustrates that well children frequently gain skills and adapt well to the demands their special sibling brings to their lives. Remarking on the positive influence of the respite nurse who comes to their home to provide care, another mother said:

When somebody is sick in this house it affects them—it affects how they do their homework, how they do in school, whatever. And having [the nurse] come here has taken some of that away from them which has been really nice. Because nowadays if you don't have an education [to] continue on or whatever, I mean you're, you're hooped.

So for this mother, nursing care at home has provided some options for her well children that ameliorate the obvious demands their sister with special needs has introduced to their lives. The overall combination of the special child's condition, its management, and respite care is not only confusing or a "hassle" for siblings, but has some advantages, such as gaining strengths, knowledge, or skills (Eiser, 1993).

✳ Reflective Questions

1. What effects on *family dynamics* might you expect when a child has a chronic condition requiring in-home care? How might this change for better or worse with nursing care being provided in the home?

2. What *family resources* might be affected when one child has a chronic condition requiring in-home care? How might the condition and its care demands affect intra-family relationships, or the relationship between the family and its community? How might this change for better or worse with respite care?

Demands at the Family Level

Recall what a mother quoted earlier said about her daughter's illness and its care affecting their *whole* family. Often the family-wide work and consequences involve extended family, godparents, close friends, and so forth. Families work constantly on adjusting to the permanency of the condition and its care, going through various phases, slipping back, and readjusting. Although internally the family may be experienced as "keyed up and tense," we observed and were told that there is a need for families to *appear* to the world to be doing fine. For example:

[Inside the family] I needed [my husband] to say to me it's not okay; once in a while, I needed for us to do that kind of talking. Whereas, whereas with people outside of our immediate close family here . . . you would put on this front. But I needed to know that he had a realistic view of what this was going to do to our life as well. And it was, it was an interesting process that . . . we had to finally discuss . . . point blank. . . . We still needed to admit to each other that it was tough and that it was a problem and that it was difficult.

Thus, we understand that internal family work is going on while the "public family

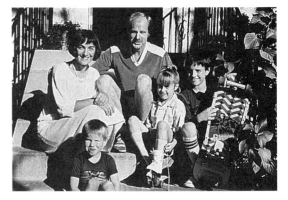

FIG. 20–4. The family may look "typical" to others, but is working hard at "Trying to Have a Life."

face" may be presented differently. One mother described this process as hard on the *"family's* self esteem."* Although inside the family may be "keyed up and tense," various members may feel that they must strive to appear near to "normal" in public, to *appear* as if they were coping well.

A compounding factor for families' "public face" is the reported tendency for health professionals, educators, and members of the general public to treat all families with a chronically ill child as if they were the same, when "Each family is totally, totally different, you know. Our family is different from the one down the street." Each family responds uniquely to its particular circumstances, and parents expressed their wish that this individuality be honored.

Other examples of family-level demands and participant responses from our data illustrate how caring for the child with a chronic illness infiltrates family life. There are fewer choices and options for members, because they must plan around caregiving (including the availability of respite), and this naturally affects spontaneity. This was graphically expressed by a father who said, "I think Desert Storm was more spontaneous than our trip to back east" (and they had taken a respite nurse with them!). Parents also alluded to losses of privacy and intimacy, and the effects that all these factors have on their sex lives.

The complex web of ways that chronicity and care operate together also affect interactions between the family and the community. Our data suggest that there are fewer extra-familial social contacts than in families without chronicity, or these may be undertaken more as individuals and less as families. Many of the families in our study could be described (and parents describe themselves) as socially isolated.

Though many families respond positively to the demands of their situations, there is no doubt they are different than "typical" families,[4] in ways they may not identify or be able to acknowledge. One father described this phenomenon as not being able to:

See the forest for the trees or the trees for the forest. And you're right in the thick of it, you just, you can't see what impact that kind of change on your family and the demands are having. He's your son and you love him and you're doing everything, naturally, for him, but you don't . . . see how it's impacting.

The interaction between the child's continuing complex health problem(s), the caregiving demands, and the pros and cons of in-home nursing care *is* complex. Families do gain, but there are many demands. They handle these demands in ways we're categorizing conceptually as Trying to Have a Life. Next, we describe some of the ways these families handle the "positives" and "negatives" in their lives, before we pass along their prescriptions for how they could be healthier—with health care professionals' help.

Responding Positively to Having a Respite Nurse in the Home

As we wish to focus on family-level health promotion in this chapter, we have selected only specific elements of the concept Trying to Have a Life, to illustrate families' responses to the demands of the children's conditions and care, and the necessity of having nurses in the home. The grounded theory data from the evaluation study provided insight into the positive consequences of in-home nursing respite services. Parents identified increases in their family time, couple time, and time for individuals to spend on themselves, on hobbies, and/or on chores. Some parents slept better (with their "radar" turned down), and some felt more rested or relaxed in other ways, although this varied broadly. They re-

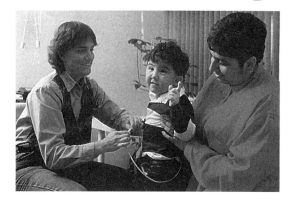

FIG. 20–5. Bradley, a home care nurse, and a care aide. Photo courtesy of *Nursing BC*.

ported feeling understood by the nurses (better than by their friends and sometimes better than by extended family members), more confident in the care *they* provided to their children, and genuinely relieved of caregiving by the care that the nurses provided. Some said they worried less. In one family, a mother was able to return to part-time work, so the father was able to quit his second job. At the family level, respite is described as decreasing family pressures, providing a needed break, helping the family respond to the unpredictable, and providing hope and support. Social contacts and connection to the communities improved in many cases. Speaking philosophically, one father noted that "once everything was up and running . . . the support that came from the [respite] program was . . . a life saver." To emphasize (added this same parent with strong agreement from his spouse),

I think it gives families the energy to keep up with the kind of care that's required, and therefore they don't slip into an acute situation with their chronic illness, if that makes any sense.

Responding Negatively to Having a Respite Nurse in the Home

In grounded theory analysis, we describe the contributing concepts as having properties (attributes or characteristics, such as color has hue, intensity, shade), and those properties as having dimensions (such as light or dark, bright or dull, etc.) (Strauss & Corbin, 1998).

---

[4]The term "typical" was used among the families in our studies, in preference to the term "normal" child or family.

As we have demonstrated, the concepts and subconcepts of this micro-theory about Trying to Have a Life do have breadth in both their variation and their substance. For example, we mentioned earlier that parents differ in their reports of changes in the amount and quality of their sleep when they receive respite services during the day or at night. Also, some family members have more difficulty than others in adjusting to having non-family members in their homes. Parents have a range of experiences with recruiting and adjusting to nurses, and find that nurses are a good fit with their families' needs in some ways, but not in others. For instance, some parents spontaneously described respite nurses who exhibited lack of caring, commitment, and professionalism, and others who seemed to treat their child's care like "business," or in a more depersonalized way than parents wished. Also, as mentioned earlier, although some parents felt relieved to have respite services at home, others felt it *increases* their overall responsibility for the management of their child's condition, that it is "more hassle than it's worth." To illustrate, a parent noted in her diary, "As is obvious, I have numerous recurring problems with the company being unable to supply nurses and with nurses canceling at the last moment." In contrast to the positive effects of in-home nursing respite care described in the previous section, one parent thought it was *more* work having respite: preparing for the nurses to come in, making coffee for her, obtaining a VCR, making her feel appreciated, and so forth.

Other significant negative aspects of having respite home care that were discovered in this study, however, were related to administrative details of service delivery. Without focusing on specific problems related to particular families' situations or to the specific respite programs we have experience with, we were able to draw a few general interpretive conclusions. Initial assessment or screening prior to starting services was often viewed as problematic for families. Parents reported that assessments were inadequate: conducted too quickly, in not enough detail, by unqualified or uninformed people. That is, personnel were not perceived to know enough about the complexity of the situations that families face, nor to make attempts to truly *understand*

families' particular circumstances, contexts, and consequences. Assessment was often seen as fragmented, with the result that an integrated, complete picture about a specific family's and child's strengths and requirements was not available as a base for accurate service planning and delivery. As well, the number of people families have to relate to was often described as overwhelming. One mother who viewed herself as the harried coordinator of her child's care said she had 16 names and telephone numbers of professionals involved in her son's care at the time of our data collection, and this was *in addition to* the five nurses she might have to call to assure her family of the respite care required.

Negative family responses were associated with the rules and regulations of program delivery. Parents are frustrated, perhaps, because they are dealing with the *particular* whereas policies and program personnel consider the *general*. Parents complained about what they perceived as a lack of flexibility in the program, such as how many, when, and for what purpose respite hours could be used. Some reported conflicts in scheduling nursing hours to fit their families' needs—both in day-to-day affairs and around their needs for employment or holidays. Obviously, these are less problematic where "good fitting" nurses can be found, trained, and available; thus, it is easier if families live in large urban centers. Those who live in small or rural communities are hampered in this regard. The up-front effort for families to institute respite care can be considerable, until "the glitches are ironed out," and again, this is worse the farther the family lives from a service hub.

In summary, although there are some definite disadvantages, family reactions to in-home nursing care range from being a huge relief to not having much impact on families' lives at all. The latter appears to occur in families that have significant resources, including a strong, available support system, and importantly, a child whose condition is relatively stable. For most, however, it is:

Such a relief. . . . That time becomes ours [because somebody is there who's trained enough] to take the responsibility. . . . And you don't feel guilty. . . . Like I couldn't have imagined, I can't imagine that things would be like they are now two years after . . . had we not tapped into the service, you know. So we don't [need to] utilize support groups per se, just the services.

✳ Reflective Questions

1. How many hours of nursing respite care do you think you would need if you were the parent of a 7-year old child who'd suffered head injuries in a motor vehicle accident three years ago, and who you care for at home on a respirator, gastrostomy feedings, and seizure monitoring?

2. What types of things would you do with your respite hours? What if there were 10 less hours per week? If there were 10 hours more per week?

Parents' Views of Promoting Family Health

Our data also illuminated family-level health promotion, that is, activities aimed to promote *family* well-being in five realms of family experience: interaction, development, coping, integrity, and health processes (Anderson & Tomlinson, 1992; see also Bomar & Baker–Word, 2001 for a review). Before our own analysis of the implications of this portion of our findings for family-level health promotion, we present parents' own suggestions on behalf of their families—about their own health, that of their children, and of their families as units. Theirs are the voices of unique and powerful first-hand knowledge and experience of living with a child's chronic condition, highly technical or complex care, and regular, in-home nursing care. We have grouped their ideas under two headings: promoting family health by minimizing negative family responses (i.e., countering the solid-head single arrows in Fig. 20–2), and maximizing the positive ones (i.e., strengthening the squared-headed arrows in Fig. 20–2), and emphasized their suggestions related to health policy development and delivery.

Minimizing the "Negatives" of Having a Respite Nurse in the Home

Referring to the negative responses that our data suggest about receiving respite care (briefly developed in the previous section), the data suggest that, to help families in Try-ing to Have a Life, health care personnel must individualize and expand assessments in order for them to fairly and meaningfully serve as a basis for making decisions about support and services. Although it is a widely stated ideal that parents are the experts about their children and their care (King, Law, King, & Rosenbaum, 1998; Letourneau & Elliott, 1996; Rosenbaum, King, Law, King, & Evans, 1998; Shelton & Stepanek, 1995), parents in our studies often report that they are not consulted or respected for their expertise. Families need options for in-home care delivery that are flexible and directly related to parents' own assessments of their families' needs. The same applies to assigning nursing hours, their distribution, and all other aspects of planning the actual home care. For example, some programs do not permit parents to work outside the home while a respite nurse is with their child, when this might be the most anxiety-relieving thing they could do with their assigned hours, because it provides a break from caregiving and allows them to generate much needed income for extra costs of having a child with a chronic condition at home. Also, consistency of nursing assignment is imperative for families' comfort, trust, rest, peace, and work, because reorienting new staff requires a great deal of family time and effort; yet agencies may not attend to this in the practicalities of booking nurses for shifts.

Parents emphasize that underneath all their suggestions is the requirement that care planners and providers have solid, "real world" understanding of childhood chronicity in general, with its impact and consequences, and enough knowledge of their child's particular health issues to ask pertinent questions, listen for and *hear* parental expertise, and be open-minded to points of view other than their own. One parent summarized beautifully:

I don't know how [assessors] can do their job. I don't think I would be able to come in [to] do an assessment without the child even being here—Blows me away. Because that has happened to another family that I know. But to come in here for half an hour or maybe an hour and go back and present your child to X amount of strangers [at a decision-making board] is—(breaks off). I don't know how you can do it, because if they were to know you—(breaks off). I could go and I could sell anybody on Alan, because I've known Alan inside out, and I can, you know, tell you the greatest things about him and I can tell you the worst things about him, you know. [But] for a stranger to go in there and try to sell strangers on [him and our needs]. . . .

(Continues) *You know, that's why . . . I've gotten them to look at changing the nursing respite program in the sense of having . . . two different boards and rotating [them] for the simple reason, I, myself, I wouldn't want to make a decision on a child, and then a week later . . . they're appealing it. . . . I've asked for . . . maybe [having] a parent with a disabled child on the board who has a nursing background. I would feel better, you know.*

This quotation provides an example of the essentially untapped insight and personal power that parents can bring to making positive changes in practices and policies applicable to families like their own.

Consider again the scenario that opened this chapter: The mother is voicing years of frustration of trying to have her families' needs met, as required supports were not available to assist the members to function healthfully. She and her husband of 15 years are now divorced; the children feel guilty, compromised, and unfairly disadvantaged; and 14 years after her son's diagnosis, she continues to feel unheard and unsupported (Kleinman, 1988). Even researchers, supposedly unbiased in their search for new understandings, are imposing *their* views about the impact of her son's chronic condition on her situation (by the preconstruction of paper-and-pencil evaluation scales), rather than seeing the real-to-her picture of what is going on in her family. This family at present is not a healthy one, or in the words of Stinnett and DeFrain (1985), a place to "enter for comfort, development, and regeneration . . . [or from which to] go forth renewed and charged with power for positive living" (p. 8). Stinnett and DeFrain observe that "strong families are made. . . . [They] have to work at it, constantly" (p. 15). This particular family's health-related work is significantly compromised because of the family work related to care of a young member with multiple sclerosis.

Maximizing the "Positives" about Having a Respite Nurse in the Home

In our data, there are also parents' views of practices and policies that serve to strengthen the positive contributions of receiving respite services: Parents urged that care *must* be planned, and actually provided, to fit with families' self-articulated structures, functioning, and values. This might translate into scheduling worker hours in creative ways, and blocking respite time to enhance parents' sleep, holidays, or out-of-home employment. Excellent communication among program personnel, between them and families, and between agencies was seen as imperative, and in this, there is need for improvement in most jurisdictions (Hayes, Hollander, Tan, & Cloutier, 1997). Families would benefit immensely from services that are organized with a central point of entry (across health social services and education), centralized recordkeeping, and family-centered care coordination (Dunst, Trivette, Gordon, & Starnes, 1994; Hayes et al., 1997).

Parents told us that home care or respite services that work well are delivered in an environment in which parents are believed to be equals, are treated as collaborators, and where they are able to function as leaders or facilitators of care if they want that role, or where they can advise or be part of program steering committees, boards, and subcommittees. In many of the families we have interacted with, parents were eloquent in their appeal for professional and social structures that bring well-trained, well-educated, committed, professional nurses to pediatric respite care, and the need for them to be well paid, well rewarded, and overtly valued. Parent informants were well aware that financial resources for services are finite, but they also knew that care provided at home is far cheaper than institutional care (Kleinman, 1988). To facilitate home care of their children with complex or medically fragile conditions, however, they emphasize that families must not be expected to absorb more than is humanly (and humanely) possible. A final quotation from a conversation with parents illustrates their awareness of the need to change policy and practices to foster healthy families:

Mother: *It's really too bad that [our nursing respite program] is so narrow that they, you know, that the requirements or how you qualify for it are so narrow and the money is so inadequate as a program. I mean, it served us fine but . . . as an overall program, you know, I can think of lots of people . . . who could benefit from it and [are] just sort of losing their minds without it. I mean we're using [non-health care] budgets to try to meet their needs when clearly it's a health issue. . . . It's a physical health issue and it becomes a mental health issue . . . especially to get these little kids out of hospital and get them home. And it's wonderful to say okay, we don't want to spend all this money (which is extraordinary, yes) in the hospital, but then there's zero at home. If only they could enhance that budget [for home care]. But it just benefits people so much more, but—[nursing respite] was a fabulous thing for us, wasn't it, Brian?*

Father: Oh yeah, yeah. . . . It appears that there's a savings with sending people home and providing a lesser, a considerably lesser degree of support [to families at home]. . . . There's perceived savings with that. . . . The stress that exists for families (and having experienced it first hand, I have a greater appreciation for it) . . . and how that's manifested in treatment of other children, and often how the social services office is called in to pick up the pieces is—It's really unfortunate for the other kids and the other family members when it gets to that point.

This couple summarized an important implication of our mini-theory: Nursing respite care that enables families to have a break from the demands of caring for their children with medically fragile or complex conditions at home is essential and appreciated, but it needs to be well-funded, with funding that is *not lost* as more and more care is transferred to family care at home. The human costs cannot be borne by families at the expense of their members' physical and mental health. Enduring unreasonable expectations result in parents burning out, and families' healthy processes becoming compromised (requiring "social services . . . to pick up the pieces").

One implication of overburdening families is that they become unavailable to supplement the formal health care system, and unable to serve society by fostering the development of healthy children to serve future communities. In our view, health, social services, and education delivery systems require a shift in focus to one that centers on "promotion of growth-producing behaviors rather than treatment of problems or prevention of negative outcomes. Emphasis [needs to be] placed on promoting and strengthening individual and family functioning by fostering the acquisition of prosocial, self-sustaining, self-efficacious, and other adaptive behaviors" (Dunst, Trivette, & Deal, 1988, p. 44). That is, families with a child with very special needs at home require supports for promotion of members' and *families'* health.

Theory Development for Family-Centered Health Promotion Practice

As Young points out in Chapter 1 of this volume, there is little theoretical knowledge to draw from in planning and delivering health promoting nursing care and services that are specifically focused on the family as the unit of care. Though there are few nursing models to guide practice, the ones that have so far appeared in the literature serve as excellent approaches to thinking "family and health promotion," as well as guiding care during a member's illness, critical period, or health crisis (Friedemann, 1995; Gilliss, Highley, Roberts, & Martinson, 1989; Hartrick, Lindsey, & Hills, 1994; Knafl, Gallo, Breitmayer, Zoeller, & Ayers, 1993; Pless, Feeley, Gottlieb, & Rowat, 1995; Whall, 1986; Wright & Leahey, 1994). The realities of practice and policymaking, however, are that nurses, other health professionals, policymakers, and bureaucrats more often target the individual for care strategies, assuming perhaps that the rest of the family will be affected "by osmosis." We would therefore argue that a first step in focusing on family health promotion is to "think family" (Rolland, 1993). "Family" is a concept, an abstract notion that includes members not physically present (in fact, perhaps very far away geographically), bonded in a unique and complex way that cannot be fully apprehended by others (Stuart, 1991).

If we seek theory to guide health promotion practice that is specifically focused on the subject of this chapter—a child with a long-term, medically fragile or complex health condition, her/his family, demanding care at home, and the regular presence of nurses in the home—then we will search a very long time! At present, the integration of knowledge pertinent to the care of this specific population of families falls to the individual nurse, who must read widely, choose thoughtfully from a broad range of resources, and integrate creatively (Hayes, 1997b). The relatively low incidence of chronic childhood conditions that require supported home care and respite care (Newachek & Halfon, 1998; Newacheck & Taylor, 1992; Perrin, Shayne, & Bloom, 1993) contributes to the paucity of practice theories (midrange or micro) in this specific area of interest. Research is hampered by the small numbers in specific diagnostic groups and the heterogeneity of potential samples.

To date, much of the research and tentative theory building concerning families and pediatric chronicity has concentrated substantively on traditional notions and popular topics: stress, burden, coping, adaptation, impact on family functioning, and "clinical" families (that is, families already identified for intervention, with emphasis on their "problems" rather than their strengths). For example, interactions and communication—between family members in the presence of chronicity and home or respite care, and between chronicity and families—require further investigation and theory development. Family members' shared experiences of living with childhood chronicity, with and without in-home professional supports, are essentially uninvestigated. We need to know much more about how families respond, develop or do not develop their use of resources and manage in the long-term, and what the human and economic costs are to individual families, communities, and society. The positive effects of living with pediatric chronicity are also ill understood (Eiser, 1993). We know very little about the interrelationships between families and health, let alone health promotion within families where children have chronic conditions (Doherty & Campbell, 1988; Ell & Northen, 1990; Keltner, 1992; Ross, Mirowsky, & Goldsteen, 1990; Stein, 1989).

There is much need for research and theory development in the general domain of family nursing that specifically targets family-level responses and health promotion to guide nursing practice. What is being missed is evidence-based direction[5] for improvement in care practices and policy development pertinent to the real lives of the often amazingly competent and resourceful families that live constantly with high-tech or complex care at home. As was stated so eloquently by some of the parents in our study: Until health professionals and policy planners get the whole picture, the home care-respite care situations for these families will not be completely, hu-

manely, or *ethically* facilitative of healthy family life.

☀ Reflective Questions

1. What specific nursing interventions do you think respite nurses are currently carrying out for children in your community who have medically fragile or complex conditions? Which are directed toward the child? The parents? The siblings? The family as the unit of care?
2. What out-of-home respite services exist in your community? What is needed?
3. What informal family supports are you aware of that families rely on? How might professionals be involved in helping to develop a network of supports built on family strengths?
4. What improvements in care would you recommend?
5. What might happen if funding for respite services were increased in your community? Consider both the advantages and the disadvantages.

Nursing Strategies and Approaches for Family Health Promotion Practice

"It is useful to consider how the nurse might practice and not simply what she [sic] should do" (Kendall, 1998, p. 76). In this section, we concentrate on our own selection of principles and approaches to family health promotion in the presence of pediatric chronicity and in-home respite services, and leave you to extrapolate the specifics of the "doing" of care. Empowering families to increase their capacities to control their situations is one general area to address, and directing efforts toward political and social change is another. Hartrick, Lindsey, and Hills (1994) summarize family nursing for health promotion as listening to and participating with the family, recognizing patterns, and envisaging action and positive change. Hartrick (1997) adds that nursing practice so directed "emphasizes the enhancement of family capacity" (p. 57).

---

[5]We define "evidence" broadly to include families' stories and nurses' accounts or reflections as well as descriptive, experimental, or quasi-experimental research designs.

Empowered Families

Nurses can use parental knowledge and skills (often significantly superior to that of professionals) in planning and changing care strategies, referrals, respite approaches, the number of hours of respite needed, and the time of day when these are most beneficial to the family. Because empowering processes must exist within the hierarchical systems of health care and society (Chinn, 1994), nurses can teach parents strategies to work as health care team partners, and encourage their use of these strategies. A place to start is for nurses themselves to reflect on what power-with interactions (Chinn) would look and feel like, rather than assuming the role of expert, leader, or facilitator, and working instead as collaborators with children and parents (Dunst, 1997). Summarized by Dunst, this includes: recognizing that the family is the constant in children's life and care; providing complete and unbiased information; honoring cultural, spiritual, socioeconomic, educational, and geographic diversity; and promoting health holistically; recognizing and respecting different methods of coping; facilitating family-to-family support and networking; assuring flexible, integrated, accessible, comprehensive care that responds to family-identified needs; and appreciating children as children and *families as families* with a wide range of strengths and concerns beyond health services and support. Thus, all family members who are able and interested can take part in decision making about their health, and are encouraged and supported in doing so. Already existing resources and skills are built upon. Family "self esteem" and self-efficacy are bolstered. Open-minded, creative, family-driven interventions and programs are designed and evaluated with the family members as active partners. It can be seen that the potential for effective and possibly very different health promoting nursing care for families is great, its scope broad, and the specifics underdeveloped and essentially undocumented.

Other Practices

How could nurses promote parental and family efforts toward health in families where the children's home care is challenging and res-

pite care is essential? Our research suggests the following: facilitating transitions from hospital to home, and from children's services to adults'; coordinating and communicating between services in the health, education, and social service sectors; home design and adaptations; improvement of transportation services; standardization and fairness in assigning and calculating the costs of equivalent services; facilitating out-of-home care and daycare while parents work for pay; improving the training of respite workers; public education about children's disabilities, health problems and their management; working in partnerships with families and care providers to evaluate existing and exemplary care programs; and communicating the findings and outcomes to policymakers and funding bodies.

✴ Reflective Questions

1. What municipal, state/provincial, federal, and world policies influence the care of children with chronic conditions and their families in your area?
2. How is funding raised and allocated for children with special needs? Who holds the purse strings?
3. What are the advantages and disadvantages of state resources being delegated to parents to hire and manage their own respite care?
4. How might nurses influence policy for families that have a child with a chronic condition and who require respite care at home?

Nurses Influencing Political and Social Change

Tones and Tilford (1994) consider it "radical" to shift focus in health promotion from traditional (prevention-focused) and empowering strategies to trying to affect the determinants of health (in this case, for children with chronic conditions and their families) from social, environmental, or political perspectives. Many nurses may not think about affecting changes in health and health care delivery at the macro level, nor may they consider themselves as having the necessary skills and power to do so. Kendall (1998) argues, however, that "nurses are in a key position to take a radical approach to health promotion. They form a very large body of professionals who ought, through their professional organizations, trade unions, and pressure groups, to be able to influence social and health policy" (pp. 92–93). The activities nurses employ in this form of health promotion are associated with lobbying, campaigning, protesting, and voting with a focus on resolving families' health issues. For example, in our local area, a strong pediatric nursing interest group joined with others to lobby provincial health care policy planners and politicians to reconsider the age of the patients for whom home care would be provided. Although formerly funded only for adults over 19, community-based home care and respite services became available for children and their families in our jurisdiction in the late 1980s. The campaign for this change, carried out publicly using various media techniques and privately in meetings and consultations with government personnel, employed case examples, parents' and nurses' stories, and strongly worded expressions of personal commitments to families' situations to achieve this goal and promote healthier families. In mere numbers of votes, nurses are a significant force at election time. As illustrated here, nurses can be effective in increasing those votes and in mobilizing public support to pressure governments to develop family-friendly policy.

Knowing how policies affect and are affected by families is an essential basis for nurses in directing their actions to effectively support others (e.g., family clients, lobby groups, community action initiatives) to affect political or social change (Bomar & Baker–Word, 2001). For example, it is critically important for nurses to know the contents of documents such as *Healthy People 2000* (U.S. Department of Health and Human Services, 1990) and the *Action statement for health promotion in Canada* (Canadian Public Health Association, 1996), and how the ideas in such documents might influence health care service planning and delivery. Families in our studies seem overdepended on by society to care for their children with chronic conditions, despite in-home nursing care, and they often struggle in the face of insufficient resources and opportunities for replenishment. In their situations, there is actual or potential oppression, and thoughtful consideration must be given to how to affect macro policy change, and how to translate these into nursing action.

Health promoting nursing strategies focused on political and social change include but are not limited to: helping parents and families to identify issues; community development and mobilization that involves families and their community at every stage; health advocacy at many levels; health education; or acting as a member of committees and action groups aimed to affect healthy public policy. Efforts could be directed to changing insurance plans and health funding legislation, action to relieve poverty, or compensating family members who stay home to care for children with complex, highly technical, or demanding care needs (Kohrman & Kaufman, 1997). We encourage you to imagine some of the innumerable ways that nurses can be active advocates for families in the social action, social justice, and political arenas.

Enhancing Family Health Promotion in the Presence of Chronicity and Nursing Respite Services

It is a family thing, and it's a family illness, and you deal with it as a family each time you have an episode, and you just carry on. . . . And you try to make everybody understand that, you know, one of you is sick and that's just the way it is.

This chapter's aim was to present an interpretation of selected data from a research project that was designed to explore the effects of respite care for families of children who have medically fragile or complex, long-term health conditions—from a whole-family point of view. Looking at the responsibilities and tasks of care coordination from within the family has illustrated some of the elements of the impact of respite care for families, and generated some ideas about how services and their guiding polices can be improved. Our constructed understanding of families' experiences of respite care is that it both helps and hinders, is a true relief and an additional burden, and provides a break but not in ways that families expect. Having a nurse partly living in your home, often awake when you are asleep, has its positive and negative outcomes, but is essential to members' healthy functioning, socialization, ability to contribute to the community, and sanity. Parents describe the process as Trying to Have a Life in the presence of significant childhood chronic illness or disability and the need for in-home nursing services. They expressed much insight into their issues: demands on individuals, demands on families, and what is required to render their lives more peaceful, at the same time as providing safe care for the special children.

Can the quality of these families' lives be improved within existing resources? We would argue that for this to happen, nurses and other health professionals, policy planners, and politicians will have to think more "out of the box." First, these families need to be seen as what they are: a valuable adjunct to the health care system, but also a fragile resource that may crumble if inadequately supported. Part of this support is high-quality respite care planned in conjunction with families, and in clearly demonstrated respect of their strengths and vulnerabilities. Nurses are good at this. Second, most health care systems for families of children with social needs are "non-systems" (Ell & Northen, 1990), and require consistent, coordinated effort to change them into seamless systems, prefer-

ably with a central point of entry and possibly centralized documentation (Hayes et al., 1997; Kannon et al., 2000). Changes of this order require combined efforts among all players—families included—and nurses have a significant role in affecting change in health care and social policy. Third, in most cases, what is *really* needed is a shift in resources to assist these families to care for their affected children in the best way possible. Fourth, these families *do* need more, better quality support from professional care delivery systems, conceived in very different ways, and organized around input from families themselves.

The ideal climate for promoting family health and development in the presence of childhood chronicity is one where families are valued and respected for what they bring to home care, and where there are no barriers to comprehensive, coordinated health, education, and social services. For us, as for Kohrman and Kaufman (1997), promoting health for families with children with demanding health conditions and complex care is to facilitate them "to achieve the remarkable benefits that home care can provide and, at the same time, . . . [assure that] all who provide that care, as well as the recipient children themselves, . . . share in those benefits" (p. 419).

✳ Reflective Questions

Returning to the scenario from Kleinman (1988) that opened this chapter:

1. In retrospect, what might have prevented this family from becoming overwhelmed?
2. What factors might have contributed to healthy outcomes for this family? What are the sources of these contributing factors?
3. How could nurses ameliorate some of the distress in this family now, 14 years after the diagnosis of muscular dystrophy?

Acknowledgement

The authors wish to thank the families and other key participants who gave unselfishly of their thoughts, time, and effort to assure that others will know more about the situations of those requiring respite care at home for a child with chronic conditions. The projects from which these ideas were drawn were funded by: the BC Medical Services Foundation; BC Ministry of Health, Public Health Nursing and Community Supports, Community and Health Programs (in kind); the Lotte & John Hecht Memorial Foundation; and the University of British Columbia Office of the Vice President for Research. The Canadian Association for Community Care and the Canadian Policy Research Networks also provided resources, consultation, and support.

REFERENCES

Anderson, K. H., & Tomlinson, P. S. (1992). The family health system as an emerging paradigmatic view for nursing. *Image: Journal of Nursing Scholarship, 24,* 57–63.

Bomar, P. J. & Baker–Word, P. (2001). Family health promotion. In S. M. H. Hanson (Ed.), *Family health care nursing* (pp. 197–219). Philadelphia: F. A. Davis.

Canadian Association for Community Care. (1996). *Best practices in respite services for children: A guide for families, policy makers and program developers.* Ottawa: Author.

Canadian Public Health Association. (1996). *Action statement for health promotion in Canada* (p. 9). Ottawa: Author.

Chinn, P. L. (1994). *Peace and power: Building communities for the future* (5th ed.). New York: National League for Nursing.

Creswell, J. W. (1998). Qualitative inquiry and research design: Choosing among five traditions. Thousand Oaks, CA: Sage.

Denzin, N. K. (1994). The art and politics of interpretation. In N. K. Denzin & Y. S. Lincoln (Eds.), *Handbook of qualitative research* (pp. 500–515). Thousand Oaks, CA: Sage.

Doherty, W. J., & Campbell, T. L. (1988). *Families and health.* Newbury Park, CA: Sage.

Dunst, C. J. (1997). Conceptual and empirical foundations of family-centered practice. In R. Illback, C. Cobb, & J. H. Joseph (Eds.), *Integrated services for children and families: Opportunities for psychological practice.* Washington, DC: American Psychological Association.

Dunst, C. J., Trivette, C. M., & Deal, A. G. (1988). *Enabling and empowering families: Principles and guidelines for practice.* Cambridge, MA: Brookline.

Dunst, C. J., Trivette, C. M., Gordon, N. J., & Starnes, A. L. (1994). Family-centered case management practices. In C. L. Dunst, C. M. Trivette, & A. G. Deal (Eds.), *Supporting and strengthening families* (pp. 89–118). Cambridge, MA: Brookline.

Eiser, C. (1993). *Growing up with a chronic disease: The impact on children and their families.* London: Jessica Kingsley.

Ell, K., & Northen, H. (1990). The social environment and family focused health care. *Families and health care: Psychosocial practice* (pp. 55–78). New York: Aldine de Gruyter.

Friedemann, M.-L. (1995). *The framework of systemic organization: A conceptual approach to families and nursing.* Thousand Oaks, CA: Sage.

Gilliss, C. L., Highley, B. L., Roberts, B. M., & Martinson, I. M. (1989). *Toward a science of family nursing.* Menlo Park, CA: Addison-Wesley.

Glaser, B. G. (1978). *Theoretical sensitivity.* Mill Valley, CA: Sociology Press.

Guba, E. G., & Lincoln, Y. S. (1994). Competing paradigms in qualitative research. In N. K. Denzin & Y. S. Lincoln (Eds.), *Handbook of qualitative research* (pp. 105–117). Thousand Oaks, CA: Sage.

Guralnik, D. B. (1970). *Webster's new world dictionary.* New York: World Publishing.

Hanson, S. M. H. (2001). *Family health care nursing: Theory practice, and research.* Philadelphia: F. A. Davis.

Hartrick, G. A. (1997). Beyond a service model of care: Health promotion and the enhancement of family capacity. *Journal of Family Nursing, 3,* 57–69.

Hartrick, G., Lindsey, A. E., & Hills, M. (1994). Family nursing assessment: Meeting the challenge of health promotion. *Journal of Advanced Nursing, 20,* 85–91.

Hayes, V. E. (1992). *The impact of a child's chronic illness on the family system.* Unpublished doctoral dissertation, University of California, San Francisco.

Hayes, V. E. (1997a). Families and children's chronic conditions: Knowledge development and methodological considerations. *Scholarly Inquiry for Nursing Practice: An International Journal, 11,* 259–290.

Hayes, V. E. (1997b). Searching for family nursing practice knowledge. In S. E. Thorne & V. E. Hayes (Eds.), *Nursing praxis: Knowledge and action* (pp. 54–68). Thousand Oaks, CA: Sage.

Hayes, V. E., Hollander, M. J., Tan, E. L. C., & Cloutier, J. E. (1997). *Services for children with special needs in Canada* (Final Report). Victoria, BC: Health Network, Canadian Policy Research Networks.

Hayes, V. E., McElheran, P. E., & Tan, E. (1997). *Evaluation of the BC Ministry of Health Nursing Respite Program: Final report* (Final Report to the Child, Youth, and Early Intervention Branch, BC Ministry of Health): BC Medical Services Foundation and BC Ministry of Health.

Kannon, E., Hayes, V. E., Radford, J., & Canadian Association of Community Care Children's Respite Project Group. (2000, June). *Best practices for respite care for children and families in three Ontario communities: Final report of Stage III of a three part project.* Ottawa: Canadian Association of Community Care.

Keltner, B. R. (1992). Family influences on child health status. *Pediatric Nursing, 18,* 128–131.

Kendall, S. (1998). Promoting health. In S. Hinchcliff, S. Norman, & J. Schober (Eds.), *Nursing practice & health care* (pp. 71–102). London: Arnold/Oxford University Press.

King, G., Law, M., King, S., & Rosenbaum, P. (1998). Parents' and service providers' perceptions of the family-centeredness of children's rehabilitation services. *Physical and Occupational Therapy in Pediatrics, 18*(1), 21–40.

Kleinman, A. (1988). *The illness narratives.* New York: Basic Books.

Knafl, K. A., Gallo, A. M., Zoeller, L. H., Breitmayer, B. J., & Ayers, L. (1993). One approach to conceptualizing family response to illness. In S. L. Feetham, S. B. Meister, J. M. Bell, & C. L. Gilliss (Eds.), *The nursing of families: Theory/research/education/practice* (pp. 70–78). Newbury Park, CA: Sage.

Kohrman, A. F., & Kaufman, J. (1997). Home care for children with technologic needs. In H. M. Wallace, R. F. Biehl, J. C. MacQueen, & J. A. Blackman (Eds.), *Mosby's resource guide to children with disabilities and chronic illness* (pp. 411–420). St. Louis, MO: Mosby.

Leonard, B. J., Brust, J. D., & Nelson, R. P. (1993). Parental distress: Caring for medically fragile children at home. *Journal of Pediatric Nursing, 8,* 22–30.

Letourneau, N. L., & Elliott, M. R. (1996). Pediatric health care professionals' perceptions and practices of

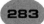

family-centered care. *Children's Health Care, 25,* 157–174.

Newachek, P. W., & Halfon, N. (1998). Prevalence and impact of disabling chronic conditions in childhood. *American Journal of Public Health, 88,* 610–617.

Newacheck, P. W., & Taylor, W. R. (1992). Childhood chronic illness: Prevalence, severity, and impact. *American Journal of Public Health, 82,* 364–371.

Patterson, J. M., Leonard, B. J., & Titus, J. C. (1992). Home care for medically fragile children: Impact on family health and well-being. *Developmental and Behavioral Pediatrics, 13,* 248–255.

Perrin, J. M., Shayne, M. W., & Bloom, S. R. (1993). *Home and community care for chronically ill children.* New York: Oxford University Press.

Pless, I. B., Feeley, N., Gottlieb, L. N., & Rowat, K. (1995). *A test of the McGill Model of Nursing with families who have a child with a chronic illness: Families' concerns, nursing strategies and outcomes* (unpublished research report). Montreal: School of Nursing, McGill University, and Montreal Children's Hospital.

Richardson, L. (1994). Writing: A method of inquiry. In N. K. Denzin & Y. S. Lincoln (Eds.), *Handbook of qualitative research* (pp. 516–529). Thousand Oaks, CA: Sage.

Rolland, J. S. (1993). Mastering family challenges in serious illness and disability. In F. Walsh (Ed.), *Normal family processes* (pp. 444–473). New York: Guilford Press.

Rosenbaum, P., King, S., Law, M., King, G., & Evans, J. (1998). Family-centred service: A conceptual framework and research review. *Physical and Occupational Therapy in Pediatrics, 18*(1), 1–20.

Ross, C. E., Mirowsky, J., & Goldsteen, K. (1990). The impact of the family on health: The decade in review. *Journal of Marriage and the Family, 52,* 1059–1078.

Selye, H. (1976). *Stress in health and disease.* Boston: Butterworth.

Shelton, T. L., & Stepanek, J. S. (1995). Excerpts from family-centered care for children needing specialized and developmental services. *Pediatric Nursing, 21,* 362–364.

Stein, H. F. (1989). Family influences on health behavior: An ethnographic approach. In C. N. Ramsey (Ed.), *Family systems in medicine* (pp. 373–392). New York: Guilford Press.

Stinnett, N., & DeFrain, J. (1985). *Secrets of strong families.* Boston: Little, Brown.

Strauss, A. L. (1987). *Qualitative analysis for social scientists.* Cambridge, MA: Cambridge University Press.

Strauss, A. L., & Corbin, J. (1998). *Basics of qualitative research: Techniques and procedures for developing grounded theory* (2nd ed.). Thousand Oaks, CA: Sage.

Stuart, M. E. (1991). An analysis of the concept of family. In A. L. Whall & J. Fawcett (Eds.), *Family theory development in nursing: State of the science and art* (pp. 31–42). Philadelphia: F. A. Davis.

Tones, B. K., & Tilford, S. (1994). *Heath education: Effectiveness, efficiency, and equity.* London: Chapman & Hall.

U.S. Department of Health and Human Services. (1990). *Health people 2000: National health promotion and disease prevention objectives* (DHHS Publication No. PHS 91–50213). Washington, DC: U.S. Government Printing Office.

Whall, A. L. (1986). The family as the unit of care in nursing: A historical review. *Public Health Nursing, 3,* 240–249.

Wright, L. M., & Leahey, M. (1994). *Nurses and families: A guide to family assessment and intervention.* Philadelphia: F. A. Davis.

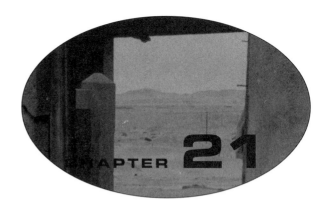

Promoting Health through Participatory Action Research: Lessons Learned from "STEPS" (Study of Environments that Promote Safety)

ELAINE M. GALLAGHER
ELIZABETH LINDSEY
VICTORIA J. SCOTT

We had an overall game plan of knowing that we wanted to get from A to B, but we realized there were many different routes to get there. What was different about this project was that we had the freedom to step back and say, "What a good idea, we hadn't thought about that so let's try it." That's not often the way research occurs and, had we been less open to input from our participants, I'm sure we would have only learned half as much in this study.

Lindsey & McGuiness, 1998, p. 45

Although nurse researchers are beginning to embrace the Participatory Action Research (PAR) approach in health promotion research, little is formally known about how to actively involve people as partners in this process. Consequently, most nurses who practice in this arena are forced to rely on trial and error in making key decisions about who, when, where, and how best to engage key stakeholders actively in research concerning issues of import to them (Lindsey & McGuiness, 1998).

Two of the authors—Elaine Gallagher and Victoria Scott—recently conducted a project entitled STEPS (Study of Environments that Pro-

mote Safety) during which the PAR process appeared to be working exceptionally smoothly and participants were expressing a great deal of satisfaction. In order to identify the factors that make a project like this satisfying for the participants, Gallagher and Scott invited two additional researchers with expertise in qualitative methods to carry out a **meta-study** of the STEPS project. In effect it became a study of a study. Both the STEPS study (Gallagher & Scott, 1997) and the STEPS meta-study (Lindsey & McGuiness, 1998) have been published separately in professional journals.

In this chapter, we introduce the topic of falls and present some of the key concepts used in the two studies, describe the original STEPS study objectives and methods, and briefly review the results of that project. We also present the methods and key findings of the STEPS meta-study, providing insight into the critical elements of the PAR process. Readers will therefore have an opportunity to see how one project simultaneously provided the following:

- a quantitative research component pertaining to the epidemiology of falls in public places

- participatory action research with seniors, empowering them to effect changes in their communities (e.g., municipal policies related to sidewalk repairs)
- a qualitative study of what the participants found enjoyable and empowering about their involvement in the PAR process

Background

The STEPS project, carried out in Victoria, British Columbia, over a two-year period, was designed as a PAR study that incorporated key principles of health promotion. PAR is based on the idea of engaging people actively in researching and affecting change on issues of relevance to them in their daily lives. PAR has a double objective: to produce knowledge and action directly useful to a group of people and "to empower people so as to see through the ways which the establishment monopolizes the production and use of knowledge for the benefit of it members" (Fals-Borda & Rahman, 1991, p.16).

The values, assumptions, and processes of PAR appear to be highly compatible with and complementary to the goals of health promotion. Even the language used to describe the two phenomena bears close resemblance. PAR concerns community involvement, **emancipation**, empowerment, and liberation (Hall, 1992; Henderson, 1995). Similarly, health promotion is described throughout this book as an emancipatory, transformative pattern of practice, which consciously attends to the valuing of people, community, and purposeful action.

PAR and health promotion also bear similarities in relation to their attention to power and power imbalances. A major underlying assumption of PAR is that knowledge is related to power and that power is related to change (Couto, 1987; Hall, 1992; Henderson, 1995). Mason and Boutilier (1996) describe participatory research as an approach that emphasizes equalization of power between researchers and research subjects. Likewise, community health promotion involves egalitarian relationships between nurses and clients and often entails increased awareness of the complexities of power relations in the broader community.

Henderson (1995) identified five qualities that may distinguish PAR from most traditional research methods.

1. PAR involves an egalitarian partnership between researchers and those who have the issue or concern in question. They work together to form research questions, to design the study, to collect data, and to analyze and disseminate the results. Many traditional research methods require the researcher to formulate the research question, design the best data collection methods, choose the subjects, and collect the data.
2. Theory is generated from experiential and popular knowledge rather than on scientifically derived knowledge. [The authors do not necessarily agree with this view as will be shown in the present study where a combination of approaches—including a scientific survey—was used to generate knowledge about risks of falling.]
3. Issues of power and power relations are examined in the course of using PAR. The end result is to encourage people to become more independently able to define their own issues and to take action to address them, so the researcher must be able to give up control and share the decision making throughout. In contrast, much traditional research requires a great deal of control on the part of the researcher.
4. PAR involves mutual education and raising of consciousness in generating data and theory. In much traditional research, the learning is often of most importance to the researcher.
5. The goal of PAR is political action or social change. Such studies do not end with the acquisition and analysis of data, as does more traditional research.

The Problem of Falls among Older People

Falling is a major health issue among older people. Although the exact incidence of falls among the elderly is difficult to determine because of underreporting of the event, approximately one of every three noninstitutionalized seniors experience at least one fall yearly and 50 percent of whom sustain a significant injury (Alexander, Rivera, & Wolf, 1992). In 1984 in Canada, falls accounted for 57 percent of accidental fatalities and the majority of severe accidental injuries for people 65 years or older (Gallagher & Scott, 1997). Many people who fall suffer physically, socially, and psychologically as a result. The cost to society is also great. For example, Ashe, Gallagher, and Coyte (2000) concluded that the cost of falls among people 65 and over to Canada's health care system was $2.9 billion in 1994. The comparable 1994 figure for the United States was $64.2 billion, of which 31.5 percent (or about $20 billion) was attributable to older Americans (Englander, Hodson, & Terregrossa, 1996).

Older people are not all equally at risk for falls and injuries. Speechley and Tinetti (1991) divided community-dwelling seniors into vigorous (healthy), transitional (in transition from vigorous to frail), and frail seniors and found that falls occurred three times more often among the frail than vigorous seniors, with about 50 percent of frail people having at least one fall a year. However, the reverse was true for injuries, with the frail having an injury rate of 6 percent and the vigorous having an injury rate of up to 22 percent. The settings of falls were found to differ between vigorous and frail seniors with the frail seniors most often falling at home during routine daily activities. Healthier seniors fell more often away from home and in the presence of environmental hazards (Speechley & Tinetti, 1991).

Women have been found to fall two to three times more often than men with correspondingly higher hospitalization rates (Prudham & Evans, 1981). It is not known why women fall more often and have more injuries, but it could be related to the fact that today's cohort of older women have not been as physically active as men and therefore have weaker legs and poorer balance. Footwear or more specifically, changes in heel height, may be a factor, as may arthritis and osteoporosis.

Tinetti, Mendes de Leon, Doucette, and Aker (1994) reported that 48 percent of people who had fallen were afraid of falling again and 26 percent had curtailed physical and social activities. Both fear and reduced activity have been identified as contributing to seniors' risks for falls. Tinetti and colleagues (1994) also suggested that falls are a common reason for loss of independence and admission to a senior's care facility.

Risk Factors for Falls

For the elderly, a fall is a serious unexpected incident that can cause injury, disability, death, fear and loss of confidence, decreased mobility, increased isolation, dependency, reduced quality of life, and reduced life satisfaction (Patla, Frank & Winter, 1990; Gallagher, Hunter, & Scott, 1999). Most falls are the result of a complex interaction of biomedical, behavioral, environmental, and sociopolitical factors (Cummings et al., 1995). These factors are summarized in Table 21–1.

As shown in Table 21–1, *biological risks* for falls include advanced age, being female, and having a chronic illness such as stroke, osteoporosis, osteoarthritis, or arthritis. Many of these conditions contribute to falls by producing gait and balance changes and reduced muscle strength. Sensory changes can also contribute to falls if a person has poor vision or hearing, wears multifocal lenses, or has reduced touch sensation—proprioception (Lord, Ward, Williams, & Anstey, 1994).

One example of a behavioral risk factor for falling is inattention. When older people are asked why they fell, they will often say, "It was because I wasn't watching where I was going or where my feet were. I was not paying attention" (Gallagher & Brunt, 1996). Increased risk-taking is also associated with falling. Examples are climbing ladders to put up Christmas lights, or going out in snowy conditions without good footwear. Choice of footwear, particularly as it relates to the height of heels, seems to be a factor in relation to falls and injuries; it has been suggested that changing the height of one's heels may be the most problematic aspect. Mobility aids themselves appear to contribute to injuries and falls, as does lack of exercise and fitness. Polypharmacy is also consistently predictive of high-risk fallers regardless of the setting (Cummings et al., 1995; Sattin, 1992; Tinetti et al., 1994).

Environmental hazards are also implicated as precursors to falls. Previous studies, focusing primarily on in-home falls, have identified hazards such as stairs, poor illumination, slippery floors, scatter mats, telephone cords, uneven sidewalks, furniture at improper heights,

TABLE 21–1

A CONCEPTUAL FRAMEWORK FOR THE STUDY OF FALL-RELATED INJURY AMONG OLDER ADULTS

Biological	Behavioral	Environmental	Socioeconomic
Advanced age	Personal health practices and coping skills	Poor building design and/or maintenance	Income
Female gender		Lack of access	Income adequacy
Chronic illness	Risk-taking or preventive behaviors	Unenforced codes or inadequate standards	Social status
Stroke			Education level
Osteoporosis	Taking multiple medications or excessive alcohol	New surroundings	Living conditions
Arthritis		Transition areas	Dwelling ownership
Cognitive impairment	Taking any of the following:	Stairs	Safe housing
Chronic disabilities	Tranquilizers	Lack of:	Living arrangements
Blindness	Sleeping pills	Handrails	Social environments
Deafness	Antidepressants	Curb ramps	Values and rules of society
Immobility	Antihypertensives	Safe access	Cohesive communities
Mobility changes	Antidiabetic agents	Rest areas	
Gait disorders	Previous fall or near-fall	Lighting	Social support networks
Poor balance		Grab bars	Caring relationships
Postural sway	Frequent falling		Social interaction
Diminished muscle strength	Fear of falling	Poor lighting or sharp contrasts	Emotional support
	Living alone	Slippery or uneven surfaces	
Sensory changes	Inappropriate footwear		
Poor vision	Mobility aids	Changes in elevation	
Wearing glasses	Not using mobility aids	Obstacles:	
Diminished proprioception		Scatter rugs	
		Clutter	
Hearing impairments		Trashcans	
		Poles	
		Sidewalk furniture	

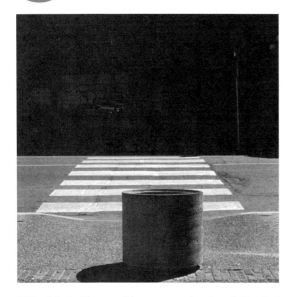

FIG. 21–1. Those with compromised mobility find obstacles a problem.

and poor fitting shoes (Gallagher & Scott, 1996; Eriksson & Lindgren, 1989). Gallagher and Brunt (1996) found that among community-dwelling elderly fallers, 78 percent of falls occurred while people were walking, and 68 percent occurred outside the home. A 1978 U.S. study of hazards noted that the limited conception of the "average" pedestrian, generally used in designing urban environments, results in unintentional discrimination against persons who are not of average mobility (Templer, Mullet, Archea, & Margulis, 1978). The urban environments they studied seemed to be designed for people who were middle-aged, of average height or weight, and who had average strength and balance.

Social and political factors are now also understood to contribute to the problem of falls. Gallagher, Hunter, and Scott (1999) linked social factors to chronic illness and falls including income inadequacy, low education levels, inadequate housing, and social isolation. Although it has long been suspected that broader social policies have an impact on this problem as well, no studies were located that make these links explicit. Such social policies include everything from national building codes for design of stairs to methods of prioritizing work by local municipal governments.

The causes of falls are therefore multifactorial and consist of complex interactions between factors specific to each individual and his or her environment. In recent years, considerable research has been conducted on biomedical and behavioral risk for falls, although even in these areas there is still a great deal more to discover. However, little attention has been paid to the contribution of environments, and no studies were reported concerning falls in public environments. In terms of methods of study, few reported studies of any sort have been reported using methods such as PAR, where older people are actively engaged as research partners.

Purpose and Methods of the STEPS Project

The overall purpose of the STEPS project was to create safer environments for those at risk of falling by increasing awareness about causes of falls in public places, increasing the likelihood of eliminating identified hazards, and promoting the development of risk management plans to reduce hazards. Using PAR methods, consultations were conducted with key stakeholders to establish project goals, develop data collection methods, and prepare for dissemination of the findings. A steering committee was formed consisting of six seniors, two people who were blind, a wheelchair-user, a physiotherapist from the local health department, and the two nurse researchers. The participants were selected on the basis of their strong and multiple connections to their respective community groups and neighborhoods, and because of their personal interest in the subject matter.

This steering committee established that the goals of the study were to:

1. identify some of the key risk factors associated with older people's fall in public places in their community
2. identify who had jurisdiction for taking action to repair identified hazards
3. establish processes whereby people could identify and report hazards that they encounter in the community in the future

For nine months, the steering committee members and other senior volunteers collected data using a telephone hotline survey. The phone line was called the "Slip, Trip and Call Hotline." The project recruited informants using pamphlets, posters, public talks, radio and television features, and newspaper stories. The Steering Committee developed a questionnaire to determine conditions under which people fell in public places, and modified it when it became clear to the volunteers that callers wanted first to simply tell their story of their fall. A total of 791 reports of slips, trips, and falls were recorded over the nine-month study period. Not all of the volunteers were equally able to handle the task of simultaneous questioning and recording as required by this methodology. Other ways were found to enable these seniors to be actively involved.

Survey Results

A call to the hotline usually began with a short historical account of the slip, trip, or fall. Here is a typical example:

I had decided to walk to the corner for a few groceries and on the way home, all of a sudden I found myself on the ground. When I hit the sidewalk, I broke my glasses, and chipped a tooth. A passerby helped me up and offered to drive me home but I said I was OK. I felt so humiliated. I limped home and later took a taxi to a clinic where I found I had a broken wrist and sprained ankle.

The majority (81%) of the reports concerned an incident the callers had had themselves. Forty-seven percent ($n = 294$) of the reports of slips, trips, and falls were about an incident that had occurred within the last month, compared to 15.5 percent ($n = 97$) concerning an event that had taken place a year or more ago. Only 29 percent ($n = 172$) of the callers said they had already reported the incident to someone who might undertake repairs. Many responded that they would have done so but had no idea who to call.

The majority of the callers were female (80%) and the average age was 65.3 (range 12–91). In relation to disabilities, 186 (35%) of those who had a fall or near fall said they had some type of physical disability. Of these,

157 (68%) said they used some type of mobility aid and 106 (47%) were using an aid when they slipped or fell. In addition, 279 (49%) of all callers said they wore glasses. Of these, 207 (70%) said they were wearing them at the time of the accident. It is important to note that of those who were wearing glasses when they slipped or fell, over two-thirds ($n = 156$) said they used bifocal or multifocal glasses.

The most frequently reported incident was a fall ($n = 68$), defined as coming to rest unexpectedly on the floor or ground. Trips, involving an obstacle and not resulting in coming to rest on the ground, were reported by 207 people. One hundred and fifteen people reported a slip involving a wet or slippery surface. Of the 538 valid cases of slips, trips, and falls, 405 (75%) said they sustained an injury from their incident. Of these, 220 (55%) people said they required medical attention. People reported having their falls or missteps at all hours of the night and day. The most frequent time period was from noon to 5:00 P.M. ($n = 180$, 45%). The most frequent type of lighting was daylight (77.7%), followed by night (10%), and twilight (6.8%).

The location of the incidents was of interest in this study. Many people reported in an open-ended question that they fell on familiar walking routes, ruling out the idea that unfamiliarity with the terrain was a contributing factor. When we examined the data by neighborhood, the hazards were often located on walking routes between seniors' residences and shopping centers, recreation centers, and health clinics. Of the 574 valid reports, 486 (84.7%) concerned outdoor locations. The outdoor sites named most frequently were sidewalks, crosswalks, and curbs. When asked about the type of surface involved, the vast majority of callers described the surfaces as uneven or cracked, with fewer callers describing wet, poorly lit, littered, or icy conditions. This would obviously be different in communities with different climates or terrain.

Concrete surfaces were overwhelmingly implicated when compared with all other types of surfaces. The single most frequently reported specific condition was broken or cracked concrete. Another category of hazard included obstacles on public walkways, brought about by competition for public

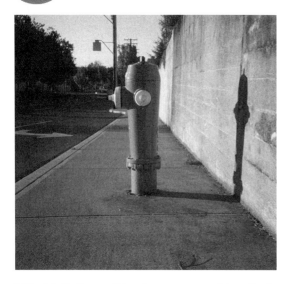

FIG. 21–2. Competition for space on sidewalks is becoming more common.

rights-of-way on sidewalks. Competing objects include power poles, garbage cans, phone booths, bus shelters, flowerbeds, and bike racks. A municipal engineer associated with the project noted the following:

It is not that we want these items in the middle of sidewalks, but simply there is no where else to put them. In trying to create more space for pedestrians, municipalities are limited in the right-of-way that can be acquired during the subdivision process by the municipal act" (Gallagher & Scott, 1997).

Taking the "Action" of the PAR Process

Concurrent with the data collection, reports of hazards were forwarded to appropriate municipalities, property managers, or property owners for consideration for repair. At the end of the survey, an estimated 30 percent of all reported hazards had either been repaired or marked with fluorescent paint to alert pedestrians.

The findings of the STEPS survey were interesting, but without a longer-term avenue for dialogue with local engineering departments, and municipal politicians, the results would have had little impact. Following the compilation and publication of the survey re-

sults, the STEPS Steering Committee hosted a symposium entitled *Risk Management of Public Hazards to Reduce Slips, Trips, and Falls.* This symposium brought together health care professionals, engineers, city planners, politicians, and others with a mandate for public safety to discuss the study findings and to compile recommendations. The members of the STEPS Steering Committee served as facilitators and group leaders at the symposium. The major recommendation that arose from the symposium was the need for municipalities and private building owners to develop a plan for prioritizing repair of uneven and slippery surfaces on sidewalks and other walkways with input from user groups, particularly seniors and persons with disabilities. It was also recommended that municipal staff review their protocols for receiving and responding to public complaints. Further, it was recommended that they publish a unique, special-purpose number in the phone directory. This number could be similar to the 911 number used for emergencies, and would provide a direct link for the public in order to report potential hazards in the community. It was agreed that all reports of hazards should be taken seriously, and callers should be made to feel appreciated for their efforts.

The STEPS project demonstrated that those with the lived experience of navigating hazardous pedestrian routes, while simultaneously dealing with a disability or age-related problem, are well suited to give advice about what is needed in terms of safety. Many of the findings and lessons learned in the STEPS project are further outlined in a video entitled "Stepping Out (1997)" and a technical manual entitled "Taking Steps (1997)," both of which were produced as further vehicles for facilitating change.

Key Elements of Community Involvement: The Meta-Study

Aside from the findings of the STEPS survey and the actions taken by civic maintenance departments, it was of interest to also examine the experiences of seniors in the PAR process itself. In order to uncover these experiences, Lindsey and McGuiness (1998) conducted a meta-study of the processes used in the STEPS project. Data collection methods

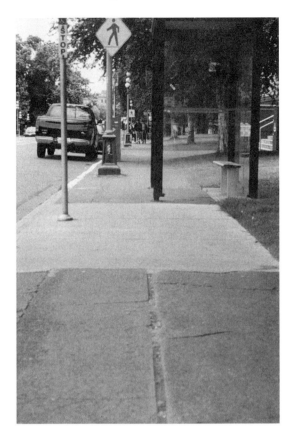

FIG. 21–3. A glass bus shelter becomes an impediment unless well marked.

included the following: a review of minutes, news releases and recorded TV and radio interviews, **participant observation**, individual interviews, and a focus group interview. Six major themes were identified. These included planning, structural components, philosophy, enhancing credibility, leadership, and personal experience and satisfaction. Each are briefly described below.

Planning: People, Power, Politics, and Purpose

The STEPS participants were adamant that advanced planning for this project was essential to its success. The PAR process had begun with a thorough assessment of the community in order to identify the various constituent groups potentially affected by unsafe public environments. Each of these groups

was then invited to have a representative at the planning table.

Power structures in the community were assessed at the outset. As a result, in order to secure funding for the study and ensure buy-in of the study findings, the 11 municipal mayors and councils in the district were asked to provide letters of support. One steering community member described this process as follows:

Our intent was to be very political, knowing the power brokers and getting them on board. We wanted to get their commitment and to recognise this as an important issue so that when we came back with the final report they would sit back and say, "Oh yes, we made a commitment to this; we endorsed this project; here's the results. Now we have some obligation to take action."

Structural Components: Respecting Diversity, Having Structure, and Encouraging Participation

The first step identified in the PAR process was to assemble all of the key players, similar to that of selecting the members of an orchestra. Just as one would not rely solely on a string section, so too the committee needed to have balance and be able to work in harmony. As one researcher noted, "We wanted people with a diversity of opinions, experiences, and skills—people who could articulate their views in a group setting." An example of the importance of this arose when a blind member of the committee described how difficult it was to tell when the sidewalk ended after city engineers made curb-cuts to accommodate people in wheelchairs. At the same time, another member who was a wheelchair-user explained how difficult it was for him to maneuver even the smallest of lips on sidewalks. One member of the committee summarized the dilemma as follows:

People who are blind and using guide dogs or canes need to know when they reach the end of sidewalk or curb. While a smooth curb corner meets the needs of someone in a wheelchair, it doesn't meet a blind person's needs at all. So we need to find some creative ways to meet the needs of both groups.

Thus the group began to search for solutions to recommend to civic officials that were a compromise of group members' diverse needs and requirements. It was necessary to not see these voices as discordant, but rather to find a common melody that both could relate to.

It was also important to the STEPS participants that Steering Committee Meetings were accessible. Participants said they appreciated the attention given to parking, access to washrooms, and accessibility for wheelchairs. As one participant noted, "Attention to these details made us feel nurtured and respected."

The processes used in setting preliminary meeting agendas, starting the meetings and providing minutes were valued by the members. They commented that they liked receiving a draft agenda ahead of time and appreciated having the opportunity to add items of interest and importance. They liked the fact that agendas were completed in the time frame allotted. They also commented on the value of a "check-in" process that helped people get focused on the business at hand and provided a brief update on members' activities since the previous meeting. Likewise, meeting minutes that were clear, succinct, and written in plain language were valued.

The Steering Committee members appreciated the flexible times of meetings to accommodate their schedules. Further, they enjoyed having some socialization time, and they valued the concern expressed for members who were ill or experiencing other stress. They appreciated the attention to verbal communication, recognizing that two of the members of the group were blind and unable to read written material.

The STEPS Steering Committee members noted how important it was to engage seniors other than themselves in the project. A number of seniors in the community had abilities and skills that they contributed to the research process, for example, distributing posters and brochures and answering the telephone hotline. One of the researchers noted that most communities have a huge untapped resource in terms of retired people who would love to be involved in projects such as this one.

Timing was also an important structural consideration in this project. First, adequate time was needed for planning and advertis-

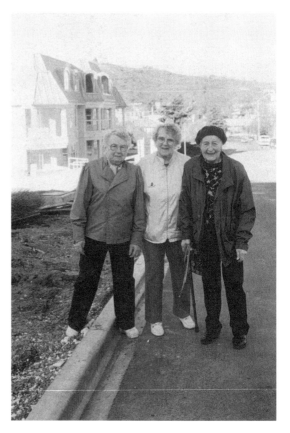

FIG. 21–4. Construction sites are hazardous for senior pedestrians.

ing. Time was needed for the Steering Committee to form good working relationships, for training of volunteers, and for charting "best courses of actions." As one person said "We had a game plan but it was more like going on a trip and having the freedom to adjust the course as conditions changed . . . having the freedom to say this sounds like a good idea, let's try it."

Participants described several strategies that helped to maintain the commitment of the many volunteers and committee members:

- having timelines with discreet, achievable tasks
- acknowledging the personal achievements of participants
- identifying goals and target that have broad appeal
- finding meaningful ways to engage the committee members

- identifying barriers before they arise and developing strategies so that barriers became opportunities
- providing updates of discrete examples of program impact

One member summed up his involvement as follows:

There's a lot of times when you're on a lot of committees and you say, "What am I doing here?" I never got that sense [with this project]. The project was always developing. There was always something that was developing that month.

Research Method: Process, Partnerships, and Power

Lindsey and McGuiness (1998) identified another theme related to the research process itself. Participants described the process of designing the study as flexible, inclusive, and creative. One researcher noted the magic of "intuitively putting together different pieces at the moment." Another participant noted the sense of appropriate fit between the research philosophy, the research methods, and the needs of the community.

The notion of partnerships was also seen to be crucial to the participants in the STEPS project. Mutual trust and respect among the researchers themselves, between the various community groups, among the members of the steering committee, and between the volunteers and study respondents were thought to be paramount. The researchers played a key role in modeling this trust and respect, "walking their talk" and carrying out promised activities. One researcher said she went into meetings "all asking, not all knowing." A steering committee member described the dynamics as "bottom-up since there was no **hierarchy** in place when decisions were being made."

It was also important to participants that they could see some short-term changes occurring as a result of the research process. Regular feedback was provided about the status of repairs undertaken by municipal public works departments throughout the project.

The participants claimed that these indicators of short-term success provided impetus for them to continue to be enthusiastic, and to realize that they were making a difference.

Credibility

The credibility of a research project is important because it helps to gain community attention, impress would-be funders, ensure access to the community, and ensure participation by members of the community. Interviews with the STEPS participants suggested that such credibility could be established in a number of ways. The reputation of the researchers was thought to lend credibility to the project. Active steps were taken to market the project to a wide range of potential stakeholders including politicians and community leaders. Well-crafted press releases reported news of the project at various stages. Television and radio interviews as well as appearances at professional conferences also helped to raise the profile of the project. Over 60 presentations were done with groups of seniors and people with disabilities. When possible, members of the Steering Committee and the researchers participated jointly in media or other speaking events.

Leadership Style

The style of leadership in the STEPS project was seen to set the tone for the successful engagement of the many participants. The skills were described as "facilitation, collaboration, and coordination" rather than "direction." Steering committee members said that the project coordinators constantly attended to issues of power relations recognizing that the true source of authority rested with the people who were experiencing the problem. Participants commented on the coordinators' flexibility and willingness to acknowledge their limitations. Other characteristics participants mentioned concerning the project leaders were "strong organizational skills" and an "ability to fully utilize resources."

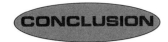

CONCLUSION

This chapter has provided details of a PAR project aimed at empowering seniors to take actions that would reduce risks in the community that contribute to falls and injuries. It is appropriate in this conclusion to speculate the extent to which Henderson's (1995) five principles described in the introduction was adhered to.

Henderson's first quality referred to the need for egalitarian partnerships between researchers and those with the issue or concern in question. This quality was only partially reflected in the present study. The researchers initially worked in isolation of the community partners to draw up the terms of reference for the grant, pose the overall research questions, hire the staff, monitor the budget, and prepare the first draft of the final report. However, they worked very closely with the community partners on deciding all aspects of how to recruit informants for the study, how to collect data, how to interpret the results, and how to present the final report. The elderly Steering Committee participants chose the colors and fonts for all publications, decided on wording of all published material, and accompanied the researchers during media interviews and conference presentations of the results.

Henderson also claimed that with PAR, theory is generated from experiential and popular knowledge rather than from scientific knowledge. In the STEPS project, new knowledge was generated using both experiential and scientific methods. In fact each helped inform the other. For example, by asking callers to tell their story before answering a questionnaire about their fall, new information emerged that may not have been expected based on published research and theory alone.

Third, Henderson claimed that issues of power and power relations are examined in the course of using PAR, the end result being to encourage people to become more independently able to define their own issues and to take action to address them. This element was evident throughout the STEPS project as steering committee members became actively involved in defining their issues and proposing solutions. A major outcome of the study was production of a video for use by seniors' groups throughout North America providing ideas for how they could become involved in identifying local issues and proposing local solutions. This outcome was in keeping with Henderson's fourth criterion, one that related to mutual education and raising of consciousness in generating data and theory.

Henderson's final defining quality of PAR is that it involves political action or social change. At the municipal and local building owner level, many changes were undertaken as a direct result of the findings of the STEPS project. Several photographs serve to illustrate the types of changes undertaken in one community as a result of this process. The authors are currently facilitating a provincial network called Adult Injury Management (AIM) that is similar to one in Florida called the Florida Injury Prevention for Seniors project (FLIPS). Both initiatives are grassroots in nature with local involvement and leadership defining injury-related issues and proposing solutions.

The outcomes of the STEPS project were thus deemed to be successful in terms of raising awareness of the importance of the environment as a contributor to falls. It was effective in improving the responsiveness of civic officials to the needs of older pedestrians and increased the likelihood that hazards would be identified and repaired.

When empowerment of the participants is also an intended outcome of research, strategies to ensure this need to be intentionally included (Gallagher, Scott, & Mills, 1999). Lindsey and McGuiness (1998) made an important contribution in identifying what these strategies might entail. This project provides support for the idea that PAR can constitute a form of health promotion practice for nurse researchers. It entailed valuing of people, the community, and purposeful action, and resulted in improved chances for risk reduction among vulnerable populations.

This study has now been replicated in at least five other cities in Canada in order to systematically uncover the subtle ways that public environments have failed to account for the needs of people who are frail or who have physical handicaps. Thus, even though this started as a research method with a goal of increased understanding of the epidemiology of falls, the process has been translated into community health promotion practice. It is akin to having a camera enabling one to take a snapshot of a town, neighborhood, or region, and providing concrete data for action in relation to enhancing safety.

✳ Reflective Questions

"Participatory Action Research" could be considered one form of a broader class of research methods known as "Participatory Research." Such methods have in common the full engagement of the researched alongside the researchers and the analysis of power relationships as integral to the research process.

1. What other social issues would lend themselves to this type of research approach?
2. Have we as nurses gone as far as possible in our thinking about how best to fully embrace and incorporate participatory research methods?
3. When might such approaches not reflect the goals of health promotion?

REFERENCES

Alexander, B., Rivera, F., & Wolf, M. (1992). The cost and frequency of hospitalization for fall-related injuries in older adults. *American Journal of Public Health, 82,* 1020–1023.

Ashe, C., Gallagher, E., & Coyte, P. (2000). *Economic impact of falls among older Canadians.* Manuscript submitted for publication.

Couto, R. (1987). Participatory research: Methodology and critique. *Clinical Sociology Review, 4,* 83–92.

Cummings, S., Nevitt, M., Browner, W., Stone, K., Fox, D., Ensrud, E., Cauley, J., Black, D., & Vogt, T. (1995). Risk factors for hip fracture in white women. *New England Journal of Medicine, 332,* 767–773.

Englander, F., Hodson, T., & Terregrossa, R. (1996). Economic dimensions of slip and fall injuries. *Journal of Forensic Science, 41,* 733–746.

Eriksson, S., & Lindgren, J. (1989). Outcome of falls in women: Endogenous factors associated with fractures. *Age and Aging, 18,* 303–308.

Fals-Borda, O., & Rahman, M. (Eds.) (1991). *Action and Knowledge: Breaking the monopoly with participatory action research.* New York: Intermediate Technology/Apex.

Gallagher, E. M., & Brunt, H. (1996). Head over heals: A program to reduce falls among the elderly. *Canadian Journal on Aging, 15,* 84–96.

Gallagher, E. M., Hunter, M., & Scott, V. J. (1999) The nature of falling among community dwelling seniors. *Canadian Journal on Aging, 18,* 348–362.

Gallagher, E. M., & Scott, V. J. (1996). *Taking steps: Modifying pedestrian environments to reduce the risk of missteps and falls.* (Available from School of Nursing, University of Victoria, Box 1700, Victoria, BC, V8X 2Y2, Canada.)

Gallagher, E. M., & Scott, V. J. (1997). The STEPS project: Participatory action research to Reduce Falls in Public Places Among Seniors and Persons with Disabilities. *Canadian Journal of Public Health, 88,* 129–133.

Gallagher, E. M., Scott, V. J., & Mills, M. (1999) *AIM: Adult Injury Management: Preventing unintentional injuries among older adults and persons with disabilities.* (Available from School of Nursing, University of Victoria, Box 1700, Victoria, BC, V8X 2Y2, Canada.)

Hall, B. (1992). From margins to center? The development and purpose of participatory research. *The American Sociologist, 23,* 15–28.

Henderson, D. (1995). Consciousness raising in participatory research: Method and methodology for emancipatory nursing inquiry. *Advances in Nursing Science, 17,* 58–69.

Lindsey, L., & McGuiness, L. (1998). Significant elements of community involvement in participatory action research: Evidence from a community project. *Journal of Advanced Nursing, 28,* 1106–1114.

Lord, S., Ward, J., Williams, P., & Anstey, K. (1994). Physiological factors associated with falls in older community-dwelling women. *Journal of the American Geriatrics Society, 42,* 1110–1117.

Mason, R., & Boutilier, M. (1996). The challenge of genuine power sharing in participatory research: the gap between theory and practice. *The Canadian Journal of Community Mental Health, 15,* 145–152.

Patla, A., Frank, J., & Winter, D. (1990). Assessment of balance control in the elderly: Major issues. *Physiotherapy Canada, 42,* 71–83.

Prudham, D., & Evans, J. (1981). Factors associated with falls in the elderly: A community study. *Age and Aging, 10,* 141–146.

Sattin, R., (1992). Falls among older persons: A public health perspective. *Annual Review of Public Health, 13,* 489–508.

Speechley, M., & Tinetti, M. (1991). Falls and injuries in frail and vigorous community elderly persons. *Journal of the American Geriatrics Society, 39,* 46–52.

Templer, J., Mullet, G., Archea, J., & Margulis, S. (1978). *An analysis of the behavior of stair users.* Washington, DC: National Bureau of Standards.

Tinetti, M., Mendes de Leon, C., Doucette, J., & Aker, D. (1994). Fear of falling and fall-related efficacy in relationship to functioning among community-living elders. *Journals of Gerontology, 49,* M140–M147.

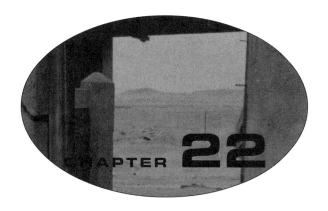

CHAPTER 22

More Than Just Questions! Implementation and Evaluation of an Arthritis Self-Management Program in Aboriginal Communities

PATRICK McGOWAN

The health status of aboriginal people in remote communities in Canada is significantly poorer than the health of the general population. The situation is even worse when aboriginal people have chronic health conditions. For example, when aboriginal people come to treatment centers, their arthritis is generally at an advanced stage with little prospect for successful rehabilitation, and contact is lost when these individuals return to their communities. Health educators have had difficulty in providing patient education in these situations.

This chapter describes what happened when a **participatory research** approach was used. Representatives from three aboriginal communities approached The Arthritis Society, British Columbia and Yukon Division, to request assistance. The health educator/researcher involved aboriginal people in the communities to design, implement, and evaluate a community arthritis self-management program. Working together, the aboriginal people and educator introduced a program specific to community needs and then used **qualitative** and quantitative research methods to test the community interventions. This participatory research process stimulated new knowledge and skills. More importantly, it em-

powered the aboriginal communities to take greater control over their health and health care.

We have more questions to ask and we're not just going to say "thank you very much for your help" and that's it, you know. We want to know why, and what, and how. This kind of program needs to be offered to elderly people, to middle aged people, to teenagers, to little people, because it's an education and education is learning. A lot of our First Nation people never asked any questions, but now we're asking questions.

First Nations Program Leader.

The World Health Organization defines health promotion as "the process of enabling people to increase control over and to improve their health" (World Health Organization [WHO], 1986). Self-help and self-care are key enabling mechanisms for health promotion (Epp, 1986). This chapter describes a self-care strategy for health promotion in an aboriginal population and evaluation of that strategy using a participatory research approach. Because self-care emphasizes community participation and personal control, participatory research is an extremely useful adjunct to help people take effective action toward improvements in their lives (Park, 1993).

The chapter also describes the four interrelated research projects conducted by the aboriginal communities with the aid of a qualified researcher to introduce, test, and determine the **effectiveness** of a self-help program.

This project was initiated when representatives of four aboriginal communities in British Columbia asked The Arthritis Society, British Columbia and Yukon Division, to work with them on the problem of arthritis. The aboriginal communities themselves had identified arthritis as a priority. An agreement was arranged whereby both parties would choose an intervention, implement it, and evaluate and interpret results.

The Arthritis Society had previously tried to meet the health care needs of native people with arthritis. The emphasis, however, had been on the education of health care professionals so they could take care of native persons with arthritis instead of enabling native people to take care of themselves. For example, in 1990, The Arthritis Society trained native Community Health Workers to implement a health education program in their communities. After 150 Community Health Workers were trained, the program was not implemented into a single community. Another issue that created a barrier to developing relationships with aboriginal communities was a history of exploitive research practices by researchers from outside the communities. All too often, investigators extracted what they needed to pursue scholarly careers but left the community with little or no benefits. Even the methodologies used left study participants concerns about misinterpretation of their data by the researchers.

This "top-down" approach to implement a program in aboriginal communities did not help people take more responsibility and control in managing their health. Meaningful participation by aboriginal community members in all program activities was needed. Fortunately, another opportunity to work with native communities was presented.

Statement of the Problem

Aboriginal people in British Columbia (BC) represent approximately 5 percent of the provincial population (BC Vital Statistics, 1997). Review of the literature shows prevalence of rheumatic disease among aboriginal people in Canada is about the same as for the general population, with the exception of a high occurrence of ankylosing spondylitis among the Haida of the Queen Charlotte Islands (Maldrom, Herring, & Young, 1995; Young, 1994). Research studies that examined how aboriginal persons live with arthritis were not found in the literature. The experience of The Arthritis Society personnel with aboriginal people indicated entry to the health care system is usually delayed and that, on entry, progressed symptoms were very common.

Early intervention and proper self-management of arthritis can result in less hospitalization and better rehabilitation. This not only helps individuals but also benefits the whole community and helps contain health care costs. The traditional approach has been to provide more information to health care workers and to educate more health care professionals. The method did not work with aboriginal people in remote communities because a service infrastructure did not exist. As well, this traditional medical method does not take into consideration cultural values and practices inherent in any community—particularly in remote Canadian aboriginal communities.

The Self-Management Approach

Self-management for chronic illness gives people the knowledge and skills needed to engage in self-care activities. Because expectation of cure is not realistic for most people with arthritis, and because medical interventions have only limited benefits, emphasis needs to be placed on bettering the patients' quality of life and degree of independence through self-management. Holman and Lorig (1992) argue strongly for the feasibility and benefits of self-management in tackling chronic illnesses. They identify seven broad skills central to self-management: (a) minimizing or overcoming physical debility; (b) forming realistic expectations and emotional responses to the vicissitudes of the illness; (c) understanding and managing the symptoms; (d) learning to judge effects of medications and to manage their use; (e) becoming proficient in techniques of problem solving; (f) communicating with health professionals; and (g) using community resources. To engage in self-management, the individual must acquire new knowledge and master new skills.

Health Promotion Approach

Health promotion focuses on broad community approaches rather than on high-risk cases or patients. The Canadian health care system reflects several health care philosophies that shape and guide the health care delivery systems. The most influential are the medical model and public health perspectives. The limitations of the medical model in dealing with chronic health conditions are well documented (Evans & Stoddart, 1994; Hewa & Hetherington, 1995; Kulbok & Baldwin, 1992; Longino, 1998; Rouge, 1998; Shannon, 1989). During the 1990s, increased emphasis was directed toward such public health and self-management strategies. In the case of arthritis, however, the public health perspective is limited because the scientific community has been unable to discover causes and important risk factors of this condition. The public health approach is justified, nevertheless, in chronic health conditions such as arthritis, when conceptualizing the entire arthritis population as the "patient." Within this perspective, clinically important minimal interventions that affect as few as 5 percent of the general population are enormously important. A minimal intervention yields therapeutic effects with small expenditures of time or money and has no side effects (Hovell & Black, 1989). Specifically, these therapeutic or preventive services and programs: (a) result in either a small effect on a large portion of the population or large effects on a small portion of the population; (b) do not require substantial quantities of money, personnel, technology, and time to provide; and, (c) involve little or no risk of side effects.

Research shows that public health programs that target all individuals with high cholesterol can be five times as effective as traditional programs that treat only those seriously ill with hypercholesterolemia (Hovell & Black, 1989). Minimal health promotion intervention strategies can help with arthritis in much the same way. For example, arthritis affects 43 percent of the population age 55 and older and ranges from mild to severe (Verbrugge, 1989; Yelin & Felts, 1990). Traditionally, only the most severe cases get treatment from practitioners, and not all patients follow that medical advice accurately; generally, such treatment involves extremely potent medications or surgery with attendant risks of serious side effects and after only modest improvements can be expected. Only a small proportion of the overall population benefits. By employing a health promotion self-management educational program in communities to stress importance of weight control, regular exercise, and appropriate medication use, a much larger proportion of those with arthritis will experience improvements—again possibly a five-fold increase.

In summary, by targeting the broader community of all potentially affected people, and including family members of those with arthritis, the health promotion approach to arthritis self-management brings about a more supportive social environment for self-care efforts. This was deemed especially important with aboriginal people because participants in the project had identified family, independence, and caring for others as major quality-of-life concerns when living with arthritis.

Health Promotion in Aboriginal Communities

A major consideration in working with communities to plan health initiatives is to incorporate prevalent conceptualizations of health and wellness. The Medicine Wheel is one of the most powerful instruments used in North American aboriginal cultures to convey the holistic character of knowledge and experience (Bobb, 1983; Bear, 1980). This ancient symbol (Fig. 22–1) was used by most First Nations peoples of North and South America, with some Canadian First Nation peoples expressing the same basic concepts using other descriptive strategies.

In recent years, healers and elders in many aboriginal communities have adopted the Medicine Wheel in teaching. It represents the circle of life. Human beings have their existence in this circle, along with other beings and the unseen forces, linked together, in a whole with no beginning and no end. The lines intersecting at the center of the circle signify order and balance. They help people

Mental

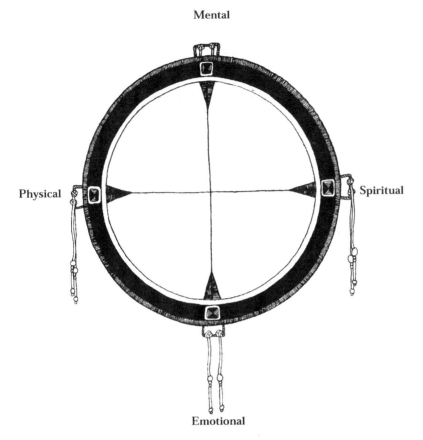

Physical

Spiritual

Emotional

FIG. 22–1. The Medicine Wheel

examine experience by breaking down complex situations into constituent parts, while reminding them not to forget the whole. The center of the wheel is the balance point where apparent opposites meet. The flags at the ends of the intersecting lines signify the four winds, whose movement is a reminder that nothing is fixed or stagnant, that change is a normal experience and transformation is always possible.

The Medicine Wheel teaches people that there are four aspects to their nature: Mental, Physical, Emotional, and Spiritual. The goal is to keep these four aspects in balance, to maintain a good rhythm, and to lead a balanced life. The *Physical* is the direction of body reality, of body awareness. The individual must learn to experience the physical presence in a healthy, wholesome way. The *Emotional* is the direction of feelings. The individual must learn to experience emotions in a

healthy manner and not suppress them due to negative reactions or feedback. It is the direction of counselors. The *Spiritual* is the direction of energy for it is an unseen concept. It is the alternate reality or mirror image of the physical. When energy levels are low, it affects all the other aspects. When someone is described as being in good spirits, she or he is happy. The *Mental* is the direction of thinking. These are the intellectual gifts an individual acquires to predict and to interpret hidden messages. The mind can be trained until it becomes a highly developed instrument. Each of these aspects can be equally developed in a healthy, well-balanced individual through the use of *volition* or *will*. Volition helps individuals make choices and act in a certain manner. Because it can direct action, volition is often placed at the center of the Wheel.

Interestingly, the four aspects of the ancient Medicine Wheel of the First Nations are similar to the World Health Organizations' definition of health developed in the late 1940s. The WHO (1948) defines health as a positive state, including physical, mental, emotional, social, and spiritual well-being and not merely absence of disease. Health care policies today are even more closely allied to the Medicine Wheel's holistic way of looking at human well-being (Epp, 1986).

The concepts in *New Perspectives on Health for Canadians* (Lalonde, 1974), which continues to direct health care policy in Canada today, are even more closely allied to the Medicine Wheel's holistic way of looking at human well-being.

Quality of Life as a Starting Point

Health promotion and participatory research differ from most biomedical and some public health approaches to planning and research in the degree to which they engage members of an affected population in assessing their own needs and they do not necessarily begin with a health problem. The Ottawa Charter (WHO, 1986) states that to achieve health "an individual or group must be able to identify and to realize aspirations, to satisfy needs, and to change or cope with the environment." This notion is particularly relevant to aboriginal people for whom health problems may be multiple and irreversible, rather than focused and curable, and for whom functions of daily living and quality of life become the paramount outcomes.

The PRECEDE-PROCEED (Green & Kreuter, 1999) health promotion model (see Fig. 22–2) makes a strong link between quality of life and health. It therefore was used to guide the planning process and to introduce the Arthritis Self-Management Model to the First Nation planners and later to the communities.

In this project, the PRECEDE model guided the development of interview questions fo-

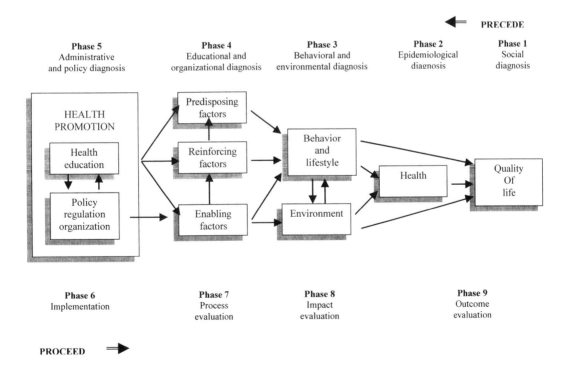

FIG. 22–2. PRECEDE-PROCEED model of health promotion planning. From *Health Promotion Planning: An Educational and Ecological Approach* (p. 35) by L. W. Green and M. L. Kreuter. Copyright © 1999 by Mayfield Publishing Company. Reprinted by permission of the publisher. Mayfield Publishing Company.

cussing on quality-of-life, arthritis beliefs, the program and type of benefits the program could facilitate, and how the community could help interpret results. Figure 22–2 shows one model of health promotion planning and evaluation that places quality of life at the beginning of the diagnostic or needs assessment process.

In the "Social Diagnosis" stage of planning in the PRECEDE-PROCEED Model, subjective assessments of conditions of living are explored with or by the affected individuals or population. The development and earliest applications and tests of this model were with issues of self-care associated with chronic diseases such as asthma (Green, 1974). Some 700 published applications of this model since 1974 have demonstrated its wide applicability to planning, implementation, and evaluation of health education, health promotion, self-care, and related areas.

With participatory research, a first principle is that those affected by the issue to be changed/studied should have influence, if not control, over the whole project, including framing the research questions in terms meaningful to them (Green, George, Daniel, Frankish, Herbert, Bowie, & O'Neill, 1995). The British Columbia Ministry of Health conducted a **Delphi** survey of First Nations leaders to assess their perception of social problems or issues facing the aboriginal populations of the province (Shannon & MacDonald, 1993). Arthritis was the only problem in the top ten priorities that was not related to alcohol or drug misuse.

Grant funding was secured for a participatory research project to adapt the Arthritis Self-Management Program (Lorig, Lubeck, Kraines, Seleznick, & Holman, 1985) specifically to the culture, circumstances, and social needs of aboriginal people. A first step in both the PRECEDE-PROCEED model (Fig. 22–2) and in participatory research is to decide jointly what matters most to the community itself. This social diagnosis is not defined biomedically, but in relation to persons' quality of life, which is defined as social, emotional, and economic well-being. Exploration with aboriginal groups concerning their quality of life and the subjective meaning they attach to arthritis included the following questions:

• You've heard people talk about quality of life. I guess this means what's really impor-

tant to you in your own life. What things are really important to you in your life?
• When you think of arthritis, what do you think about?
• What about other people in your community? What are their experiences with arthritis?
• If the First Nations Arthritis Self-Management Program were to have any effects on the people who take it, what kinds of effects would they be?

These inquiries led to a set of social or quality-of-life meanings attached to arthritis, representing desired outcomes other than biomedical that could serve as criteria for success of the program. This proved particularly valuable in making the program more relevant to this elderly population of aboriginal people with arthritis because of both generational and cultural differences in how they view health and arthritis symptoms.

Social Meaning of Arthritis

When allowed to range beyond biomedical perspectives on a health problem, people generally discuss health in terms of meaningfulness to their social lives and their quality of life. For aboriginal participants in the planning and research process, the six most important themes or meanings associated with arthritis were: pain, fear, inability "to do the things I used to do," crippling, problems with medications and treatments, and needing to learn how to deal with it. These themes in the qualitative analysis phase of these four projects helped to formulate and adapt outcome measures and program content that would give the program relevance and the participants a greater sense of owning it. Other dimensions of quality of life touched by arthritis that were of concern and interest to the participants included family, culture, independence, and caring for others.

Also reflected in this stage of the participatory planning and research were desired effects of the program besides those reflected in the social meanings attached to arthritis. Concretely, participants in the project wanted better understanding of arthritis, to "learn how to take care of myself," to learn

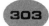

about diets, medications, and exercises, and to learn to deal with stress, anger, and frustration.

Outcome Measures Chosen

The foregoing social diagnosis and epidemiological diagnosis of the symptoms and consequences of arthritis (Phases 1 and 2 of the PRECEDE-PROCEED model, Fig. 22–2) produced the criteria of success for the program. These included **visual analog scales** (Polit & Hungler, 1995) measuring pain, stress, fear, and anger, and standardized measures of disability (functional limitation scale), depression, and **self-efficacy.** Self-efficacy has been found in a series of studies with the Arthritis Self-Management Program to be an intervening variable between program participation and program outcomes (Lorig & Holman, 1993). This brings us to a second major distinguishing feature of the health promotion and participatory research approaches to planning and evaluation.

Determinants of Health beyond the Medical and Behavioral

Participation of a wider range of research collaborators introduces a wider range of variables for consideration as outcomes, and as causes, determinants, or barriers to the desired outcomes. Behavioral scientists have added richly to the biomedical models of causation, specifying variables represented in Phases 3 and 4 of the PRECEDE-PROCEED model (Fig. 22–2) as predisposing and reinforcing factors. The behavioral sciences contributed enormously to the development of health education interventions and programs that could be demonstrated by experimental design to affect behavioral changes conducive to health. Other social scientists have extended these concepts into social, economic, political, and cultural domains, elaborating the concepts and variables of lifestyle, environment, and enabling factors shown in Phases 3 and 4 of Figure 22–2. As a case in point, Social Learning Theory (Bandura, 1977) and its concept of self-efficacy straddle several disci-

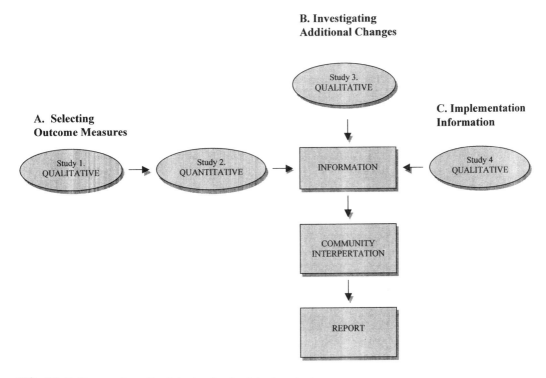

FIG. 22–3. Research methodologies in aboriginal project

plinary perspectives about health and social behavior.

Combining Quantitative and Qualitative Methods

Both quantitative and qualitative data are needed to further the adaptation and application of health promotion for special populations (Steckler, McLeroy, Goodman, Bird, & McCormick, 1992; Greene, Caracelli, & Graham, 1989). Figure 22–3 shows the several ways and the sequence in which qualitative and quantitative data served in this project.

At the initial participatory stages ("A" in Fig. 22–3), qualitative data helped to select the quantitative outcome measures. Then outcome questionnaires were chosen with information elicited from 18 interviews with leaders from eight rural communities. The information was analyzed in two ways: a group process involving the First Nations Advisory Committee, and by the project investigator using a standard methodology for developing themes and stages in conducting content analysis. When compared, results from both methods showed a high degree of congruency and provided a basis for choosing the outcome measures: health status (Medical Outcomes Study [Stewart, Hayes, & Ware, 1988]); visual analogue scales for pain, stress, fear, and anger; functional ability (Health Assessment Questionnaire [Fries, Spitz, Kraines, & Holman, 1980]); depression (Center for Epidemiologic Studies Depression Scale [Radloff, 1977]); and self-efficacy (Arthritis Self-Efficacy Scale [Lorig, Chastain, Ung, Shoor, & Holman, 1989]). A pre-post and four-month follow-up design was used to obtain the data. Cultural sensitivity, education level, and comfort with self-administered paper-and-pencil tests were considered in preparing the questionnaire containing the selected outcome measures, which was completed by 150 persons.

At later stages of the research, qualitative data were used to investigate additional changes ("B" in Fig. 22–3) not tapped by the quantitative measures. Aboriginal leaders indicated that additional changes were taking place as a result of the program. They defined what they felt these changes were and developed interview questions to investigate the nature and scope of the changes. The leaders then traveled to involved communities and interviewed other persons who had participated in the project. During and after program implementation by trained aboriginal leaders (who took the program into their own communities), we used further qualitative investigation to understand the process and problems of application (Phase "C" in Fig. 22–3). Project staff interviewed the aboriginal leaders who had provided the program in their communities.

In this project, qualitative and quantitative methods were combined with participatory research processes to facilitate a collaborative research partnership. The combination of research methods provided a meaningful opportunity for collaborative and participatory program planning and evaluation with the aboriginal communities.

Design and Focus of Evaluation

Health promotion and participatory research, as characterized above, do not lend themselves easily to some canons of randomized experimental design. The active participation in planning by those who would be subjects of experimental programs precludes their blinding, if not their random, assignment. Their informed involvement in identifying the criteria and measures of success precludes their serving as subjects for pre-tests and post-tests of knowledge, attitudes, and beliefs. Their investment in designing the program makes them suspect as evaluators of their own programs. It is possible, however, to select a new cohort of members of the affected community as subjects for the evaluation, or take research conducted elsewhere on the **efficacy** of the basic contents of the programs as warranting simplified designs for adaptation and implementation of these programs in new populations.

Generations of Research and Evaluation

Ideally, knowledge development in the biomedical or social sciences progresses from theory to clinical trials or other experimental

ABORIGINAL PARTICIPANTS

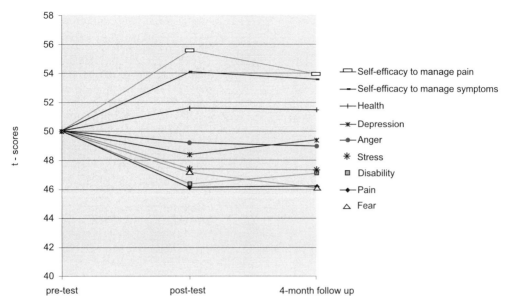

**Figure 4. Pre-test, post-test, and 4-month follow-up
t-scores for outcome measures**

FIG. 22–4. Pre-test, post-test, and four-month follow-up *t*-scores for outcome measures

studies to test the efficacy and effectiveness of innovations. Those found effective are then submitted to research that demonstrates their applicability to disease management, and results are disseminated (Green et al., 1995). Much of the work that has been done at the levels of basic science and controlled trials remains to be applied and disseminated widely, however, especially to marginalized populations (Nutbeam, Smith, & Catford, 1989; Farquhar, 1996; MacLean, 1996). The basic efficacy and effectiveness questions have been answered for more innovations than have been effectively implemented by practitioners or applied to or by aboriginal people. The research most needed in health promotion for aboriginal people is at the demonstration and dissemination end of the spectrum. Here the research questions have more to do with adaptation, implementation, sustainability, and diffusion of innovations.

Pre-Test and Post-Test Design

We adapted the First Nations Arthritis Self-Management Program from the foundation of a program that had been extensively tested with controlled trials among nonaboriginal people. We settled, therefore, with an evaluation design based on significant pre-post differences within the new populations as sufficient evidence of the effectiveness of the adapted program, as long as the difference was greater than that observed in pre-post tested control subjects in the previous trials. We based this assumption on the now highly standardized measurement instruments used to assess outcomes in arthritis treatment and self-management, and the further assurance that the pre-testing effect on post-test scores is similar for different populations (Lorig & Holman, 1993). Accepting these assumptions,

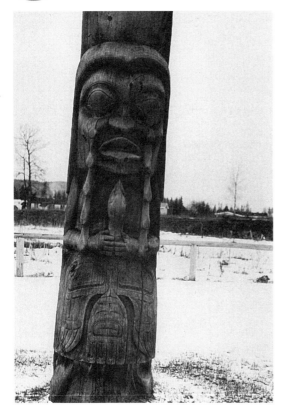

FIG. 22–5. Ceremonial totem pole at Hazelton, British Columbia, one of the many sites of the program. *Photographed by Patrick McGowan, used with permission.*

We've always thought of our elders to be our books of knowledge . . . because they've lived for so many years . . . you're kind of taking the native and non-native traditions and kind of putting them on a equal path, you know, and kind of living side by side.

Treatments . . . there's a lot of [elders] who have their ideas about things that have been handed down for generations . . . they like to pass them on.

I think we as First Nations people are very . . . sociable kind of people, human beings, where you come together at a gathering. . . . This was a kind of potlatch feeling where you came together and witnessed what each other had to put up with on a day-to-day basis in regard to their arthritis, and witnessed what people had to say and listened. It was a time to be together and be happy about something that was bad. So it was a kind of a gathering of . . . family and friends, and it was a gathering of human beings coming together and talking about something that affected them all . . . sharing your knowledge with each other and not outdoing each other because you are all at the same level in dealing with something that affected your life.

These quotes were included in a full report on the project and the four evaluations that was made available to the funding agency (McGowan & Green, 1995).

Preliminary Results of the First Nations Project

Figure 22–4 presents the results of the first set of outcome measures. The improvements from pre-test (at the beginning of the program) to post-test (at the end of the program) for 73 participants who were experiencing arthritis disability are significant for pain level and the two self-efficacy subscales of pain and other symptoms ($p < .001$). Findings were also significant for health status, stress, and anger levels ($p < .05$). We used repeated measure **analysis of variance tests (ANOVA)** in both sets of measures. The changes for the other outcome measures (i.e., fear, disability, and depression) were in the right direction, but not statistically significant.

The self-efficacy measures were highly responsive to the program as suggested by significance levels ($p < .0001$) and the absolute values of scores compared with other studies. The self-efficacy changes accounted for most of the variance in a multivariate ANOVA with

simple pre-test–post-test designs combined with qualitative observations can serve far more efficiently to answer the research questions of adaptation, implementation, and dissemination for those program approaches that have been validated in previous controlled trials. The alternative that might serve where participatory research circumstances preclude pre-testing is a randomized or other equivalent control group design with post-tests only (Green & Lewis, 1986).

Excerpts from the qualitative data from these four studies illustrate some of the kinds of changes that can come about through **self-help** programs and participatory research.

We made them all involved. . . . They were communicating and sharing . . . about their pain, how they were feeling.

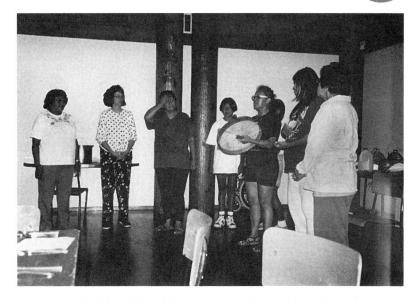

FIG. 22–6. Traditional First Nations ceremonies, such as drumming, were included in group meetings as participants explored strategies for an arthritis self-management program. *Photographed by Patrick McGowan, used with permission.*

all nine outcome measures. This was significant ($p < .0001$) with 73 participants for whom we had complete measures at pre-test and post-test.

Concerning the sustainability of the results, the program sought an effect that participants could maintain beyond the end of the program. The results of a four-month follow-up survey of 62 participants showed no significant change in scores on the nine outcomes between post-test and follow-up survey.

Discussion

This experience of extending and adapting the Arthritis Self-Management Program among a sample of aboriginal people in British Columbia offers some insights into those national and provincial or state health promotion policies urging attention to self-governance in health issues at the local level and use of self-care, especially in aboriginal populations.

We initiated this study when four native communities in British Columbia requested help from The Arthritis Society to work with them on the problem of arthritis, which they had identified themselves as a priority. To negotiate appropriate methods that included the native community as full partners, we employed participatory research processes using both quantitative and qualitative methods and guided by a health promotion planning model (Fig. 22–2). With grant funds supporting our collaboration, the communities defined their experience with the problems of arthritis, thus specifying the desired outcomes and the research questions. They then participated in the adaptation of the Arthritis Self-Management Program, the training of leaders, the recruitment and implementation of local groups, and the evaluation of the intervention. Health promotion seeks not only the immediate impact on reductions in behavioral risks, symptoms, or voluntary changes in environmental conditions, but also, and equally important, participants more empowered to engage effectively in their community's affairs.

Using a health promotion planning framework that starts with the aspects of the problem or goal considered most important to the community and defined in relation to the members' quality of life (Green & Kreuter, 1999), working as partners in all the plan-

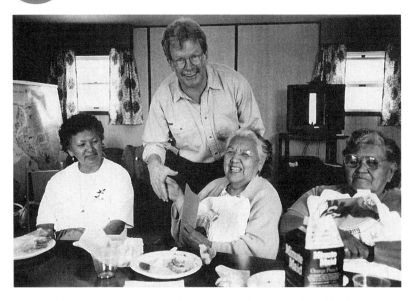

FIG. 22–7. A qualified researcher who worked closely with the groups conducted formal evaluations of the program. *Photographed by Patrick McGowan, used with permission.*

ning, implementation, and evaluation activities (Green et al., 1995), and using a sequential combination of qualitative and quantitative methodology, partners were able to realize both health and social or quality-of-life benefits.

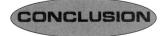

CONCLUSION

This chapter describes a case study illustrating the use of methodological diversity in a collaborative research project with aboriginal communities. Participatory research combining qualitative and quantitative methodologies enriched and made more comprehensive the findings of this study. It also provided the opportunity for extending the benefits of science to populations who have not fully benefited from new health knowledge and innovations available through self-care. We have illustrated some of the advantages and problems in participatory research approaches with aboriginal populations. The communities of aboriginal people identified specific quality-of-life concerns such as coping with the daily problems related to arthritis as *their* priorities for adaptation of the Arthritis Self-Management Program. The process and the results of this study may apply to other populations with arthritis, or possibly other chronic conditions. Preliminary results from our First Nations Arthritis Self-Management study illustrate how participatory research can be applied within a specific population or demographically defined group. They also demonstrate promising outcomes for the adaptability of the health promotion strategies inherent in a participatory research approach to planning, implementing, and evaluating self-care programs.

✳ Reflective Questions

1. What do you imagine are the gains that various participants from this project experienced? (e.g., elders, community health nurse(s) on the reserves, members of the communities who had arthritis, members of the families or communities-at-large who did not have arthritis themselves, research team members, researchers, and so forth)

2. What elements of the way in which this project was conducted would you say were participatory research methods ? Can you imagine any ways that the project might *not* have been fully participatory?

3. Discuss the rationale for using a combination of quantitative and qualitative research methods.

4. Can these research and program implementation methods be classified as health promoting in and of themselves? Why or why not?

5. Describe the advantages of using a public health perspective in planning health education programs.

6. How might a program that interests you be implemented using similar methods? Would you evaluate the implementation? How? Why?

REFERENCES

Bandura, A. (1977). Self-efficacy: Towards a unifying theory of behavior change. *Psychological Review, 84*(2), 191–215.

Bear, S. (1980). *The medicine wheel: Earth astrology.* New York: Prentice Hall.

Bobb, J. (1983). *The sacred tree: Four winds development project.* Lethbridge, AB: Four Worlds Development Press.

British Columbia Vital Statistics Agency. (1997). *Analysis of Status Indians in British: Updated Report, 1991–1996.* Victoria, BC: BC Ministry of Health and Ministry Responsible for Seniors.

Epp, J. (1986). Achieving health for all: A framework for health promotion. *Health Promotion (International) 1,* 419–428.

Evans, R. G., & Stoddart, G. L. (1994). Producing health, consuming health care. In R. G. Evans, M. L. Barer, & T. R. Marmor (Eds.), *Why are some people healthy and others not? The determinants of health of populations* (pp. 27–64). New York: Aldine de Gruyter.

Farquhar, J. W. (1996). The case for dissemination research in health promotion and disease prevention. *Canadian Journal of Public Health, 87,* (Supp.), 44–49.

Fries, J. F., Spitz, P., Kraines, R. G., & Holman, H. R. (1980). Measurement of patient outcomes in arthritis. *Arthritis and Rheumatism, 23,* 137–145.

Greene, J. C., Caracelli, V. J., & Graham, W. (1989). Toward a conceptual framework for mixed method evaluation designs. *Educational Evaluation and Policy Analysis, 11,* 225–274.

Green, L. W. (1974). Toward cost-benefit evaluations of health education: Some concepts, methods and examples. *Health Education Monograph, 2*(2), 34–64.

Green, L. W., George, M. A., Daniel, M., Frankish, C. J., Herbert, C. J., Bowie, W. R., & O'Neill, M. (1995). *Participatory research in health promotion.* Ottawa: Royal Society of Canada.

Green, L. W., & Kreuter, M. W. (1999). *Health promotion planning: An educational and ecological approach* (3rd ed.). Mountain View, CA: Mayfield Publishing.

Green, L. W., & Lewis, F. M. (1986). *Measurement and evaluation in health education and health promotion.* Mountain View, CA: Mayfield Publishing.

Hewa, S., & Hetherington, R. W. (1995). Specialists without spirit: Limitations of the mechanistic biomedical model. *Theoretical Medicine, 16*(2), 129–139.

Holman, H., & Lorig, K. (1992). Perceived self-efficacy in self-management of chronic disease. In R. Schwarzer (Ed.), *Self-efficacy: Thought control of action* (pp. 305–323). Washington, DC: Hemisphere.

Hovell, M. F., & Black, D. R. (1989). Minimal intervention and arthritis treatment: Implications for patient and physician compliance. *Arthritis Care and Research, 2,* 565–570.

Kulbok, P. A., & Baldwin, J. H. (1992). From preventive health behavior to health promotion: Advancing a positive construct of health. *Advances in Nursing Science, 14*(4), 50–64.

Lalonde, M. (1974). *A new perspective on the health of Canadians.* Ottawa: Information Canada.

Longino, C. F. (1998). The limits of scientific medicine: Paradigm strain and social policy. *Journal of Health & Social Policy, 9*(4), 101–116.

Lorig, K., & Holman, H. (1993). Arthritis self-management studies: A twelve year review. *Health Education Quarterly, 20,* 17–28.

Lorig, K., Chastain, R., Ung, E., Shoor, S., & Holman, H. (1989). Development and evaluation of a scale to measure perceived self-efficacy in people with arthritis. *Arthritis and Rheumatism, 32,* 37–44.

Lorig, K., Lubeck, D., Kraines, R. G., Seleznick, M., & Holman, H. R. (1985). Outcomes of self-help education for patients with arthritis. *Arthritis and Rheumatism, 28,* 680–685.

MacLean, D. R. (1996). Positioning dissemination in health policy. *Canadian Journal of Public Health, 87,* (Supp.), 40–43.

Maldrom, J. B., Herring, D. A., & Young, T. K. (1995). *Aboriginal health in Canada: Historical, cultural, and epidemiological perspective.* Toronto: University of Toronto Press.

McGowan, P., & Green, L. W. (1995). *First Nations Arthritis Self-Management Program.* Vancouver: Unpublished report to the British Columbia Health Research Foundation.

Nutbeam, D., Smith, C., & Catford, J. (1989). Evaluation of health education: A review of the progress, possibilities, and problems. *Journal of Epidemiology and Community Health, 44,* 83–89.

Park, P. (1993). What is participatory research? A theoretical and methodological perspective. In P. Park, M. Brydon-Miller, B. Hall, & T. Jackson (Eds.), *Voices of change: Participatory research in the United States and Canada* (pp.1–19). Toronto: OISE Press.

Polit, D. F., & Hungler, B. P. (1995). Nursing research: Principles and methods. Philadelphia: Lippincott.

Radloff, L. (1977). The CES-D Scale: A self-report depression scale for research in the general population. *Applied Psychological Measurement, 1,* 385–401.

Rouge, A. (1998). Prevention—limitations of the medical model. *Psychiatrie, 90,* 25–31.

Shannon, M. T. (1989). Health promotion and illness prevention: A biopsychosocial perspective. *Health & Social Work, 14,* 32–40.

Shannon, W., & MacDonald, M. (1993). *A Delphi survey of aboriginal health priorities.* Victoria, BC: Ministry of Health and Ministry Responsible for Seniors.

Steckler, A., McLeroy, K. R., Goodman, R. M., Bird, S. T., & McCormick, L. (1992). Toward integrating qualitative and qualitative methods: An introduction. *Health Education Quarterly, 19,* 1–8.

Stewart, A. L., Hayes, R. D., & Ware, J. E. (1988). The MOS short-form general health survey: Reliability and validity in a patient population. *Medical Care, 26,* 724–735.

Verbrugge, L. M. (1989). Recent, present, and future health of American adults. In L. Breslow, J. E. Fielding, & L. Lave (Eds.), *Annual Review of Public Health, 10,* 333–361.

World Health Organization. (1948). *Inaugural Constitution.* Geneva: Author.

World Health Organization. (1986). The Ottawa Charter for Health Promotion. *Health Promotion, 1,* 3–5.

Yelin, E. H., & Felts, W. R. (1990). A summary of the impact of musculoskeletal conditions in the United States. *Arthritis and Rheumatism, 33,* 750–755.

Young, T. K. (1994). *The health of native Americans: Toward a biocultural epidemiology.* New York: Oxford University Press.

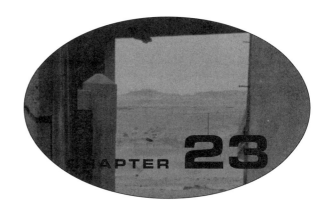

CHAPTER 23

Enhancing Nursing Health Promotion through Cooperative Inquiry

MARCIA D. HILLS
JENNIFER MULLETT

How did it get to be that nurses look after four, five, or six patients at one time? And how can a nurse assure good care when she has five other patients? After doing three intravenous medications in a row I couldn't see how I could do that plus look after other patients. When I asked the nurse about flushing the intravenous before each of the medications, she said that she never flushes the line and she had been practicing for 20 years. She said, "It takes too much time!" I see things done differently by staff RNs because they know they can't do it all within their shift so they cut corners. Why doesn't someone say "I am not going to do this anymore. I can't possibly give quality care to five or six patients." When will all nurses take a stand? . . . I don't want to be in a profession where the demands of the system are so high that the patient is forgotten in the process. . . . Because patients know when their nurse doesn't care. But I do care. And I want to be able to give quality care. I don't want to rush or cut corners. I don't want to be so stressed that all that I am worrying about is the job at hand and forgetting what I am there for . . . to care for the person.

This student's story highlights the dilemma presented to new graduates who have been educated from a health promotion perspective as they enter the current workforce. They are confronted with the contradiction between what they have learned as best practices and what they see happening in the workplace. This story frames the research question for this chapter. How can we change the nursing practice to be more congruent with the emerging paradigm of health promotion?

In recent years nurses have been encouraged to consider their potential role in health promotion and to reorient their practice to be more consistent with the principles of health promotion (Hills & Lindsey, 1994; Maglacas, 1990; MacLeod Clark, 1993). Although evidence suggests that nursing is committed to do so, the research also indicates that achieving such a reorientation is a formidable task indeed! Nursing has long been steeped in a culture of oppression and subordination. This culture is characterized by an emulation of physicians' practices, by a focus on technical aspects of care, and by horizontal violence inflicted among colleagues when they attack rather than support one another (Lovell, 1981; Robinson, 1995). An analysis of the culture further suggests that, "in pursuing their practice, nurses maintain a focus on mastery of specific tasks or competencies which must be performed according to strict rules, with penalties for creativity, and where compliance is measured" (Robinson, 1995, p. 66). Tradition lies as an obstacle on the path to change.

A reorientation to health promotion principles requires a significant shift from a natural science paradigm, with its emphasis on disease, to a human science paradigm, with its recognition of the primacy of people and their experiences. It is critical and timely to transform the current practice of nursing.

Because of its transformative and empowering nature, cooperative inquiry, a form of participatory action research, is ideally suited to assisting nurses to examine their practice and to develop new and innovative ways of practicing. Empowerment is a cornerstone of both participatory action research and health promotion practice. Therefore, engaging in participatory action research while focusing on health promotion can catalyze both nursing culture and nursing practice.

This chapter introduces, describes, and provides examples of cooperative inquiry. The chapter also promotes its use as a catalyst in transforming nursing health promotion practice.

Nurses' Approach to Health: Moving to Empowerment and Participation

The evolution of nursing practice in general and health promoting nursing practice in particular has been influenced by prevailing approaches to health upon which these practices have been based. Labonte (1993) described three approaches to health, each of which contains "a template of differing health conceptualizations, program strategies and success criteria" (p. 1). An analysis of these approaches illuminates nurses' present struggle to practice from a health promotion perspective.

The Biomedical Approach to Health

Labonte (1993) reiterated that a biomedical approach to health is founded upon a disease-treatment model of care and incorporates a definition of health as the absence of diseases or infirmity. Although this medical definition of health was challenged by the World Health Organization over 50 years ago, the disease-treatment model of care continues to be the predominant model used by health professionals, including nurses (Labonte, 1993). When taking a biomedical approach, promoting health amounts to preventing disease. The focus is on reducing physiological risk factors with a view to preventing a serious

disease from arising due to less than optimal physical functioning. For example, a biomedical approach to heart health would emphasize the use of cholesterol-lowering medications.

The Behavioral Approach to Health

In the second approach, the behavioral approach, health is conceptualized as physical well-being and health care moves slightly beyond disease prevention. This behavioral perspective adds education, marketing, and policy theories to medical theory and incorporates secondary and primary prevention. The principal strategies within the behavioral approach target lifestyle change. The major criticism of the approach is that clients may feel blamed for their behaviors, and thus their illnesses, because consideration is seldom given to other factors, such as the environment or socioeconomic issues, which might contribute to their health (Raeburn, 1992; Whyte & Berland, 1993). Using the heart health example again, a behavioral approach would focus on smoking cessation, exercise, and distribution of information about healthy lifestyles.

The Socioenvironmental Approach to Health

The third approach to health outlined by Labonte (1993) incorporates socioenvironmental factors and expands the definition of health to include the concept of health promotion. Health is conceptualized as "a resource for living . . . a positive concept . . . the extent to which an individual or group is able to realize aspirations, to satisfy needs, and to change or cope with the environment" (World Health Organization, 1986, p. 2). The socioenvironmental approach to health is qualitatively different from the biomedical and behavioral approaches because it mediates societal and individual responsibility for health by considering the context of a person's life.

A social view of health implies that we must intervene to change those aspects of the environment that are promoting ill health rather than continue to simply deal with illness after it appears, or continue to exhort individuals to change their attitudes and lifestyles when, in fact, the environment in which they live and work gives them little choice and support for making such changes. (South Australian Health Commission, 1988, p. 3)

To go back to the example of heart health, a socioenvironmental approach would consider, among other factors, the social and environmental contexts of a person's life (e.g., their socioeconomic status, social networks, living conditions, and responsibilities).

From a socioenvironmental perspective, health promotion is defined as "the process of enabling individuals or communities to increase control over and to improve their health, and is viewed as a mediating strategy between personal and environmental issues affecting one's health" (World Health Organization, 1986, p. 2). The concept of empowerment is embedded in this definition of health promotion. To practice health promotion, nurses and other health professionals must relinquish their traditional "power over" relationships with clients allowing the development of collaborative partnerships with them and with communities—the ultimate goal being health for all. The socioenvironmental perspective thus has introduced the notions of empowerment, participation, and partnerships—the central tenets of the Ottawa Charter (World Health Organization, 1986) definition of health promotion.

Nurses' Health Promotion Practice: From Rhetoric to Reality

Nursing Practice

Several British studies of nursing health promotion practice have found that, although nurses may espouse the virtues of a socioenvironmental approach to health and its inherent valuing of health promotion, empowerment, and participation, their nursing practice does not reflect their ideals (Gott & O'Brien, 1990; Kendall, 1993; McBride, 1994; Wilson-Barnett & MacLeod Clark, 1993). The methods used in these studies were designed to capture the actual behavior of practitioners and ranged from observation to taped interactions and interviews. The researchers consistently found that nurses' health promotion practices were congruent with the biomedical and behavioral approaches to health, with the nurses' attitudes and activities focused primarily on individual and lifestyle change. The concept of participation was not put into practice. In addition, nurses were maintaining the traditional unequal balance of power between nurse and patient characteristic of the medical model of care. There was little evidence of clients initiating an active stance or nurses promoting client participation; patients were not treated as equals in care but as subordinates.

Furthermore, nurses did not appear to be involved in empowering patients, fostering self-esteem, or encouraging decision-making skills. One researcher concluded: "both perception and practice are characterized by an illness-oriented, one-to-one approach with a lack of recognition or enactment of many of the central tenets of current health education and health promotion philosophy" (Latter, 1993, p. 78). Another referred to nursing as being a dominant style of interaction between nurses and patients, indicative of sick nursing not health nursing (MacLeod Clark, 1993).

A Canadian study (Berland, Whyte & Maxwell, 1995) seemed more promising than the British studies in that it demonstrated that nurses play an active role in promoting health through teaching patients, supporting families and caregivers, and contributing to a healthful hospital environment. The researchers used a survey design to examine the knowledge, attitudes, and practices of acute care nurses in relation to health promotion. The researchers designed a questionnaire from the focus group data of the previous study. They report that hospital nurses perceive health promotion as an "essential, independent, attractive, and indeed integral part of nursing" (p. 21). However, this study was based on self-report and revealed inconsistencies between what the nurses reported as their values and what they reported as their actions. For example, nurses in this study expressed a strong belief in health promotion, but only 52 percent of them reported that they had altered hospital rules or routines to accommodate patients' control. The authors concluded that, although respondents' definitions of health promotion were consistent with the WHO conceptualization that promotion efforts increase control over health-related circumstances, the hospital environment does not support nurses' health promotion practice.

Nursing Education

Some of these studies recommended reorienting nursing education to teach future nurses to practice with a health promotion perspective (Gott & O'Brien, 1990; Wilson-Barnett & MacLeod Clark, 1993). This strategy is being implemented by programs in Canada, Australia, Britain, New Zealand, and the United States (Bevis & Watson, 1989; Hills & Lindsey, 1994). The Collaborative Nursing Program of British Columbia, Canada, uses health promotion as a framework for a program implemented at 10 educational institutions throughout the province (Hills, Lindsey, Chisamore, Bassett-Smith, Abbot, & Fournier-Chalmer, 1994).

A phenomenological study conducted with students from the British Columbia program revealed that students were indeed practicing with a health promotion perspective as a guide to their practice (Hills, 1998). But the data also revealed that students were repeatedly concerned about their ability to practice from this perspective, in a system that seemed to militate against socioenvironmental health promotion practice. Students cited several instances of registered nurses not understanding this approach. (See Chapter 17 in this volume.) An issue therefore remains: Even if graduating students ascribe to a health promotion perspective, will it be difficult for them to maintain this perspective while working in an environment that is entrenched in a biomedical approach to health?

For change to occur in the practice of nursing, practicing nurses themselves must be involved in bringing about the change. Cooperative inquiry is a methodology that has proven to be an ideal catalyst for transforming practice (Reason, 1988; Traylen, 1994).

Cooperative Inquiry: A Catalyst in Transforming Practice

Pushing the Boundaries of Participatory Action Research

Participatory action research is gaining recognition (in health promotion and primary health care) as a viable alternative to more traditional research approaches (Green, George, Daniel, Frankish, Herbert, Bowie, & O'Neil, 1995). One reason for its popularity is that "it is built on a recognition of the inextricable links between research and practice" (Carr & Kemmis, 1986, p. 162).

Cooperative inquiry is a form of participatory action research. Because of its focus on bringing about change rather than on prediction or theoretical/empirical understanding alone, it is particularly well suited to addressing the challenge of transforming nursing practice to be more congruent with health promotion. By engaging in cooperative inquiry and its intrinsic cycles of action and reflection, nurses develop new models of practice and experiment with them in their day-to-day work. It is an empowering process that allows nurses to actually change their practices at the same time that they are developing their knowledge about it. As Reason and Rowan (1981) explain, "because of the emphasis on self-reflective agency, this is a method particularly suitable for practitioner research and for the development of innovative approaches to practice" (p. 144). And, as required for social relevancy, this methodology brings about change by doing research *with* people, not *on* them or *about* them. This requires that nurses, who would be considered "subjects" in most traditional research projects, must actually join the "initiating researchers" (Reason, 1988, p. 20) to form an inquiry group and engage in the inquiry process as co-researchers. As part of the research team, the nurses develop research questions, collect and analyze data, and make recommendations.

This research process differs from traditional research by removing the boundaries between researcher and subject, engaging all participants as co-researchers and co-subjects. "If research is to reflect a health promotion perspective, the emphasis must be on working with people as equal partners, involving them in the research process and acknowledging their expertise in it" (Wass, 1994, p. 64). Further, "to generate knowledge about persons without their full participation in deciding how to generate it, is to misrepresent their personhood and to abuse by neglect their capacity for autonomous intentionality. It is fundamentally unethical!" (Heron, 1996, p. 21). By participating in the research process, including decision making, and critical reflection of their practice, nurses are in an excellent position to know how best to change their practice.

Central Assumptions of Cooperative Inquiry

Cooperative inquiry is based on three fundamental assumptions that guide the research process.

1. *Persons are self-determining.* People behave as they do out of intelligent choice and intention. They are the "authors of their actions" (Reason, 1994, p. 41). In order to interpret and understand human action, those engaged in the action must be involved in making decisions about how they will participate in the inquiry and what meaning can be interpreted from their actions. Traditional research methods purposely exclude "subjects" from the decision making in the research process. "Such exclusion treats the subjects as less than self-determining persons, alienates them from the inquiry process and from the knowledge that is its outcome, and thus, invalidates any claim the methods have to a science of persons" (Reason, 1994, p. 325). From a cooperative inquiry perspective, what people do and experience as part of the research must, to some degree, be determined by them.

2. *There are at least four types of knowledge.* Cooperative inquiry is based on an epistemology, which includes four types of knowledge: experiential knowledge, which is gained by direct experience with people, places, or things; practical knowledge, which is knowing how to perform some skill or task; propositional knowledge, which is knowledge about something usually expressed in statements or theories; and presentational knowledge, which is the way we represent our experiences through spatio-temporal images such as drawing, writing, dancing, or story telling. In Cooperative Inquiry, propositional knowledge has to be grounded in the experiential, presentational, and practical knowledge of the subjects in the inquiry. For example, propositional knowledge (theory) about

health promotion should be considered in relation to the nurses' experiences of health promotion (experiential knowledge), their way of describing health promotion (presentational knowledge), and their ability to practice health promotion (practical knowledge).

3. *Critical subjectivity is required.* As part of the inquiry process, participants have the opportunity to develop "critical awareness of the theories and ideas that they bring to their actions in the world" (Reason, 1994, p. 42) and to see the extent to which their experiences are congruent with these theories. In this way, both theory and practice are refined. The subsequent form of consciousness that arises from this process is called critical subjectivity (Torbert, 1991, p. 221). Schon (1983), in describing reflection in action, explains the process thus:

When we go about the spontaneous, intuitive performance of actions in everyday life, we show ourselves to be knowledgeable in a special way. Often we cannot say what it is that we know. When we try to describe it, we find ourselves at a loss or we produce explanations that are obviously inappropriate. Our knowing is ordinarily tacit, implicit in our pattern of action and in our feel for the stuff with which we are dealing. It seems right to say that our knowledge is in our action. (p. 49)

Within the research context, as nurses reflect on their practice, they expose and critique their own and each others' assumptions underlying their actions.

Phases of Cooperative Inquiry: The Research Process

Based on these assumptions, the process of cooperative inquiry engages participants in rigorous iterations of action and reflection that result in the integration of systematic inquiry and human experience. Cooperative inquiry consists of three phases: initiating and planning the research, putting the model into practice (action), and reflecting on experiences and making sense (reflection). These phases are repeated in subsequent cycles between action and reflection. For instance, in the clinical evaluation study described later in the chapter, nurse educators engaged in four cycles of action and reflection to develop an evaluation strategy that would be consistent with health promotion.

Phase One: Initiating and Planning the Research

During the initial phase, the inquiry group is established and explores in depth the phenomena under study. The research questions are clarified and the research methodology is learned by those not familiar with it. It is helpful to pose conditional questions at this phase. For example, in the nursing evaluation study described next, the conditional question was, "What would it look like if we evaluated students from a human science, health promotion perspective?"

Also in Phase One, a *conceptual* model or framework is created that articulates the group's collective best understanding, at the time, of the critical elements of a human science model/framework for health promotion practice. The relationship among the elements may also be described. Experiential knowledge is often complemented with propositional knowledge by various group members sharing articles, readings, or books.

The group completes this phase by developing an action plan for the next phase, including deciding how the group members will observe and record their own and each other's experiences. The methods chosen tend to be naturalistic (Guba & Lincoln, 1984) and include observations, keeping journals, interviewing each other, collecting critical incidents, and audiotaping or videotaping interactions.

Phase Two: Action—Putting the Model into Practice

The action phase takes place in the day-to-day lives of the practitioners. The members of the inquiry group, considered co-researchers in Phase One, now become co-subjects as they engage in practice and monitor their experiences. During this phase, the model developed in Phase One is vetted in relation to practice experiences. It is imperative that the members of the inquiry group not become committed to the recently conceived model but rather hold it tentatively to test its validity in practice. Practitioners need to be aware of the key components constituting their conceptual model so that they can recognize these components if and when they occur but without imposing their new knowledge on

their experiences. In this way, they are open to seeing how practice is similar to or different from their original conceptualization. This is a time for "thinking past the limitations of current practice towards the truly creative" (Reason, 1994, p. 33). At some point practitioners usually become deeply engaged in the experience of their practice. Some may experience remarkable insights or discover new awareness of themselves or their practice. In the clinical evaluation study described later, the nurse educators became co-subjects as they experimented with their newly developed evaluation strategy in their day to day work with students in the clinical area. Through this experimentation, they became more aware of the limitations of their earlier evaluation methods and revised their tentative model based on these insights.

Phase Three: Reflecting on Experiences and Making Sense

At a prearranged time, the group reconvenes to begin the process of making sense of each members' experiences. This phase is characterized by a reconsideration of the tentative model developed in Phase One in light of the members' experiences while experimenting with their conceptualizations in practice. These considerations direct the future cycles of action and reflection. The group may decide to continue to pursue their original notions or they may decide to alter their conceptualizations because of their practice experiences. New questions may be raised and different actions may be planned.

Subsequent Cycles

These three phases are repeated, cycling six to ten times for a predetermined duration. The duration varies depending on the issue being studied, but it usually ranges from 6 to 18 months. Greater understanding is developed with each cycle. The information generated about practice is considered in light of the original frameworks and research questions. In this way, propositional knowledge is considered in relation to experiential, presentational, and practical knowledge. Refinements are made to the framework or model and to the data collection methods that are established for the next cycle of action. Practitioners return to their work and continue to generate data about their practice using the methods determined by the group and their new understanding of their practice. Subsequently, the new data that are generated are again analyzed using the appropriate methods and another cycle begins. Each cycle develops further knowledge about the phenomena being studied.

Empowering and Transformative Processes of Cooperative Inquiry

Cooperative inquiry is a catalyst in changing nursing practice because it engages nurses in three critical empowering processes that encourage transformation: creating collaborative relationships, engaging in critical dialogue, and reflecting in action.

Creating Collaborative Relationships

Collaborative relationships are created within the cooperative inquiry group. Collaborative relationships are egalitarian relationships; these relationships are based on trust, mutual respect, and shared power. All participants are viewed as having different, but equally valued, perspectives to contribute to the research process.

Establishing these types of relationships is much more difficult and complex than is often realized. It is difficult for people who have more power by virtue of their education, status, or rank, to value the contributions of others with different experiences and knowledge. For example, it is difficult for a nurse administrator, educator, or researcher to equally value the contribution of a nurse who has recently graduated. But if cooperative inquiry is to be successful in transforming nursing practice, all nurses engaged in the inquiry must value the contribution of all participants. As an example, it may be helpful to establish ground rules for group participation and discuss the ways that power may influence group process. The role of establishing these relationships usually falls first to the initiating researcher. Ideally, this responsibility is shifted early to the whole group, requiring that all participants protect and advance the synergistic alliance that is created by developing these types of relationships.

Engaging in Critical Dialogue

Engaging in critical dialogue promotes critical thinking, critical reflection, the creation of new knowledge, and the discovery of personal meaning (Hills, 1998). This type of dialogue demands that participants challenge their own and each others' assumptions, engage in critical debate, and demonstrate respect—all at the same time! Participants can feel overwhelmed, disillusioned, or exhilarated. Most importantly, at the end of such dialogue, participants should feel that their ideas were challenged but that their self-esteem is still intact (Hills, 1998). Freire (1972) contends that, through the process of critical dialogue, people can become "masters of their thinking by discussing the thinking and views of the world explicitly or implicitly in their own suggestions and those of their comrades" (p. 95). The act of finding one's voice can be a very empowering experience.

Reflecting-in-Action

Reflection is sometimes thought of as an internal process that occurs within us. Thinking of reflection in this way, separating thought from action, neglects the dialectical nature of the process. Viewed as a dialectic, reflection means that people can consider their actions and at the same time consider their thoughts about those actions—they develop insight. This has been referred to as reflection-in-action (Carr & Kemmis, 1986). Reflection-in-action is fundamental to transformation because change will not occur without insight.

Cooperative inquiry engages people in reflection-in-action by having them constantly reexamine their knowledge about the subject of the inquiry. And, as stated, cooperative inquiry assumes that there are four types of knowledge: propositional, presentational, experiential, and practical. Group members move through cycles of action and reflection, considering their practical and experiential understanding of phenomena in relation to their empirical or theoretical understanding. Through this process they develop insight.

When nurses engage in cooperative inquiry, they develop insight by reflecting on their actions and making choices about how to change their practice. For example, in one study, nurses examined their experiences of health promotion practice in acute care settings (described later), they discovered that their values of health promotion were intrinsic to their job satisfaction. They explained that the hegemony of the institution often made it difficult for them to practice in a way that was consistent with their values. Through the process of reflection-in-action, they are developing strategies for change. Connor (1998) suggested that engaging in this type of reflective inquiry would advance the discipline of nursing and would facilitate bridging the gap between theory and practice.

Exemplars of Cooperative Inquiries from Other Disciplines

This methodology has been used extensively and with great success by many disciplines in Britain (Archer & Whitaker,1994; DeVenney-Tiernan, Goldband, Rackham, & Reilly, 1994; Marshall & McLean, 1988; Reason, 1988; Traylen, 1994) and is gaining recognition in Australia and in North America (Whitmore, 1994; Treleaven, 1994) as a useful research methodology to bring about change.

Youth Care

DeVenney-Tiernan and colleagues (1994) demonstrated that cooperative inquiry is a useful catalyst in changing practices of training and qualifying youth care workers. By examining the role of reflection in the process of learning for these workers, the researchers/ workers were able to identify 10 norms that influenced workers' taking ownership for their learning. The youth care workers were able to implement many changes as they discovered them and also made recommendations about alternative routes to qualification.

The research team concluded that, although many of the group members were not academics, many of the skills needed to conduct cooperative inquiry were present in the various group members. Further, their experience with the methodology strengthened their conviction to collaborative research and they "believe that any group of people committed to a particular area of research can employ a full blown collaborative inquiry method" (p. 137).

Government

Marshall and McLean (1988) used cooperative inquiry to examine organizational cul-

ture in a government district in England. Through a series of structured reflective processes, the inquiry group identified several themes that were apparent in the organizational structure. Although the authors raised some questions about the full participatory nature of the inquiry, they concluded that:

Their organization is using the analysis as a basis for future action and policy. What is more, the learning generated in this exercise is still alive and present within the organization, not just in the form of a report and presentations but carried and kept alive by the members of the research group who participated in the original study. (p. 220)

In contrast to "traditional" research that often does not lead to change, many cooperative inquiries result in ongoing change processes that are reflected in the day-to-day work of practitioners. It is reasonable to assume that a similar benefit could be derived by nurses who engage in cooperative inquiry.

University

Treleaven (1994) demonstrated that cooperative inquiry was an effective methodology to bring about organizational change in a university setting. This project challenged the assumptions of many staff development managerial programs. Incorporating a collaborative research process made it possible to move away from both the university's outdated training model and its traditional approaches to management training. Further, this process enabled the group to examine ways in which a gendered culture was produced and reproduced in its workplace. In the same way, nurses engaged in cooperative inquiry could create their own vision of nursing practice, despite the pressures of tradition.

Physicians

A study conducted with a group of physicians in England (Reason, 1988) was influential in conceptualizing the studies with groups of nurses that are described later in this chapter. A physician inquiry group systematically explored the theory and practice of holistic medicine. The group was committed to providing a better service to patients and to increasing the personal satisfaction that the physicians experienced in their work. The group engaged in six cycles of action and reflection, consisting of two-day reflection meetings followed by six-week intervals of application and data generation. The most common ways of recording experiences consisted of keeping diaries, observing each others' work, and recording interactions with patients. A five part model of holistic medicine was developed and formed the basis of the inquiry through the six stages of action and reflection. The holistic medicine study demonstrated that:

It is possible to inquire systematically and rigorously into a complex field of human action, and do justice to its wholeness without distorting or fragmenting it; it is possible to link inquiry and action in fruitful and illuminating ways; it is possible to co-opt busy practitioners into committed inquiry into their own professional and personal processes; it is possible for co-researchers to descend into the confusion of chaos and order that is real life without the protective clothing of questionnaires, experimental designs, and other forms of defensive armour, and to emerge with worthwhile understandings. (p. 125)

This study provides a successful analogy for transforming nursing practice and demonstrates in particular that busy practitioners can change their own practice through a thoughtful approach.

Transforming Nursing Practice

The following exemplars demonstrate how the cooperative inquiry methodology has been used with respect to nursing practice. The first two demonstrate how cooperative inquiry can be used to transform practice. The last exemplar is an ongoing research project and pays particular attention to how cooperative inquiry can be used specifically to focus nursing practice on health promotion.

Cooperative Inquiry with Health Visitors

This study was conducted in England and explored the sources of stress in public health nursing (health visitor) practice (Traylen, 1994). The researchers came to understand that much of the stress that they were ex-

periencing originated from hidden agendas in their work. The stress was related to the nurses' unexpressed and unexplored suspicions about problems within the families that they were visiting. Through the cooperative inquiry process the nurses experimented and learned ways to confront these hidden agendas and they implemented the new strategies in their practice. Following several action and reflection cycles, the nurses wrote a report to share their learning with others. They concluded that this methodology not only helped the nurses express their feelings about real problems but also enabled them "to move towards more open and constructive relationships with their clients, with each other, with other agencies and with their managers. It provided . . . a means of finding a better and more effective way of practising as health visitors" (Traylen, 1994, p. 81).

Clinical Evaluation Study

Several members of the faculty of a university-based school of nursing formed an inquiry group with 24 students to explore issues related to evaluating student performance in a way that held true to the principles of health promotion (see Chapter 17 of this book). The school had reoriented its curriculum to be consistent with the philosophy and principles of health promotion and recognized that an evaluation method that was consistent with a health promotion perspective needed to be developed.

Viewing evaluation from a health promotion perspective required a shift in thinking from the traditional biomedical approach that endorses the use of behavioral objectives and outcomes to a focus on students' abilities to understand people and their experiences of health and healing and on their abilities to work from an ethic of caring (Chap. 17 of this book, p. 229).

The inquiry group completed the three phases of cooperative inquiry and engaged in several iterations of planning, acting, and reflecting. By engaging in critical dialogue, the inquiry group members were able to think differently about student evaluation. A transformative perspective was created when they came to understand the importance of considering evaluation in terms of accessing students' thinking about their practice.

After several cycles of action and reflection, an evaluation methodology was developed that was consistent with the principles of health promotion and included the following critical components: Students wrote narrative accounts from their practice; students reflected on their accounts from practice using an analytical framework designed for this purpose; teachers read the students' accounts and critiques and posed critical questions to encourage further exploration; and students responded to teachers' comments and questions.

Nurses' Experiences of Health Promotion Practice in Acute Care Settings

Recently, five practicing nurses, educated in the nursing program referred to in the previous section, formed a new inquiry group to explore ways to practice health promotion in acute care settings. The nurses work in different clinical areas but they all agree that they are facing a similar challenge: How do they (and other nurses) practice from a health promotion perspective when they are situated in a system that militates against, and places no value on, this type of practice?

In the planning phase, the inquiry group held several meetings to deepen its members' understanding of nursing health promotion practice. It soon became clear that, because this way of practicing differs greatly from traditional models, descriptions for this model of practice have yet to be developed. Thus the model development aspect of cooperative inquiry was particularly useful in this study in that it allowed critical analysis of existing practices while at the same time it furthered the evolution of a new approach to nursing.

The group decided on the research question: "What would it look like if we practiced nursing from a health promotion perspective?" It was hoped that if models of practice could be articulated, the group could more readily describe nurses' health promotion practices to others. Through critical dialogue and reflection, a model for health promotion practice was developed and articulated. It contains the following eight key components: valuing everyone's experience; understanding the patient's perspective; including the family; acknowledging that people are entitled

to be in control (they have a right to choose and to make decisions); recognizing the value of taking time with patients; understanding the context of peoples' lives (where they come from and where they are going); recognizing teachable moments; creating emancipatory-empowering environments; and having a voice. Because the members of the group wanted to remain open to their experiences in the clinical area, they chose neither to define the key components too specifically nor to articulate the relationship among them too concretely. "In this way, the really significant issues can emerge from creative interaction with a domain, rather than be imported into it from the outset" (Heron, 1996, p. 75).

The group discussed possible methods that could be used to generate data from practice and decided to collect narrative accounts of their practice over a five-week period. All the narratives were transcribed and distributed to each group member for initial analysis. The group members met to discuss their perspectives and to reflect on what was learned from the analysis in order to refine the model of practice. In this way, propositional knowledge was considered in relation to experiential and practical knowledge embodying the essence of cooperative inquiry.

From this analysis, it became apparent that nurses need to feel satisfied with the way that they work with their clients in particular situations. This major component of the participants' practices was reflected in their narratives but not in their original conceptualization of a model for health promotion practice. In addition, it was noted that very little medical terminology or disease pathology was described in the narratives. The model of practice was revised based upon these new understandings. It was decided that the group members would continue to collect narrative accounts of their practice.

The group members entered the next action phase as they returned to practice to experiment with and generate data about the new conceptualizations of health promotion nursing practice. It is anticipated that, through several iterations of reflection and practice, the evolution of a health promotion nursing practice model will continue.

CONCLUSION

It is timely for nurses to face the challenge of transforming their practice in ways to be more aligned with the emerging trends of health promotion. Physicians and nurses share many characteristics, not the least of which is intransigence. But just as the physicians in Britain were able to transform their practice through the use of cooperative inquiry, so too can nurses.

Nurses can be leaders in bringing about change in the health system by systematically addressing the issues arising out of nursing culture and medical and behavioral approaches to health. From the preliminary studies conducted with nurses about their health promotion practices, it is reasonable to conclude that nurses can engage with clients in ways that both promote client control and create an emancipatory, empowering environment. Clients can participate fully in the decisions that affect their health and nurses can base their care on the client's perspective and experiences without undermining professional judgement, knowledge, and skills. It is possible to transform nursing practice.

✳ Reflective Questions

1. How will you participate in the transformation of nursing practice?
2. How could you initiate a process in your workplace to form an inquiry group to focus on transforming nursing practice?
3. Where would you begin?
4. Who would you need to involve?

REFERENCES

Archer, L., & Whitaker, D. (1994). Developing a culture of learning through research partnership. In P. Reason (Ed.), *Participation in human inquiry* (pp. 163–186). London: Sage.

Berland, A., Whyte, N., & Maxwell, L. (1995). Hospital nurses and health promotion. *Canadian Journal of Nursing Research, 27*(4), 13–31.

Bevis, E., & Watson, J. (1989). *Toward a caring curriculum: A new pedagogy for nursing.* New York: National League of Nursing.

Carr, W., & Kemmis, S. (1986). *Becoming critical.* Lewes: Falmer Press.

Connor, M. (1998). Expanding the dialogue on praxis in nursing research and practice. *Nursing Science Quarterly, 11*(2), 51–55.

DeVenny-Tiernan, M., Goldband, A., Rackham, L., & Reilly, N. (1994). Creating collaborative relationships in a co-operative inquiry. In P. Reason (Ed.), *Participation in human inquiry* (pp. 120–137). London: Sage.

Freire, P. (1972). *Pedagogy of the oppressed.* London: Penguin Books.

Gott, M., & O'Brien, M. (1990). The role of the nurse in health promotion. *Health Promotion International, 5,* 137–143.

Green, L., George, M., Daniel, M., Frankish, J., Herbert, C., Bowie, C., & O'Neil, M. (1995). *Study of participatory research in health promotion.* Ottawa: The Royal Society of Canada.

Guba, E., & Lincoln, Y. (1984). *Naturalistic inquiry.* Beverly Hills, CA: Sage.

Heron, J. (1996). *Co-operative inquiry.* London: Sage.

Hills, M. (1998). Student experiences in nursing health promotion practice in hospital settings. *Nursing Inquiry, 5,* 164–173.

Hills, M., & Lindsey, L. (1994). Health promotion: A viable curriculum framework for nursing education. *Nursing Outlook, 42*(4), 158–162.

Hills, M., Lindsey, L., Chisamore, M., Bassett-Smith, J., Abbot, K., & Fournier-Chalmers, J. (1994). University-college collaboration: Rethinking curriculum development in nursing education. *Journal of Nursing Education, 33*(5), 220–225.

Kendall, S. (1993). Client participation in health promotion encounters with health visitors. In J. Wilson-Barnett & J. Macleod Clark (Eds.), *Research in health promotion research and nursing* (pp.107–118). London: Macmillan.

Labonte, R. (1993). Health promotion and empowerment: Practice frameworks. In *Issues in Health Promotion 3.* Toronto: Centre for Health Promotion, University of Toronto.

Latter, S. (1993). Health education and health promotion in acute ward areas. In J. Wilson-Barnett &

J. Macleod Clark (Eds.), *Research in health promotion research and nursing* (pp. 61–71). London: Macmillan.

Lovell, M. (1981). Silent but perfect partners: Medicine's use and abuse of women. *Advances in Nursing Science, 3,* 25–40.

McBride, A. (1994). Health promotion in hospitals: The attitudes, beliefs, and practices of hospital nurses. *Journal of Advanced Nursing, 20,* 92–100.

Macleod Clark, J. (1993). From sick nursing to health nursing: evolution or revolution? In J. Wilson-Barnett & J. Macleod Clark (Eds.), *Research in health promotion research and nursing* (pp. 249–255). London: Macmillan.

Maglacas, A. (1988). Health for all: Nursing's role. *Nursing Outlook, 36,* 66–71.

Marshall, J., & McLean, A. (1988). In P. Reason (Ed.), *Human inquiry in action* (pp. 199–220). London: Sage.

Raeburn, J. (1992). Health promotion research with heart: Keeping a people perspective. *Canadian Journal of Public Health, 83,* 20–24.

Reason, P. (Ed.). (1988). *Human inquiry in action.* London: Sage.

Reason, P. (Ed.). (1994). *Participation in human inquiry.* London: Sage.

Reason, P., & Rowan, J. (Eds.). (1981). *Human inquiry: A sourcebook of new paradigm research.* London: John Wiley & Sons.

Robinson, A. (1995). Transformative "cultural shifts" in nursing: Participatory action research and the "project of possibility." *Nursing Inquiry, 2,* 65–74.

Schon, D. (1983). *The reflective practitioner.* Boston: Basic Books.

South Australian Health Commission. (1988). *Health for the nation.* South Australia: Ministry of Health.

Torbert, W. *The power of balance: Transforming self, society and scientific inquiry.* Newberry Park, CA: Sage.

Traylen, H. (1994). Confronting hidden agendas: Co-operative inquiry with health visitors. In P. Reason (Ed.), *Human inquiry in action* (pp. 59–81). London: Sage.

Treleaven, L. (1994). Making space: A collaborative inquiry with women as staff development. In P. Reason (Ed.), *Participation in human inquiry* (pp. 138–162). London: Sage.

Wass, A. (1994). *Health promoting.* Marrickville, Australia: Harcourt Brace.

Whitmore, E. (1994). To tell the truth: Working with oppressed groups in participatory approaches to inquiry. In P. Reason (Ed.), *Participation in human inquiry* (pp. 82–98). London: Sage.

Whyte, N., & Berland, A. (1993). *The role of hospital nurses in health promotion.* Vancouver: Registered Nurses Association of British Columbia.

Wilson-Barnett, J., & Macleod Clark, J. (1993). *Research in health promotion research and nursing.* London: Macmillan.

World Health Organization. (1986). *The Ottawa charter for health promotion.* Copenhagen: Author.

SECTION FIVE

A Critique of Transformative Health Promotion Practice

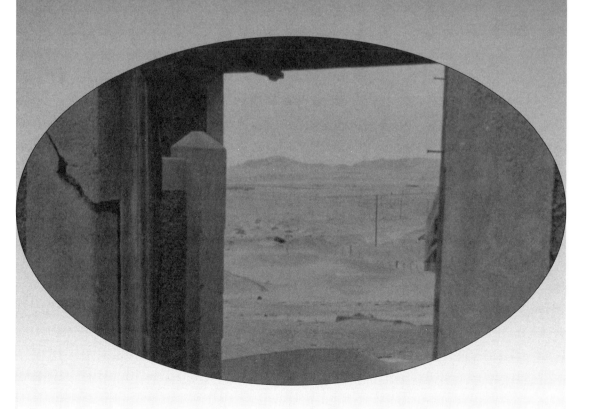

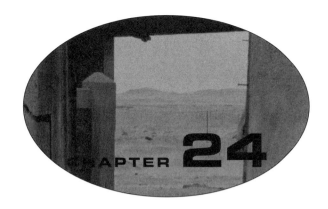

CHAPTER 24

Transforming Practice, Dodging False Dichotomies, and Avoiding Ideological Quicksand

LAWRENCE W. GREEN
MARK DANIEL

Coming to this final chapter, we glance back at the initial chapters to try to tie a thread between the history told there, through the concepts and experiences reported in the intervening chapters, to a door here that could help launch the young professionals reading this into a transformed practice. The student might despair at this point that anything short of massive change at the institutional level, with reduced disparities between social groups, with equalized socioeconomic opportunities, and with each intervention justified by a transformed practice based on a unique participatory research project, will be fruitless.

The radical vision of transformed practice that emerges from these chapters, inspiring as it might be at one level, could also have a numbing effect. It could make the practical methods that students and young professionals are learning in their day-to-day preparation, and the skills they have the opportunity to practice in the institutions that employ them, seem futile. We seek in this final chapter to encourage the vision while acknowledging the importance—indeed the growing centrality—of some traditional nursing practices in the emerging epidemiologic and demographic circumstances of the 21st century.

The Individual and the Collective Good

In Chapter 1 Young suggests that transforming health promotion practice will require working with the client at the individual level, but taking into more active consideration the meaning that client attaches to health constructed as a social, historical, cultural, "gendered," and economic phenomenon. In Chapter 2 MacDonald recounts and celebrates the 1960s turning point from the era of neoliberal individualism toward greater concerns for social justice. Her vision of a transformed practice might be seen as a shift from individual patient care to population health concerns.

We subscribe to a community-oriented, population-based notion of health promotion, and we relish the task of weaving a thread through this stimulating series of chapters that would help nurses connect to that broader, ecological enterprise (Green, 1990). But we do not believe that each practitioner must be personally responsible for interventions outside the sphere of individual patient or client care. We must ask whether

325

the critiques of current practice warrant a radical leap from the individual patient care roles to some form of transformed practice that the more ambitious reader might imagine. Does the transformed practice really have to hold itself accountable for community-wide impact, and influencing distal rather than proximal determinants of health, as the population health and social-determinants orientations would argue, for example? We believe that a community-wide, ecological effect is achieved not by each practitioner, but by the combined effect of many practitioners working on many different levels.

Even the Ottawa Charter, for all its transformational rhetoric, as chronicled by Young's and MacDonald's chapters, acknowledges that personal health care, self-care, and chronic disease self-management for individuals remain important points of intervention in health promotion. Interventions in any of these settings, in support of any of these processes in traditional health care practice, qualify as health promotion by most of the more balanced perspectives on health promotion (Poland, Green, & Rootman, 2000). The authors and editors of this book have taken pains to locate health promotion in a broad range of settings besides the broad community and primary prevention reach of population health. They have included examples of health promotion in critical care, chronic illness care, and long-term care, as well as the settings identified with community health promotion.

Are nursing and other health care professions prisoners of the individualistic focus of the institutions in which they practice? Does their patient care setting for practice mean they cannot "do" ecological approaches? Does it mean they are inexorably destined to tinker at the margins of family, community, and policy approaches to health promotion? The unfortunate false dichotomy of individual and ecological approaches has made such questions necessary to address because so many practitioners feel marginalized by the rhetoric of health promotion. Ecology consists not of something outside and beyond the individual, but of an interaction between the individual and his or her environment, a reciprocal relationship between behavior and environment (Bandura, 1986). The ecological contribution of health care practitioners working in clinical settings can be just as important as that of community health practitioners working in public health departments. An ecological approach is not something anybody "does" single-handedly. It is the sum of the many practitioners' efforts contributing to a community's health (Green, Richard, & Potvin, 1996). Each practitioner working with individuals, families, institutions, or neighborhoods is contributing to an ecological approach so long as there is some coordination and harmonization of the efforts made at each of these levels.

Young, in Chapter 1, captures at the cognitive, interpersonal, and experiential levels the ecological notion of reciprocal interaction between person and environment. "Health promotion practice founded on these assumptions is a transformative process in which the nurse as partner engages clients in a consciousness raising process characterized by a respect for the dynamic relatedness between people and the environment." MacDonald, in turn, raises the ante and the challenge to nursing by invoking the Ottawa Charter's call for health promotion that takes "action on the social determinants of health and illness, social responsibility for health, and collective action." We hope nursing as a profession can find ways to contribute to the latter without neglecting the former, and without leaving its entry-level practitioners feeling like failures if they have little opportunity in their day-to-day practice to participate directly in the collective action.

The Individual and the Structural

Another false dichotomy, similar to the individual versus the collectivity, might arise in reading the tendency of some of the chapters to overwork the distinction between health promotion directed at individuals and that directed at structural changes. This dichotomy is more complicated, because, unlike the individual-collectivity or individual-population dichotomy, it is not just a matter of scale or aggregation. It amounts to nearly the same thing in operational terms for health promotion, however, insofar as the usual assumption about interventions to affect population health or the collective good is that they must be directed at structures, not individuals. This assumption flies in the face of the reality in democratic societies that structural changes require considerable public awareness, informed consent, or assent and cooperation. Most changes in policy require political support. If they are passed legislatively or by administrative decree, with the intent of affecting behavior, the history of seat belt laws, tobacco control laws, alcohol abolition, motorcycle helmet laws, and others tell us that inadequate preparation of the public through health education predicts widespread noncompliance. Attempts to enforce such structural changes passed against the will of the public often results in the laws or policies being overturned.

Even if we could have structural change without individuals giving their assent at the point of passing the policies or at the point of complying with them, we could not have widespread individual change without some structural modification. Making the personnel available to affect an individualistic behavioral change strategy such as smoking cessation, weight control counseling, or any other complex behavior modification program would require structural changes in personnel policy at the very least. It also might require structural changes in health insurance or health system reimbursement policies. Even with these elements of structural change in place, behavior modification requires attention to the environmental cues, barriers, and rewards that predispose, enable, and reinforce the old and the new behavior. These cues, barriers, and rewards require structural changes of some kind for effective change even of the most individualistically directed behavior.

Proximal and Distal Determinants of Health

The individual-structural dichotomy has greater meaning to most practitioners when cast as a metaphor of upstream and downstream interventions (McKinlay, 1975). Upstream refers to interventions on the more distal determinants of health. These include the genetic, fetal, and early childhood conditions of the individual or group, the socioeconomic conditions that expose the individual to differential risks, the commercial or industrial positioning of products conducive or harmful to health, and the government poli-

cies that make health resources more or less accessible (Kuh & Ben-Shlomo, 1997). What characterizes most upstream or distal determinants is that they are largely beyond the control of the individual by the time their inevitable effects on health trajectories become apparent. Downstream refers to the more proximal determinants that present themselves as target opportunities for the practitioner trying to help individuals or groups cope with a presenting or immediately threatening health problem or need.

The focus on proximal determinants of health would seem to be what Young in Chapter 1 and MacDonald in Chapter 2 object to most in what they characterize as the "individualistic," "behavioral," and "lifestyle" approaches or traditions of health promotion practice. Yet, the proximal becomes central to the transformational practice outlined in Hartrick's Chapter 3 on the significance of relationships, and in Thorne's Chapter 4 on promoting health at the client-professional interface. People who live with a chronic condition deserve the best that practitioners can offer in understanding the "here and now" of their life circumstances and in relating to them as co-participants in coping with the proximal determinants of their symptoms or course of the disease (Daniel & Green, 1999). They do not need political posturing, system blaming, guilt-arousing victim blaming, or parent-blaming moralization about the distal determinants of their health condition.

Participatory Principles

One theme or thread that emerges throughout this book is the importance of the patient, client, or population as active participants in their care or the promotion of their health. MacDonald in Chapter 2, Thorne in Chapter 4, Starzomski in Chapter 5, Northrup's Chapter 9 on self-care, and Berland and Young's Chapter 16 with their emphasis on the patient's role in defining quality, all drive home a message of participation. Starzomski questions the sincerity of some token forms of client participation. Thorne cautions against simplistic acceptance of "compliance" models of self-care, noting instances in which patients actively identify themselves as noncompliant to signal "their active resistance against what they deem to be inappropriate authority over their lives." Northrup examines the myth of self-care that merely suits the needs of the health care system to offload some of its responsibility. VanderPlaat's Chapter 6 calls into question notions of empowerment that fail to transfer power from an agent to a subject.

In all of these, the essential element of active as opposed to passive participation calls for a degree of emancipation from the provider-consumer, provider-patient relationship in which the term provider implies a holder of powers that cannot be commanded by the other. The core of that power is information or knowledge. It follows that a core of health promotion should be the transfer of "knowledge power" or "information power." Making this transfer primarily through patient teaching is simply another form of the same provider-consumer relationship, insofar as the transfer depends on the provider possessing the knowledge and being in a position to control the amount and type of information transferred.

One antidote to this is what Hartrick in Chapter 3 calls "the mutuality of health promoting relationships" in which health practitioners are no longer the ones in charge of the relating, but are engaged in a mutual process of engagement. This is not a new concept, having been developed rather systematically under the notion of the "activated patient" (Sehnert & Eisenberg, 1975; Roter, 1977) in the 1970s. Hartrick puts the notion on a more theoretically grounded basis with complexity theory and the "butterfly effect," giving greater credence to the power of small changes to affect more substantial changes.

Another approach to the power imbalance is to place the patient, family, or community in a direct role as active participants in collecting the data that go into the knowledge construction (Green, George, Daniel, Frankish, Herbert, Bowie, & O'Neill, 1995; George, Daniel, & Green, 1999). This falls more clearly under the rubric of participatory research, a concept that has a growing following within health promotion because of its consistency with many of the principles and methods of health promotion. As applied in patient care settings, it may involve participation in the diagnosis, in self-monitoring of vital signs or behavioral and environmental determinants, and in evaluation of the interventions. Thorne in Chapter 4 gives some

ways in which health care professionals stand to gain from greater attention to "consumer analyses."

The Post-Modern, Deconstructed Science Invoked

This book, in some chapters, seems inclined to build a post-modern health promotion on the ashes of science. For all our enthusiasm in tracing some of the ideas described earlier, we find ourselves most uncomfortable in following the more radical lines of deconstruction as the rationale for a new health promotion. As Goethe (1855) warned in Faust:

Scoff at all knowledge and despise
reason and science, those flowers of mankind.
Let the father of all lies
with dazzling necromancy make you blind,
then I'll have you unconditionally.

We would not expect Goethe to know what was to come to the minds of 20th century scholars, much less the 21st century nursing scholars, in their critiques of conventional reason and science. But his admonition not to let loathing of science blind us seems as relevant to health promotion as some authors' admonitions in this book not to let the conventions of science blind us. At the same time that we face growing pressure to justify our budgets and best practices on scientific evidence, we find in this book a thread of antagonism to traditions of science and scientific reasoning.

In Chapter 1, Young leads the attack with her historical account of the professional and scientific literature of the 1970s having a destabilizing effect on the "hallowed assumptions of science formulated in the 16th century through a re-envisioning of what counts as knowledge and reality." This characterization of science in the 1970s, both as a direct extension of science in the 1500s, and as a destabilized force in society, seems overdrawn to us. The science of the 1970s was a distant reflection of the nascent scientific stirrings of the 16th century. The historical thread worthy of note from 16th century science to the present is the demand that scientists at least make observations of nature rather than appeal and respond to the dogma of faith or hierarchical authority. This shift from the 15th century tendencies was, in Young's own words, "critical" and "emancipatory," in its liberation of people to achieve *reasoned* understandings of their environments, each other, and their relations to each other and their environments. This was the beginning of ecological thinking, relatively unencumbered by ideology or theology. Thus, the critical and emancipatory role of science itself began with the Enlightenment, not with the 1970s.

Latter-day criticisms of scientific methods and reasoning have added new dimensions to ways we can know our reality (or realities). They have, indeed, called into question the existence of a single reality, but these challenges to science have coexisted with science in philosophical writing since the earliest scientific writing. The debates between Plato and Socrates were on this very question, long predating the Dark Ages, the Renaissance, and the Enlightenment periods. How important are these challenges to scientific methods, reasoning, or data, in fashioning a transformed practice of health promotion? This would seem to depend on whether the task is to transform traditional, biomedically dominated practices in health care settings to make them more health promoting, or to transform existing health promotion practices to make them fit a new, post-modern paradigm (Daniel, Green, & Sheps, 1998). The editors' view is that the latter is needed to create a new playing field—one that might overcome "the relative invisibility of nurses' health-related work."

Having practiced health promotion largely in community settings reaching beyond or initiated outside health care institutions, we perhaps have less of the authors' sense of urgency for a paradigm overhaul. Our work in health promotion has not been quite so dominated by the biomedical paradigm; our health-related work has not been rendered so invisible as that of nurses.

The post-modern critique has perhaps served nursing more than some other health professions because of the greater urgency nurses might have felt to challenge the prevailing scientific methods employed in human sciences. Their practice might have placed them in closer, more intense, client relationships than many other professions so that they were more inclined to call into question the subject-object relationship of biomedical and behavioral sciences. They might be in a better position than others to see the need for a more participatory way of conducting research in partnership with those for whom the issues are a concern, and to take context and values into consideration. Their gender demographics might make them more receptive to the feminist critique and feminist approaches.

Acknowledging these reasons to appreciate the perspectives that nursing can bring to a more balanced understanding of health promotion, we approach our comments on some of the other chapters with diffidence and caution. We offer our observations and questions in the spirit of looking for a way to preserve the best of what past theory and science have given us in the health and service professions while hoping to draw on the special insights and experiences that nursing can bring to bear.

Some Cautious Comments and Questions on . . .

Chapter 3

Hartrick reaches beyond the assumptions underlying health promotion practice in the disease-care legacy of nursing in search of a phenomenological, rather than physical, basis for relating to clients or patients. She finds it in an "emancipatory health promotion" as "a *way-of-being* that is relational." It seeks a more "egalitarian, participatory form of alliance . . . practitioners do not just *act* collaboratively, they become collaborators." She urges a "mutuality of health promoting relationships" that is not "under the power of health practitioners." This does challenge the professional's assumption of relationships as a "means to an end" but in substituting the patient's assumptions and values, it might deny the needs or hopes of some patients to have the practitioner take control. Health promotion and communication skills might need to bring the patient or client to a more centered self-efficacy. Hartrick puts the onus on practitioners to get to an "in-relation" connectedness with the client, but there might be as much of a need, instrumental as it might necessarily be, to help the client get "in" the in-relation.

Chapter 4

Thorne builds a compelling case for practitioners to pay greater attention to the worldview, values, and understanding of consumers, patients, or clients, especially those living with chronic diseases. In doing so, she also makes a case, without naming it, for participatory research. She refers to her approach as "consumer analysis" by which we understand that she uses the chronic illness perspective and insights of her patients or consumers of health care to "understand our own ideological underpinnings and challenge us anew to re-examine and deconstruct them." She does this by "synthesizing insights from the interpretations of consumer research into chronic illness experience." The accounts she provides of health care interactions from her sources are, indeed, fascinating and full of insights and implications for nursing and its potential for a transformed practice of health promotion. Some of the insights must be time-, place-, condition- and culture-specific, limiting their generalizability. We suspect that the average practitioner would not have the training to replicate the methods used by Thorne and her colleagues in arriving at these new understandings. This leaves us to encourage nursing to employ participatory research (George, Daniel, & Green, 1999) more routinely in academic-practitioner-patient partnerships to update and particularize such useful knowledge.

Chapter 5

Starzomski takes a similarly critical view of the ways in which health care decision making tends to exclude "consumers" and ways in which the poorly conceptualized notions of consumer participation conspire against effective involvement. She acknowledges that participation can have untoward effects. From experience in British Columbia, we can also point to some instances of efforts to increase the participation of poor and other underrepresented segments of the population in health planning producing very unsatisfactory results for very good reasons from the point of view of the poor (Wharf-Higgins, Vertinsky, Cutt, & Green, 1999).

Chapters 6, 7, and 8

VanderPlaat presents "emancipatory approaches" to health promotion as theory and philosophy, and as social activism. She challenges nurses to view themselves as both practitioners and as social activists who can bring about social change. This challenge has much to recommend it for those whose careers have brought them to a point of recognizing the limits and the sources, causes, or reasons for the limitations of the health care systems in which they work. It might be viewed somewhat with some caution, however, by students whose careers are just beginning, who will be vulnerable in their first jobs. They might well be advised to support change through their professional associations, but one might argue that the professors and senior nurses should be the ones expected to take the risks associated with social activism. In arguing that nurses should examine "how our own privilege may disempower others . . . [and] use this privilege to challenge the disciplinary and institutional barriers that stand in the way of meaningful social change," the author might be viewed as more privileged than the students reading this chapter, and part of the institutional structure of nursing education that disempowers them. That this author is a sociologist and not a nurse might also make the reading of this chapter less compelling for student nurses. For these reasons, Chapter 6 provides a perfect opening to the next section in which Chapters 7 and 8 offer concrete examples of situations (three countries) and roles (transformational leadership) in which nurses can aspire to make a difference beyond the clinical level of intervention.

Chapters 9 and 22

Northrup takes a decidedly skeptical view of how the self-care movement has been managed and manipulated by commercial and professional interests. This chapter should be read in conjunction with McGowan's Chapter 22 on the implementation and evaluation of an arthritis self-management program in native communities of Canada. If Chapter 9 left you doubtful about the potential value to patients or consumers of self-care programs,

Chapter 22 will restore your hope that they can be done in a way that does not substitute expert values and knowledge for indigenous ones. McGowan offers an antidote, complete with quantitative and qualitative evaluation, for each of the toxins Northrup laments having crept into most self-care initiatives. If Northrup's main concerns are with the commercialization and professionalization of self-care, McGowan demonstrates how these aspects can be circumvented, especially if the request comes initially from the community, and the people who seek guidance in developing their self-management program remain involved in and in control of its development. McGowan's case example also illustrates another instance of participatory research.

Chapter 10

Liaschenko worries that health and health promotion, as morally charged concepts that have historically assumed individual responsibility and blame for good or bad health, also set up health care systems and institutions that become instruments of social control. She illustrates her thesis with paintings and posters depicting Hygeia and images of health in past and present eras. Her interpretations of the paintings and poster images run the usual risks of artistic interpretation, and she acknowledges that she "may be too harsh in my interpretation. . . ." One is tempted to consider other interpretations of the same paintings and posters and to draw a less worrisome conclusion, but the author's admonitions about the potential conflict between the aims of health care institutions and the aims of nursing might be equally supported by other sources of evidence.

Chapter 11

Kearney states her purpose to review from qualitative studies of women using the grounded theory approach, to provide a window on "the effect of practical and intangible conditions and constraints on health promoting behaviors." She begins with women's views on health itself and staying healthy, and then examines how beliefs are enacted in some common health issues faced in the

course of development and aging. She states her intention that the developmental order of presentation should serve to show how women modify the learning from earlier life points when new issues emerge as they age. A major limitation of Kearney's review, however, is that the studies reported on are apparently all cross-sectional, specific to a given point in time, not representative of change over time.

Some of the work is her own, other work is not. Kearney does not articulate her version of grounded theory. Although her reporting strategy is consistent with the intent of grounded theory—to represent concrete situations in their complexity—her descriptive exposition does not attempt to synthesize, nor to produce, nor to test, abstract theory. Her narrative understandings of women's experience are, however, poignant and insightful, rich in details relevant to better understanding factors influencing women's health-related behavior. It is unclear, though, why and how Kearney selected the studies she reviewed.

On views of health from within women's lives, Kearney reviews separately and contrasts health issues for women outside the European-origin majority with health issues for women in the American majority culture. Within the first grouping she also contrasts perspectives between Mexican-American and African-American women. Her sampling includes studies from across the United States as well as Canada. Of special note in this section is the extent of variation in cultural perspectives and health-related values.

The next section, on how women cope with body changes and attempt to defend against health risks across the lifespan, is notable for its breadth of focus on issues from menstruation and sexual risks to caregiving, menopause, and the vulnerability to chronic disease and functional losses that accompany aging. Racism, sexism, and "lookism" are addressed; however, although ethnic perspectives are represented, they are not contrasted.

The conclusion, even though acknowledging the diversity of experience and the effect of context on women's lives, is nevertheless rather sweeping in its recommendations for improving health-related opportunities for women across the life course. It is also unclear whether the object of Kearney's critique is the biomedically oriented health care system, public health education or outreach for health promotion and disease prevention, or broad social policy influencing women's health. Given the specificity of the material reviewed on health values and culturally shaped health orientations, it would seem that strategies for more effectively addressing women's health issues could be better brought into line with the specific needs of particular ethnic and age group combinations, toward reducing existing disparities in health outcomes, as well as access to health-related resources.

Chapter 12

Willinsky and Pape revisited the Canadian Mental Health Association's and Health Canada's attempt in the late 1990s to construct a general model of mental health promotion. They identified through literature reviews and focus groups the key elements of mental health promotion to include participation, choice, control, empowerment, and social support. They also note the commonalities in seeking to "address the population as a whole, including persons experiencing risk conditions, in the context of everyday life." These mirror some of the core concepts of the Ottawa Charter, as outlined in Chapter 2 by MacDonald. True to the Canadian and Ottawa Charter approaches to health promotion and population health, their approach to mental health promotion also orients them "towards taking action on the determinants of health, such as income and housing, rather than focusing on risk factors and conditions." This use of the term "determinants of health" in Canada has taken on a meaning of its own, somehow exclusive of the "risk factors and conditions" that are by most evidence the most dependable determinants of health, at least in the sense of more direct determinants. The more distal determinants mentioned here such as income and housing might be more important in the end, but they are indirect in most of their influences on health and they operate through risk factors, for the most part. They might, indeed, be referred to more appropriately as "risk conditions" (Green & Kreuter, 1999, p. 10).

Chapter 13

The extreme stereotypical case study "exemplar" of an aboriginal youth injured in a motorcycle accident admitted to an intensive care unit, and the actions of his rude and uncouth family members in the waiting room afterwards, provides a jarring opening for Chapter 13. Richardson rapidly presents her problem—a gap between knowledge from research carried out on the needs of the family members of critically ill persons and the application of that knowledge in nursing practice. She introduces her *Nursing Support Model* (referencing two unpublished papers) as a framework to guide nursing actions to promote the health of family members so that they in turn can be helpful to their critically ill relative. She then returns to the case study to use it as an example of how the attending nurse's actions were insufficient in providing support to the boy's family.

Chapter 13 then reviews the origins of support, nursing support specifically, and other types of support, before returning to the need for a framework to help practitioners choose actions and interventions to meet critical care needs as given by family members. In staking her claim (e.g., "Most recently, Hupcey & Morse (1997) posed the critical question I have been addressing for some time") and terminology (e.g., "'Instrumenting,' a term I coined"), Richardson allows that her model derives from earlier work by others, notably in ethics, and that she is pursuing development of the ethical framework, in terms of a concept analysis of nursing support, and a "meta-review" of the critical care literature.

The Nursing Support Model is described as composed of core concepts, informing theories, and practice theories. These are illustrated in a figurative portrayal of the model as a clover plant, with roots, a stalk, and a cloverleaf having germinated from the Human Caring Seed. The leaflet depicts dimensions of support focused on critical care family members by nurses: connecting, empowering, finding meaning, and instrumenting. Root forks underground are labeled with the names of theories: conservation theory, loss and grief theory, family systems theory, general systems theory, resiliency model, stress and coping theory, and crisis theory. Three sprouting buds are labelled as nurse integrity, family integrity, and patient integrity.

Richardson then reviews dimensions of support. She does not explain why she selected the theories that she did, and she does not relate the components of the model to the preceding review of the critical care literature. Nor does she discuss relations among constructs, or empirical work informing theoretical development or directly supporting her use of the theories chosen. She allows that her approach is "eclectic," and asserts its validity on the basis that the theories overlap and "no one theory ever encompasses every element of the critical care experience of families." The primary support or justification for her model is that it is "based on the literature."

In thinking about the empirical utility of the nursing support model, looking for procedures or plans for validating it, we come to the final section, to the first of two clinical exemplars, "a contrary case." The situation painted is of an infant on total life support after a serious head injury. Parental abuse is suspected. Richardson guides us through what happens when the model is not applied. The staff's behavior toward the parents is abhorrent. We proceed to the next exemplar, "a model case." The situation: Mr. Gee, a 46-year-old divorced, childless, and unemployed computer technician, is admitted to an ICU after being attacked by a relative at a family reunion. His blood alcohol level is high, and he is unconscious. The attending nurse applies the model. This ICU's nurse is an angel of goodness, described at length in the text. A medical resident commenting harshly on the patient's blood alcohol level, and labeling him an alcoholic on the basis of a CAT scan showing brain atrophy, is expertly rebuked by the nurse who, on the basis of having applied the model, knows better. Mr. Gee's family is meek and humble (in stark contrast to the pushy and foul-mouthed aboriginal family in the first exemplar). The model works in this case example, but awaits data to verify it in practice.

Chapter 14

Purkis begins Chapter 14 with an epigram by Norbert Elias, author of "Symbol Theory." She interprets the epigram as supporting her argument that "practice *is* theory." Her concern with "the theory-practice gap" leads her to question why theory should come first, acting to inform subsequent practice. Purkis does not comment explicitly on the Western tendency to separate subject from object, but she draws attention to such dualism in our conceptions of theory and practice and their perceived relationship to each other. She seems to favor practice over theory. She strives to convey the idea that practice, in and of itself, *is* theory, and that we might not try so hard, perhaps, to *impose* theory *on* practice. We would agree that even when practice (or research) is not founded on explicit theory, neither theory nor practice (or research) can be judged independently of the other. Readers of this chapter, however, will need to consult the source of the epigram to discern *how* Elias's notions of structures of language, and their meaning, are relevant to bridging the theory-practice gap.

Elias's sociolinguistic model of language argues that we need to approach the study of language and theory in terms of their social functions. We found it difficult to see how Elias's epigram can be construed as support for rendering theory and practice as inseparable. Whether Purkis has misread Elias the reader of both would have to judge.

Purkis introduces Michel Foucault's notion of "governmentality" (a link to the title of the chapter). Foucault is invoked regularly by deconstructivist/post-modernist theorists. He is considered to be among the most important social theorists of the 19th century. His work is frequently used to support "critical" critiques of science. We find it curious *why* Foucault tends to be interpreted and used as a "threat" to science, except that he drew strongly on history in his social theorizing. This had the effect of highlighting that science is "socially constructed." These days, most social scientists, at least, accept that science cannot help but be socially constructed, for it is the activity of communities of scientists, not individuals. Foucault saw science as a part of society, contributing to social actions in ways that were not always consistent with what scientists claimed science was doing, and he drew on history to illustrate this point. Foucault's notion of "governmentality" characterized the sociopolitical changes Western Europe was undergoing in the 18th and 19th

centuries, and referred to a growing appropri-
ation of strategies of social organization and
control previously contained primarily in mon-
astic traditions, the military, and hospitals. He
viewed his place and time as *reflecting* through
discipline the foundations of governance, in
the *processes* by which people had learned to
govern themselves rather being ruled in a hierarchical system. Foucault saw his era in terms
of a historic movement to self-governance, and
he saw bureaucratic organization as an enabling factor in this process.

Purkis uses "governmentality" to support
her notion that "practice is theory," but she
does not state why, or how, Foucault's historical perspectives on governmentality are important or relevant to her focus on the
context of nurse-parent-child interactions in
a present-day clinical setting. Beyond brief
mentions of how the clinical encounter acts
to encourage parents to "self-enforce" certain
state-approved parenting behavior, it is also
unclear to us how such actions can be construed as relating to the health of *populations.*
Her material on parent-nurse interactions is
intriguing and provocative in thinking about
these relationships in terms of governmentality and discipline. Indeed, her material might
prompt us to ask if these state-mandated behaviors are about health at all.

Purkis's data serve to situate the nurse clinician as the more powerful actor in the nurse-
parent dyad. In the role the nurse is fulfilling
via practice her theoretical purpose is that of
an instrument of governance, in gaining
entry to an emic understanding of family relationships that affect the health of the child,
and then intervening on health matters. The
historical linkage and the degree to which
nurses themselves are controlled and regulated bureaucratically by protocols, administrators, medical and facility rules, insurance
rules, and even by parent "clients" seem to be
missing in this discussion.

Although we question here exactly how
Foucault is relevant to Purkis's thesis, we do
realize that it is important to recognize how
"social control" is implicated in many contemporary "health management" practices. If
one looks to the ways in which Foucault has
been appropriated in sociology, cultural studies, and anthropology, then his work may
indeed be relevant to discussions such as
Purkis's. We should ask, however, to what
degree and in what sense Foucault's historical
work on 18th and 19th century sociopolitical
changes in Western Europe is relevant to specific cases in the 21st century. We should also
bear in mind that Foucault himself recognized his contemporary Gilles Deleuze as the
theorist of "the present," a time when social
regulation is characterized by diffuse forms of
"control" rather than by confined architec-
tures of discipline.

Chapter 16

Berland and Young ask what is quality of
care, a question central to health promotion
practice because it concerns itself with outcomes beyond the biological changes and the
structures or processes typically used to measure quality in health care. They answer that
quality must be understood from the patient's
perspective, and illustrate how this can be
measured in terms of patient satisfaction.
They offer the results of surveys of nursing
practice (Berland, Whyte, & Maxwell, 1995)
and patient satisfaction in hospitals (Charles
et al., 1994), and the Johari Window model
from cognitive psychology as approaches to
analyzing quality of care. They also consider
how working collaboratively with patients,
fostering mutual aid, and education can enhance communication between patients and
providers, and how research can contribute
to a better understanding of quality from patients' perspectives.

Chapter 17

Hills's chapter on "Perspectives on Learning
and Practicing Health Promotion in Hospitals:
Nursing Students' Stories" begins with an excerpt from a nursing student's narrative on
her first-year training experience. Hills then
introduces the focus on the Collaborative
Nursing Program in British Columbia (the
"B.C. Program"). She states that the purpose
of the chapter is to demonstrate that nursing
students educated from a health promotion
perspective do in fact "practice in a way that
reflects the central tenets of health promotion
on which the B.C. Program is based."

Hills states that the B.C. Program is "based
in its entirety on the philosophy and principles of health promotion [and that] students
are steeped in the rhetoric and discourse of

health promotion. . . ." One would hope that the students are immersed and educated in something more substantial than simply the rhetoric and discourse of health promotion, such as, for example, theory and theory-informed, evidence-based practice perspectives, planning, research and evaluation methods, skills in communication and community organization, and, of course, clinical skills.

Hills states that, in the context of her chapter, health promotion has a specific meaning and that it "is seen as being distinct from lifestyle change, illness prevention or health education." The definition given is that of the Ottawa Charter on Health Promotion (1986): "A process of enabling people to increase control over and to improve their health." We have difficulty seeing how lifestyle change, illness prevention, and health education can be made distinct from and not encompassed by the Ottawa Charter. This rhetorical attempt to distance one philosophy of health promotion from most of the practical, evidence-based grounding of health promotion has not served the field especially well if measured by the persistence of policy initiatives. Canadian leadership in this line of argument for a distinct health promotion independent of lifestyle change, disease prevention, and health education, for example, has not fared well in the latest round of reorganization in Health Canada. The term "health promotion" no longer exists in the bureaucratic structure, and most of the initiatives under the former Health Promotion Directorate are now encompassed by population health. Even in British Columbia, the Health Promotion Directorate disappeared from the Ministry of Health's organization chart six years after the Ottawa Charter and has not reappeared in the nine years since then.

Hills asserts that "three pillars of health promotion are embedded by the Ottawa Charter definition": (1) health promotion is primarily about people and secondarily about health (later labelled "the primacy of people"); (2) health promotion is about empowerment; and (3) health promotion is about enabling. She cites Labonte (1993), Raeburn (1992), Raeburn and Rootman (1997), and Wallerstein and Bernstein (1994) in support of this interpretation, and proceeds to discuss each "pillar." We have applauded Raeburn and Rootman's (1997) book on "the primacy of people" (Green, 1997). It is about valuing

and respecting people, respecting differences, and viewing the world, human relations, and individuals, holistically. These align well with Hills's B.C. Program, but Raeburn and Rootman do not put health in a less important place in health promotion. Nor do they build their case for a people-centered health promotion on the ashes of reductionist perspectives, as Hills seems bent on doing, though they clearly see the whole as more than the sum of its parts. Hills asserts the B.C. Program to be informed by a phenomenological theoretical orientation, in which context is central. Phenomenology is a mental construct; it refers to the ways individuals see the world. The founder of phenomenology, German philosopher Edmund Husserl, defined phenomenology as the study of structures of consciousness that enable consciousness to refer to objects outside itself. His method of studying it involved reflection on the content of the mind to the exclusion of everything else. He called such reflection phenomenological reduction. He identified the abstract content of activities such as remembering, desiring, and perceiving, which he called meanings. Phenomenology was, and remains, quintessentially reductionist to the individual, and to perception and lifestyle.

The holistic and phenomenological orientations need not be cast as contrary to reductive analyses. The two complement each other in understanding the micro, internal workings and the macro, contextual interactions. An ecological approach to health promotion, the essence of the holistic approach, requires an understanding of the reciprocal determinism of individuals and their environments (Green, Richard, & Potvin, 1996).

Hills's section on empowerment gives power and control, and their relations, a central place in the B.C. Program. "Power over" relations, where the nurse is in change, are contrasted with "power with" relations, where the nurse negotiates an exchange of power with the patient. Labonte's (1993) conception of hegemonic power is featured: "Nursing students are taught to recognize the prevailing hegemony within the health care system and to create a counter hegemony by understanding the systemic nature of some issues and the impact of this institutional ethos on people who work in the system."

Hills contends that students "learn health promotion strategies that seek to empower and emancipate," and that "empowerment comes from the act of finding one's voice and that can occur only in conditions of justice and equity." No evidence of these assertions is offered. We cannot agree that one can only find one's voice in conditions of justice and equity and, therefore, that empowerment can only occur in conditions of justice and equity. Greater justice and equity may indeed be *outcomes* of empowerment, and they may be *conducive* to empowerment, but if empowerment *required* justice and equity as pre-conditions, then we might find ourselves in less need of empowerment, because we would already have justice and equity.

The section on "enabling" states that, "to increase control over and to improve one's health, one must not only be empowered to do so but also able to do so" (underlines in original) and that "to be able, one must possess the requisite skills, resources and knowledge." This contradicts the earlier assertion that lifestyle change, illness prevention, and health education are separate from health promotion. It also implies that empowerment is something that is given to or handed over to a person, to be used together with other resources and knowledge also conceded to affect greater control over and to improve health. Hills's own charge was that this conception is reductionistic and even disempowering in its implications.

Hills states that, "from a health promotion perspective, people are viewed as experts about their bodies and their experiences." This is a sweeping and simplistic statement to make about all people, and it hardly speaks for all of health promotion. It might be more applicable to most people and most health promotion professionals if it said that health promotion accords people the opportunity to use their knowledge of their bodies and their experience as enabling their control over their health.

In the following paragraph, Hills states that "health promotion can be thought of as a paradigmatic approach to health and health care [involving] an acceptance of certain beliefs, values, assumptions, and central tenets that results in a particular 'way of being'." Beyond defining her three health promotion tenets (primacy of people, empowerment, and enabling), Hills does not articulate the beliefs, values, and assumptions that adherents of health promotion allegedly accept. Where

she attempts to do so, as in the previous paragraph, she sometimes speaks for the field with a particular perspective that cannot claim to be as widely accepted as she would wish.

We cannot help but ask, on what basis are people assumed to accept these beliefs, values and assumptions?" *Is there any concern with evidence?* Is it simply a matter of claiming that "health promotion is good" or that "we know good health promotion (or good nursing practice) when we see it"? It would seem so, because the next section progresses to describe Hills's research study of 24 nursing students enrolled in their 2nd or 3rd semester of the B.C. Program. The description of the qualitative method used is supported by citations to four unpublished papers (three of them by Hills). The introduction to the Results section advises that "the analysis successfully found that the three central tenets of health promotion that are intrinsic to the B.C. Program are reflected in students' narrative accounts of their clinical experiences." Excerpts follow to support this claim. One of them repeats in full the narrative exemplar given at the outset of the chapter. Beyond our concern with how these data were produced—and how the excerpts were selected—is the issue of claims that the students "gave up their power" in negotiating relations with patients. As students with two six-hour days per week (over a 14-week semester) devoted to clinical training, we cannot see how they had much "power" to give up. Indeed, beyond the one student who challenged an anaesthetist and a senior nurse, the others kept their feelings about inappropriate patient relations to themselves, as least in the clinical practice setting.

The conclusion maintains that "the evidence of the three tenets in students' narrative accounts suggests that students who are educated with a health promotion perspective do value and attempt to practice in that way." The quality of the "evidence" and its limitations are not considered. Potential bias by students' self-selection (they volunteered to participate) and desirability to be perceived favorably by Hills through their narratives is not taken into consideration. The assumption that the students had or conferred control to patients is not documented. It seems that the study sought only to provide a favorable judgement about the success of the program. There may, indeed, be no universal "scientific method." Yet for all the concern of this book with knowledge being "socially produced," this account of reforming the training of nurses is remarkably unconcerned with the validity and subjectivity of the author's own work.

Chapter 19

Banister reports on her own research. She quickly gets to the heart of the matter: a need for venues by which women can share the midlife knowledge and expertise, where "the truth of female experience emerges." Banister does a nice job framing the issues with an informative review of the literature. She states her research question explicitly: "What are midlife women's perceptions of their changing bodies?" She rationalizes her use of ethnography because it "would enable me to study the influence of the social and historical context upon the women's experience." She then describes her convenience sample of 11 women and how she conducted two interviews with each woman, plus three group interviews with the entire sample, over a one-year period. The interviews were taped and transcribed and a well-used method of analysis applied. She comments on the richness of the data, and states that her chapter focuses on the group interviews, given the insights achieved in "facilitating an empowerment process that provided groundwork for social and political action." Banister's setting of the stage is complete and logical.

Banister's first task is to define "empowerment" as it relates to her chapter. She states that, in the health promotion field, the term has *two* meanings, quoting Young (1994, p. 48): (a) the individual's development of autonomy and self-control, and (b) the development of collective influence on the social conditions of one's life.

This definition of empowerment might benefit from some harmonization with another: "The process and outcome of gaining control and influence in one's life and in community participation, through shared experience, analysis and influence in achieving and utilizing resources and strategies to enhance community control" (adapted from Lord & Hutchison, 1993). This is similar to Wallerstein's (1992) definition of empowerment as "a social-action process that promotes participation of people, organizations,

and communities towards the goals of increased individual and community control, political efficacy, improved quality of community life, and social justice" (p. 198).

It can be helpful to conceive of empowerment as a process and an outcome, as a multidimensional construct implying individual change as well as change in the social setting itself. This is because of the implication that health promotion initiatives may be more effective if undertaken in combination with, or in the context of, broader social actions supporting self-determination. Banister writes of "an empowerment process" and her definition implies but is not explicit about empowerment being limited to a process and not also an outcome.

As Banister works through her data, she characterizes the level of empowerment rising in the context of women talking in the group interview. This ostensibly occurred when Banister's agenda for the meeting was hijacked by the participants to serve their needs to talk about their own issues. Gaining control through this very limited group experience may be necessary but, in our opinion, is not sufficient to qualify as empowerment, because resources and strategies have not been developed and used to achieve broader social or environmental, or even behavioral, change.

In subsequent pages, Banister presents several instances of the group disparaging physicians (both male and female) over their management of menopausal issues. This venting of frustrations is rather euphemistically referred to as "consciousness raising." As most, if not all, participants participate, does this collective venting qualify as consciousness raising? The participants' consciousness were already raised.

In drawing meaning from the data, Banister might overstate her conclusions, given the limitations of her data and method. She speaks of having illustrated an assortment of many characteristics of empowerment, when such characteristics were not defined *a priori* or made explicit in her reporting. Further, given that she couches her interpretations in terms of "most of the women," one cannot help but wonder about the perspectives of those participants whose perspectives were not consistent with majority tendencies. These women are silent in Banister's analysis. The reader may want to know more about them, what they thought, and why the emancipatory benefit received by other participants did not apply to them.

In considering the implications of her work for health promotion, Banister states that health promotion practitioners "hope that clients attain empowerment within enabling conditions that are co-created between ourselves and our clients." She stops just short of claiming that her research project was empowering, advising that the "process that occurred during this study exemplifies the co-creation of an enabling condition within which the movement toward empowerment was facilitated."

A more critical stance toward empowerment might have fit the critical stance of other chapters toward more conventional concepts in health care. The chapter might have considered, for example, the counterpoint from which empowerment evolves; that is, as a sense of powerlessness (Cargo, 1998; Daniel, 1997). Kieffer (1984) summarized this as "an attitude of self-blame, a sense of generalized distrust, a feeling of alienation from resources for social influence, an experience of disenfranchisement and economic vulnerability, and a sense of hopelessness in socio-political struggle" (p. 16). Powerlessness concerns the expectancy that one cannot determine the occurrence of the outcomes that one seeks (Seeman, 1959). Friere (1970) conceives powerlessness similarly as passive acceptance of oppressive cultural "givens," where one becomes powerless in assuming the role of "object" acted on by the environment, rather than "subject" acting in and on the world. Gaventa (1980) conceives of it as loss of sense of control over one's place in a system of social relations. Given Young's focus in Chapter 1 on Friere, it might be illuminating to reflect on whether the participants in Banister's study perceived themselves as lacking agency. In this regard, Lerner's work is relevant.

Lerner (1986) distinguished "real" powerlessness from "surplus" powerlessness. "Real" powerlessness, he argued, reflects economic, political, and social arrangements that prevent people from actualizing their human capacities. In contrast, "surplus" powerlessness reflects the contribution of people to "real" powerlessness to the extent that they do not believe they are capable of actualizing possibilities that exist within the context of "real" powerlessness. The latter might be akin to what Bandura (1986) refers to as a lack of self-efficacy.

Chapter 20

This chapter offers insights and guidance to nurses seeking a transformed practice of health promotion in the difficult circumstances of families with children having complex, chronic conditions being cared for at home.

Hayes and McElheran grapple with the dual task of providing in-home nursing respite care to a child while helping the family remain integrated and functional. They focus in this chapter on the "stories" of families, from a larger study that evaluated the effectiveness of a nursing respite program. They acknowledge that the complexity and demands of the evaluation compromised the theoretical sampling for their grounded theory approach to the qualitative part of the study reported in Chapter 20, but the stories are poignant and moving. The analysis should provide the nurse in preparation for such circumstances of practice with fair warning that families are complex, but also that one can work with such families in ways that minimize the negative aspects of coping with a child's chronic condition while maximizing some positive aspects. The authors also appeal, as every chapter could, for policy support to make this arena of practice more ethical and humane than contemporary systems allow.

Chapter 21

This chapter provides a good example of how principles of participatory research (PAR) can be applied by nurses outside of the clinic or hospital, in the community, to address behavioral and social and physical environmental influences on falls in the elderly. Gallagher, Lindsey, and Scott emphasize power and its relationship to knowledge in the context of participatory research. They use a paper by Henderson (1995) as their framework for PAR. Henderson's tenets align reasonably well with our guidelines based on an international literature review and an assessment of Canadian health promotion experience (George et al., 1999; Green et al., 1996).

The paper flows from an introductory background on PAR to a problem statement on how little we know about methods of involving people actively as partners in the process of PAR. The STEPS project is introduced as a case study example illustrating Henderson's tenets in melding health promotion and PAR to "improve client health and impact on public policy." Improved "client health" was not truly the outcome assessed, although individual risk of falls may have been reduced by changes at the community level, through lobbying efforts and consequent efforts to reduce social and physical environmental risks.

The authors' review of the literature established falls as a substantial problem in the elderly. They divided risk factors for falls into biological, behavioral, environmental hazard (i.e., physical environmental), and social and political categories. In covering the basics, they did not define their community, and they asserted that they were "using PAR methods" without ever saying what the research methods were. In our review, we sided with the more common view that PAR is neither a method nor a collection of methods. It is an approach to partnering in research that seeks to ensure education and change, but any research method can be applied in PAR.

It would probably be more to the point to drop the phrase "using PAR methods" in favor of reporting their systematic "consultations with stakeholders to establish goals, develop data collection methods, and prepare for dissemination of the findings." Beyond that, one looks fruitlessly for a specification of who those stakeholders were, what was the local population in terms of geography and parameters, or the age range of people to whom the project might be relevant, and what were the research methods employed.

The steering committee is described as "consisting of six seniors, two people who were blind, a wheelchair user, a member of the local health department, and two researchers." This description leaves ambiguous whether the total number of participants was six or twelve. We infer that it might have been six, all of them seniors, including the two researchers. Members of the steering committee and other elderly volunteers collected data on falls using a telephone hotline survey over a nine-month period. Callers were encouraged using media messages. The hotline recorded "slips, trips, and falls" over the nine months it ran. The survey results are presented as a narrative, blending percentages and numbers in such a way that the reader must strain to imagine a table of the types of incidents and related perceived hazards, and of callers' ages and gender.

The steering committee took action in forwarding reports of hazards to various authorities. An "estimated" 30 percent of hazards were reportedly addressed by some form of action by the end of the project. The committee also hosted a symposium to disseminate to a diverse audience their findings and to focus attention on hazards for falls.

The next section presents the results of a "meta-study"—what is described as a study of the study—to assess key elements of community involvement in PAR activities of the project. Diverse methods were used to collect data: review of minutes, news releases, TV/radio interviews, participant observation, and a focus group interview. Six major themes were identified: planning, structural components, philosophy, enhancing credibility, leadership, and personal experience and satisfaction. Each theme is reviewed. The conclusions about PAR and health promotion assert that the chapter provides evidence of a PAR project aimed at empowering seniors to take actions that would reduce risks in the community that contribute to falls and injuries. The authors then discuss the extent to which Henderson's "qualities" of PAR were "adhered" to. They conclude that the project embodies each of Henderson's qualities of PAR, and admirably itemize the ways. This chapter is exemplary in its relative clarity, consistency, balance, thoroughness, and restraint from libellous or simplistic generalizations. It lies in unenviable placement between two chapters (17 and 23) that would impugn its relevance to health promotion because it addresses a specific health problem, seeks to prevent specific injuries, and encourages individual lifestyle changes.

Chapter 23

Hills and Mullett hit readers hard with a student's narrative on the contradiction between what she learned as best practice, and the realities of hospital practice. They then posed a "research question" for the chapter: how to change nursing practice to be more congruent with the emerging paradigm of health promotion?

We find their phrase "emerging paradigm of health promotion" discomforting both in its use of "emerging" *and* its use of "paradigm." The *notion* or the *perspective* of health promotion, not to put too fine a point on what they call a paradigm, was retreating rather than emerging in Canada and British Columbia governments at the time they wrote this chapter, as evidenced in our review of Chapter 17. The authors assert that a reorientation to health promotion principles would require a substantial shift from a natural science paradigm emphasizing diseases, to a "human science" paradigm, with its recognition of the primacy of people and their experiences. Among the many models of health promotion, used widely in the published literature as guides to planning and evaluating programs, training students, and advocating policy, none would qualify as a paradigm, but most of the viable ones among them contain elements of both natural and social or "human" sciences.

Hills and Mullett propose that, because of its "transformative and empowering" nature, "cooperative inquiry," a form of PAR, is ideally suited to assisting nurses to examine their practice and to develop new and innovative ways of practising. They assert that engaging in PAR while focusing on health promotion can catalyze nursing culture and practice, and describe the purpose of their chapter as to introduce and promote cooperative inquiry "as a catalyst in transforming nursing health promotion practice." They then draw heavily on Labonte (1993) in describing and contrasting the biomedical, behavioral, and socioenvironmental approaches to health, aligning with the last, because it enables a focus on empowerment, participation, and partnerships.

The next section takes a critical look at whether nursing rhetoric on the merit of the socioenvironmental approach translates into observable effects on nursing practice. The evidence would suggest so, but to a limited degree only. The following section on nursing education suggests that the prevailing system in which most nurses practice does not enable progressively trained nurses to apply and maintain a broader perspective. Hills and Mullett proceed to describe cooperative inquiry, which seems to us much like PAR.

Hills and Mullett label as unethical the generation of "knowledge about persons without their participation in deciding how to generate it," because this misrepresents their "personhood" and abuses by neglect their capacity for "autonomous intentionality." Their appropriate moral outrage is lost in this postmodern jargon. They invoke Peter Reason's "central assumptions of cooperative inquiry" but turn his positive principles into attacks on "traditional research methods" as a basis for some "new method." They assert that "cooperative inquiry is based on an epistemology that includes four types of knowledge: experiential . . . , practical. . . , propositional. . . , and presentational. . . ." The line between research as knowledge development, human therapy, and social reordering becomes far too blurred. As a consequence, we descend in a spiral of relativism, where anything and everything is valid, and the right of science to assert its claim as a standard is no longer unique. It may well be that science does provide just one possible view of the world among others that are equally legitimate. But the claims of detractors of science that it is no standard at all does not seem to pose a problem for their proposals to cede epistemological authority to alternative methodologies of their choosing. Science, at least, has a concern with evidence. Independent of the nature of evidence, and the explanatory and predictive utility of a theory evaluated on the basis of evidence, we might also consider questions about the benefits or harms of pursuing inquiries of various sorts, in terms of what is done with the evidence. These are different questions, no less important, but different. Some of the post-modernist criticism and rhetoric completely confounds the issues.

Hills and Mullett work through the phases of cooperative inquiry, now referred to as a *methodology*. We wonder what is meant by the question, "What would it look like if we evaluated students from a human science, health promotion perspective?" We fail to see how claims of "testing validity" can be accomplished in practice in this instance because the details are missing. This goes beyond PAR as an approach to research and asserts itself as a methodology for knowledge development. The purpose of this knowledge development process is ostensibly to create collaborative relationships, to engage in critical dialogue, and to do "reflecting-in-action."

What *happens* to the knowledge developed? It seems to have as its sole purpose to act as a catalyst, as Hills and Mullett claim, being essentially consumed in the process of empowering and transforming the research participants. They seem to be saying that the mass application of cooperative inquiry to nursing practice might act to change the culture to bring it into better alignment with what they call the socioenvironmental approach to health promotion. This has little with to do with the goals of science and research. The knowledge produced by application of the method at the level of the nurse is not the point as much as the impact of the process on nursing culture. It would be mass therapy, social engineering, or exploitation to impose this widely and indiscriminately on nursing, patients, clients, or communities. What about nurses who want to remain the dedicated, caring practitioners they are now, willing to be seen as dinosaurs, but determined to provide the care they were trained to provide? What about a systematic approach of considering factors that might predispose, enable, and reinforce change within the nursing, patient, and community cultures? What about research on dimensions of the problem and its antecedents, and actions targeting behavioral interventions for voluntary change, with enabling environmental supports for individual behavioral change, and structural environmental change? Again, for a discipline so outwardly concerned with context and holism, the lack of attention in this proposal to broader issues is disappointing.

Subsequent sections report on uses of the cooperative inquiry approach in other settings, ending with Hills's study involving the same 24 students reported on in Chapter 17. This report has a different focus, however, describing how the 24 students are part of an inquiry group with faculty members, which has completed all phases of cooperative inquiry over multiple iterations of reflection and action.

We are left in this chapter with the uneasy impression that nursing training could be transformed not toward a more health promoting practice, but toward a more labor-intensive cooperative research mode. We subscribe passionately to participatory research, but as described in this chapter, it seems to be offered not a research proposal but a routine nursing practice mode. As routine nursing practice, it is unsupportable by a health care system that can ill afford the release of precious nursing skills for such research activity, and would be imposed on many patients and clients who cannot afford the time or emotional energy to participate in the research.

CONCLUSION

In attempting to highlight the themes and uncover the threads running through the chapters of this book, we have quibbled with some of the authors' claims and conclusions, especially where they seem to have overworked their criticisms of the past. We have urged the preservation of some foundations on which we believe health promotion is well grounded, rather than torching them to transform health promotion practice on the ashes of the research that has gone before. We have, as our title suggests, counseled against the construction of false dichotomies and the tendency sometimes to wallow in ideological quicksand. Ideals are good. Ideology can give energy to a profession and an organization's mission. But when pursued so passionately or single-mindedly that facts and history are distorted, the professions and the cause of health promotion can lose their grounding in previous research and development that have taken decades to accrue.

It is not just the credibility of health promotion in the eyes of the health sciences and professions that is at stake. If that were all, we could hope that false dichotomies would find their equilibrium of truth somewhere between the false constructions of the past and the yet untested constructions of the present. We could hope that the ideological rhetoric would gain enough converts to maintain a progressive movement toward a reformed practice. If the vision of that reformed practice, however, is based on poorly developed concepts, unfounded assumptions, belittled experience and data from the past, or invalid data from new research, then it cannot lead clearly to reforms that improve either practice or outcomes.

Nursing cannot afford, for example, to dismiss its own practitioners and past researchers as misguided and misinformed stooges of a scientific establishment that has exploited and duped them. Nursing, as one of many professions practicing health promotion of various types in various populations, also cannot afford to isolate itself from the mainstream of scientific and evidence-based practice emerging from those other fields of science and practice. It should be critical of the mainstream, but not with a voice so shrill and antagonistic that it alienates its potential allies. A respectful blending and reconciling of the science of the past with the new concepts and ideals of the present will serve the cause better than a radical schism and partitioning of the reform movement, wrapped in loosely formulated ideologies and paradigms.

In short, we applaud the authors and editors of this book for their vision, courage, and commitment to improving nursing practice and education. We would hope the intended audience will be sufficiently stimulated and inspired by the perspectives and stories contained in these pages to appreciate and strive for a *balanced* transformation of nursing practice, one that benefits specific individuals in clinical care settings as much as the greater population. We promote a critical understanding of nursing as historically and socially situated, one that seeks to understand and analyze not only for contextual effects acting *upon* nursing, but sociopolitical tendencies acting from *within* nursing itself. In this sense, a critical awareness of interconnectedness within and between nursing, the other health professions, and the larger social system, is at the heart of what nursing can offer to lead the emergence of truly post-modern health promotion practice and research. "Post-modernism" need not necessarily be a synonym for deconstructive, cynical, even nihilistic perspectives, which, carried to extremes, may more truly represent modernism extended to its limit. Rather, as some of the perspectives contained in this book attest, the commitment to a positive, grounded transformation of nursing practice can embody the emergence of a *reconstructive* post-modernism based on concern for a sustaining system of relationships between individuals, the health professions, and society.

REFERENCES

Bandura, A. (1986). *Social foundations of thought and action.* Englewood Cliffs, NJ: Prentice Hall.

Berland, A., Whyte, N., & Maxwell, L. (1995). Hospital nurses and health promotion. *Canadian Journal of Nursing Research, 27*(4): 13–31.

Cargo, M. D. (1998). *Partnering with adults as a process of empowering youth in the community: A grounded theory study.* Ph.D. Thesis. Vancouver, BC: University of British Columbia, Department of Health Care and Epidemiology.

Charles, C., Gauld, M., Chambers, L., O'Brien, B., Haynes, R. B., & Labelle, R. (1994). How was your hospital stay? Patients' reports about their care in Canadian hospitals. *Canadian Medical Association Journal, 150*: 1813–1822.

Daniel, M. (1997). *Effectiveness of community-directed diabetes prevention and control in a rural aboriginal population.* Ph.D. Thesis. Vancouver, BC: University of British Columbia, Department of Health Care and Epidemiology.

Daniel, M., & Green, L. W. (1999). Community-based prevention and chronic disease self-management programmes: Problems, praises and pitfalls. *Disease Management and Health Outcomes, 6*(4): 185–192.

Daniel, M., Green, L. W., & Sheps, S. B. (1998). Paradigm change and uncertainty about funding of public health research: social and scientific implications. *Journal of Health and Social Policy, 10*(2): 39–56.

Friere, P. (1970). *Pedagogy of the oppressed.* New York: Seabury Press.

Gaventa, J. (1980). *Power and powerlessness.* Urbana, IL: University of Illinois Press.

George, M. A., Daniel, M., & Green, L. W. (1999). Appraising and funding participatory research in health promotion. *International Quarterly of Community Health Education, 18*(2): 181–197.

Goethe. (1855). *Faust.* Translated by Carlyle F. MacIntyre. Norfolk, CT: New Directions, 1941.

Green, L. W. (1990). The revival of community and the public obligation of academic health centers. In R. E. Bulger & S. J. Reiser (Eds.), *Integrity in health care institutions: Humane environments for teaching, inquiry and healing,* pp. 148–164. Des Moines, IA: University of Iowa Press.

Green, L. W. (1997). Foreword. In J. Raeburn & I. Rootman (Eds.), *Understanding people-centred health promotion.* Chichester: John Wiley & Sons, Ltd.

Green, L. W., George, M. A., Daniel, M., Frankish, C. J., Herbert, C. J., Bowie, W. R., & O'Neill, M. (1995). *Study of participatory research in health promotion: Review and recommendations for the development of participatory research in health promotion in Canada.* Ottawa: The Royal Society of Canada.

Green, L. W., & Kreuter, M. W. (1999). *Health promotion planning: An educational and ecological approach* (3rd ed.). Mountain View: Mayfield.

Green, L. W., Richard, L., & Potvin, L. (1996). Ecological foundations of health promotion. *American Journal of Health Promotion, 10*: 270–281.

Henderson, D. (1995). Consciousness raising in participatory research: Method and methodology for emancipatory nursing inquiry. *Advances in Nursing Science, 17*, 58–69.

Hupcey, J. E., & Morse, J. M. (1997). Can a professional relationship be considered social support? *Nursing Outlook, 45*, 270–276.

Kieffer, C. H. (1984). Citizen empowerment: A developmental perspective. *Prevention in Human Services, 3*(16): 9–36.

Kuh, D., & Ben-Shlomo (Eds.). (1997). *A life course approach to chronic disease epidemiology: Tracing the origins of ill health from early to adult life.* New York: Oxford.

Labonte, R. (1993). Health promotion and empowerment: Practice frameworks. In Issues in Health Promotion. Toronto: Centre for Health Promotion University of Toronto.

Lerner, M. (1986). *Surplus powerlessness.* Oakland, CA: The Institute for Labor and Mental Health.

Lord, J., Hutchinson, P. (1993). The process of empowerment: Implications for theory and practice. *Canadian Journal of Community Mental Health, 12*, (1): 5–22.

McKinlay, J. B. (1975). A case for refocusing upstream-the political economy of illness. In A. J. Enelow & J. B. Henderson (Eds.), *Applying behavioural science to cardiovascular risk.* New York: American Heart Association.

Ottawa Charter on Health Promotion (1986). *Health Promotion, 1* (4): iii–v.

Poland, B. D., Green, L. W., & Rootman, I. (Eds.). (2000). *Settings for health promotion: Linking theory and practice.* Thousand Oaks, London, New Delhi: Sage.

Raeburn, J. (1992). Health promotion research with heart: Keeping a people perspective. *Canadian Journal of Public Health, 83*, (1) 19–24.

Raeburn, J., & Rootman, I. (Eds.). (1997). *Understanding people-centred health promotion.* Chichester: John Wiley & Sons.

Roter, D. L. (1977). Patient participation in the patient-provider interaction: The effects of patient question-asking on the quality of interaction, satisfaction and compliance. *Health Education Monographs, 5*: 281–315.

Seeman, M. (1959). On the meaning of alienation. *American Sociological Review, 24*: 783–791.

Sehnert, K., & Eisenberg, H. (1975). *How to be your own doctor sometimes.* New York: Grosset & Dunlap.

Wallerstein, N. (1992). Powerlessness, empowerment, and health: Implications for health promotion programs. *American Journal of Health Promotion, 6*: 197–205.

Wallerstein, N., & Berstein, E. (1996). Introduction to [special issue on] community empowerment, participatory education, and health. *Health Education Quarterly, 21*: 141–148.

Wharf-Higgins, J., Vertinsky, P., Cutt, J., & Green, L. W. (1999). Using social marketing as a theoretical framework to understand citizen participation in health promotion. *Social Marketing Quarterly, 5*(2): 42–55.

Young, I. M. (1994). Punishment, treatment, empowerment: Three approaches to policy for pregnant addicts. *Feminist Studies, 20*, 33–57.

Ageism Negative attitudes toward the aged (Unger & Crawford, 1992).

Analysis of Variance (ANOVA) A complex statistical analytic procedure used to test mean differences among a set of research variables. When this sophisticated technique is used, one variable is held constant while many other covariates are tested to find their effects (Polit & Hungler, 1995).

Baby Boomers The group of individuals born between 1947 and 1966 during the post-war reestablishment of nuclear families (Foot, 1996).

Constructivism An approach to research in which all attempts are made to understand/reconstruct participants' realities by collecting data via interactions between informants and researchers. One basic premise is that realities are apprehensible in the form of multiple, intangible constructions that are socially and experientially based. The methods used are conversations and observations, compared and contrasted through interpretive, dialectical interchange between and among the investigator and the participants (Guba & Lincoln, 1994).

Critical Theory An approach to social theory concerned with analyzing the objective structures that constrain imagination. Critical theory can be an empirical enterprise concerned with the simultaneous critique of society and the envisioning of new possibilities (Morrow, 1994). Critical theorists aim to destabilize entrenched thought patterns as a first step in the social change process.

Delphi Method A method of sampling the opinions or preferences of a small number of experts, opinion leaders, or informants, whereby successive questionnaires are sent by mail and the results are summarized for further refinement on subsequent mailings.

Effectiveness The extent to which a specific intervention, procedure, regimen, or service, when employed in the field, does what it is intended to do for a defined population.

Efficacy The extent to which a specific intervention, procedure, or service produces a beneficial result under ideal conditions. Ideally, the determination of efficacy is based on the results of a randomized, controlled trial.

Emancipation A state in which people know who they are and collectively determine the direction of their existence.

Expectancy-Value Theory Posits that a person is likely to engage in a particular action if she or he positively values the outcome of taking action, and if the person believes that a particular action will achieve the outcome. Thus, individuals are unlikely to take action that does not have value to them, nor will they work toward goals that they perceive as impossible to achieve (Feather, 1982; Pender, 1996).

Grounded Theory A qualitative research approach through which the researcher(s) generate(s) an abstract analytic schema of a phenomenon. This approach is best suited to description of social actions, interactions, or processes, particularly when little is known about them. Data may be conversational, observational, or derived from artifacts. During data analysis, data are synthesized into theory by a specific set of techniques (Strauss & Corbin, 1998).

Health Health is more than the absence of disease; it is total physical, psychological, and social well-being, and is a resource for living (Ottawa Charter, 1986; World Health Organization [WHO], 1981).

Health Promotion Health promotion is a process that enables people to address cultural, social, and political factors to increase control over and to improve their health (WHO, 1984). It is a transformative process in which the nurse as partner engages clients in consciousness raising, a process characterized by a respect for the dynamic relatedness between people and the environment.

Hierarchy Relations based on ranking roles according to perceived importance.

Individualism A social philosophy that views society as existing only for the sake of its members as individuals. This philosophy justifies the private interests of individual persons above collective or public interests. Several assumptions underlie individualism, including the notions that (a) to be human is to be free from dependence on others, (b) individuals are free from any relations to which they do not enter voluntarily, (c) individuals own and control their own capacities, for which they owe nothing to society (Williams, 1989).

Liberalism A political philosophy that emphasizes individual freedom and the idea that human beings can improve themselves and society through systematic and rational action. It emerged in Europe in the period between the Reformation and the French Revolution. Liberalism sought to expand civil liberties and to limit political authority in favor of constitutional representative government. Liberalism promotes rights to property and religious tolerance. Classical liberalism (sometimes called neoliberalism) is markedly opposed to state intervention and views the free market as the solution to all ills. Liberal thinking shifted in the 20th century to support a greater role for government in promoting individual freedom and protecting the public good. Today, free-market traditional liberals are often classed as conservatives (Baum & Saunders, 1995; Williams, 1989).

Mental Health Promotion The concept of fostering, protecting, and improving mental health.

Meta-Study A research project in which the findings of several studies on a given phenomenon are reanalyzed together to provide knowledge that would not have been discernable from single studies alone (Polit & Hungler, 1995; Schreiber, Crooks, & Stern, 1997).

Midlife That period of life between the ages of 40 to 55 years (Berkun, 1983).

Neo-Marxism Encompasses a broad array of reformist Marxist theories that reject the classical Marxist notion of economic or class determinism. In other words, there is a deemphasis on "class" as the central category for critique that considers race, gender, and ethnicity as distinct forms of disadvantage that do not reduce entirely to the dynamics of class. Neo-Marxist theory stresses the importance of culture in the workings of capitalist society and the basic belief that social phenomena cannot be understood except in relation to the total political-economic-cultural context in which it is situated (Morrow, 1994; Stevens, 1989; Stevens & Hall, 1992).

Paradigm A way of viewing phenomena, or a worldview.

Participant Observation The researcher's role in the field that requires that he or she participate in the social world and reflect upon the products of that participation (Hammersley & Atkinson, 1983).

Participatory Research The process of a group taking an active role in defining their own health needs, setting their own priorities among health goals, controlling the application of health-enhancing methods in their own lives, and evaluating efforts to improve their own health.

Population Health Population health is an approach to health that aims to improve the health of the entire population and to reduce health inequities among population groups. In order to reach these objectives, those using a population health approach consider and act upon the broad range of factors and conditions that influence health. Population health, as an approach to addressing health-related issues, recognizes that health is a capacity or resource rather than a state, a definition that corresponds more to the notion of being able to pursue ones goals, to acquire skills and education, and to grow. This broader notion of health recognizes the range of social, economic, and physical environmental factors that contribute to health. The best articulation of this concept of health is "the capacity of people to adapt to, respond to, or control life's challenges and changes" (Frankish et al., 1996; http://www.population-health.com).

Praxis The dialectic between thought and action, theory and practice, values and behavior. Reflection on practice refines theory, which in turn enhances practice (Thorne, 1997). Action and reflection on the world to change it (Freire, 1992).

Reflexivity A means of reflecting on and accounting for a researcher's input into qualitative analysis. Based on the assumption that the scientific observer is part of the phenomenon he or she is trying to understand and represent, self-reflection and self-criticism are used (and usually recorded), and accounted for in analyses and concepts that are reported from the research (Altheide & Johnson, 1994).

Qualitative Research A broad category of research methods in which data are collected in the form of words and text rather than numerical indicators or measures, data that is analyzed with attention to the perspectives of participants and the context of their responses.

Self-Care The decisions and actions taken by someone who is facing a health problem in order to cope with it and improve his or her health.

Self-Efficacy A construct from social learning theory referring to an individual's perception that he or she is capable of performing a specific behavior.

Self-Help A process of sharing common experiences, situations, or problems. It is participatory in nature and involves getting help, giving help, and learning to help oneself, as well as sharing knowledge and experience.

Sexism Refers to the belief that women are valued in terms of their physical attractiveness and use to men (Unger & Crawford, 1992).

Social Learning Theory (or **Social Cognitive Theory**) This theory describes an interactional model of causation in which factors in the environment, personal factors, and individual behavior act as reciprocal determinants of each other. Perceived self-efficacy is a particularly important determinant of behavior, in which judgements about one's ability to carry out a particular action are important influences on that action (Bandura, 1986).

Train-the-Trainer A method of transferring knowledge by training a core group of people who, in turn, teach the content to others. Appropriate teaching/learning strategies are modeled during the original training for the participants to experience and then apply to their own teaching situations. This approach is particularly well suited to primary health care because it allows for wide dissemination of health knowledge and builds local capacity through education of the trainers.

Triangulation Using two or more data sources, methods, theories, or investigators to shed light on the phenomenon of interest (Creswell, 1998).

Visual Analog Scale A visual scale designed for numeric assessment of an experience, often clinical symptoms such as pain, fatigue, or stress. These scales are frequently graphic, like a thermometer, and the experience may be indicated anywhere on a line (continuous data) or at pre-demarcated intervals (interval data) (Polit & Hungler, 1995).

Index